PUBLIC HEALTH AND PREVENTIVE MEDICINE IN CANADA

CHANDRAKANT P. SHAH

FIFTH EDITION

Elsevier Canada is extremely pleased to publish this fifth edition of *Public Health and Preventive Medicine in Canada* by Dr. Chandrakant Shah. Dr. Shah's work on this and previous editions has resulted in a book that is regarded with well-deserved esteem by health sciences professionals, instructors, and students throughout the country. We are very proud to include this prestigious publication in Elsevier's health sciences publishing program.

Ann Millar
Acquisitions Editor

PUBLIC HEALTH AND PREVENTIVE MEDICINE IN CANADA

Chandrakant P Shah
MD, DCH, MRCP (Glas), FRCPC, SM (Hyg), FACPM, FAAP

Professor Emeritus
Department of Public Health Sciences
Faculty of Medicine
University of Toronto
and
Honorary Staff, The Hospital for Sick Children,
Courtesy Staff, St. Michael's Hospital
Staff Physician, Anishnawbe Health Toronto

Fifth Edition

iv

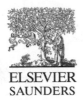

ELSEVIER
SAUNDERS

National Library of Canada Cataloguing in Publication
Shah, Chandrakant P. (Chandrakant Padamshi), 1936-
Public health and preventive medicine in Canada / Chandrakant P. Shah. — 5th ed.

Includes bibliographical references and index.
ISBN 0-9205-1393-X

1. Public health—Canada. 2. Medical care—Canada. 3. Medicine, Preventive—Canada. I. Title.

RA449.S48 2003   362.1'0971   C2003-903279-5

Printing and Binding: The Maple-Vail Book Manufacturing Group

Elsevier Canada
1 Goldthorne Avenue., Toronto, ON, M8Z 5S7
Phone: 1-866-896-3331
Fax: 1-866-359-9534

Printed in The United States of America

1 2 3 4 5   07 06 05 04 03

Dedicated to those who have cared
for me and awakened my spirits:
My wife, Sudha, my sons, Sunil and
Rajiv, my daughter-in-law, Kausha, my
grand-daughters, Anita and Neha, and the
Aboriginal peoples of Canada

ABOUT THE AUTHOR

Dr. Chandrakant Shah, Professor Emeritus at the University of Toronto is a pracitising physician, a public health practioner and an advocate for improving the health and well-being of marginalized groups in Canadian society. He was a Professor in the Department of Public Health Sciences, University of Toronto from 1972–2001. He was instrumental in developing the Endowed Chair in Aboriginal Health and Wellbeing at the University – the first of its kind in Canada. He held cross appointments in the departments of Health Policy, Management and Evaluation, Paediatrics, Family and Community Medicine in the Faculty of Medicine and also in the Faculties of Social Work and Nursing at the University of Toronto.

He is the recipient of the **John Hastings Award** (1997) from the Faculty of Medicine for his excellent services to the University of Toronto and communities. In 1999, he received the highest award of the Canadian Public Health Association, the **R. D. Defries Award and Honorary Life Membership** for his contribution to furthering medical education in public health as well as his advocacy for disadvantaged populations such as the homeless, unemployed and poor. He is the recipient of the **Eagle Feather**, the highest award given by First Nations House at the University of Toronto for his lifetime work with the aboriginal community, and particularly for developing an annual *Visiting Lectureship on Native Health* program series. He received the **25th Anniversary Race Relations Award** from the Urban Alliance on Race Relations in 2000 for his work in creating racial harmony; a **Certificate of Recognition** by the City of Toronto Public Health Department for outstanding commitment and dedication towards the pursuit of Access and Equity at the University of Toronto in 2001; an **Honarary Life Membership** from the Ontario Medical Association in 2002 and designation of **Senior Member** from the Canadian Medical Association in 2003, for his lifetime devotion to improving the health of Canadians and particularly the marginalized population. In 1987 the University of Toronto established an annual prize and a scholarship in his name, **The C. P. Shah Award** is to be granted to the Community Medicine Resident for his/her best work in the field of public health. In July 2001, the University also established **The C. P. Shah, Government of Ontario/Public Health Sciences Graduate Scholarship in Science and Technology**, which will fund $15,000 per year for a doctoral stream student in Public Health Sciences. He was nominated for the Ontario New Democratic Party's **J. S. Woodsworth Award for Human Rights** in 2001 and an **Alumni Award of Merit** by the Harvard School of Public Health Alumni in 2002. He has been listed in *Who's Who in Ontario* and *Who's Who in Canada* from 1995– 2003.

TABLE OF CONTENTS

CHAPTER 13
Federal and Provincial Health Organizations 395

CHAPTER 14
Funding, Expenditures, and Resources 425

LIST OF TABLES AND FIGURES

FOREWORD

I am honoured to write the Foreword to the fifth edition of Public Health and Preventive Medicine in Canada. My colleagues, my students, and I have come to rely on earlier editions of this book as a standard resource. Chandrakant Shah has been diligent in updating previous versions of the text, thus making each edition essential reading for Canadians and their international colleagues who want to learn about health and health care in Canada. This edition is no exception. The book is an excellent primer for beginning healthcare professionals and an important reference for administrators and practitioners who must understand health and the health system in order to work effectively within it.

A unique feature of this text is that it connects health promotion and prevention models with the policy and history of the healthcare system. Dr. Shah leads the reader through the complex determinants of health and its measurement to the development of contemporary health care in Canada. The assiduous attention to detail ensures that the most current legislation, policy recommendations, and reports are included. Dr. Shah describes past and present thoughts and events that will influence the future development of health and health care in Canada. People will refer to this book for years to come as a key to understanding Canadian healthcare policy as it evolves.

Readers can progress one chapter at a time, or can easily reference facts about individual topics by referring to the detailed table of contents or the index. This comprehensive work about the Canadian healthcare system should be required reading for students in all health disciplines, including medicine and nursing.

Andrea Baumann, RN, PhD
Associate Dean Faculty of Health Sciences (Nursing), McMaster University
Co-Director, Nursing Effectiveness Utilization and Outcomes Research Unit
Director, World Health Organization Collaborating Centre in Primary Health Care
Nursing and Health Human Resources

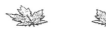

PREFACE TO
THE FIFTH EDITION

When I published my first edition, I never anticipated that I would be doing a fifth edition. I am grateful to the many teachers who have adopted this book as required or reference reading for their courses and to the students who have challenged and inspired me. This book is now used by both undergraduate and a graduate courses for many different health sciences disciplines, such as medicine, nursing, health record administrators, chiropractors, optometrists, pharmacy, and dentistry, in colleges and the universities from St. John's in the east to Victoria in the west and from The Pas in the north to Windsor in the south. While this is inspiring to me as an author, my task has become daunting.

The purpose of this book is to help readers learn about their role as healthcare professionals, administrators, or policy makers by understanding the extent of health and disease in Canada and about the functions and challenges of our healthcare system. It is also intended for those members of the general public who are interested in participating in the ongoing debate on these issues by providing the fundamentals about the health and health care of Canadians.

Preparing for this edition has been challenging, as has been in previous four editions. First, there have been drastic changes in the healthcare system in all provinces and territories over the past four years. Strapped with increasing debt and a poorly performing economy in early 1990s, governments at all levels reduced or capped their healthcare budgets by restructuring and reforming the system to allow the private sector to take more and more functions of healthcare and social services delivery previously provided by them. Second, the public has voiced concerns about long waiting times to receive certain health services, such as elective surgery, emergency services, CAT scans or MRIs, and specialized services for cancer. Concerns have also been expressed about increasing drug prices, unavailability of certain homecare services, and the very sustainability of a publicly funded healthcare system. To alleviate these concerns, the federal and the provincial and territorial governments appointed number of healthcare commissions and their reports have recommended many needed changes. Third, a large number of population-based studies on health status have been carried out by most provinces and federal governments, which provide data on health indicators even at sub-regional levels. Even though many of these studies are available on the Internet, the barrage of new data makes it increasingly difficult to judge what is essential knowledge for book of this nature.

In revising the book, I have attempted to incorporate latest available information and have been mindful not to expand the size. Chapters 3 to 8, 13, 14, and 18 are almost completely rewritten, and the remainders have gone through extensive revisions. Chapter 17 is a new addition describing unique nature of Quebec's healthcare system and was written by two leading public health experts from Quebec. Appendix B outlines educational objectives, and a detailed index is again provided.

There are some deliberate omissions in this book as far as detail is concerned, as excellent textbooks on subjects such as biostatistics and epidemiology are available. The first two chapters of the book are dense and synoptic in nature and are not intended to replace any standard textbooks on the subjects covered. In other instances, details are omitted because of different legislation in different Canadian jurisdictions. However, the general principles are covered. Anyone who wants to study a particular topic in greater depth is advised to consult one of several comprehensive textbooks of community health that already exist. To ensure that the information is current, each chapter was reviewed by experts too numerous to list here (see page xxi) but to whom I am most grateful for their diligence.

I am also indebted to many individuals across the country for their support and comments. While this list does not include everyone who has contributed, I would like to express special thanks to Drs. Karen Lee, Doug Manuel, Roohi Qureshi, Julia Rackal, and Brent Moloughney, and to Ms. Brenda Gamble and Monali Varia, for their contributions in researching material, and to Dr. Rose Bilotta for her helpful suggestions. I also thank Drs. Pierre Bergeron and Jean-Frédérick Lévesque for their contribution on the Quebec healthcare system. I am indebted to Madeline Koch for editing, Christopher Blackburn for indexing, Don O'Shaughnessy for formatting, graphics, and prepress production, Lorna MacPhee for proofreading, and Jewell Kennedy and Ann Millar from Elsevier Canada. I also thank Dean Andrea Baumann for writing the Foreword. Finally, I thank my children, Sunil, Rajiv, and Kausha, for their understanding, and my wife, Sudha, for her patience and silent endurance during the entire process.

C.P. Shah
University of Toronto
Toronto, Ontario
March 2003

CONTRIBUTING AUTHORS

Jean-Frédéric Lévesque
Institut national de santé publique du Québec

Pierre Bergeron
Institut national de santé publique du Québec
and the Département de médecine sociale et préventive, Université Laval

REVIEWERS

Chapter 1
Dr. Ian Johnson, Professor, Department of Public Health Sciences,
University of Toronto
Dr. Suzanne Jackson, Professor & Director, Centre for Health Promotion,
Department of Public Health Sciences, University of Toronto
Chapter 2
Professor Mary Chipman, Professor, Department of Public Health Sciences,
University of Toronto
Dr. Bernard Choi, Senior Research Scientist, Centre for Chronic Disease Prevention
& Control, Health Canada
Chapter 3
Dr. Kue Young, Professor, Department of Public Health Sciences,
University of Toronto
Dr. John Millar, Senior Advisor, Strategic Development,
Canadian Institute for Health
Chapter 4
Dr. Doug Manuel, Scientist, ICES Assistant Professor, Department. of Public
Health Sciences, University of Toronto
Dr. George Pasut, Medical Officer of Health, Simcoe County District Health Unit
Chapter 5
Dr. Isra Levy, Director, Office for Public Health, Canadian Medical Association
Dr. George Pasut, Medical Officer of Health, Simcoe County District Health Unit
Chapter 6
Dr. Kue Young, Professor, Department of Public Health Sciences,
University of Toronto
Dr. Sudeep Gill, Post Doctoral Research Fellow, Division of Geriatric Medicine,
University of Toronto
Dr. John Millar, Senior Advisor, Strategic Development,
Canadian Institute for Health
Dr. W. G. De Marchi, Chief Medical Advisor, Ontario Disability Support Program
Branch, Ministry of Community, Family and Children's Services

Chapter 7

Dr. Matthew Hodge, Former Senior Medical Consultant,
Ministry of Health & Long Term Care, Government of Ontario
Dr. Gregory Taylor, Director, Centre for Chronic Disease Prevention & Control,
Health Canada
Dr. Catherine McCourt, Director, Centre for Healthy Human Development,
Health Canada

Chapter 8

Dr. Linda Panaro, Director, Field Epidemiology Training Program,
Centre for Surveillance Coordination, Health Canada
Dr. Donna L. Reynolds, Associate Medical Officer of Health,
Durham Region Health Department

Chapter 9

Dr. Edward Ellis, Chief, Tuberculosis and Bacterial Respiratory Diseases,
Division of Immunization and Respiratory Diseases, Health Canada
Dr. Donald Cole, Professor, Department of Public Health Sciences,
University of Toronto
Mr. John Wellner, Director, Environmental Health, OMA

Chapter 10

Dr. Gary Liss, Medical Consultant, Ministry of Labour, Government of Ontario
Dr. Ronald House, Professor, Occupational Health,
Department of Public Health Sciences, University of Toronto

Chapter 11

Dr. Ross Upshur, Professor, Department of Family & Community Medicine,
University of Toronto

Chapters 12, 13, 15, 16

Mr. Owen Adams, Director, Health Policy, Canadian Medical Association
Dr. Paul Williams, Professor, Department of Health Policy, Management &
Evaluation, University of Toronto

Chapters 14, 18

Mr. Owen Adams, Director, Health Policy, Canadian Medical Association
Dr. Raisa Deber, Professor, Department of Health Policy, Management & Evaluation,
University of Toronto

Chapter 17

Mr. Owen Adams, Director, Health Policy, Canadian Medical Association
Dr. Suzanne De Blois, Medical Consultant, Regional Health Board,
Montreal Centre

"The primary determinants of disease are mainly economic and social, and therefore its remedies must also be economic and social. Medicine and politics cannot and should not be kept apart."

Geoffrey Rose, The Strategy of Preventive Medicine

PART
ONE
HEALTH AND DISEASE

For healthcare professionals, it is vital to understand what makes people healthy. Part I deals with the definitions of health, illness, and disease, and includes synopses of the scientific methods used in determining the factors that influence health and disease. These indicators provide evidence that there are factors beyond traditional health care that influence our health. Canada has led the world in this regard, since publishing the Lalonde Report in 1974 and Ottawa Charter for Health Promotion in 1986.

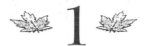

1

CONCEPTS, DETERMINANTS, AND PROMOTION OF HEALTH

In Canada, many diseases, particularly infectious diseases, have been controlled or almost eradicated with the advent of better living conditions, the availability of antibiotics, and public health interventions such as immunization, new technology, and universal health care. Mortality in the population has been drastically reduced and life span has increased. However, chronic diseases and infectious diseases such as acquired immunodeficiency syndrome (AIDS) have emerged as important health concerns. With these changes, our concepts of health and disease have also changed. The focus of health care is shifting toward disease prevention, health promotion, and caring rather than curing. In this chapter, we describe modern concepts of health and disease or illness, the determinants of health and disease in the population, death and dying, and new approaches to promoting and maintaining the health of the population.

1. CONCEPTS OF HEALTH AND DISEASE

1.1. CONTEMPORARY DEFINITIONS OF HEALTH

Health is multidimensional: it is not merely the presence or absence of disease but also has social, psychological, and cultural determinants and consequences. In 1948, the World Health Organization (WHO) acknowledged this multidimensional nature. The WHO defined health as "a complete state of physical, mental and social well-being and not merely the absence of illness" (1). More recently, the WHO has developed a new definition of health that recognizes the inextricable links between an individual and the environment. According to this socio-ecological definition, **health** is defined as "the ability to identify and to realize aspirations, to satisfy needs, and to change or cope with the environment. Health is therefore a resource for everyday life, not the objective of living. Health is a positive concept emphasizing social and personal resources, as well as physical capacities" (2). Measures of health must incorporate these distinct dimensions of human experience. Determinants are more than biological. Health, therefore, involves more than just bodily integrity; it encompasses social and political concerns and the relationship of individuals to their environment. From this perspective, it is the responsibility not only of the traditional healthcare sector, but also of all the sectors, institutions, and organizations that may influence the well-being of individuals and communities. In infectious diseases, the influence of other sectors in the control of disease and prevention of epidemics is recognized (e.g., trade policies, housing regulations, restaurant inspection); nonetheless, there remains much to do in acknowledging the roles of non-health sectors in the prevention and control of chronic diseases.

Furthermore, this new definition provides the foundation for the concept of health promotion articulated at the First International Conference on Health Promotion in Ottawa in 1986. The Ottawa Charter for Health Promotion defines health promotion as "the process of enabling people to increase control over, and to improve, their health" (2). Health promotion efforts attempt to increase the degree of control that individuals and communities have over their health and the determinants of health.

1.2.   CONCEPTS OF DISEASE AND ITS CONSEQUENCES

The strength of this broad definition of health is that it includes psychosocial as well as biophysical dimensions. **Disease** refers to abnormal, medically defined changes in the structure or functioning of the human body; **illness** (or sickness) refers to the individual's experience or subjective perception of lack of physical or mental well-being and consequent inability to function normally in social roles.

Disease and illness have their consequences. A useful systemic taxonomy was developed for the WHO, which defines three concepts related to human experience in the context of disease (3). **Impairment** is defined as any loss or abnormality of psychological, physiological, or anatomical structure or function. **Disability** is any restriction or lack of ability to perform an activity in a manner or within the range considered normal for a human being. **Handicap** is the disadvantage for an individual with an impairment and disability that limits or prevents the fulfilment of a role considered normal (depending on age, sex, and social and cultural factors) by society. Thus, impairment refers to changes in the individual's body, disability to changes in what the individual can and cannot do, and handicap to changes in the individual's relationship with the physical and social environment. Handicap can only be understood through sociological inquiry. These concepts are linked dynamically in Figure 1.1.

The relationships among impairment, disability, and handicap are not necessarily direct. Disability and handicap may result from impairment, and handicap may be the outcome of disability, but these are not always necessarily the case. Nor is there any necessary relationship between the severity of impairment and disability and the extent of handicap experienced. For example, a study of people with multiple sclerosis found that the psychosocial handicaps they experienced were not related to the severity of the underlying disease (4). Similarly, a study of individuals with chronic respiratory disease found that clinical measures of lung function were not good predictors of disability and that there was considerable variation in the extent of handicap associated

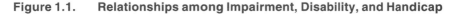

Figure 1.1. Relationships among Impairment, Disability, and Handicap

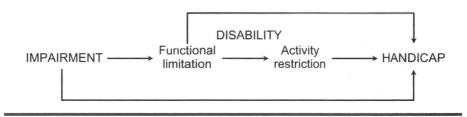

with a given level of disability (5). This highlights the fact that these relationships are mediated by social, cultural, and other factors.

These conceptual distinctions point to the many ways in which the well-being of people with various kinds of disorders may be improved. Clinical medicine focuses on the limitation of impairment. Rehabilitation is concerned with limiting disability and maximizing independent functioning, and social welfare mechanisms modify the disadvantage experienced by people with impairments and disabilities. For many people with chronic and disabling disorders, minimizing the social impacts of their disease is the primary route to improving the well-being of both patient and family. The WHO recently proposed an integrative model called International Classification of Functioning, Disability, and Health (ICF), which incorporates perspectives of both social and medical models and uses a biopsychosocial approach, illustrated in Figure 1.2 (6).

The following definitions help clarify the interrelationship of medical model and social model.

- **Body functions** are the physiological functions of body systems (including psychological functions).
- **Body structures** are anatomical parts of the body such as organs, limbs, and their components.
- **Impairments** are problems in body function or structure such as a significant deviation or loss.
- **Activity** is the execution of a task or action.
- **Participation** is involvement in a life situation.
- **Activity limitations** are difficulties in executing activities.
- **Participation restrictions** are problems experienced in life situations.
- **Environmental factors** make up the physical, social, and attitudinal environment.

In essence, this model takes into account various medical, psychological, social, and environmental factors that could influence an individual's ability to function or participate in life situations. For example, paraplegic individuals could participate in the workforce only if they can access the building in which they work or they could work from home via electronic devices. Accommodating all the factors listed above improves the meaningful integration of individuals with activity limitations or restricted participation in society. The population health model that is described in a

Figure 1.2.   Interactions between the Components of the International Classification of Functioning, Disability, and Health

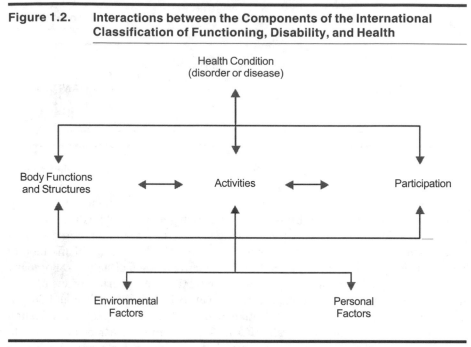

Source: World Health Organization. 2002. *International classification of functioning, disability, and health.* <www.who.int/icidh> (January 2003).

later section and the conceptual model of health indicators described in Chapter 3 take similar approaches to the multidimensionality of health.

Illness behaviour is any activity undertaken by individuals who perceive they have a potential health problem for the purpose of defining their state of health and undertaking an appropriate remedy. The study of illness behaviour addresses the question of what a person does in the presence of signs and symptoms, and why. Often, but not always, this involves the use of medical care. Illness behaviour is significant because it determines the volume of professional services used, as they are currently provided by the healthcare system.

Research shows that people do not bring most of their signs and symptoms to the attention of a medical professional but deal with them in alternative ways (see Chapter 5, Figure 5.1). This phenomenon, referred to as the clinical iceberg, means that there is a permanent and irreducible gap between the need for medical care and the demand for it. The clinical iceberg is important for two reasons. First, many people tolerate symptoms that may be painful or otherwise distressing but may well respond to medical treatment. Second, cases of a particular disorder presenting for medical treatment may not represent cases of that disorder in the population. It is crucial to distinguish between factors related to the onset of the illness and factors related to the seeking of medical care. Illness behaviour depends on the level of medical knowledge, the perception of the costs and benefits associated with a medical consultation (which can be influenced by accessibility of care), and the influence of lay-referral networks.

Another important factor is cultural variation in perception of illness. What may be regarded as part of the normal pattern of everyday life by one cultural group may indicate illness to another. There are also cultural differences in managing health problems of various kinds. Some cultural groups have highly developed systems of ethno-medicine; traditional and professional healers may be consulted according to the nature of the problem and whether it is recognized by scientific medicine. Culture is likely to play an important role in the formation and expression of health beliefs. The beliefs about health and illness held by individuals and groups are now considered very important with respect to the seeking of medical care, patient-practitioner communication, patient responses to consultation, and the degree of patient compliance with medical advice (see Chapter 18).

Compliance has been defined as "the extent to which a person's behaviour (in terms of taking medications, following diets, or executing lifestyle changes) coincides with medical or health advice" (7). This concept implies that practitioners unilaterally pronounce which regimen patients should follow, and patients who do not adhere to those recommendations are perceived as non-compliant. Whether the individual follows advice depends on many psychological, behavioural, personal, and social characteristics; the nature of the health problem; the type, length, side effects, and cost of the regimen; the personality of the individual; and the pattern of communication between the provider and the individual. However, all these factors conceptualize compliance as a characteristic of individual patients and seek to increase it by modifying patient behaviour to fit with the demands of the medical system.

Current research endorses reconceptualizing compliance in terms of **adherence** to reflect the need to address the social and economic limitations that prevent patients from following regimens, instead of attributing differences to individual disobedience. Adherence improves when patients are asked what parts of their regimens are most challenging to follow and what they would like to see. A broad interpretation of how to think about patient behaviour creates more opportunities for healthcare practitioners to respond productively to patients instead of labelling them non-compliant and lowering treatment goals.

The Measurement Iterative Loop framework breaks compliance into two types in determining the effectiveness of interventions. **Provider compliance** is the extent to which the healthcare provider complies with appropriate diagnostic and management actions, and **patient compliance** is the extent to which patients comply with the recommendations made by healthcare providers and treatment (8).

There are some general assumptions about the rate of adherence to a treatment regimen among the patient population. The rule of one third states that about one third of patients totally adhere with treatment, one third partially adhere, and the remaining third do not adhere. Models that explain or predict the likelihood of adherence with health education efforts are described later in this chapter.

Figure 1.3:   **Epidemiological Triangle**

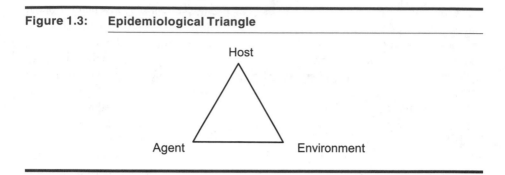

1.3.   THEORIES OF DISEASE CAUSATION

Just as definitions of health have changed over time, so have theories about the nature and causes of disease. Recently the role ascribed to social and psychological factors in the causal processes leading to disease has received increasing attention. Underlying much of what constitutes medical practice is the **biomechanical/ biomedical model**. This has its roots in the 17th-century Cartesian revolution in which mind and body were seen as separate entities, the body being a physical entity activated by mental processes. According to this view, the body is akin to a machine, which can be corrected when things go wrong by procedures designed to repair damage or restore functioning by neutralizing the specific sources or modifying the responsible pathological processes. Thus the model focuses on the causes and treatment of ill health and disease in terms of biological cause and effect. This approach ignores the part played by social, psychological, spiritual, and economic factors in disease onset and recovery. Even in a specialty such as psychiatry, the biomedical model has played a large role in explaining abnormal behaviour. Genetic abnormalities and problems with the biochemistry or physical structure of the brain are popular explanations for psychiatric disorders from the biomedical perspective.

The biomechanical/biomedical model is fully compatible with the **germ theory of disease**, which emerged at the end of the 19th century. Although the idea that disease was caused by a transmissible agent had existed since the 16th century, it was verified only in the late 19th century. Louis Pasteur and Robert Koch showed that these agents were living organisms that enter the body via food, water, or air. From this theory emerged the doctrine of specific **etiology**: the idea that each disease has a single and specific cause.

The germ theory suggests that the mere introduction of an organism into a community is sufficient to cause disease. This is usually not the case; we are exposed to a wide variety of organisms yet rarely succumb to disease. Consequently, it is incorrect to designate an organism or other noxious agent as the sole cause of disease.

From an epidemiological point of view, such an agent is necessary but not sufficient, because suitable conditions for the host and the environment must be present for disease to develop (9). The epidemiological triangle in Figure 1.3 portrays the interaction between agent, host, and environment. The agent may be chemical (e.g., lead), biological (e.g., bacteria), or physical (e.g., violence); host factors may be genetic or acquired, and influence susceptibility to disease; environmental factors may be biological, social, or physical, and may affect exposure and susceptibility. Thus, all diseases are multifactorial and preventable by procedures that modify either the host or the environment. In fact, successful control of diseases requires both.

Often, in chronic degenerative disorders such as heart disease, no single agent can be identified. One explanation is the web of causation (10): diseases such as heart disease develop through the interactions of many factors that form complex, interwoven chains. These factors may be biophysical, social, or psychological, and may promote or inhibit the development of the disease. For example, diet, smoking, physical inactivity, work and life stress, type A personality, obesity, cholesterol levels, hypertension, and diabetes are all implicated in heart disease. Some of these factors are also associated with other disorders such as cancer. More recently, the **theory of general susceptibility** has been developed to explain why some social groups are more vulnerable to disease in general. In this theory, non-specific social and psychological factors are associated with a variety of health outcomes. For example, single, divorced, or widowed men have consistently higher mortality rates than married men. One explanation is that marital status is associated with a wide variety of psychological and lifestyle factors, some of which are related to the risk of disease and death. There is also accumulating research that shows that a lack of social support or close social and emotional ties increases vulnerability to disease and death. Research in many societies has shown that lower socioeconomic status is associated with a higher risk of death, regardless of the cause of death (11, 12). This work directly challenges the doctrine of specific etiology.

2.   DETERMINANTS OF HEALTH

Traditionally, healthcare providers in hospitals, such as doctors and nurses, have been concerned primarily with diagnosing and treating existing disease in individuals (13). The quantity and quality of their services are widely seen as the chief factors in determining the health of the population. Thus, the biomedical model has been pre-eminent. Furthermore, significant changes in health outcomes (such as decreasing morbidity and mortality rates) have been attributed to improvements in medical interventions. More recently, however, this view has been challenged and gradually replaced by more comprehensive concepts of health. The impetus for this broader view comes from two main sources.

First, a critical assessment of the history of disease reveals that major infectious diseases such as tuberculosis and cholera, the leading causes of death in western societies at the turn of the last century, began to decline long before the introduction of effective therapy. Improvements in sanitation, nutrition, and general living conditions are now thought to be important factors in reducing the mortality due to these scourges (14). Second, the evaluation of the factors underlying today's major causes of death and disability has been illuminating. For example, motor vehicle collisions, which constitute the major cause of death and potential-years-of-life-lost in young adults, are largely the result of risk-taking behaviour and the broader socioeconomic and psychosocial factors that influence such behaviour. Mortality caused by motor vehicle collisions cannot be reduced by traditional forms of medical treatment, but requires behavioural changes, such as increased caution, sobriety, the use of seatbelts, and changes in the conditions that lead to that behaviour (e.g., social norms, laws affecting access to alcohol, engineering in cars such as standard inclusion of seatbelts). Therefore, a concept of health must include other factors in addition to traditional curative medicine.

In Canada, the health field concept put forward in 1974 by Marc Lalonde, Minister of Health, offers a more comprehensive view. In *A New Perspective on the Health of Canadians,* he outlined four elements that determine the health of Canadians: human biology, environment, lifestyle, and the healthcare organization (15). More recently, these definitions have extended to psychosocial factors such as gender, ethnicity, and socioeconomic status (16).

2.1.   HUMAN BIOLOGY

Human biology encompasses those aspects of health (both mental and physical) that are determined by the organic structure and physiological functioning of the human body. An individual's genetic make-up determines the likelihood of inherited disorders and predisposition to diseases acquired later (see Chapter 4). That person's constitution also determines susceptibility to risk factors that can arise from certain lifestyles and environments; however, biological factors can also change in response to the environment. Changes in the human body due to maturation and aging can interact with the other three health field elements in determining the individual's state of health. Science has made great progress in understanding the complex processes of the human body and mind, but much remains to be elucidated.

2.2.   THE ENVIRONMENT

The physical environment includes all physical factors external to the human body that may affect health. More recently, the concept of environment has expanded to include the psychosocial environment. Individuals often have little or no control over the presence of environmental risk factors but may be able to exercise some control over the degree of exposure. Society, however, may be able to exert control over the presence of hazards in the environment through legislation, regulations, and policies.

2.2.1.   The Physical Environment

Factors in the physical environment include the quality of air, water, and soil; the safety of food, drugs, and other products that humans consume or are exposed to; the physical handling and disposal of waste; the control of excessive noise; and the control of animal and insect vectors that can transmit diseases (see Chapters 9 and 10). The physical environment is both outdoors and indoors, and involves factors such as workplace ergonomics and indoor air quality (e.g., sick building syndrome). The physical environment can affect human health directly, for example, by exposure to potentially hazardous agents such as chemicals or radiation, or indirectly, for example, by global warming, which is predicted to diminish food production. A major challenge is the development of economic production methods that sustain a healthy environment (sustainable development) as a legacy for our children.

2.2.2. The Psychosocial Environment

The psychosocial environment — the social and physical environments, the places where people live and work, education, and income and social supports — has a major impact on health. Many researchers have adopted a historical perspective and investigated changes in the health of population over time. For example, one analysis has shown that the massive decline in mortality from infectious disease during the 18th and 19th centuries was the product of social and environmental progress rather than any specific medical intervention (14). Improvements in agricultural production led to better nutrition and a population more resistant to infectious disease. Improvements in sanitation and clean water supplies reduced the exposure of the population to infectious organisms. By the time medicine had developed specific therapies for diseases such as tuberculosis, for example, 90% of the decline in mortality from that disease had already occurred.

Other researchers have focused on specific factors that predispose an individual to illness, such as bereavement, social mobility, migration, cultural change, income, unemployment, and work hazards. This research applies a systematic approach on the assumption that life changes, particularly those involving some form of loss, are stressful and render an individual vulnerable to health problems via a variety of mechanisms including biological explanations, for example, processes affecting feedback inhibition of cortisol (17-19). The human body adjusts to chronic stress by altering its physiological characteristics and processes, which leads to what are referred to medically as risk factors such as hypertension, lipid alterations, and insulin resistance.

However, whether life stress leads to some form of illness can depend on the presence of one or more mediating factors. Personality characteristics, coping styles, and the presence of social support are the main variables shown to influence the response to life stress. Social support can provide a sense of belonging and intimacy and can help people to be more competent and self-efficacious. A review of eight population-based cohort studies conducted over the last 20 years indicates that people who are isolated have an increased risk of death from a number of causes (20). This is a complex area conceptually and methodologically, but current research indicates that an individual's social circumstances frequently exert a significant influence over health status.

The group characteristics of a society can also be important in the health of a population. **Social cohesion** is defined as the networks, norms, and trust that bring people together to take action: "the glue that binds people together" (21). The two most commonly used indicators are trust and the number of memberships in voluntary organizations. Several studies have examined the association between social cohesion and health. All have found significant associations (after statistical adjustment for potential risk factors for ill health that are unrelated to social cohesion) (18).

Like life stress, work stress has been shown to be an important determinant of health. **Job strain** — a combination of high job demands and low job control — and the imbalance between the efforts put into a job and the rewards in terms of pay, status, recognition, and job security have been found to be strongly and consistently associated with diseases such as coronary heart disease and hypertension (22-24). Job strain has also been shown to be associated with depression, workplace injuries, and sickness absence (25). A recent study of Japanese men also found that working long working hours was associated with an increased risk of developing type 2 diabetes, independent of the traditional risk factors such as smoking, physical activity, body mass index, and family history (26). In Canada, moving to longer working hours was found to be associated with unhealthy weight gain for men, an increase in smoking for both men and women, and increased drinking in women (27).

Socioeconomic status has been consistently found to be an important determinant of health and an important source of inequalities in health. Some social groups have markedly better health than others, with lower death rates and less illness and disability. For example, the British Whitehall study demonstrated a clear relationship between place in the social hierarchy (as determined by position in the civil service in the United Kingdom) and mortality risk (28). Inequities may be horizontal, with unequal distribution of resources, or vertical, for those at a disadvantage without the resources to reduce differentials. Differences in health can also be connected to geographic location, gender, race, or ethnic origin, and employment status.

Canada's federal and provincial governments have identified social inequities as a major health policy issue (29). There are now documented statistical links between health and socioeconomic status (30, 31). At each rung up the income ladder, Canadians have less sickness, longer life expectancies, and improved health. Data from other countries have also shown a clear inverse relationship between socioeconomic status and a wide range of health indicators, including acute and chronic illness rates, days of restricted activity, psychiatric symptoms, high blood pressure, height, obesity, low birth weight, prematurity, ability to conceive, and self-perceived health (32). Moreover, there is evidence to show that these differences have widened over the past four decades in spite of universal access to health care in many developed countries.

A number of explanations account for the association between socioeconomic status and health. The **artifact explanation** claims that such differences are a product of attempts to measure complex social entities such as socioeconomic status and health using inadequate instruments. However, the evidence concerning health inequities is overwhelming. Systematic gradients exist whether objective or subjective measures of health are used and whether socioeconomic status is measured by income, education, or occupation.

The **theory of natural and social selection** argues that inequities in health are created and maintained by a process of social mobility, whereby healthy individuals move up the socioeconomic scale and less healthy individuals move down. Some studies confirm that conditions such as schizophrenia and chronic bronchitis often lead to a downward occupational drift, with the affected individual ending up in low-paid, unskilled manual labour, or unemployed. Other studies have shown that healthy women were more likely to be upwardly mobile at marriage, marrying men from a socioeconomic group higher than the one they were born in, while less healthy women tended to be downwardly mobile. However, longitudinal studies tracing people from birth show that health clearly affects social position, but that the effect is relatively small and cannot, on its own, account for the observed relationship between social position and health (33).

The **materialist explanation** suggests that inequities in health originate in material deprivation. That is, groups at the lower end of the socioeconomic scale lack adequate financial and other resources to maintain their physical and psychological well-being and to protect themselves from hazardous physical or social environments. Most of the supporting evidence focuses on differences in income and wealth, working conditions, the quality of housing, and the nature of communities where people live. Lower socioeconomic groups are frequently disadvantaged in terms of all four of these factors. Evidence from numerous studies has demonstrated an inverse relationship between material deprivation and health. For example, differences in the health of children from different socioeconomic groups have been linked to poor quality housing and hazardous domestic environments. Overcrowding, damp conditions, and inadequate heating are associated with increased rates of respiratory illness and deaths from accidents in the home. As well, people from lower socioeconomic groups often work in more hazardous environments, which is reflected in data on deaths from unintentional injuries at work or from occupationally related disease. The argument against the materialist explanation is that the relationship between income and health status follows a **gradient**, with each successively lower income grouping having successively lower health status. There is no absolute level of poverty below which health status suffers and above which health status is unaffected (21). The **neomaterialist mechanism** ascribes the gradient in health status across income levels to individuals at each income level having, for example, less well-balanced diets, less adequate housing, more exposure to hazardous working conditions or environmental toxins than individuals at the next highest income level, and less access to social infrastructure (34).

A **psychosocial mechanism** ascribes the gradient in health status across income levels to powerful psychosocial connotations of material differences, not the material differences themselves. This mechanism is a host of factors commonly grouped together under the term "psychoneuroendocrinology" or "psychoneuroimmunology" (17). Psychological processes arising from perceptions of one's status, economic insecurity, relative deprivation, or stress translate into important changes in the nervous, endocrine, and immune systems, which, in turn, lead to deterioration in mental and physical health.

The Canadian National Population Health Survey data for 1994–95 reveals a clear gradient for chronic stress levels across the social hierarchy. Only 15% of Canadians with a university education reported high levels of chronic stress, compared to 25% with college education, 28% with high school education, and 31% with less than high school education (29). For many types of undesirable events (e.g., income loss, ill health, separation/divorce, and death of a loved one), people with lower socioeconomic status have been found more likely to experience the event than their more socially advantaged counterparts (35). In addition, persons of lower socioeconomic status were found to be more vulnerable to or more strongly affected by such events.

Cultural or behavioural theories seek explanations in reference to differences in knowledge, attitudes, and behaviour. Individuals in lower socioeconomic groups are considered less healthy because they consume health-damaging substances such as tobacco and alcohol at higher rates, have diets high in sugars and fats and low in fibre, are less likely to exercise regularly, and make less use of preventive health services (36). This explanation is valid to the extent that lifestyles and consumption patterns are related to socioeconomic status and, in turn, are associated with the onset of conditions such as heart disease or cancer.

However, the Whitehall study shows that although people in lower grades of employment were more likely to smoke, less likely to be physically active in their leisure time, and more likely to be obese, after taking these factors into account, a social gradient in the incidence and mortality rate of coronary heart disease remained (33). The social gradient in mortality applies not only to the lifestyle-influenced diseases such as this example but also cut across most conventional causes of death, such as most cancers, respiratory disease, renal disease, gastrointestinal disease, and violent death.

It remains to be seen which of these theories best explains the social inequalities in health. The materialist theory suggests that widespread social change is necessary to ensure that all individuals have equal opportunities for maintaining and improving their health. This involves a fundamental redistribution of resources in society in order to ensure that all have access to those goods and services necessary to produce health. The cultural theory more narrowly suggests that the remedy lies in health education to change health-damaging attitudes and behaviour; however, it assumes such attitudes and behaviour are freely chosen, rather than environmentally induced, and carries a tendency to blame individuals for situations over which they have relatively little control. Cultural and behavioural patterns deleterious to health are rooted in the material conditions of life of people in the lowest socioeconomic groups, a fact recently demonstrated by a Toronto study that showed that welfare payments would not cover the costs to purchase and consume a healthy and nutritious diet (37).

Efforts to change attitudes and behaviour are likely to fail if such material conditions are not addressed at the same time. This is embodied in the socioecological approach to health promotion, which regards social change as a prerequisite for changes at the individual level (38). Health-related behaviour does not occur independently of the influence of the surrounding physical and social environment. In *The Strategy of*

Figure 1.4.   Risk Continuum of Alcohol Consumption

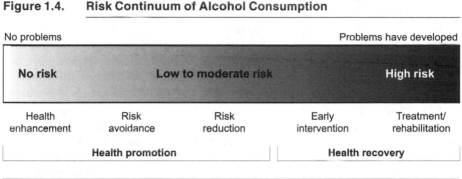

Reproduced from: The Ontario Ministry of Health: *A framework for the response to alcohol and drug problems in Ontario,* 1988.

Preventive Health Care, Geoffrey Rose concludes that "the primary determinants of disease are mainly economic and social, and therefore its remedies must also be economic and social. Medicine and politics cannot and should not be kept apart" (39).

Another factor that may contribute to differences in health status is access to and use of medical services. There is evidence from a number of Canadian jurisdictions that low income groups use fewer family practitioner services in relation to need than their high-income counterparts.

2.3.   LIFESTYLE, BEHAVIOUR, AND RISK FACTORS

Lifestyle involves aspects of individuals' behaviour and surroundings that they control; it must take into account that behaviour is influenced by the social, physical, and economic environment in which people live and work. A **healthy lifestyle** must incorporate elements of social responsibility as well as individual responsibility and can be defined as "comprising patterns of health-related behaviour, values, and attitudes adapted by groups of individuals in response to their social, cultural, and economic environment" (40). The decisions that individuals make result in favourable or adverse consequences for health and play an important role in today's major health problems (41).

The level of risk is significant in balancing health promotion with disease treatment (health recovery). Figure 1.4 shows the risk continuum of alcohol consumption, an example of a substance abuse lifestyle factor (42). For individuals and groups at minimal or no risk, further enhancement of health is appropriate, as is avoidance of risk (e.g., by consuming 14 or fewer drinks per week for men and 9 or fewer drinks per week for women) (43). For individuals at moderate levels of risk (e.g., those consuming more than 14 drinks per week but who may not be experiencing health or social problems yet), reduction of risk is appropriate. Those with significant health problems will require treatment and rehabilitation (health recovery).

2.4.   THE HEALTHCARE ORGANIZATION

The healthcare organization is what is traditionally defined as the healthcare system. It includes medical and dental practice, nursing, hospitals, homecare, chronic care facilities, rehabilitation, drugs, public health services, and health services provided by allied and complementary healthcare professionals such as chiropractic, podiatric, optometric services, and naturopathic. The Canadian healthcare system is discussed in detail in Chapters 12 to 18.

Although the healthcare system primarily alleviates or remedies the problems associated with ill health, it also contributes to morbidity and mortality. A New York hospital study found that 4% of patients had suffered an iatrogenic complication that prolonged hospital stay or resulted in measurable disability. Medication errors were common, occurring in 14% of patient stays, although not usually resulting in serious harm. Missed or incorrect diagnoses were also problematic (44). The extent of the problem in Canada needs further systematic study (see Chapter 18).

2.4.1.   Alternative Health Care

As the Canadian population becomes more cosmopolitan and heterogeneous, many individuals seek to enhance their health by pursuing alternative healthcare modalities. A large number of traditions and practices are covered under this umbrella term. Homeopathy, naturopathy, acupuncture, Ayurvedic medicine, herbology, and Aboriginal healing practices are just a few examples. Epidemiological studies have indicated that many Canadians seek alternative healthcare practices (45, 46). Critics of alternative health care assert there is little or no evidence to support the efficacy of these modalities (47) and argue that they should not be funded by a public healthcare system. However, systematic analysis is ongoing, and the scientific demonstration of benefit cannot be ruled out for all practices.

As more and more Canadians visit complementary therapists and make use of herbal and other alternative medicines, there is a growing concern about the need to evaluate the effectiveness of alternative therapies as well as the interactions between therapies (29). Responding to increasing public demand for governments to protect consumers by setting standards and controls on the manufacturing and sale of alternative medicines, Health Canada has established the Natural Health Product Directorate, which is legislated to carry these functions (see Chapter 13).

2.5.   EXPANDING THE DETERMINANTS OF HEALTH MODEL: POPULATION HEALTH

Population health is variously defined as the study of the determinants of health and disease, health status, and the degree to which health care affects the health of the community. The Canadian Institute of Advanced Research's population health program has extended the study of population health to include the broad determinants of health, detailed in *Why Are Some People Healthy and Others Not?* (48). This research framework seeks to explain how societal influences exert a profound influence on health and well-being throughout the life cycle. The current research focuses on the integration of physical responses into social stimuli (psychoneuroimmunology) and the consequences of deprivation in early childhood development. The framework expands the Lalonde health field concept by synthesizing the vast empirical literature on diverse determinants and health outcomes. In broad terms, the population health model recognizes the influence of various determinants of health (49) and is summarized in Table 1.1.

2.6.   SPIRITUAL DIMENSIONS OF HEALTH

Spirituality encompasses the practices, beliefs, and values a person holds concerning his or her place in the cosmos. Spiritual people are often at peace with themselves or have what is called "inner peace"; they feel connected with their fellow human beings and other creatures in a meaningful and caring way through their practice, beliefs, and values. Spirituality is related to, but not entirely synonymous with, religion. Its impact on health may be through a psychoneurohumoral mechanism that reduces stress and through social connectedness, which increases one's social network. The spiritual model incorporates a holistic approach in which healing plays a central role. Healing is different from treatment. Treatment focuses on discrete physical abnormalities in order to mitigate them or cure the body. Healing applies to all dimensions of a person's existence; correcting a physical abnormality is but one aspect of a healing approach. In healing, how an illness affects the psychological and spiritual dimensions of the afflicted person's life must be considered. The use of sweat lodges in some Aboriginal healing practices illustrates this distinction. Prayers have been used in many cultures for healing. One double-blind, randomized, placebo-controlled clinical trial of prayer on 393 coronary care patients found that the treatment group required less ventilatory support and less treatment with antibiotics or diuretics (50).

2.7   DEATH AND DYING

Technology has resulted in a range of techniques to prolong life. Such life-sustaining technologies have provoked concerns about their appropriate use, and more Canadians are reflecting upon the need to consider end-of-life care. Most provinces have introduced legislation regarding the use of advance directives, which permit individuals to document their preferences for the use of life-sustaining technologies while they are still competent. People may also nominate a proxy to make end-of-life decisions on their behalf. Related to this issue is the debate concerning euthanasia and physician-assisted suicide. The case of Susan Rodriguez, who had a chronic life-threatening and disabling condition known as amyotrophic lateral sclerosis (ALS) and was assisted in terminating her life, brought the issue to the forefront of the Canadian consciousness in 1994 and stimulated vigorous debate that will no doubt continue for the foreseeable future. Euthanasia was legalized in the Netherlands in 2000.

Table 1.1.   Determinants of Health

Determinant	Relevance
1. Income and social status	the most important determinant of health nationally. However, it is the distribution, rather than the actual amount of wealth that is associated with healthier people amongst the population.
2. Social support networks	the effects of social support may be as important as identified risk factors such as smoking, physical activity, obesity, and high blood pressure. It is not the quantity of relations that matter but the quality.
3. Education	provides skills useful for daily tasks, employment (income and job security) and community participation
4. Employment and working conditions	health status is improved with increased control of work circumstances and lower levels of stress. Unemployment is highly correlated with poorer health as well.
5. Physical environment	factors in the natural environment, such as air, water and soil quality are key influences on health. Human-built factors such as housing, workplace, community and road design are also important. Many of the writings from a PHP do not account for environmental implications.
6. Biology and genetic endowment	the functioning of body systems and genetic endowment contribute to health status as well as the process of development.
7. Personal health practices and coping skills	psychological characteristics such as personal competence, locus of control, and mastery over one's life contribute to mental and physical health; however, the focus on personal health practices has been characterized as blaming the victims instead of societal factors.
8. Healthy child development	a wide range of chronic conditions seem to have their origins in fetal and infant life. Prenatal and early childhood experiences are also important in the development of coping skills and competence.
9. Health and social services	contribute to healthier people. However, increased expenditures on health care seem to be less successful in improving the health of Canadians.
10. Gender	biological differences in sex and socially constructed gender influence health and health service use.
11. Culture	may influence the way people interact with health care systems, participation in prevention activities, health-related lifestyle choices, and understanding of health and illness. Racism, language barriers, prejudice and misunderstandings may reduce access to health care.
12. Social environment	low availability of emotional support and low social participation have a negative impact on health and well-being. Questions have been raised about any value added in including "social environment" as a health domain, since it already exists within at least seven of the determinants.

Source: *Chronic Diseases in Canada,* 23(4):124, Health Canada, 2002© Reproduced with the permission of the Minister of Public Works and Government Services Canada, 2003.

3.   APPROACHES TO ACHIEVING HEALTH

Previous sections have described a shift in the concept of health from a predominantly biomedical view to a multidimensional concept. Inter-related components of many aspects of life may affect health and are viewed as a resource for living. The following section moves on to a discussion of the implications for the prevention of disease and the attainment of health.

3.1.   TRADITIONAL MODEL OF PREVENTION

Traditionally, there have been three approaches to disease prevention: primary, secondary, and tertiary. **Primary prevention** aims at preventing disease before it occurs, thereby reducing the incidence of disease. Examples include immunization programs, dietary recommendations, avoidance of initiating smoking, and the use of seatbelts and other protective devices. **Secondary prevention** involves the early detection of disease and the treatment that may accompany screening. **Tertiary prevention** attempts to reduce death and disease by treatment and rehabilitation of diseased individuals, and is carried out by the existing healthcare system.

Many primary and secondary preventive measures for individual patients of health practitioners are incorporated in the periodic health examination, which is fully described in Chapter 11. The remainder of this chapter concentrates on primary prevention and population health and emphasizes approaches that are more appropriate for the community.

3.2.   HEALTH PROMOTION: THE OTTAWA CHARTER

The Lalonde Report was crucial in drawing the attention of Canadians to the determinants of health outside the healthcare sector. With the explicit recognition that human biology, environment, and lifestyles are also important in determining health, a new framework for making impacts on the health of Canadians was necessary.

The 1978 Declaration of Alma Ata on Primary Health Care set the international stage for numerous initiatives in health promotion (51). In particular, in 1984 the WHO's *Targets for Health for All by 2000* (52) proposed improvements in health, specified the locus of action, and provided tools to monitor progress toward health goals. The United States began to develop health goals based on health promotion and disease prevention with the publication of *Healthy People: The Surgeon General's Report on Health Promotion and Disease Prevention* in 1979 (53), followed by the development of 226 specific objectives with target dates for achievement (54). Since then the U.S. has monitored and revised these goals several times, with the most recent version being *Healthy People 2010* (53).

In Canada, although traditional models of prevention in public health and the clinical world had addressed the modification of biology (developing antibodies by vaccination), the environment (clean water supply), and the healthcare organization (screening for breast cancer), the concept of health promotion served as a basis for a reformulation of national and provincial health policies. At the national level, in 1986 Jake Epp, Minister of National Health and Welfare, released *Achieving Health for All: A Framework for Health Promotion* (55). Subsequently, Health and Welfare Canada, the European Region of the WHO, and the Canadian Public Health Association endorsed the Ottawa Charter for Health Promotion (2), which provides a clear vision of current concepts of health promotion and calls on all concerned to join forces to introduce strategies for health promotion that affect the moral and social values that support the Ottawa Charter. The charter defines **health promotion** as follows:

> *the process of enabling people to increase control over, and to improve, their health. To reach a state of complete physical, mental and social well-being, an individual or group must be able to identify and to realize aspirations, to satisfy needs, and to change or cope with the environment. Health is, therefore, seen as a resource for everyday life, not the objective of living. Health is a positive concept emphasizing social and personal resources, as well as physical capacities. Therefore, health promotion is not just the responsibility of the health sector, but goes beyond healthy lifestyles to well-being.*

3.3. HEALTH PROMOTION STRATEGIES

A number of strategies have been developed or adapted for the promotion of health. Many aim at influencing healthy behaviour and the social and environmental conditions that influence such behaviour. Methods that involve changes in lifestyle and social conditions include a number of approaches directed at the levels of the individual, community, and policy. Health promotion approaches in general, as articulated in the Ottawa Charter, involve five main components: **reorienting health services, enhancing personal skills, strengthening community action, creating supportive environments, and building healthy public policy**. Specific strategies include education, communication, legislation, fiscal measures, community organizational change, community development, and local community action (56). Legislation and fiscal measures may affect policy not traditionally under the purview of health (e.g., physical education time in schools, costs associated with nutritious foods, incomes associated with the ability to afford nutritious and healthy foods, costs associated with access to recreational spaces) and are part of building a healthy public policy. Communication and education, in conjunction with community organizational change and community development, can help enhance personal skills, facilitate community action, and create supportive environments. No one strategy is effective on its own — used together, they can promote health and prevent disease.

3.3.1. New Directions

The framework for population health has been combined with health promotion concepts in *Population Health Promotion: An Integrated Model of Population Health*

Figure 1.5.   An Integrated Model of Population Health and Health Promotion

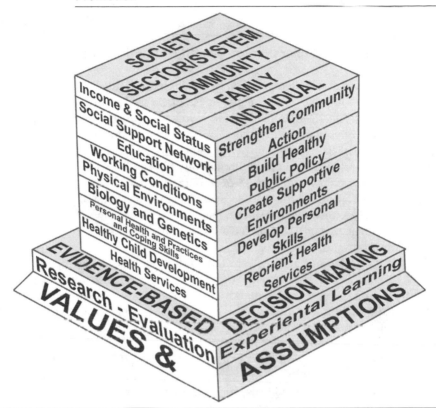

Source: *Population health promotion: an integrated model of population health and health promotion,* Health Canada, 1996.© Reproduced with the permission of the Minister of Public Works and Government Services Canada, 2003.

and Health Promotion (57). This document describes the elements of the population health approach to the broad determinants of health with the strategies and techniques of health promotion as outlined in the Ottawa Charter and Epp's framework. Figure 1.5 shows the interrelationship of the elements of the population health promotion framework. Each element can be extracted so that health promotion strategies can be developed at the social, sectoral (e.g., the agricultural industry), local community, family, or individual level. The framework is also explicit in noting that the choice depends on values and assumptions about desirable health-related goals that must be mediated through evidence and evaluation. The model provides a synoptic view of the manner by which health promotion strategies can be conceived and implemented.

In the U.S., the Institute of Medicine Committee on Capitalizing on Social Science and Behavioral Research to Improve the Public's Health recently endorsed the use of a **social ecological model** that takes a social and environmental approach to health and health interventions. It emphasizes the important influence of biology and genetics as well as social and familial relationships, the environment, and broader social and economic trends on health. Thus, multilevel interventions addressing these health determinants at different life stages and within different settings (e.g. work, school, community) are called for (38).

3.3.2. The Jakarta Declaration on Health Promotion into the 21st Century

The fourth International Conference on Health Promotion, titled "New Era: Leading Health Promotion into the 21st Century in Jakarta," was the first to be held in a developing country in 1997, and the first to involve the private sector in supporting health promotion. Subsequent conferences were held in Australia (on healthy public policy) and Sweden (on supportive environments).

The Jakarta Declaration on Health Promotion offers a vision and focus for health promotion, calling on the widest range of resources to tackle health determinants in the 21st century (58). It asserts that the **prerequisites** for health are peace, shelter, education, social security, social relations, food, income, the empowerment of women, a stable ecosystem, sustainable resource use, social justice, respect for human rights, and equality. Above all, poverty is the greatest threat to health.

The Jakarta Declaration acknowledges that infectious diseases and mental health problems require an urgent response. Transitional factors, such as the integration of the global economy, financial markets and trade, and access to media and communication technology, also have a significant impact on health, as does environmental degradation due to the irresponsible use of resources. The declaration expands the ideas set forth in the Ottawa Charter with the following priorities.

1. *Promote social responsibility for health.* Both the public and private sectors should promote health by: a) pursuing policies and practices that avoid harming the health of other individuals; b) protecting the environment and ensuring sustainable use of resources; c) restricting production and trade in inherently harmful goods and substances such as tobacco and armaments; d) limiting unhealthy marketing practices, safeguarding both the citizen in the marketplace and the individual in the workplace; e) and including equity-focused health impact assessments as an integral part of policy development.

2. *Increase investments for health development,* in particular for women, children, older people, the indigenous, and poor and marginalized populations.

3. *Strengthen existing partnerships and explore the potential for new partnerships* between different sectors at all levels of governance and society.

4. *Increase community capacity and empower the individual.* Improving the capacity of communities for health promotion requires practical education, leadership training, and access to resources. Empowering individuals demands more consistent, reliable access to the decision-making process and the skills and knowledge essential to effect change.

5. *Secure an infrastructure for health promotion.* New mechanisms of funding health promotion at the local, national, and global levels must be found. Incentives should be developed to influence the actions of governments, non-

governmental organizations, educational institutions, and the private sector to make sure that resources for health promotion are maximized.

After Jakarta, the fifth conference was held in Mexico in 2000, where the declaration focused on getting countries to commit to support health promotion at all levels. The theme of "Bridging the Equity Gap" addressed health determinants related to economically and socially disadvantaged populations. Eighty-seven countries, including Canada, signed the Mexico Ministerial Statement for the Promotion of Health — From Ideas to Action, which affirms that health promotion strategies contribute to the sustainability of local, national, and international health activities. The signatories commit to draw up country-wide health promotion plans (59). In particular, this commitment has led to an expansion of the healthy cities movement in Latin America. Since 1984, there has been a worldwide movement toward healthy cities, communities, schools, and workplaces. These elements share a common focus on using comprehensive health promotion strategies to define processes for community participation to create a healthy future (59).

3.3.3. Health Education

Health education can be any combination of learning experiences designed to facilitate voluntary actions conducive to health. The aim is to encourage people to modify their lifestyles positively while encouraging them to resist reverting to bad habits. People who have adopted unhealthy lifestyles often find it difficult to change their behaviour even if they want to. It is increasingly recognized that social and economic influences affect behaviour. Without reinforcement from change in social norms and economic incentives, health education is less effective in producing a change in behaviour (41).

Several theoretical views of behaviour change underlie the types of programs developed for health education. One unifying concept proposed states that behaviour is a result of predisposing, reinforcing, and enabling factors (60). Predisposing factors comprise knowledge (for example, the health consequences of smoking), attitudes, beliefs, and values. Researchers have found that the intention to change behaviour is also a strong predictor (61). Reinforcing factors (such as those provided by the social context of family, society, or healthcare professionals) involve reward or feedback for the discontinuation or adoption of behaviour. Enabling factors include skills such as behaviour modification techniques as well as the availability of relevant supports such as reasonably priced, low-fat foods that support dietary change.

An influential **theory of social learning** has been constructed from a number of related concepts that must be addressed in lifestyle education (62). There is a strong correlation between social learning principles and some health-related actions. The essential concept is of reciprocal determinism, which is recognition that social environment influences behaviour, which in turn affects environment. Behaviour is the result of personal and environmental factors. The importance of the social environment as the context for learning has been developed in the social influences model.

Apart from components of behavioural capability (the acquisition of skills and knowledge), reinforcements, and supportive social and economic environments, there are other components of social learning theory. These are observation (such as with role models), expectations of positive results from behaviour change, expectancies (such as an improved appearance following weight loss, which may be a more potent motivator than the expected health benefits), perceptions of an individual's situation (e.g., what the consequences of pregnancy might be), and emotional factors that may pose barriers to behaviour change (such as anxiety associated with the anticipation of giving up a lifestyle habit).

Self-efficacy and self-control are components of behaviour change that are increasingly being incorporated into health education for sustained behaviour change. **Self-efficacy** refers to the cognitive state when one is confident that one can achieve a behaviour change. This may be reached by the achievement of short-term goals. **Self-control** relates to decision-making capacities for healthy choices and self-monitoring, such as those used in guided self-management programs for smoking cessation.

An important model, the **health belief model** attempts to explain the factors influencing compliance (see Figure 1.6) (63). This model suggests that behaviours undertaken by individuals in order to remain healthy, including the use of preventive services, are a function of a set of interacting beliefs. In order to be motivated to take action to avoid illness, an individual must be in a state of readiness to take action and must believe that the action will have positive consequences. In order to be ready to act, the individual needs to feel susceptible to the disease in question and to believe that it would have some significant impact on his or her life. Beliefs about the benefits of the action in question involve consideration of barriers to action such as time, cost, and inconvenience.

Current formulations of the health belief model include the role of cues and modifying factors. Cues are specific events that stimulate preventive health behaviours. Modifying factors are sociodemographic variables such as age, sex, and race, sociopsychological variables such as personality and peer group pressure, and other variables such as knowledge of, and prior experience with, the disease. All these factors influence the individual's perception of susceptibility to disease and seriousness, as well as perception of the benefits of health-related actions. This model has provided the foundation for many health education and awareness programs. One of its implications is that these programs must be carefully targeted at specific social and cultural groups and must be based on a detailed understanding of their health beliefs.

More recently, a model based on the stages of change has provided a useful framework to understand how changes of lifestyle behaviour can be facilitated (64) (see Figure 1.7). In studies of cigarette smokers, four different stages were identified: the precontemplation stage, when the individual was unaware of a behaviour-related health problem; the contemplation stage, when change was considered; the action stage, when initial attempts at change were made; and maintenance, or long-term change. Individuals may not move through these stages in a linear fashion. There are barriers to change at each stage, as well as facilitative processes.

Figure 1.6. Health Belief Model

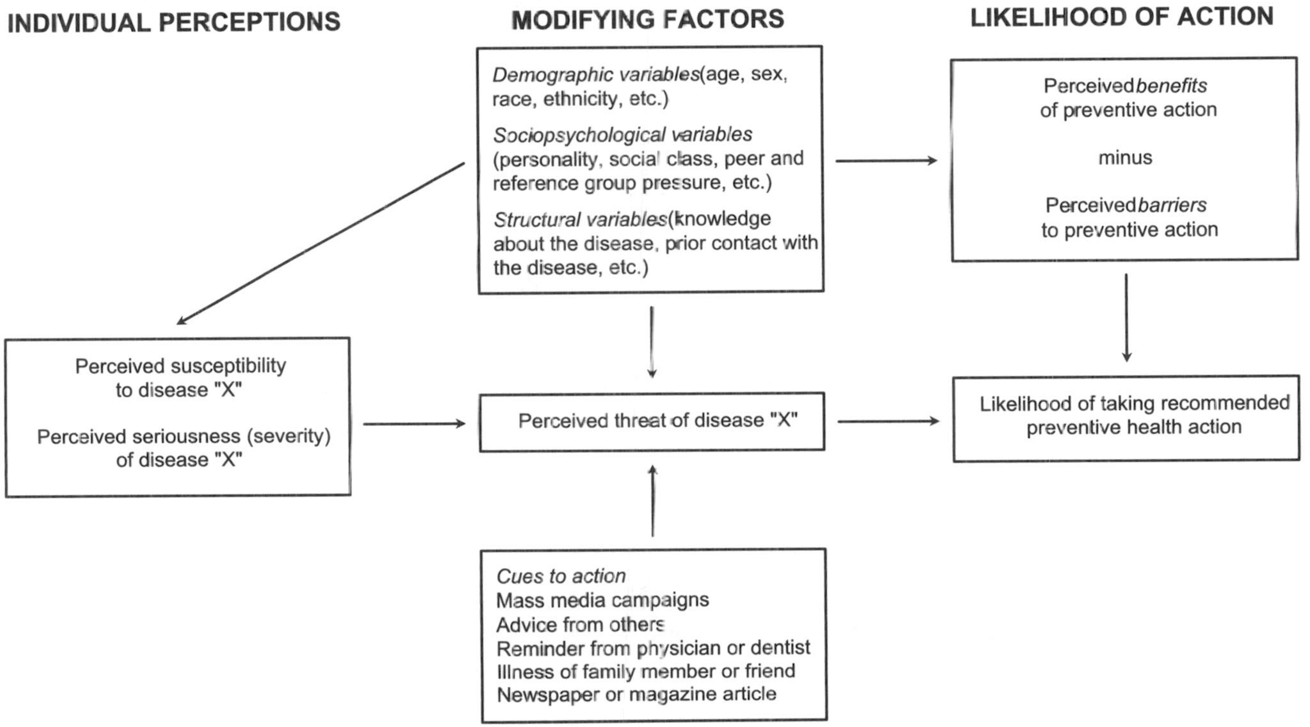

INDIVIDUAL PERCEPTIONS

Perceived susceptibility
to disease "X"

Perceived seriousness (severity)
of disease "X"

MODIFYING FACTORS

Demographic variables(age, sex,
race, ethnicity, etc.)

Sociopsychological variables
(personality, social class, peer and
reference group pressure, etc.)

Structural variables(knowledge
about the disease, prior contact with
the disease, etc.)

Perceived threat of disease "X"

Cues to action
Mass media campaigns
Advice from others
Reminder from physician or dentist
Illness of family member or friend
Newspaper or magazine article

LIKELIHOOD OF ACTION

Perceived*benefits*
of preventive action

minus

Perceived*barriers*
to preventive action

Likelihood of taking recommended
preventive health action

Source: Reproduced with the permission of the publisher, from MH Becker, DP Haefner, and SV Kasl, et al. Selected psychosccial models and correlates of individual health-related behaviours. Medical Care 15:27-46, 1977.

Figure 1.7.   **The Five Stages of Change**

Precontemplation: an individual is not seriously considering change (for all kinds of reasons) and isn't interested in any kind of intervention.

Contemplation: the individual begins to seriously consider making the change within the foreseeable future (often defined as six months).

Preparation: the individual begins experimenting, making small changes. He or she resolves to make a serious attempt in the near future (usually defined as 30 days).

Action: the individual is actively involved in making the change, using different techniques.

Maintenance: the individual must learn to successfully cope with temptations to return to the previous behaviour pattern.

Adapted from: JO Prochaska, CC DiClemente, and JC Norcross, *In search of how people change. Applications to addictive behaviors.* American Psychologist 47(9):1102-1114, 1992.

The Stages of Change Model. Models such as this one have been applied to enhance compliance. The stages-of-change model can successfully aid the design of effective compliance strategies (65). Strategies that allow personal control over decision-making also facilitate changing behaviour and increasing compliance.

Evaluation of health education programs has shown that effectiveness depends heavily upon target group and setting, as well as the content of programming and the method of delivery of the health education messages. For example, a meta-analysis of 33 school-based drug-use prevention programs found significant changes in knowledge and attitudes but none on drug behaviour overall. However, peer-based programs, which used older peers to deliver the messages, had a significant impact on drug-use behaviour. Interactive programs that taught skills to resist behaviour and peer pressure were more effective than non-interactive programs, and large programs were less effective than smaller ones (66). Effectiveness was also affected by whether the health education messages delivered to specific target groups were consistent with larger community norms for specific target groups (e.g., school and community). For example, the effects of school-based smoking prevention programs appear to be sustained when the behaviour promoted by these programs complies with larger community norms but not when health education messages and social norms are inconsistent (38).

Health education alone is usually insufficient in producing sustained behaviour change. A systematic review of randomized controlled trials of multiple risk factor interventions to prevent coronary heart disease concluded that although personal counselling and education appeared to reduce risk factors and mortality in high-risk hypertensive populations, "standard health education methods have limited use in the general population" (67).

Instead, behaviour change in the population requires attention to the **4 E's: education, environmental supports, economic levers, and enforcement of regulations and legislation**. For example, effective prevention of teen smoking requires health education measures combined with changing the norms in the larger social environment (using mass media communications and social marketing strategies), price controls through tobacco taxation (as part of healthy public policy), and legislation and regulations restricting access to cigarettes (also as part of healthy public policy) (38). The use of fiscal and legislative measures to prevent disease is also referred to as health protection (67).

3.3.4. Risk Reduction Strategies

An important concept of harm reduction is emerging from the risk continuum that some behaviour cannot be eliminated by current knowledge and techniques (68-70). For example, harm reduction does not seek to eliminate drug use; it focuses instead on minimizing the personal and social harms and costs associated with substance abuse. Some controversial harm-reduction strategies include methadone maintenance programs, needle exchanges, and illegal-drug dispensing under controlled conditions.

Five basic principles have been identified for **harm reduction**:

1. It offers a practical alternative aimed at the consequences of harmful behaviour rather than whether the behaviour is morally right or wrong.
2. It accepts alternatives to abstinence such as needle-exchange and methadone programs.
3. It is based on consumer input and demand rather than a top-down policy.
4. It supports low-threshold access to treatment and user-friendly approaches in order to reduce barriers to treatment.
5. It is based on compassionate pragmatism and not on moral idealism.

3.3.5. Communications and Behaviour Change

Information can be communicated effectively in a strategy to promote knowledge of health and its determinants. Mass media constitute an important tool for influencing awareness, knowledge, attitudes, and behaviour. The Stanford Five-City Study used mass media to affect behaviour in relation to cardiovascular risk factors on a community-wide basis (71). The prevalence of risk factors increased in the control city (which was comparable to the experimental community on a sociodemographic basis), while risk behaviour was reduced in the community in which the intensive mass media campaign was used. There have been conflicting views about mass communication programs; some suggest that while they do affect attitudes and knowledge levels, behaviour frequently remains unchanged. However, others have indicated that behaviour changes were influenced (72). Mass media form one modality that assists in setting and framing the public agenda and are most effectively used in conjunction with other health promotion measures.

3.3.6. Social Marketing

Social marketing is another health promotion strategy and is defined as "the application of commercial marketing technologies to the analysis, planning, execution, and evaluation of programs designed to influence the voluntary behaviour of target audiences in order to improve their personal welfare and that of society" (73).

Social marketing combines the best elements of the traditional approaches to social change in an integrated planning and action framework. It uses advances in communication technology and marketing to generate discussion and promote information, attitudes, values, and behaviour. By doing so, it helps to create a climate conducive to social and behavioral change.

3.3.7. Healthy Public Policy

Despite awareness of risk-taking behaviour and associated health hazards, many people still resist change. Various adverse behaviour patterns appear more desirable and attractive by the use of sophisticated advertising techniques. For example, even though early models of cars had seatbelts and the general public was aware of their benefit, few people used seatbelts. Compliance improved when legislation imposed a fine on passengers found not wearing seatbelts. The implementation of legal deterrents to individual behaviour such as seatbelt legislation, anti-smoking bylaws, or legal drinking age is an approach to overcoming these barriers to change. Government control is also mediated by tax and pricing policies aimed at reducing the accessibility of certain commodities (such as cigarettes and alcohol) by raising prices. The effectiveness of these economic policies depends on the amount of the individual's disposable income. Programs based on personal motivation and behavioural change take much longer to effect change and involve a smaller percentage of the participating public than do public policy changes. Thus, although health education programs that change behaviour based on individual knowledge, attitudes, and motivation are important, healthy public policy plays a significant role in supporting and sustaining such changes.

Public and private policies shape how money, power, and material resources flow through society and therefore affect the determinants of health. As a society, creating healthy public policies is the most important strategy for acting on the determinants of health. For example, social welfare, day care, and unemployment insurance can have a big effect on individual health (74).

The Ottawa Charter, the Adelaide Recommendations (75), and the Jakarta Declaration call for building healthy public policy: for healthcare professionals to put health on the agenda of policy makers in all sectors and at all levels, directing them to be aware of the health consequences of their decisions and to accept their responsibilities for health.

According to the Canadian Public Health Association, healthy public policies are required in order to:

- reduce inequalities in income and wealth;
- ensure that economic activity contributes to human development and is environmentally and socially sustainable;
- protect people and the earth from toxic pollution, resource depletion, and systemic global effects;
- create safe, secure, and meaningful work opportunities;
- create opportunities for meaningful activities beyond the workplace (i.e., at home and in the community);
- create safe, supportive environments in schools, workplaces, and the community;
- support the active participation of people significantly affected by a particular policy in discussing, choosing, and implementing the best option;
- ensure that individuals and families have access to the recreation opportunities and other programs needed to stay healthy; and ensure that individuals and families have access to the resources necessary to choose and sustain healthy lifestyles, including sufficient incomes that can support the affording of healthy and nutritious diets and the availability of healthy and nutritious foods at affordable prices (74).

3.3.8. Community Organization and Community Development

Enhanced public participation is a major strategy in Epp's framework (55). The nature and extent of public participation can be conceptualized along a spectrum of increasing community capacity to respond to issues of community concern.

Community efficacy represents the state of community confidence necessary to bring about desired social change (76). Mechanisms include lobbying, coalition building, and political action. **Community development** refers to the process of community members identifying issues and problems affecting their community, and developing and acquiring the planning skills and capacity to bring about the implementation of change. Healthcare organizations, such as public health departments, may facilitate this community-initiated and directed process.

Community organization also involves the identification of problems within a community and the mobilizing of resources for change (77). However, the process is driven to some extent by the goals and strategies established by the healthcare sector, and assists the community to achieve the change. There are three elements of community organization: social planning, which is the rational solution of problems using the existing power structure; community locality development, or the development of a community for an organized approach to a given problem; and social action, which is a shift in power structures in the community. Organizing occurs when interest focuses on a concern by the development of leadership, commitment, bargaining, protest, education, and persuasion. This may result in changes within administrative structures themselves, or "inter-organizing" the development of joint structures for community problem solving.

These strategies can be integrated into a concept that views an entire community as the focus of health promotion. In the healthy cities framework, health-enhancing strategies are integrated into urban planning and community design (77). Elements of a **healthy city** include a clean and safe physical environment, a sustainable ecosystem, the meeting of basic human needs, and a strong and supportive community in which decision making is shared by all. The strategy involves including health promotion issues on the political agenda so that key decision makers and the community at large make prevention and health promotion highly visible and community supported. This strategy was emphasized at the WHO's Mexico Conference and has strengthened the healthy municipalities and communities movement in Latin America.

3.3.9. Community-Based Prevention

Recognition of the prevalence of multiple preventable factors in communities and the widespread distribution of some risk factors has resulted in the emergence of the community-based or population-based approaches that complement, or replace, a high-risk approach focusing on special high-risk groups. **Population approaches** aim at the general public at large while **high-risk approaches** target intervention at individuals at high risk of developing a disease. Population approaches seek to shift the distribution of risk factors across the entire population to lower levels (39, 78).

The Canadian Heart Health Initiative has piloted population-based, multifactorial pilot projects that combine communication-behaviour change, community organization, and social marketing (79). Other community-based intervention projects have included the North Karelia Project in Finland, the Stanford Five-City Project, the Minnesota Heart Health Program, and the Community Intervention Trial for

Smoking Cessation (COMMIT) (80). Initial evidence supporting the effectiveness of community-wide prevention came from the North Karelia Project in Finland, which showed a reduction in cardiovascular mortality subsequent to a community-wide prevention program, and the Stanford Five-City Project, in which cardiovascular risk factors decreased after five years (71, 81). However, there is also evidence of differential effectiveness among community subgroups in the Stanford Five-City Project and COMMIT (80).

3.3.10. Innovation-Diffusion Theory

Complementary theories have developed to explain the process by which health promotion innovations spread in communities and to identify the most effective ways to encourage people to adopt a different behaviour. **Roger's theory of diffusion** conceptualizes a population as composed of innovators, early adapters, an early majority, a late majority, and those who resist most efforts for change (82). Community leaders tend to be early adapters and can be effective as project advisors. Other characteristics of an innovation affecting its adoption are whether it is simple, workable, reversible, flexible, advantageous, cost-effective, low risk, and compatible with value systems.

4.   PUBLIC HEALTH ETHICS

Concern for ethical issues in public health has increased in light of evidence of systematic problems of accountability in Canada's public health system. These concerns relate for example to water safety in the aftermath of Walkerton, Ontario, and North Battleford, Saskatchewan, to the importation of serious infectious disease in contaminated food, to access to health information for public health surveillance, to the justification of coercive measures for disease control, and to the communication of environmental risks. The conclusions of the Krever Commission inquiry into the contamination of the blood supply by blood-borne pathogens clearly outlined the ethical responsibilities of public health practitioners and the consequences of the failure to uphold those responsibilities (83).

The focus of ethics in public health differs from that of clinical medicine (84). In clinical medicine, four principles — autonomy, beneficence, non-malfeasance, and justice — are well recognized. In public health, the focus is on populations, communities, and the social determinants of health, which are not neatly analogous to a focus on individual patients. There is no set of common principles for public health ethics. The scope of ethical issues in public health is also broader, reflecting the wide range of issues involved (85, 86).

The central issues in public health ethics revolve around concerns for weighing individual rights versus community rights. The origins of public health are intimately tied to the application of utilitarian thought (the ethical theory that holds that the criterion for determining the worth or goodness of an action is the maximization of happiness or the greatest good for the greatest number of people). Concerns for equitable distribution of goods and providing for the most vulnerable of society are also concerns of public health and can be supported by egalitarian concepts of justice.

In most western countries, legislation supports public health action against individuals. It sets out the justification for communicable disease surveillance, mandatory reporting, detention, and quarantine. The ethical justification rests in the necessity of the community to be able to protect itself from health threats.

There are also important ethical issues raised by screening programs, health promotion programs, privacy and confidentiality of health information, and research ethics (84). Global issues relating to environmental health, emerging infectious diseases, and population control, and economic disparities also require systematic analysis (87). A newly sparked interest in public health ethics has seen the creation of an international task force to develop courses for inclusion in public health curricula.

5. SUMMARY

This chapter outlines the concepts of health and disease, determinants of health, and approaches to achieving health.

Health has been defined in various ways. In this book, the World Health Organization's definition is used: *health* is the ability to identify and to realize one's aspirations, to satisfy one's needs, and to change or cope with one's environment. Thus, health is a daily resource rather than the objective of living, and emphasizes social and personal resources and physical capacities.

Impairment is any loss or abnormality of psychosocial, physiological, or anatomical structure or function. *Disability* is any restriction or inability to perform an activity in a way considered normal, whereas *handicap* is the disadvantage experienced by someone with an impairment or disability that limits or prevents the fulfilment of a role that is normal for that person.

Illness behaviour can be any activity undertaken by someone who perceives a potential health problem for the purpose of defining his or her state of health and for undertaking an appropriate remedy. Illness behaviour depends on many factors, including cultural background.

There are several theories of disease causation. One, the *biomechanical/biomedical model*, holds that the body is like a machine that can be corrected by procedures designed to repair damage or restore functioning. According to the *germ theory of disease*, a living organism enters the body via food, water, or air, and hence each disease has a single and specific cause. The most recent is the *theory of general susceptibility*, which holds that broad, non-specific social and psychological factors are associated with increased susceptibility to a variety of health outcomes.

The *determinants of health* include the individual's human biology (those aspects of both mental and physical health that arise out of the basic biology of humans or are due to the individual's organic make-up); the individual's physical environment (factors include food, drugs, air/water/soil quality, waste disposal, and animal and insect vectors) and psychosocial environment; lifestyle, behaviour, and modifiable risk factors (aspects of an individual's behaviour and surroundings over which the individual has some control, although these are shaped by the social and economic environmental conditions within which the individual lives); and the healthcare organization.

Approaches to achieving health include prevention and health promotion strategies. There are three levels of *prevention*: primary, secondary, and tertiary. Primary prevention aims at preventing disease before it occurs. Secondary prevention involves early detection of disease and the treatment that may accompany screening. Tertiary prevention attempts to reduce complications by treatment and rehabilitation. A number of *health promotion strategies* have been developed or adapted for the promotion of health and include education, risk reduction, communication-behaviour change, social marketing, healthy public policy (including fiscal measures and legislation), community development and organization, community-wide prevention, and diffusion of innovations.

In recent years, there is increased concern for ethical issues in public health and a demand for more accountability in Canada's public health system. In public health, the ethical focus is on populations, communities, and the social determinants of health, which are not neatly analogous to a focus on individual patients. The scope of ethical issues in public health is broad, and reflects a concern for weighing individual rights versus community rights.

6.   REFERENCES

1.   Culyer A. *Health indicators*. Oxford: Martin Robertson, 1983.
2.   Canadian Public Health Association, World Health Organization. *Ottawa Charter for Health Promotion*. Ottawa: Health and Welfare Canada, 1986.
3.   Wood P. The language of disablement: A glossary relating to disease and its consequences. *International Journal of Rehabilitative Medicine* 1980; 2(2):86-92.
4.   Harper A, Wood P, Chambers L, *et al*. An epidemiological description of physical, social and psychological problems in multiple sclerosis. *Journal of Chronic Disease* 1986; 39(4): 305-10.
5.   Williams S, Bury M. Impairment, disability, and handicap in chronic respiratory illness. *Social Science and Medicine* 1989; 29(5):609-16.
6.   World Health Organization. 2002. *International classification of functioning, disability, and health*. <www.who.int/icidh> (January 2003).
7.   Lutfey K, Wishner W. Beyond "compliance" is "adherence": Improving the prospect of diabetes care. *Diabetes Care* 1999; 22(4):635-9.
8.   Tugwell P, Bennett K, Sackett D, *et al*. The measurement iterative loop: A framework for the critical appraisal of need, benefits and costs of health interventions. *Journal of Chronic Diseases* 1985; 38(4):339-51.
9.   Rothman KJ, Greenland S. *Modern epidemiology*. 2nd ed. Haggertown, MD: Lippincott-Raven, 1998.
10.   MacMahon B, Pugh T. *Epidemiological principals and methods*. 2nd ed. Boston: Little, Brown and Co., 1996.
11.   Evans R, Barer M, Marmot M, *et al. Why are some people healthy and others not?* New York: Aldine de Gruyter, 1994.

12.   Syme S, Balfour J. Social determinants of health. In Wallace R, editor. *Maxey-Rosenau-Last public health and preventive medicine*. 14th ed. Stamford, CT: Appleton & Lange, 1998.

13.   Bunker J, Frazier H, Mosteller F. *The role of medical care in determining health: Creating an inventory of benefits*. Society and Health. New York: Oxford University Press, 1995.

14.   McKeown T, Record R, Turner RD. An interpretation of decline mortality in England and Wales during the twentieth century. *Population Studies* 1975; 29(3):391-422.

15.   Lalonde M. *A new perspective on the health of Canadians*. Ottawa: Ministry of Supply and Services, 1975.

16.   Federal, Provincial, and Territorial Advisory Committee on Population Health. *Towards a healthy future: Second report on the health of Canadians*. Ottawa: Health Canada, 1999.

17.   Brunner E, Marmot M. Social organization, stress, and health. In Marmot M, Wilkinson R, editors. *Social determinants of health*. Oxford: Oxford University Press; 1991. p. 17-43.

18.   Kawachi I, Kennedy B, Wilkinson R, *et al. The society and population health reader: Income inequality and health*. New York: New Press, 1999.

19.   Wilkinson R. *Unhealthy societies: The afflictions of inequality*. London: Routledge, 1996.

20.   Berkman L. The role of social relations in health promotion. *Psychosomatic Medicine* 1995; 57:245-54.

21.   Lavis J, Stoddart G. *Social cohesion and health*: McMaster University Center for Health Economics and Policy Analysis Working Paper Series, 1999.

22.   Bosma H, Peter R, Siegrist J, *et al.* Two alternative job stress models and the risk of coronary heart disease. *American Journal of Public Health* 1998; 88:68-74.

23.   Hemingway H, Marmot M. Psychosocial factors in the aetiology and prognosis of coronary heart disease: systemic review of prospective cohort studies. *British Medical Journal* 1999; 318:1460-7.

24.   Siegrist J. Adverse health effects of high-effort/low-reward conditions. *Journal of Occupational Health Psychology* 1996; 1:27-41.

25.   National Institute of Occupational Safety and Health Working Group. *Stress at work*. Cincinnati: National Institute of Occupational Safety and Health, 1999.

26.   Kawakami N, Araki S, Takatsuka N, *et al.* Overtime, psychosocial working conditions, and occurrence of non-insulin dependent diabetes mellitus in Japanese men. *Journal of Epidemiology and Community Health* 1999; 53:359-63.

27.   Shields M. Long working hours and health. *Health Reports* 1999; 11(2):33-47.

28.   Marmot M. Socioeconomic determinants of coronary heart disease mortality. *International Journal of Epidemiology* 1989; 18(suppl 1):196-202.

29.   Federal, Provincial, and Territorial Advisory Committee on Population Health. 1999. *Statistical report on the health of Canadians*. Ottawa. <www.statcan.ca/english/freepub/82-570-XIE/free.htm> (November 2002).

30.   Wilkins R, Berthelot J, Ng E. Trends in mortality by neighbourhood income in urban Canada from 1971 to 1996. *Health Reports* 2002; 13(Suppl):1-28.

31.   Mustard C, Derkson S, Berthelot J, *et al.* Age-specific education and income gradients in a Canadian province. *Social Science and Medicine* 1997; 45(3):383-97.

32.   MacIntyre S. The Patterning of Health by Social Position in Contemporary Britain: Directions for Sociological Research. *Social Science and Medicine* 1986; 23(4):393-415.

33.   Marmot M. Social determinants of health: From observation to policy. *Medical Journal of Australia* 2000; 172(8):379-82.

34.   Lynch J, Kaplan G. Understanding how inequality in the distribution of income affects health. *Journal of Health Psychology* 1997; 2(3):297-314.

35.   McLeod J, Kessler R. Socioeconomic status differences in vulnerability to undesirable life events. *Journal of Health and Social Behaviour* 1990; 31:162-72.

36.   Manga P. *Equality in Access and Inequalities in Health Status*. Health and Canadian Society. Markham: Fitzhenry and Whiteside, 1987.

37.   Vozoris N, Davis B, Tarasuk V. The affordability of nutritious diet for households on welfare in Toronto. *Canadian Journal of Public Health* 2002; 93(1):36-46.

38.   Smedley B, Syme S, editors. *Promoting health: Intervention strategies from social behavioural research*. Washington DC: National Academy Press; 2000.
39.   Rose G. *The strategy of preventive medicine*. New York: Oxford University Press, 1992.
40.   Conway J. With gun and camera in darkest Ontario: Searching for elusive health lifestyle concept. *Public Health and Epidemiology Reports Ontario* 1992; 3(16):268-9.
41.   Lyons R, Langille L. 2001. *Healthy lifestyle: Strengthening the effectiveness of lifestyle approaches to improve health*. <www.hc-sc.gc.ca/hppb/phdd/docs/healthy/index.html> (February 2003).
42.   Ministry of Health. *Understanding AIDS and HIV infection: Information for hospitals and health professionals*. Toronto: Government of Ontario, 1988.
43.   Centre for Addiction and Mental Health. 2002. *Low-risk drinking guidelines*. <www.camh.net/addiction/pims/low_risk_drinking.html> (November 2002).
44.   Leape L. Error in medicine. *Journal of American Medical Association* 1994; 272(23):1851-7.
45.   Buske L. Looking for an alternative. *Canadian Medical Association Journal* 1999; 161(4):363.
46.   Verhoef M, Russel M, Love E. Alternative medicine use in rural Alberta. *Canadian Journal of Public Health* 1994; 85(5):308-9.
47.   Brigden M. Unproven cancer therapies: A multi-headed Hydra. *Annals of Royal College of Physicians and Surgeons of Canada* 1998; 31(1):9-14.
48.   Evans R, Hodge M, Pless I. If not genetics, then what? Biological pathways and population health. In Evans R, Barer M, Marmor T, editors. *Why are some people healthy and others not?* New York: Aldine de Gruyter; 1994. p. 161-88.
49.   Tonmyr L, MacMillan H, Jamieson E, *et al*. The population health perspective as a framework for studying child maltreatment outcomes. *Chronic Disease in Canada* 2002; 23(4):129-32. <www.hc-sc.gc.ca/pphb-dgspsp/publicat/cdic-mcc/23-4/a_e.html> (February 2003).
50.   Astin J, Harkness E, Ernst E. The efficacy of "distant healing": A systemic review of randomized trials. *Annals of Internal Medicine* 2000; 132(11):903-10.
51.   World Health Organization. *International Conference on Primary Health Care, Alma Ata, USSR, 1978*. Geneva: World Health Organization, 1978.
52.   World Health Organization. *Targets for health for all by the year 2000*. Copenhagen: World Health Organization Regional Office for Europe, 1984.
53.   U.S. Department of Health Education and Welfare. 2000. *Healthy people 2010: The Surgeon General's report on health promotion and disease prevention*. <www.health.gov/healthypeople> (February 2003).
54.   Centers for Disease Control. *Healthy people 2000: National health promotion and disease prevention objectives — Healthy people review 1998–99*. Hyattsville: U.S. Department of Health and Human Services, 1999.
55.   Epp J. *Achieving health for all: A framework for health promotion*. Ottawa: Ministry of Supply and Services, 1986.
56.   Noack H, McQueen D. Health promotion indicators. *Health Promotion* 1988; 3(1):1-125.
57.   Hamilton N, Bhatti T. *Population health promotion: An integrated model of population health and health promotion*. Ottawa: Health Promotion Development Division, Health Canada, 1996.
58.   World Health Organization. 1997. *The Jakarta Declaration on health promotion into the 21st century*. <www.who.int/hpr/archive/docs/jakarta/english.html> (September 2002).
59.   World Health Organization, Pan American Health Organization, Ministry of Health of Mexico. 2000. *Health promotion: Bridging the equity gap — Conference report*. <www.who.int/hpr/conference> (February 2003).
60.   Green L, Kreuter M. *Health promotion planning: An educational and environmental approach*. 2nd ed. Toronto: Mayfield Publishing Company, 1991.
61.   Fishbain M, Aizen I. *Beliefs, attitudes, intentions, and behaviours: Introduction to theory and research*. Reading MA: Addison-Wesley Press, 1975.

62.   Bandura A. *Social learning theory*. New York: General Learning Press, 1971.
63.   Becker M, Hafner D, Kasl S. Selected psychosocial models and correlates of individual health-related behaviors. *Medicare* 1977; 15(5):27-43.
64.   DiClemente C, Prochaska J, Fairhurst S, *et al*. The process of smoking cessation: An analysis of precontemplation, contemplation, and preparation stages of change. *Journal of Consulting and Clinical Psychology* 1991; 59(2):295-304.
65.   Butler C, Rollnick S, Stott N. The practitioner, the patient, and resistance to change: Recent ideas on compliance. *Canadian Medical Association Journal* 1996; 154(9):1357-62.
66.   Schuster C, Kilbey M. Prevention of drug abuse. In Wallace R, editor. *Maxey-Rosenau-Last public health and preventive medicine*. 14th ed. Stamford, CT: Appleton & Lange; 1998.
67.   Ebrahim S, Davey Smith G. Systemic review of randomized controlled trials of multiple risk factor interventions for preventing coronary heart disease. *British Medical Journal* 1997; 314:1666-74.
68.   Canadian Centre on Substance Abuse: National Working Group on Policy. *Harm reduction: Concepts and practice*. Ottawa, 1996.
69.   Des Jarlais D. Harm reduction: A framework for incorporating science into drug policy. *American Journal of Public Health* 1995; 85(1):10-1.
70.   Hilton A, Thompson R, Moore-Dempsey L, *et al*. Harm reduction theories and strategies for control of human immunodeficiency virus: A review of the literature. *Journal of Advanced Nursing* 2001; 33(3):357-70.
71.   Shea S, Basch CA. Review of five major community-based cardiovascular disease prevention programs. Part 1: Rationale, design, and theoretical framework. *American Journal of Health Promotion* 1990; 4(3):203-13.
72.   Hastings G, Haywood A. Social marketing and communication in health promotion. *Health Promotion International* 1991; 6(2):135-45.
73.   Health Canada. 2001. *Social marketing: Primer*. <www.hc-sc.gc.ca/hppb/socialmarketing/resources/primer.html> (October 2002).
74.   Canadian Public Health Association. *Action statement for health promotion in Canada*. Ottawa, 1996.
75.   World Health Organization. 1998. *The Adelaide recommendations: Conference statement of the 2nd International Conference on Health Promotion*. <www.who.int/hpr/archive/docs/adelaide.html> (February 2003).
76.   Wallerstein N. Powerlessness, empowerment, and health implications for health promotion programs. *American Journal of Health Promotion* 1992; 6(3):199-205.
77.   Kickbusch I. Healthy cities: A working project and growing movement. *Health Promotion* 1989; 4(2):77-82.
78.   Rose G. Sick individuals and sick populations. *International Journal of Epidemiology* 1985; 14:32-8.
79.   Health and Welfare Canada. 1992. *Heart health equality: Mobilizing communities for action*. Cat. H39-245/1992 E. <www.hc-sc.gc.ca/hppb/ahi/hearthealth/pubs/equal/eqa01.htm> (November 2002).
80.   Ferguson J. Community intervention programs. In Wallace R, editor. *Maxey-Rosenau-Last public health and preventive medicine*. 14th ed. Stamford, CT: Appleton & Lange; 1998.
81.   Shea S, Basch CA. Review of five major community-based disease prevention programs. Part 2: Intervention strategies, evaluation methods, and results. *American Journal of Health Promotion* 1990; 4(4):279-87.
82.   Rogers E. *Diffusion of innovations*. 14th ed. New York: The Free Press, 1995.
83.   Krever H. *Commission of Inquiry on the Blood System in Canada (Krever Commisssion Report)*. Ottawa: Health Canada, 1997. <www.hc-sc.gc.ca/english/protection/krever> (October 2002).
84.   Upshar R. Principles for justification of public health intervention. *Canadian Journal of Public Health* 2002; 93(2):101-3.

85.   Darragh M, McCarrick P. Public health ethics: Health by numbers. *Kennedy Institute of Ethics Journal* 1998; 8(3):339-58.
86.   Gostin L. Public health law in a new century — Part I: Law as a tool to advance the community's health. *Journal of the American Medical Association* 2000; 283:2837-41.
87.   Bantar S. Global disparities in health and human rights: A critical commentary. *American Journal of Public Health* 1998; 88:295-300.

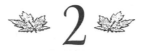

2

MEASUREMENT AND INVESTIGATION

As indicated in Chapter 1, the concepts of health and disease are changing and are multidimensional. To assess health, both quantitative and qualitative data are used. The science of epidemiology has been widely used for its quantitative approaches to studying the health of populations. This chapter provides an overview of the principles of epidemiology and some basics of statistics. Standard epidemiology texts offer an in-depth treatment of this subject (1-4).

1. EPIDEMIOLOGICAL STUDIES

Epidemiology is "the study of the distribution and the determinants of health-related states and events (such as diseases) in specified populations, and the application of this study to the control of health problems" (5). The distribution of disease is studied in terms of person, place, and time. **Person** attributes include age, sex, socioeconomic status, race, and ethnicity. **Place** factors include location of residence, work, and school, and can involve comparisons between urban and rural, between north and south, and among different countries. **Time** factors describe the occurrence of health events per specified unit of time, for example seasonal or diurnal variations, trends over an extended period. The **determinants** of diseases may be studied in terms of at-risk (demographic) groups, lifestyle and behavioural factors (e.g., diet, smoking), occupation, and environment (physical, psychosocial, political, and economic).

In recent years, the science of epidemiology has been well recognized for investigating epidemics and identifying new health problems in populations. Examples include infectious diseases (e.g., AIDS, Lyme disease, Legionnaires' disease, toxic shock syndrome), exposure to environmental and occupational hazards (e.g., ozone pollution, pesticides, asbestos), and diseases for which no agent has yet been identified (e.g., Reye's syndrome, Kawasaki disease). Epidemiologists use certain methodologies to identify and evaluate the causal or contributing factors to disease, their distribution, and possible means of prevention.

1.1.   DESCRIPTIVE STUDIES

An epidemiological descriptive study describes the presence (prevalence) of disease or other phenomena in terms of person, place, and time. Prevalence studies in specific sociodemographic groups, geographic areas, or over a particular period that do not look for associations between variables are examples of descriptive studies. **Prevalence rates** are calculated by dividing the number of individuals who have an attribute or disease at a particular time by the total population at the same point in time. Most data obtained in surveys, including census data, report prevalence rates. One cannot make any causal attribution from descriptive studies; these studies, however, may generate hypotheses that could be further investigated. For example, a study of children in the care of child welfare agencies revealed that 400 per 1,000 such children were disabled. Based on the high rate of disabled children within the care of child welfare agencies compared to the rate of disabled children in the general population, one may hypothesize that children with disabilities are more likely to come into public wardship than those with no disabilities. This hypothesis may be tested in an analytic study.

1.2.   ANALYTIC STUDIES

In analytic studies, a hypothesis is tested to discover if there is an association between a given disease, health state, or other dependent variable (outcome), and possible risk or causative factors. Analytic studies are of two types: observational and experimental.

1.2.1.   Observational Studies
There are four types of observational studies: ecological, cross-sectional, case-control, and cohort studies.

Ecological Studies
Ecological studies differ from other observational studies in that the method of analysis involves an aggregate rather than individuals. Commonly, geographical areas, such as countries or census tracts, are used as units of analysis, and differences in exposures and outcomes of interest are compared between the geographical areas. The recent interest in dietary epidemiology stems from the comparison of disease rates among countries with varying diets. Such studies suggest a possible role of dietary differences in the differences in disease rates found among countries. However, one cannot infer that a specific type of diet is associated with a disease within an individual. Additionally, because of potential confounders, one cannot be certain from such studies that diet is in fact the causal factor in question.

Because they are usually quick and easy to do and make use of readily available data, ecological studies are useful for generating hypotheses. However, they cannot be used for the direct assessment of causal relationships between risk factors and health outcomes in individuals because the individual is not the unit of analysis. Interpretation of ecological studies must avoid the **ecological fallacy**, whereby inferences about relationships between a risk factor and outcome at the individual level are made inappropriately (6). Ecological data can provide accurate descriptions of the average exposure or the average risk of disease for populations, but nothing can be inferred about any particular individual in the population. Additionally, it is often difficult to draw conclusions regarding causal relationships at the population level because full control of all confounding variables is difficult to achieve. However, when a variable in question (e.g., income distribution) is either only measurable at the population level or most appropriately measured at this level, then the ecological study may become necessary. A new technique in epidemiology and biostatistics, known as **multilevel modelling**, may allow for the assessment of individual and ecological level data concomitantly and thus increase the strength of the evidence obtained for population level variables.

Cross-Sectional Study

In this type of study, the prevalence of diseases, disability, and risk factors is examined simultaneously in a defined population at one particular time (5). The population is divided into those with the disease and those without it, and then various characteristics of the two groups are compared. The total population can also be divided according to different variables such as age or sex and the disease prevalence rates can be compared among the groups. Although cross-sectional studies allow for a determination of association between variables, they do not allow for the assessment of the temporal relationship between the variables.

Case-Control Study

The **case-control study** is a type of observational study in which persons with a disease of interest (cases) are compared to similar persons without the disease (controls) for exposure to the presumed risk factors. It is sometimes called a **retrospective study** because it looks for exposures occurring in the past. Investigators collect data by examining medical and other relevant records, and by interviewing cases and controls. If a presumed risk factor (variable) is present in cases significantly more frequently than in controls, then an association exists between this variable and the disease. This association is expressed by the **odds ratio**, which is the ratio of the odds of exposure among cases to the odds of exposure among non-cases (the next section describes how to calculate odds ratio).

Case-control studies are less costly and time consuming than cohort studies, but they may suffer from **recall bias**; people with a disease may be more prone to recalling, or believing, that they were exposed to a possible causal factor than those who are free of disease. Because case-control studies start with an identification of individuals with and without disease, they are good for studying rare disease outcomes. When the disease outcome is rare, the odds ratio is a good estimate of the relative risk. As with other types of observational studies, case-control studies may also show a spurious association between a factor and a health outcome because of unrecognized confounding. **Confounding** occurs when a variable (confounder) is related to both the exposure and the outcome but either is not measured or is distributed unequally in the comparison groups. If not corrected, a false association between the confounder and the outcome may occur because the confounder is associated with both the outcome and the exposure. For example, a study that sought to investigate the relationship between coffee drinking and heart disease found a strong relationship between increased coffee consumption and heart disease but did not measure cigarette smoking. In this case, it is likely that the association between coffee drinking and heart disease is confounded by cigarette smoking, since cigarette smoking is associated with coffee drinking and with heart disease. Thus, because cigarette smoking was not measured and controlled for, the association seen between coffee drinking and heart disease may be deceptive, arising from the association between increased cigarette smoking in coffee drinkers and heart disease. One method commonly used to attempt to control for confounding is to match controls to cases on potential confounding characteristics such as age, sex, socioeconomic status, and other potential or known risk factors.

Cohort Study

A **cohort** is a group of people with a common characteristic such as year of birth, residence, occupation, or exposure to a suspected cause of disease that may be followed forward in time by investigators. This type of study may be considered an organized observation of a natural experiment. Although cohort studies look forward in time, there are two types: retrospective and prospective. In **retrospective cohort studies**, the whole period of observation is historical; in **prospective cohort studies**, the period of observation starts now and continues for a period of time into the future. In both types, a cohort that becomes exposed to the hypothesized risk factor is chosen from a defined population free of the disease under study, along with a "control cohort" that ideally has the same characteristics except that it is not exposed to this factor. Both groups are followed for a certain period of time (e.g., 5, 10, or 20 years) and the observed rates of disease or other outcomes in the two cohorts are compared.

Cohort studies provide an estimate of the **incidence rate**, the rate at which a new disease or other events in a defined population at risk of having that disease or event occur over a given time. The numerator consists of the number of new events (e.g., new cases of a disease diagnosed or reported) over a given period, and its denominator is the number of people in the defined population who do not have the disease or event at the beginning of the follow-up period. Cohort studies allow the determination of a **relative risk**, also known as the **risk** or **rate ratio**, which is the ratio of the incidence rate of a health outcome among the exposed to the incidence rate of the health outcome among the unexposed. Cohort studies also allow for the determination of **attributable risk,** the risk or rate of a health outcome attributable to the risk factor in question. Incidence density can also be calculated from cohort studies and is defined as the number of new cases that occur per unit of population-time (for example, person-years at risk). At times, it is difficult to follow a cohort that is exposed to an agent for an extended period. In such cases, the total length of time that each person is exposed becomes the denominator for the calculation of incidence density (i.e., the number of new cases divided by time at risk of developing the disease). An example is the incidence rate of lung cancer expressed in terms of 1,000 person-years exposed to smoking.

Table 2.1.   Comparison of Cohort and Case-Control Studies

	Cohort study	Case-control study
Advantages	Provides incidence rates, relative risk, and attributable risk Less bias Can get natural history of disease Can study many diseases	Small number of subjects Quick to do Suitable for rare diseases Inexpensive Can study many factors
Disadvantages	Large number of subjects Long follow-up Attrition Costly Changes over time Locked into factor under investigation	Recall bias Provides only odds ratio Problems in control group selection Does not provide incidence rate Incomplete recall Locked into disease

Cohort studies have the great advantage that possible risk factors are identified and recorded before the disease appears, thus reducing the possibility of many sources of bias (systematic error in making inferences and recording observations). However, these studies are expensive, pose great difficulty for studying very rare diseases, and take many years before results can be analyzed. As with other observational studies, uncontrolled confounding factors may also lead to a false association between the exposure factor and the health outcomes under study. Table 2.1 summarizes the advantages and disadvantages of case-control and cohort studies.

The Calculation of Relative Risk, Odds Ratio, Attributable Risk, and Attributable Fraction/Population Attributable Risk

The risk of disease for individuals may be measured by either a relative risk or odds ratio. To calculate these risk measures requires the number of persons with and without disease, as well as the number of people with and without exposure to the suspected causal or risk factor.

	DISEASE (cases)	NO DISEASE (control)
POSITIVE	a	b
NEGATIVE	c	d

Exposure

The **relative risk (RR)** of those exposed having the disease, compared to the unexposed is:

$$\left(\frac{a}{a+b}\right) \div \left(\frac{c}{c+d}\right)$$

The **odds ratio (OR)** of a case having been exposed, compared to a control, is $(a \times d) \div (b \times c)$. For rare diseases, for example, where the values of a and c are small, the formula for RR approximates $(a \div b) \div (c \div d)$, which equals $(a \times d) \div (b \times c)$. Thus, for rare diseases, the OR (derived from a case-control study) is a suitable estimate of the RR (otherwise derived from the more costly cohort study).

The attributable risk is calculated by subtracting incidence rate of exposed minus incidence rate of unexposed:

$$\left(\frac{a}{a+b}\right) - \left(\frac{c}{c+d}\right)$$

Attributable fraction is the fraction of disease associated with an exposure within the population. **Population attributable risk (PAR)** is a measure of the excess incidence of disease associated with an exposure within a population. PAR can be derived by subtracting the incidence density in the unexposed group from the incidence density in the total population. PAR can also be calculated directly from the relative risk (RR) and the prevalence of exposure (Pe) to the risk factor in the population:

$$PAR = Pe\,(RR - 1) \div \{1 + [Pe\,(RR - 1)]\}$$

1.2.2.   Experimental Studies

Unlike observational studies, **experimental studies** are those in which conditions of the study are under the direct control of the investigator. Observational studies are the best types of studies possible for the study of exposures to risk factors, since it would be unethical to expose healthy people intentionally to risk factors. However, experimental studies are possible when trying to assess the effects of an intervention to improve health outcomes, either by providing a new treatment to those already ill or by providing an intervention to attempt to prevent a disease. In a **randomized controlled trial (RCT)**, people with a disease or at risk of a disease are randomized into two or more groups. Randomization is expected to equalize the distribution of all major demographic characteristics, such as age, sex, and socioeconomic status. To ensure that this is the case, known confounders should still be measured. However, because of randomization, with a large enough sample size, unknown confounders will likely distribute themselves equally among the groups and thus play little role in the results obtained. One group is subjected to the intervention being evaluated, usually a treatment, while all other groups (controls) are given either an inactive treatment (placebo) or current standard treatment. When subjects are blinded to (unaware of) their treatment status, this procedure is called a **single-blind** trial. The effectiveness of the treatment is best evaluated when there is a comparison group, because the health status of individuals or groups changes constantly. Outcomes for both groups are ideally assessed by an individual who does not know which group each trial participant belongs to, thus reducing the possibility of bias in the observer. Trials where neither participant nor observer knows the group assignment are called **double-blind** clinical trials. If the health outcomes in the treatment group are statistically significantly better than those in the control group, then the treatment is considered to have been effective in this trial. **Triple-blind trials** are those where blinding occurs with the participants, the assessors of health outcomes, and those reviewing and analyzing the data collected.

Although many clinical trials evaluate new drugs or operations, alternative forms of healthcare delivery can also be studied in this way. For example, Shah et al. (7) examined the attitudes of parents whose children were sent home after minor surgery rather than kept in hospital. Children scheduled to have surgery were randomly assigned to two groups: the experimental group, whose members were discharged within eight hours after surgery and received home care, and the control group, whose members were kept in hospital for the usual one to three days. The groups were similar in age, sex, socioeconomic status, and type of surgery. After the children had recovered from surgery, the parents were asked about their child's symptoms and their satisfaction with the treatment. Parents were also asked about their preference for care (i.e., whether they would prefer their children to be hospitalized for minor surgery or prefer them to return home on the same day as surgery). There were 116 children in each group. Most parents of the control children (66.4%) preferred hospitalization, but the parents of experimental subjects favoured home care (78.4%). Thus, it appears that such home care is well accepted by those who have experienced it.

Although trials can yield reliable and valid results, there are many situations in which trials cannot be carried out on humans. If a treatment is already known to be superior to the control treatment, it would not be ethical to deprive people in the control group of the treatment. If a factor is thought to cause or predispose a person toward a disease, ethical considerations forbid deliberately exposing humans to such risk. Furthermore, recent experience with trials for new treatments for AIDS has shown that personal desire to have the new treatment can result in contamination of the trial. **Contamination** occurs when members of the control group receive the treatment meant for the intervention group; this can occur, for example, as a result of patients visiting and obtaining the treatment from physicians not participating in the trial. This has led to innovative new strategies such as **open-arm** trials in which some of the participants can choose the therapy they wish to receive. With the open-arm trial, however, randomization and its advantages are lost. Two other important issues that can affect the results of a RCT after randomization are compliance and co-intervention. **Compliance** refers to the degree with which patients in the intervention or control group adhere to the treatment regimen they are given. **Co-intervention** refers to interventions other than the one being studied that patients from either the intervention or the control group may receive that may affect their disease outcome (2).

Community trials of preventive health interventions are delivered to whole populations. One community is given an intervention (mass regimen) while another serves as a control. This methodology was used, for example, to evaluate the effects of naturally fluoridated water supplies on the prevalence of dental caries. There are intrinsic reasons why community trials are more likely than randomized controlled trials to produce equivocal results. Community trials are quasi-experimental, because allocation of the intervention is not randomized among individuals in the communities. It is particularly difficult to control for contamination, which occurs when the comparison communities also receive some of the intervention, and **confounding** from unmeasured factors is also a concern. Frequently, the outcomes observed are changes in the risk behaviour of the population, which are intermediate rather than "final" health outcome data.

1.2.3. Systematic Reviews and Meta-analysis

As the scientific literature grows and numerous studies are published on each health topic, it is increasingly difficult to make sense of the sometimes conflicting results of multiple studies. In recent years, systematic reviews and meta-analyses have become important tools for addressing this issue. A **systematic review** is a summary of research evidence that relates to a specific question. It attempts to overcome biases that might occur through rigorous and systematic methods for searching for papers, retrieving, rating relevance and quality, extracting the data, synthesizing the data, and writing up the review. Criteria for the inclusion of studies, including for rating relevance and quality of the studies, are preset. Two people independently conduct each stage of the review, compare their results, and discuss the discrepancies. **Meta-analysis** takes systematic reviews one step further and quantitatively combines the results of the studies to get an overall summary statistic that represents the combined effect of an intervention across different studies (8). The purposes of meta-analyses include increasing statistical power for outcome assessment and sub-group evaluation, resolving uncertainty or conflicting results, improving estimates of effect by increasing sample size, and providing answers to questions not posed by the original trials.

Although it is always appropriate and desirable to review the literature systematically in order to answer a question about a health topic, it is not always appropriate to combine the results quantitatively and statistically. Thus, even though systematic reviews should always be done, meta-analyses are not always applicable. Although this can be true for both experimental and observational studies, it is particularly relevant for observational studies. Unlike randomized controlled trials, where unmeasured confounders should be distributed equally among the study groups, observational studies cannot guarantee that unmeasured confounders do not bias the results due to some unaccounted process of self-selection. There are concerns in the scientific community that the current methods of meta-analysis, when done on observational studies, can actually increase the precision of estimated results that are biased. In other words, a result that is less precise and biased through meta-analysis may become more precise but still biased. Better research methods for combining the results of observational studies are currently being sought (9).

There are several sources of systematic reviews. An international effort to collect and collate all randomized controlled trials relevant to clinical medicine was started when the Cochrane Centre was opened in Oxford, England, in 1992. The **Cochrane Collaboration** is an international collaboration of healthcare researchers that undertakes systematic reviews and meta-analyses, and maintains a central and accessible database of all evidence related to healthcare delivery. At present, there are 49 Cochrane review groups internationally, organized by topic. Five are located in Canada: the Back Review Group, the Hypertension Review Group, the Inflammatory Bowel Disease Review Group, the Musculoskeletal Review Group, and the Neonatal Review Group. The Cochrane Collaboration also has 10 fields (with the child health field located in Canada) that compile specialized databases of reviews relevant to the field and 12 method groups that work on methods development and improvement. For systematic reviews related to the practice of public health, there are several other sources in addition to the Cochrane Collaboration. These include the Effective Public Health Practice Project, which is an initiative of Ontario's Public Health Research, Education, Development (PHRED) Program, the Health Development Agency funded by the United Kingdom's National Health Service, and published systematic reviews in scientific journals. Many of these databases can be accessed through their websites.

1.2.4. Clinical Epidemiology

An important source of information on the natural history, prognosis, and outcome of disease states comes from the observations and actions of practising physicians. Clinical epidemiology represents the application, modification, and refinement of epidemiologic techniques to individual patient care; its purpose is to collect systematic information from the practice of medicine in order to increase the accuracy, reliability, validity, and effectiveness of clinical care. An important facet of this process is the development of clinically relevant disease and outcome taxonomies, known as **clinimetrics** (10, 11).

One of the concerns of clinical epidemiology is the accuracy of diagnostic strategies. Clinical epidemiology uses a variety of statistical techniques such as **decision analysis** and **Bayesian analysis** to study the most efficient use of diagnostic technology. Statistical techniques are also used to study the natural history and prognosis of diseases, with a particular emphasis on the extent to which medical intervention improves outcomes.

Closely related to clinical epidemiology is the technique of **critical appraisal**, which has been defined by Sackett et al. (3) as the "application of certain rules of evidence to clinical (symptoms and signs), paraclinical (laboratory and other diagnostic tests), and published data (advocating specific treatment manoeuvres or purporting to establish the etiology or prognosis of disease) in order to determine their validity (closeness to the truth) and applicability (usefulness in one's own clinical practice)." A series of articles outlining the principles and methods of critical appraisal of different types of studies has been published (12-15), and is available on the Web sites.

The application of the techniques of clinical epidemiology and critical appraisal constitute **evidence-based medicine**. The aim of evidence-based decision making (EBDM) is to ensure that decisions about health and health care are based on the best available knowledge (16-18). To use EBDM one must first assess what constitutes evidence, both in relation to health-enhancing interventions and to organizational or policy-level decision making. One also needs to explore the availability and accessibility of reliable information and knowledge that identifies how interventions, practices, and programs affect health outcomes. EBDM is also used to explore the causes that prevent change from taking place in the health system (in practice and policy) when there is clear evidence that change is necessary and desirable. An EBDM framework also examines the length of time the health system takes to adopt existing information about the interventions that work, and their degree of success. Canadian researchers are pioneers in developing levels of evidence to include or exclude manoeuvres for clinical prevention, which deal with screening and counselling for asymptomatic individuals in clinical settings by primary care health practitioners (19). The methodology for this has been described in Chapter 11. Practice guidelines for clinical encounters and interventions aimed at individuals and populations rely heavily on the evidence. The Cochrane Collaborative centres and Canadian Medical Association are useful sites for different guidelines (20, 21).

1.2.5.   Causal Associations

The types of studies outlined in the previous sections are frequently undertaken in a step-wise fashion, with the overall objective of identifying and establishing associations between exposure to factor(s) and disease. Each type of study has its strengths and limitations. Descriptive studies, such as prevalence studies, can identify potential risk factors in a specific population and generate hypotheses about potential risk factors, which can be further investigated by analytic studies such as case-control studies and cohort studies. By comparing the odds of exposure in cases of disease with individuals who are free of the disease, case-control studies are able to determine an odds ratio, i.e., an indirect estimate of the relative risk when a disease outcome is rare. Cohort studies take more resources and time as large numbers of subjects are followed over a long period; however, the relative risk of disease following exposure to a putative risk factor, as well as attributable risk, can be directly determined. Randomized controlled trials give the highest calibre of information about the effect of an intervention on individuals. Community intervention studies, although only quasi-experimental, provide intervention effectiveness information for communities.

Although analytic studies are able to draw associations between exposures and specific health outcomes, the determination of causation is more challenging. In 1965, Hill (22) published the following criteria for determining whether a causal association exists between an exposure and a disease:

- **Consistency of the association:** Do the findings of studies of the same design as well as different designs in different populations demonstrate the same association?
- **Strength of the association:** How large is the relative risk of the outcome in relation to exposure?
- **Dose-response:** Does the severity or the likelihood of the outcome increase as the amount, intensity, or duration of the exposure increases?
- **Temporal relationship:** Did the exposure occur before the onset of the disease?
- **Plausibility:** Is the association with a risk factor specific, given the existing basic science and clinical knowledge about the disease?
- **Coherence:** Does the association make sense in terms of the theory and knowledge

about the disease process?

- **Analogy:** Do other established associations provide a model for this type of relationship?
- **Experimental evidence:** Is there experimental or quasi-experimental evidence that removal of the putative causative factor results in reduction of disease incidence?
- **Specificity:** Is the association specific for a particular disease or group of diseases? (In practice, however, this criterion often is not satisfied, particularly with many chronic diseases that can have multiple causes).

1.2.6. Qualitative Research

Many important issues in public health cannot be adequately addressed by quantitative methods. Issues relating to the attitudes and beliefs of community members or healthcare practitioners may be best explored using qualitative research techniques. **Qualitative research** uses interpretive and naturalistic approaches to study research questions. Studies are carried out in natural non-experimental situations. Unlike the quantitative approach, which places a high value on quantitative measurement and analysis, qualitative research focuses on explaining and understanding the particular process. Narrative accounts replace statistical summaries (23); specific qualitative research techniques are used to capture and analyze the narrative accounts in a reliable and valid manner.

A variety of qualitative research techniques, developed in the social sciences, have found applications in the healthcare field. Examples of data-gathering methods include focus groups, key informant interviews, and Delphi and nominal groups. **Focus groups** use group interviews to generate data for thematic analysis. In-depth interviews, such as **key informant interviews**, seek to garner information from individuals with special insight into health issues. Consensus methods such as **Delphi** and **nominal groups** seek to establish the extent of agreement, often among experts, in cases of unclear evidence.

2. INVESTIGATION OF DISEASE IN POPULATIONS

The above section provided an overview of different epidemiological methods in studying health and disease in the population. The following describes several situations in which these methods are applied to investigate non-communicable disease in populations.

2.1. CLUSTERS OF DISEASE

One of the most frequent problems faced by local health units or a provincial department of health is the concern of local residents and practising physicians about apparently excessive numbers of a relatively rare health problem or disease in their community. For example, residents may express concern about an apparent excess number of cancer deaths or birth defects in their community and wish for an investigation into the cause. The excess number of cases is often referred to as a cluster. Caldwell (24) defines a **cluster** as "a number of like or similar things occurring together in time and space." This definition includes the notion of disease aggregation and its etiology. In common usage in epidemiology, the term "cluster" tends to be used for uncommon non-infectious diseases, while the terms "epidemic" and "outbreak" tend to refer to infectious diseases (see Chapter 8). There are different types of disease clusters including clustering of possibly related diseases within the same person, clustering within families or other interpersonal networks, clustering in time (i.e., cases of the same disease within a short period), clustering in space (i.e., within close geographical proximity), or clustering in both time and space.

Although it is important to gather as much information as possible about the potential cluster — including suspected health events, suspected exposures, number of cases, time period of concern, and geographical area of concern — a hasty cluster investigation is often not useful. The reasons for this include the following: often what is reported as a cluster of one disease actually involves multiple diseases with multiple causes and so is not a cluster of a specific disease (e.g., "cancer" is not one disease but many different diseases with vastly different etiologies); the diseases reported are often not rare diseases — and so are expected to be seen (e.g., "cancer" occurs in a large percentage of the population as they age; birth defects, although less common than cancer, occur in 1–2% of live births); numbers reported are frequently small and therefore do not allow for an appropriate epidemiological study; exposures are poorly characterized, in low concentration, or difficult to measure; and an unexposed similar population that is needed for comparison in an epidemiological study is not available. Thus, before proceeding to investigate the causes of a potential cluster, two major issues must be assessed: the probability that a true cluster (i.e., a real excess of cases of a disease) exists and, if it does, then whether an epidemiological study is even possible.

An excess number of cases of a particular disease over a particular period or within a specific geographical area is usually confirmed by comparing the rates found in the population in that period or area with the rates seen in a reference population. By means of statistical tests, the observed number of cases in the population at risk can be compared to the expected number in the reference population. If a statistically significant excess of cases (a true cluster) is found, then the feasibility of appropriate epidemiological studies must be assessed. If feasible, epidemiological studies assess the degree of exposure to the suspected causal factor (e.g., a chemical or physical agent) and test the hypothesis that this agent is indeed a cause of, or significant risk factor for, the disease in question. The U.S. Centers for Disease Control has published a comprehensive guide to the analysis of clusters in populations (25).

2.2.   SCREENING

Prior to the development of symptoms or physical signs, diseases may be present in affected people without their knowledge (asymptomatic disease). Diabetes, hypertension, and cancer (such as breast or cervical cancer) fall into this category. The commonly used method for detecting asymptomatic disease in a population is screening.

Screening is defined as "the presumptive identification of unrecognized disease or defect by the application of tests, examinations or other procedures which can be applied rapidly" (26). Thus, the goal of screening is early detection — identifying which asymptomatic people in the community probably have the disease and which probably do not — so that early intervention may be instituted and better health outcomes achieved. Examples of screening procedures are blood pressure checks for hypertension, mammography for breast cancer, and Papanicolaou (Pap) tests for cervical cancer.

2.2.1. Types of Screening

Three types of screening can be applied to a community.

Mass screening is the application of a screening test to an entire population. For example, screening for tuberculosis by chest x-ray or sputum microscopy is done in many developing countries where the disease is still highly prevalent. It is not widely performed in developed countries where the prevalence is low.

Selective screening is performed on selected sub-groups of a population at increased risk of developing certain diseases. Maple syrup urine disease (transmitted by a recessive gene, resulting in mental retardation and premature death) is quite common among French Canadians in some parts of Quebec. Thus, screening for carriers coupled with genetic counselling may be worthwhile in this population.

Multiphasic screening programs include multiple screening modalities such as a medical history, physical examination, and various measurements and investigations. The objective is to detect as many diseases as possible with one screening intervention. Screening of this nature is done by large organizations, especially U.S. organizations (such as Kaiser Permanente and the Health Insurance Plan of New York) that operate prepaid group health plans.

It is important to distinguish screening from case finding. **Screening** refers to looking for asymptomatic disease in a defined population, including selective screening in defined high-risk populations. **Case finding** in context of screening refers to looking for asymptomatic disease in individual patients because, in the opinion of their clinician, the individual is thought to be at higher risk of a disease based on an individual set of risk factors.

2.2.2. Characteristics of Screening

People with positive screening tests do not always have the disease (see Figure 2.1). Screening tests are not diagnostic tests. People with positive or questionable results must be referred for diagnostic evaluation. For screening to be ethical and to fulfill its intended purpose, there should be adequate, effective, and accessible methods of diagnosis and early treatment for diseased individuals.

Screening tests are evaluated in terms of their validity, reliability, and yield. The **validity** is measured by the frequency with which the result of the test is confirmed by an accurate diagnostic method and is often expressed in terms of its sensitivity and specificity. **Sensitivity** is the proportion (percentage) of truly diseased persons identified as diseased by a screening test. **Specificity** is the proportion (percentage) of truly non-diseased persons who are so identified by the test (see Figure 2.1). Both sensitivity

Figure 2.1.   Mass Screening

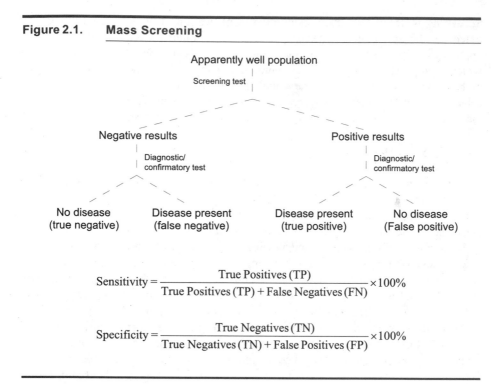

$$Sensitivity = \frac{True\ Positives\ (TP)}{True\ Positives\ (TP) + False\ Negatives\ (FN)} \times 100\%$$

$$Specificity = \frac{True\ Negatives\ (TN)}{True\ Negatives\ (TN) + False\ Positives\ (FP)} \times 100\%$$

and specificity are characteristics of a given test, and do not change when applied to populations with varying prevalence of disease.

Tests with low sensitivity and specificity (i.e., low percentages of correctly identifying those who have and those who do not have the disease) are poor screening tests. To have high sensitivity, screening tests must produce few false negative results; for high specificity, few false positive results should arise. A screening test is never 100% sensitive and specific. High sensitivity is gained at the expense of specificity and vice versa. Raising test sensitivity will increase false positives and therefore result in a loss of specificity. This trade-off between sensitivity and specificity is often expressed and demonstrated by a **receiver operator characteristic (ROC) curve**. Tests that discriminate well crowd toward the upper left corner of the ROC curve where sensitivity is plotted on the y-axis and one minus specificity on the x axis (2).

Whether sensitivity or specificity is more important will determine the test chosen to screen for a particular disease. When there is an important penalty for missing a disease, a highly sensitive test should be chosen. Highly specific tests should be chosen when false positive results can harm the patient physically, emotionally or financially (2). When available screening tests have low specificity or sensitivity but it is important to screen for a disease, multiple tests can sometimes be used to help increase specificity or sensitivity. **Parallel testing** — running multiple tests at the same time and looking for any positive test result — can be used to increase sensitivity.

Figure 2.2.   **Result of a Hypothetical Screening Test**

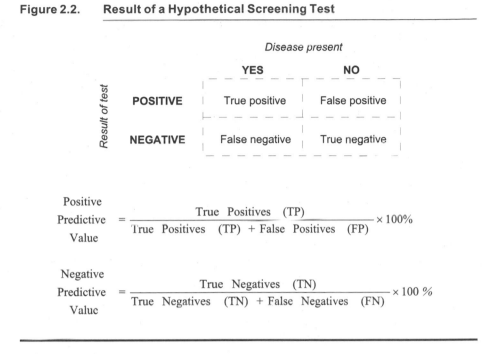

$$\text{Positive Predictive Value} = \frac{\text{True Positives (TP)}}{\text{True Positives (TP) + False Positives (FP)}} \times 100\%$$

$$\text{Negative Predictive Value} = \frac{\text{True Negatives (TN)}}{\text{True Negatives (TN) + False Negatives (FN)}} \times 100\%$$

Serial testing — running a series of tests in sequence and stopping at the first negative test as a sign of no disease — can be used to increase specificity (2).

The **positive predictive value** is measured as the proportion of true positives in all test positives (i.e., the proportion of cases who truly have the disease among those with positive tests) (see Figure 2.2). The predictive value of a positive test tends to be higher when the disease is more prevalent (see Table 2.2). The **negative predictive value** is the test's ability to identify all those who truly do not have the disease among all those who tested negative. The predictive value of a negative test decreases with increasing disease prevalence.

The **reliability** of a screening test refers to its ability to produce consistent results when applied to different populations or repeatedly to the same individual. The **yield** from a screening test is the amount of previously unrecognized disease detected in the population; it depends on the sensitivity of the screening test as well as the prevalence of unrecognized disease in a population. For example, the yield from the Pap smear is very low among women who have never had sexual intercourse but is much higher among sexually active females.

2.2.3. Biases

Two types of biases are particularly important when determining whether screening and early intervention actually lead to improved outcomes. **Lead-time bias** refers to the appearance of a longer survival time or longer time to morbidity with the use of a

Table 2.2.   **Predictive Values of a Positive Test with 99% Sensitivity and 95% Specificity at Three Levels of Prevalence**

Item	Level of prevalence		
	1 percent	**10 percent**	**20 percent**
a) Number in population	1,000	1,000	1,000
b) Diseased	10	100	200
c) Not diseased	990	900	800
d) True positive [b x 0.99]	10	99	198
e) False positive [c x (1 - 0.95)]	50	45	40
f) Total positive [d + e]	60	144	238
g) Predictive value of a positive test [d/f]	17%	69%	83%

screening test, occurring because the disease has been detected at an earlier stage in the asymptomatic period but not because of an actual improvement in disease outcome. **Length-bias** is the appearance of improved disease outcomes with screening occurring as a result of the screening test picking up milder forms of the disease with better prognoses rather than any real beneficial effect from screening and early intervention (2, 27)

2.2.4.   Criteria for the Population-Based Screening Program

As new tests or procedures emerge for screening for a disease, there are pressures on healthcare professionals and the healthcare system to adopt and institutionalize them. However, screening of a defined population can only be justified if the following disease, test and health system criteria are met (28, 29):
- **Disease:**
  - The disease must cause significant morbidity and/or mortality.
  - There is an asymptomatic stage of the disease that is detectable by a test.
  - The natural history of the disease is understood, and early detection and intervention are known to affect health outcomes favourably.
  - Early treatment is effective and acceptable.
  - The disease is not too common and not too rare.
- **Test:**
  - Screening tests should have high sensitivity and specificity; screening must be safe, rapidly and easily applied, relatively inexpensive, and acceptable to healthcare providers and the screened population (for example, chest radiographs or a blood test may not bother most individuals, but the discomfort produced by sigmoidoscopy may be unacceptable).
  - Ideally, there is randomized control trial evidence of effectiveness.

- **Healthcare system:**
  - There should be adequate capacity within the healthcare system for diagnostic follow-up of all those who screen positive and treatment of those diagnosed with disease.
  - Screening and early intervention has been shown to be cost effective.
  - The screening program is sustainable over time.
  - The program will reach those who will benefit from it.
  - Other relevant operational issues have been considered such as a clear policy on the population to be screened, who is responsible for screening, what constitutes a positive test, and how findings will become part of the medical record.

Beyond these accepted criteria, there are issues that must be considered before instituting a provincial or national program (30), such as the following:

- Are the screening program requirements for time, money, and costs appropriate for the community?
- Are other equally worthy procedures and efforts being given equal consideration or are existing resources being redirected unnecessarily?
- Does the procedure create new medical risks, and how are these assessed in relation to the procedure?
- Does the procedure place additional strain on healthcare resources in a disproportionate manner to the magnitude of the health problem being studied?
- What are the limitations of using screening assessments as a widespread diagnostic tool in relation to other diagnostic approaches?
- Are there specific ethical or moral issues raised by the program?
- How will the objectives of the screening program be communicated to the various target populations at risk?

The introduction of various forms of screening can be effective in secondarily preventing illness and improving the health of populations. A consideration of possible harms must also be addressed before instituting a screening program, as summarized by Marshall in a series of articles (31-33).

3. RELEVANT STATISTICAL CONCEPTS

Statistics are frequently used in studying the health and disease of populations. Statistics deal with the collection, classification, description, analysis, interpretation, and presentation of data and are the backbone of all epidemiologic research. A brief summary is provided here; more detailed discussion is available in standard statistical textbooks (34-36).

In general, statistics can be either descriptive or inferential. **Descriptive statistics** are counts of events or other characteristics of interest and give information about the nature of a group. For example, census data can provide a description of the population by age or region. **Inferential statistics** are used to compare and look for differences between groups and regions, and to make inferences on potential causes of differences.

A population can consist of individuals grouped by a specific characteristic of interest (e.g., geographical area, susceptibility to disease). Data can be derived from an entire population or from a sample. In epidemiology, data are usually available only on a sample of the population. Sampling may involve random selection, systematic selection, stratified selection, or cluster selection, or may be non-random (convenience) in nature. The sampling strategy influences the amount of bias likely to be encountered in the data; it also influences making generalizations based on the observations from the sample to the whole population.

Data collected can be grouped or ungrouped, qualitative or quantitative. In quantitative epidemiology, data are collected on variables. A **variable** is a category of measurement that can take on a variety of values. Data can be either continuous or discrete. A **continuous variable** is measured on an unbroken scale; e.g. blood pressure (mm of mercury), age, and time are examples of continuous variables. **Discrete variables**, also known as categorical variables, are chosen from a limited number of possible values but there is no possibility of a value between the other values and the distance between the values cannot be measured. There are three types of discrete variables depending on measurement characteristics: **nominal,** which are named categories with no measurement implied (e.g., religion, country of birth, sex); **ordinal,** which are ranked so that measurement is implied but not explicit (e.g., scales of agreement in a questionnaire, cancer staging, scale of colour on a test strip); and **integral**, which is an explicit measurement limited to counts (e.g., parity, gravidity, frequency of asthma attacks in past six months). Health data consist of sets of numerical information about anything related to health. This information constitutes the basic scientific tools for measuring and studying health and disease, but, like any tools, they must be of suitable quality to do the job expected. First, data must be **reliable** — when the same group of people is measured more than once, similar values must be obtained. Second, data must be **valid** — the findings must accurately capture the problem being studied. For example, hospital admissions can be expected to provide a valid assessment of the incidence of third-degree (very severe) burns, but not to measure the incidence of type 2 diabetes, since most people with early type 2 diabetes are not hospitalized. Validity reflects the degree to which a measurement measures what it purports to measure. Also, data in the health field must have sufficient resolution to give the answers being sought; like a microscopist, the epidemiologist may need to see one part of the problem in great detail. For example, a report of a slight increase in the national incidence of tuberculosis would not indicate where the cases were or in what groups of people they occurred. No action could be taken until these details were determined by using epidemiological and statistical techniques. Third, data must be **precise** — the measuring instrument defines how "sharply" it can provide a value. For example, a measurement of four decimal places is more precise than two decimal places. Unfortunately, very precise data may be neither valid nor reliable.

Data can be analyzed to determine the distributional characteristics. Common methods of presenting data are **bar graphs** for discrete data and **histograms** for continuous data. The frequency with which values occur is referred to as a **distribution**. The most common and well-known distribution is the **normal** or **Gaussian** distribution,

Figure 2.3.   **Distribution Curves**

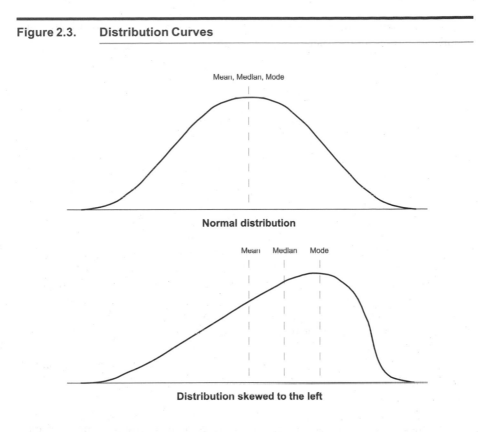

Normal distribution

Distribution skewed to the left

which is shaped like a bell (see Figure 2.3). Distributions can often be succinctly summarized mathematically by numeric values called **parameters**. For normal distribution, **measures of the central tendency** (the mean, median, and mode) and **measures of the variation of the data** in the distribution (the variance and standard deviation) are most commonly used to summarize the distribution. The **mean**, or average, is calculated by summing all the observations and dividing by the number of observations. It is expressed mathematically as follows:

$$\bar{x} = \frac{\sum x_i}{n}$$

The variation in a normal distribution, as related to the mean, consists of the variance and the standard deviation. The **variance** expresses the amount of dispersion in the data and is calculated by taking the sum of the squares of the deviations from the mean value and dividing by the sample size subtracting one observation. It is represented mathematically as follows: note:

$$s^2 = \frac{\sum(x-\bar{x})^2}{n-1}$$

The **standard deviation** is merely the square root of the variance:

$$s = \sqrt{\frac{\sum(x-\bar{x})^2}{n-1}}$$

The **median** is a measure of central tendency that describes the value above and below which 50% of the values lie. The **mode** describes the data value that is observed most frequently. Another measure of the variability of data is the range, which reflects the difference between the highest and lowest values in the distribution.

Statistical techniques are used to test hypotheses and determine the degree to which an effect or difference exists between two or more comparison groups. Tests of statistical significance are chosen on the basis of the type of data being analyzed. Statistical tests also differ on the type of distribution the data is thought to approximate.

Statistical testing requires the statement of a null hypothesis and an alternative hypothesis. A **null hypothesis** states that there is, in fact, no real difference between the groups being compared, and that the differences seen are due to chance. Thus, a **significance level** is a statistical value arbitrarily set as the cut-off point at or below which one rejects the null hypothesis and selects the alternative hypothesis (i.e., concluding that there is, in fact, a real difference between the groups being compared). A **p-value** represents the probability that a difference seen between the groups being compared is due to random variation or chance. The significance level of 0.05 is frequently used; however, even at a significance level of 0.05, there is still a small chance (5% or 1 in 20) that random variation may be responsible for the observed difference (i.e., that the difference seen between the groups being compared is not a real difference but merely due to chance). When a p-value is at or below the set cut-off, for example 0.05, the difference between the groups is said to reach **statistical significance**.

Figure 2.4 indicates the type of errors that can occur in the interpretation of data. The truth, or gold standard, is whether the intervention confers benefit or not. A type 1 or alpha error occurs when a real difference does not exist but the study results find it as a statistically significant difference. Based on the table below, an alpha error occurs when there really is no difference, but the study rejects the null hypothesis, and hence concludes that there is a difference. In other words, the incorrect rejection of a null hypothesis or asserting that there is a difference between treatments when in fact there is not. Thus, in a situation of p=0.05, there is a 5% chance, or 1 out of 20 chance, of rejecting a null hypothesis that should not be rejected.

Figure 2.4.   Type I and Type II Error Probabilities

		Truth	
		Treatment benefits (H_1)	No benefit (H_0)
Result from the study	**Positive: Difference exists (reject H_0)**	**True positive** Correctly reject H_0 $p = 1 - \beta$ (power)	**False positive** Type I error Incorrectly reject H_0 $p = \alpha$ (level of significance)
	Negative: No difference (do not reject H_0)	**False negative** Type II error Incorrectly fail to reject H_0 $p = \beta$	**True negative** Correctly accept H_0 $p = 1 - \alpha$

A **type II** or **beta error** occurs when the null hypothesis is not rejected when it should be or when there is a failure to recognize a difference in the result of an intervention when it is actually present.

The chance of a type II error occurring is used to determine the **power** of a study, which is 1 minus β. The power of a study is the probability that a difference will be detected when there is indeed a difference. Power is a function of the sample size of the study and increases with sample size. A small study may fail to reject the null hypothesis because the numbers were too small to detect a significant difference. Therefore, it is crucial to consult a statistician before commencing a study to ensure that the sample size is adequate.

Study results are usually reported by either a p-value or confidence interval.

Confidence Interval

A set of observations or measurements can be used to calculate means or proportions of some characteristic. This is called an **estimate** of the true value of the mean or proportion, the value that applies to the entire population. Usually this true value is unknowable, often because the entire population is infinite, or includes elements that exist in the past or in the future and cannot be measured in the present (e.g., the population of people who die of lung cancer in Canada).

The best one can do is make estimates on a sample that is representative of the underlying population. The confidence interval is a statistical device that indicates how close to the truth the result is likely to be, by providing a range of values within which the unknowable truth "probably" lies. Often the probability used is 95%; i.e., there is a 95% chance that the calculated confidence interval actually contains the true population mean. Other probabilities, such as 90% or 99% are sometimes used.

A confidence interval takes the form:

$$\text{estimate} \pm \text{margin for error}$$

The confidence interval for a mean or proportion always has the estimate in the centre of the interval. Some estimates, notably estimates of a relative risk or odds ratio, will not be in the centre of the confidence interval. This is because the interval is calculated using a logarithmic, or proportional scale rather than the simple arithmetic scale used above.

The size of the margin for error depends on the variability in the population (measured by the standard deviation), the number of observations used to calculate the estimate, and the level of confidence desired. Less variable populations (e.g., the mean height of some occupational groups will be less variable, because of height restrictions, than for the general population of working adults) will have narrower confidence intervals. Estimates based on larger sample sizes will also have narrower intervals than small sample sizes. A higher level of confidence will also require a wider range of values.

Sometimes, the confidence interval can be used in place of a test of significance. If the 95% confidence interval for a difference in the means of two groups excludes 0, for example, then the difference is significant at the 5% level.

For a relative risk or odds ratio, a confidence interval that excludes 1.0 is considered to be statistically significant. If the confidence interval exceeds 1.0, the factor being studied can be considered to be associated with an increased probability of the health outcome being studied; if it is below 1.0, the factor can be considered to be associated with a decreased probability of the health outcome being studied. For example, if a study reports a p-value of 0.01, one can conclude that it is statistically significant, but cannot infer the magnitude of effect or the precision of the estimate. If the same study yields a relative risk of 1.6 with 95% confidence levels of 1.2 to 1.8, one can infer that the sample size was large enough to give a precise estimate that the effect was consistent with a 20% to 80% increase in risk and that the effect was statistically significant. A wide confidence interval indicates a small sample size and is an imprecise quantification of effect indicating uncertainty about the estimate. Medical journals often require both p-values and confidence intervals (37).

Statistical significance is distinct from **clinical significance**, also known as clinical relevance or importance. While **statistical significance** refers to the probability that the results seen are real and not due to chance or random variation, clinical significance refers to the clinical importance of the results. For example, a study may show that an intervention is capable of reducing systolic blood pressure by 1 mm Hg in healthy people with normal blood pressure. Although the result may be statistically significant between the intervention and the control groups, the result is not clinically significant since a systolic blood pressure reduction of 1 mm Hg in those who are healthy and have normal blood pressure is unlikely to make any difference to their overall health or risk of disease. A wide variety of statistical techniques exists in the literature. With the advent of powerful computers, multivariate analysis has become increasingly common. Whereas **univariate analysis** involve analysis of single variables, although the comparison may be between two or more groups (one independent and one dependent variable), **multivariate analysis** allows for a number of relevant independent variables to be related to an outcome of interest. The most common form of multivariate analysis is **regression analysis**. Regression (one y and one x) involves two variables, one dependent variable y, and one independent variable x. Multiple regression involves a number of independent variables, x_1, x_2, x_3, etc., although there is still only one dependent variable y. Multiple regression can take a number of forms, depending on whether the dependent variable is continuous or discrete. Linear regression is used when the dependent variable is continuous while logistic regression is used when the dependent variable is dichotomous. Commonly, an outcome such as mortality is related to a set of potential risk factors such as smoking status, age, gender, blood pressure, and blood cholesterol level. Multiple regression analysis provides an estimate of the contribution each factor makes when the potential confounding effects of the other variables are controlled.

3.1. RATIOS, PROPORTIONS, AND RATES

Usually, health data take into account the population where the events have occurred. Hence, in most situations, one needs a numerator, that is, the frequency of occurrence of an event under observation, and a denominator, that is, size of population where the event occurred. As disease is relatively rare, rates are expressed in terms of per 100, 1,000, 10,000, or 100,000 population. More common phenomena, such as risk factor prevalence, may be expressed as a percentage. For example, the smoking prevalence for a given population may be expressed as 40% whereas death rates are expressed as 7 deaths per 1,000 people per year. For example, lung cancer in males, which is rare, is expressed as 55 per 100,000 population per year. Similarly, use of hospital days is often expressed as days per 1,000 population.

Three commonly used measures of data expression are ratio, proportion, and rate. A **ratio** is an expression of the relationship between two items that are usually independent of each other. If there are 6 males and 12 females in a particular situation, then the ratio of males to females in that situation is 1:2. Another public health example is the maternal mortality ratio, which expresses the number of maternal deaths per year relative to the number of live births in that year. These are not independent (a large number of live births is more likely to produce more maternal deaths than a small number would), but it is a ratio nevertheless.

A **proportion** is the relationship of a part to its whole and is generally expressed as a percentage. If there are 25 ill persons out of 100 persons, then the proportion of ill persons is 25% or 0.25.

A **rate** is an expression of the probability of an occurrence of an event in a defined population at risk during a specific time period. If five cases of bladder cancer occur among factory workers who have accumulated 5,000 person-years since they were first employed, the rate of bladder cancer in this group is 5/5,000 or 1 per 1000 person-years.

3.2. OTHER MEASURES OF EFFECT ON SIZE

Clinical trials are traditionally reported in terms of the reduction of the outcome measure associated with the intervention in comparison to a placebo or alternative treatment. There are three equivalent statistical measures of trial data: the relative risk reduction, the absolute risk reduction, and the number needed to treat. It is important to note that framing results in these different but mathematically equivalent ways influences practitioners and planners in their willingness to employ an intervention (32, 38).

These concepts can be illustrated with the following example. A randomized trial shows a rate of 34% reduction in the placebo group and a rate of 28% in the treatment group. This is equivalent to a relative risk reduction of 18% (i.e., $[1 - RR] \times 100\%$ or $[1 - 0.28 \div 0.34] \times 100\%$) and an absolute risk reduction of 6% (i.e., 34% – 28%). The number needed to treat shows how many individuals would need to comply fully with the intervention to prevent one outcome (39). It is the inverse of the absolute risk reduction, in this case 1/0.06, or 17 individuals (15). Practitioners' willingness either to accept or recommend a therapy can be influenced by the way these numbers can be presented.

3.3.   AGE STANDARDIZATION

In descriptive studies of health problems, one often relies on comparisons of rates between countries, provinces, or communities, or in the same jurisdiction followed over time. However, populations change over time, and different populations have different proportions of young and old, or male and female, that make simple comparisons difficult. If the prevalence of Alzheimer's disease is much higher in one community than in another, is it because the proportion of people over 65 is higher or is there some (more interesting) explanation? Epidemiologists rely on techniques of standardization to remove or reduce the influence of these demographic differences from comparisons. Age-, or sex-, or age- and sex-standardized rates exist. Standardized rates are also known as adjusted rates.

There are two methods of standardization: direct and indirect, which will be briefly described below. For more detail, one is advised to consult a standard epidemiological textbook (40).

Direct Method
If the age- or sex-specific rates are available for each population under study, the direct method is appropriate. The existing rates are applied to an arbitrary "standard" population to give the number of events (new cases of the disease for incidence rates, deaths from the disease for mortality rates) one would expect in this arbitrary population. Such rates, based on the specific rates of different populations, will be more comparable, because the differences in age- or sex-distribution have been removed.

Indirect Method
Sometimes the groups to compare are too small to produce reliable, stable age- or sex-specific rates on which to calculate directly standardized rates. In this situation, indirect standardization is appropriate. Here, the specific rates come from the standard population and are applied to each group to calculate the expected number of cases in

the group and compare it to the number actually observed. The ratio of observed to expected is called the standardized mortality ratio (SMR) for death data and the standardized incidence ratio (SIR) for incidence data. Each group may have a different SMR. Multiplying the SMR from each group by the crude rate in the standard population will produce indirectly standardized rates for each of the groups being compared. If the SMR is greater than 1, the rate within that population is higher than expected; if it is less than 1, the rate is lower than expected. Through their SMRs, the rates in the different populations being compared can be deemed either higher than expected or lower than expected. The magnitude of the rates above or below what is expected can also be ascertained for each population.

4. SUMMARY

This chapter examined the data quality, epidemiological studies, investigation of diseases in populations, and some relevant statistical concepts. Health data consist of sets of numerical information about anything related to health and are compiled from many sources. These data must meet three criteria: they must be reliable, be valid, and have sufficient resolution or precision.

Epidemiological studies are commonly used for data collection and analysis. **Epidemiology** is the study of the distribution (in terms of person, place, and time) of determinants of disease, health-related states, and events in populations. Epidemiology can be applied to control of health problems. The two types of epidemiological studies are descriptive and analytic.

A **descriptive study** investigates the occurrence of a phenomenon in relation to person, time, and place. Prevalence studies are one type of descriptive studies. Causal associations should not be drawn from the results of a descriptive study; however, the results may lend themselves to hypotheses for investigation of an association or causal relationship within an analytic study. In **analytic studies**, a hypothesis is tested to find out if there is an association between a given disease, health state, or other dependent variable, and possible risk or protective factors. There are two types of analytic studies: observational and experimental.

Observational studies include **ecological studies**, which can compare aggregated variables between different geographical areas, and **cross-sectional studies**, which examine the relationship between diseases and other variables of interest as they exist in a defined population at one particular time. In a cross-sectional study, the population is divided into those with and without the disease and then various characteristics of the two groups are examined. This type of study reveals the prevalence of measured health outcomes and risk factors in a given population at one point in time. Associations can also be made regarding the risk factors and health outcomes. However, because risk factors and health outcomes are measured at the same point in time, the temporal relationship between them cannot be determined.

A third type of observational study is the **case-control study**, in which people with the disease (cases) are compared with similar people without the disease (controls) who have also had the opportunity for exposure. Hence, the study begins after the disease has appeared and attempts to ascertain exposures in those with the disease and in those without disease. As a result, there is a risk that those with disease will be biased in their recall of potential past exposures compared with those without disease, leading to recall bias. In **cohort studies**, a cohort (a group of people with common characteristics) with a specific exposure is identified, and the initial characteristics and health status are compared to those of a control cohort (chosen on the same basis as the original cohort, except for exposure to the suspected cause of disease); both groups are followed for a certain time period to observe for evidence of disease or other outcomes, yielding incidence rates, attributable risk, relative risk, and incidence density.

Experimental studies are those in which conditions are under the direct control of the investigation. These studies include randomized controlled trials and community trials. In a randomized controlled trial, subjects with a disease are randomized into two or more groups. One group is subjected to the intervention being evaluated, usually a treatment, while the control group is given either an inactive treatment (placebo) or current standard treatment. Subjects are usually unaware of their treatment status, in a procedure called a single-blind trial. Trials where neither the participant nor observer knows the group assignment are called double-blind clinical trials. Triple-blind trials are trials where the participants, the observers/assessors of clinical outcomes, and the analysts of the results are blinded. If the final outcomes show a statistically significant difference between the study group and the controls, then the results obtained are usually attributed to the treatment. The community trial is used when a comparison study of two communities is desired in order to see what effects a variable or intervention has on the health of a community rather than an individual. One community is given an intervention while the other serves as a control.

Although observational and experimental studies allow for the determination of associations between risk and protective factors and health outcomes, the determination of causation is more complex. For a **causal association**, there must be sufficient consistency of association, strength of association, dose-response, correct temporal relationship, plausibility, coherence, analogy, experimental evidence, and specificity.

As the scientific literature grows and numerous studies are published on each health topic, it has been increasingly difficult to make sense of the sometimes conflicting results of multiple studies. In recent years, systematic reviews and meta-analyses have become important tools for addressing this issue.

Clinical epidemiology represents the application, modification, and refinement of epidemiological techniques to individual patient care. The purpose of clinical epidemiology is to collect and evaluate information systematically from the practice of medicine in order to increase the accuracy, reliability, validity, and effectiveness of clinical care. An important facet of this is the development of clinically relevant disease and outcome taxonomies. This field is known as clinimetrics.

Critical appraisal has been defined as the "application of certain rules of evidence to clinical (symptoms and signs), paraclinical (laboratory and other diagnostic tests), and published data (advocating specific treatment manoeuvres or purporting to establish the etiology or prognosis of disease) in order to determine their validity (closeness to the truth) and applicability (usefulness in one's own clinical practice)" (3).

The application of the techniques of clinical epidemiology and critical appraisal constitute evidence-based medicine. Evidence-based medicine emphasizes the following for clinical decision-making: precisely defining a patient problem, efficient literature searching, selection of the best of the relevant studies and the critical appraisal of these studies, in addition to sound pathophysiological rationale and sensitivity to patients' emotional needs.

Qualitative research uses interpretive and naturalistic approaches to study research questions. Studies are carried out in natural non-experimental situations. Narrative accounts replace statistical summaries; specific qualitative research techniques are used to capture and analyze the narrative accounts in a reliable and valid manner. A variety of qualitative research techniques, developed in the social sciences, have found applications in health care.

Screening is commonly used for detecting asymptomatic disease in populations. It is intended to detect early stage disease when early identification and treatment lead to more favourable outcomes than detection after symptoms occur. Two types of biases that are particularly important to consider when determining whether screening and early intervention actually lead to improved outcomes are lead-time bias and length bias. In order to institute a screening program for a disease, a number of criteria must be met for the disease, test, and healthcare system. There are various types of screening that can be carried out within a community, such as mass screening and selective screening. Screening tests are evaluated in terms of their validity, reliability, and yield. The validity of a screening test is measured by the frequency with which the result of the test is confirmed by an accurate diagnostic method, and is often expressed in terms of its sensitivity and specificity. The sensitivity of a test is the proportion of truly diseased who are identified as diseased by a test. Specificity is the proportion of truly non-diseased persons who are so identified by the test. Tests with low sensitivity and low specificity are poor screening tests. However, no screening test is 100% sensitive and 100% specific, and high sensitivity is gained at the expense of specificity and vice versa. The reliability of a screening test refers to its ability to produce consistent results when applied to various screened populations or even repeatedly on the same individual. The yield from a screening test is the amount of unrecognized disease that is detected in the population, and thus depends on the sensitivity of the screening test as well as the prevalence of unrecognized disease in a population.

Statistics deal with the collection, classification, description, analysis, interpretation, and presentation of data, and are a crucial aspect of epidemiological research.

In general, statistics can be either descriptive or inferential. **Descriptive statistics** are counts of events or other characteristics of interest and give information about the nature of a group. For example, census data can provide a description of the population by age or region. **Inferential statistics** are used to compare and look for differences between groups and regions, and to make inferences on potential causes of differences.

Data collected can be grouped or ungrouped, qualitative or quantitative. In quantitative epidemiology, data are collected on variables. A **variable** is a category of measurement that can take on a variety of values. Data can be either continuous or discrete. A **continuous variable** is measured on an unbroken scale. **Discrete variables**, also known as categorical variables, are chosen from a limited number of possible values but there is no possibility of a value between the other values, and the distance between the values cannot be measured. There are three types of discrete variables depending on measurement characteristics: **nominal**, which are named categories with no measurement implied; **ordinal**, which are ranked so that measurement is implied but not explicit; and **integral**, in which measurement is explicit but limited to counts.

Health data consist of sets of numerical information about anything related to health. This information constitutes the basic scientific tools for measuring and studying health and disease, but, like any tool, they must be of suitable quality to do the job expected.

Data can be analyzed to determine its distributional characteristics by **mean**, or average, **variance,** and **standard deviation**.

Statistical testing requires the statement of a null hypothesis and an alternative hypothesis. The **null hypothesis** states that there is no real difference between the groups being compared, and that the differences seen are due to chance. A **type I** or **alpha error** occurs when there is no real difference but the study result finds a difference and rejects the null hypothesis. A **type II** or **beta error** occurs when the null hypothesis is not rejected when it should be or when there is a failure to recognize a difference in the result of an intervention when it is actually present.

The **confidence interval** is a statistical device that tells how close to the truth the results are likely to be by providing a range of values within which the unknowable truth probably lies. **Clinical significance**, also known as clinical relevance or importance, refers to the clinical importance of the results. **Statistical significance** refers to the probability that the results seen are real and not due to chance or random variation.

When comparing health status of populations, epidemiologists rely on techniques of standardization to remove or reduce the influence of the demographic differences from comparisons. There are two methods of comparison: **direct standardization** and **indirect standardization**.

5.   REFERENCES

1.   Beaglehole R, Bonita R, Kjellstromm T. *Basic epidemiology*, 1st ed. Geneva: World Health Organization, 1993.
2.   Fletcher R, Fletcher S, Wagner E. *Clinical epidemiology*, 3rd ed. Philadelphia: Williams and Wilkins, 1996.
3.   Sackett D, Haynes R, Tugwell P. *Clinical epidemiology: A basic science for clinical medicine*, 2nd ed. Toronto: Little, Brown and Co., 1991.
4.   Coggon D, Rose G, Barker D. 1997. *Epidemiology for the uninitiated*. <www.bmj.com/epidem/epid.html> (September 2002).
5.   Last J. *A dictionary of epidemiology*, 3rd ed. New York: Oxford University Press, 1995.
6.   Kelsey J, Thompson W, Evans A. *Methods in observational epidemiology*. New York: Oxford University Press, 1986.

7. Shah C, Robinson G, Kinnis C, *et al.* Day care surgery for children: A controlled study of medical complications and parental attitudes. *Medical Care* 1972; 10(5):437-50.

8. Ciliska D, Thomas H. Why would I bother? And which ones should I use? Toronto. *Public Health and Epidemiology Report Ontario* 2001:232-5.

9. Egger M, Ebrahim S, Davey Smith G. Where now for meta-analysis? *International Journal of Epidemiology* 2002; 31:1-5.

10. Elwood M. *Critical appraisal of epidemiological studies and clinical trials*, 2nd ed. London: Oxford University Press, 1998.

11. Feinstein A. *Clinimetrics.* New Haven, CT: Yale University Press, 1987.

12. Oxman A, Sackett D, Guyatt G. Users' guide to the medical literature: How to get started. *Journal of American Medical Association* 1993; 270(17):2093-95.

13. Oxman A, Sackett D, Guyatt G. Users' guide to the medical literature: How to use an overview. *Journal of American Medical Association* 1994; 272(17):1367-71.

14. Guyatt G, Sackett D, Cook D. Users' guide to the medical literature: How to use an article about therapy or prevention — Are the results valid? *Journal of American Medical Association* 1993; 270(21):2598-601.

15. Guyatt G, Sackett D, Cook D. Users' guide to the medical literature: How to use an article about therapy or prevention — What were the results and will they help me in caring for my patients? *Journal of American Medical Association* 1994; 271(1):59-63.

16. National Forum on Health. 1995. *Evidence based decision making: A dialogue on health information.* <wwwnfh.hc-sc.gc.ca/publicat/evidence/idxebdme.htm> (February 2003).

17. Evidence-Based Medicine Working Group. Evidence-based medicine: A new approach to teaching the practice of medicine. *Journal of American Medical Association* 1992; 268(17):2420-25.

18. Friedland D, editor. *Evidence-based medicine.* Stamford, CT: Appleton & Lange, 1998.

19. Canadian Task Force on Preventive Health Care. 1997. *History and methods.* <www.ctfphc.org> (October 2002).

20. Canadian Cochrane Network and Centre. 2002. *Promoting evidence-based health care in Canada.* <cochrane.mcmaster.ca/default.asp?u=4> (November 2002).

21. CMA Infobase. 2002. *Clinical practice guidelines.* <mdm.ca/cpgsnew/cpgs/index.asp> (February 2003).

22. Hill AB. The environment and disease: Association or causation? *Proceedings of Royal Society of Medicine* 1965; 58(295-300).

23. Pope C, Mays N. Reaching the parts other Methods cannot reach: An introduction to qualitative methods in health and health services research. *British Medical Journal* 1995; 311:42-5.

24. Caldwell G. Time-space clusters. *Health Environment Digest* 1989; 3(5):4-5.

25. U.S. Centers for Disease Control. Guidelines for investigating clusters of health events. *Morbidity and Mortality Weekly Report* 1990; 39(RR-11):1-23.

26. Whitby L. Screening for disease: Definitions and criteria. *Lancet* 1974; 2(3):819-21.

27. Wallace R. Screening for early and asymptomatic conditions. In Wallace R, editor. *Maxey-Rosenau-Last public health and preventive medicine.* 14th ed. Stamford, CT: Appleton & Lange, 1998.

28. Wilson J, Jungner F. *Principles and practice of screening.* Geneva: World Health Organization, 1968. Public Health Report No. 34.

29. Cadman D, Chambers L, Feldman W, *et al.* Assessing the effectiveness of community screening programs. *Journal of American Medical Association* 1984; 251(12):1580-5.

30. Task Force on the Use and Provision of Medical Services. *1989-1990 Annual report.* Toronto: Government of Ontario and Ontario Medical Association, 1990.

31. Marshall K. Prevention: How much harm? How much benefit? 1. The influence of reporting methods on perception of benefits. *Canadian Medical Association Journal* 1996; 154(10):1493-9.

32.   Marshall K. Prevention: How much harm? How much benefit? 3. Physical, psychological, and social harm. *Canadian Medical Association Journal* 1996; 155(2):169-76.
33.   Marshall K. Prevention: How much harm? How much benefit? 4. The ethics of informed consent for preventive screening programs. *Canadian Medical Association Journal* 1996; 155(4):377-83.
34.   Altman D. *Practical statistics for medical research.* London, UK: Chapman and Hall, 1991.
35.   Pagano M, Gauvreau K. *Principles of biostatistics*, 2nd ed. Belmont, CA: Duxbury Press, 2001.
36.   Rosner B. *Fundamentals of biostatistics.* Belmont, CA: Duxbury Press, 2001.
37.   Walter S. Methods of reporting statistical results from medical research studies. *American Journal of Epidemiology* 1995; 141:896-906.
38.   Naylor CD, Chen E, Strauss B. Measured enthusiasm: Does the method of reporting trial results alter perceptions of therapeutic effectiveness? *Archives of Internal Medicine* 1992; 117:916-21.
39.   Laupacis A, Sackett D, Roberts R. An assessment of clinically useful measures of the consequences of treatment. *New England Journal of Medicine* 1988; 318:1728-33.
40.   Kahn H, Sempos C. *Statistical methods in epidemiology*, 2nd ed. London: Oxford University Press, 1997.

PART TWO

THE HEALTH OF CANADIANS

Evidence and facts are essential for building and developing an effective healthcare system. Healthcare professionals working in the field need to know the overview picture. This part provides facts about health and the diseases that exist in Canadian society and the factors that influence them. It covers morbidity, mortality, and the economic burden of disease, including communicable and chronic diseases, as well as the health of disadvantaged groups, and it discusses health in relation to the environment and to occupation. It finishes with a discussion of evidence-based facts about the type of preventive practice recommended for individuals, a field pioneered by Canada.

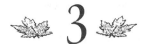

3

HEALTH INDICATORS AND DATA SOURCES

The planning and evaluation of services to meet the health needs of a population must be based on the health status of that population and how it evolves. As government involvement in the provision of health care has increased, so have interest in the measurement of health and demand for data on the health of the population for which governments are responsible. Many contemporary trends reinforce and consolidate that interest, particularly demographic changes, patterns of disease and illness, and medical practice, as well as changes in technology, the need for meaningful outcome measures, and the increasing costs of health care.

The measurement of health dates from the 17th century, when governments first began to collect information on death and its causes. Mortality statistics continue to be a major source of information, and are useful primarily in developing countries, where death rates remain high. In industrialized countries, where death rates are much lower, mortality statistics and associated measures such as life expectancy are no longer adequate indicators of health; they do not take into consideration illness that does not result in death or the often-profound disability and distress that may accompany such illness. As seen in Chapter 1, the very concept of health has changed and a number of other non-medical determinants have been recognized. Hence, there has been a rethinking of the data required for Canada (1, 2). Chapter 2 outlined the various ways in which data, once collected, can be summarized and analyzed by various statistical techniques. This chapter describes the various types of health indicators and the variety of data sources used for the health status of Canadians, with examples of indicators and descriptive statistics derived from these sources.

1.   HEALTH INDICATORS

Health indicators are qualitative and quantitative statistical summaries that describe the health of a population. An **indicator** is a statistic that gives a meaningful indirect depiction of the health of a community. For example, mortality rates are an endpoint indicator of the burden of illness in a population. Comparing rates between communities can reveal underlying differences between these communities. Mortality rates alone do not suffice to describe the health of a community, because they address only one dimension. An **index** is the weighted average of related indicators designed to describe a phenomenon. An example of this is the Health Utility Index (HUI), a generic health status index that synthesizes both quantitative and qualitative aspects of health (3). The HUI is based on a set of questions and provides a summary index of the health of each respondent and a quantitative measure of a population's overall health status, as opposed to focusing on narrowly defined health indicators, risk factors, or diseases. Indicators and indices are useful for depicting trends over time and giving capsule summaries of various aspects of community health. Ideally, indicators are derived from data that are reliable and valid, collected frequently, and sensitive to changes in the community so that planning and intervention strategies can be promptly implemented when warranted.

Table 3.1 shows a useful framework for health indicators, which addresses health in its broad sense, that has been developed by Statistics Canada and Canadian Institute for Health Information (CIHI) (4). This framework is the basis of many recent reports on health of Canadians (5).

These indicators are organized into four categories: health status (including health conditions, mortality rates, measures of well-being), non-medical determinants of health (socioeconomic characteristics and health behaviour), health system performance (measures of accessibility, appropriateness, effectiveness of healthcare services), and community and health system characteristics (contextual information). The notion of equity spans all dimensions of the framework, and can apply equally to any construct or dimension. Therefore equity is not included as a fifth dimension of the Health Indicators Conceptual framework, but is presented as a crosscutting element of the framework that applies to each of the four dimensions. Detailed definitions of indicators and sources for obtaining such data are available from the CIHI (2, 4, 6).

The following section provides specific definitions and methodologies for deriving some representative common health indicators as they pertain to health status in Table 3.2. A description of commonly used health indicators for Canada is presented in Chapters 4, 5, and 6, which are organized to reflect the relationship between different health influences and their consequences.

It is important to note that there is no ideal taxonomy of indicators. This framework is only a guide to categorizing information on many aspects of health. Additionally, there are few indicators for some aspects that are considered important and for which further research is needed. Health promotion activities are a case in point, although some progress has been made in this direction. Ease of access to health services is another health indicator, which may in itself only be an indirect, proxy measure for the underlying concept.

1.1. HEALTH STATUS

Health status is defined as the degree to which a person is able to function physically, emotionally, socially, with or without aid from the healthcare system (7). **Quality of life** is defined as the degree to which persons perceive themselves able to function physically,

Table 3.1.   **Health Indicator Framework**

Health Status				How healthy are Canadians? Health Status can be measured in a variety of ways, including well-being, health conditions, disability, or death.	
Health conditions	Human function	Well-being	Deaths		
Determinants of Health				These are factors that are known to affect our health and, in some cases, when and how we use health care.	**E** **Q** **U**
Health behaviours	Living & working conditions	Personal resources	Environmental factors		
Health System Performance				How healthy is the health care system? Those indicators measures various aspects of the quality of health care	**I** **T**
Acceptability	Accessibility	Appropriateness	Competence		
Continuity	Effectiveness	Efficiency	Safety		
Community & Health System Characteristics				These measures provide useful contextual information but are not direct measures of health status or the quality of health care	**Y**
Community	Health system		Resources		

Source: Adapted from Table 1: Health Indicators Conceptual Framework. *Health indicators conceptual framework: Background paper*, Prepared for ISO/TC 215, March 14, 2001.
secure.cihi.ca/cihiweb/en/downloads/infostand_ihisd_e_ISO_background.pdf> © 2003, CIHI. Reprinted with permission, Canadian Institute for Health Information, Ottawa, Canada.

emotionally, and socially (7). As one can see, health status is objective measure whereas quality of life is a subjective measure. Often, health status, health-related quality of life (HRQOL), quality of life, and morbidity are concepts that are often used interchangeably as measures of health (8, 9). Quality of life is generally considered a generic term that refers to aspects outside the usually defined boundaries of health, such as access to recreational parks and public transportation. Health status is usually defined as any measures of health, including negatively valued aspects such as death or disease. Likewise, morbidity is a negatively defined term of HRQOL. In determining health status, the World Health Organization (WHO) uses the concepts of function, activities, and participation (10), which include the dimension of objective and subjective health

Table 3.2.   Health Indicators

Health Status			
Well-being	**Health conditions**	**Human function**	**Deaths**
➢ Self-rated health ➢ Self-rated esteem	➢ Body mass index ➢ Incidence and prevalence of: arthritis, diabetes, asthma, high blood pressure, chronic pain, depression ➢ Cancer incidence, age standardized rates: all cancer, lung, colorectal, breast, and prostate ➢ Injuries hospitalization Food & waterborne diseases ➢ Low birth weights	➢ Functional health ➢ Disability days ➢ Condition causing activity limitations ➢ Disability-free life expectancy ➢ Disability-adjusted life expectancy ➢ Disability-adjusted life years ➢ Health expectancy	➢ Infant mortality ➢ Perinatal mortality ➢ Life expectancy ➢ Mortality crude counts/rates, age-adjusted rates for all major causes of deaths ➢ Potential years of life lost (PYLL): total & for cancer, circulatory, suicide respiratory, unintentional injury
Non-Medical Determinants of Health			
Health behaviours	**Living & working conditions**	**Personal resources**	**Environmental factors**
➢ Smoking status, initiation and quitting rates ➢ Frequency of heavy drinking ➢ Physical activity ➢ Breast feeding ➢ Dietary practices	➢ High school and post-secondary graduates ➢ Unemployment rate ➢ Low-income rate ➢ Children in low-income families ➢ Housing affordability ➢ Decision-Latitude at work ➢ Income inequality ➢ Government transfer income ➢ Owner-occupied dwellings	➢ School readiness ➢ Social support ➢ Life Stress	➢ Exposure to second-hand smoke

Health System Performance			
Acceptability	**Accessibility**	**Appropriateness**	**Competence**
	➢ Influenza immunization, 65+ years ➢ Screening mammography, women aged 50-59 years ➢ Pap smear, women aged 18-69 years ➢ Childhood immunization	➢ Vaginal birth after caesarean ➢ Caesarean sections	
Continuity	**Effectiveness**	**Efficiency**	**Safety**
	➢ Disease incidence: pertussis, measles, Tb, HIV, chlamydia and pneumonia and influenza hospitaliz-ations ➢ Deaths due to medically-treatable diseases, age standardized rates: bacterial infections, cervical cancer, hypertensive disease and pneumonia & unspecified bronchitis ➢ Ambulatory care sensitive conditions ➢ 30-day AMI in-hospital mortality ➢ 30-day stroke in-hospital motality ➢ Readmission rates: AMI, asthma, prostatectomy, hysterectomy	➢ May not require hospitalization ➢ Expected compared to actual stay	➢ Hip fracture hospitalization

Community and Health System Characteristics		
Community	**Health System**	**Resources**
➢ Population: characteristics, population density, dependency ratio, urban, aboriginal, lone-parent families, immigrants, visible minorities and 1&5 year mobility	➢ Inflow/outflow ratio ➢ Selected surgical operations: coronary artery bypass graft, hip and knee replacement and hysterectomy ➢ Contact with: health professionals, mental health professionals, dental and alternate health care providers	➢ Health expenditures ➢ Doctors ➢ Nurses ➢ Other health professionals

Source: Table 2: Health Indicators confirmed at the Consensus Conference. *National Consensus Conference on Population Health Indicators*, © 2003, CIHI. Reprinted with permission, Canadian Institute for Health Information, Ottawa, Canada.

described in Chapter 1. The health status indicators below, which are used by CIHI, capture the essence of this duality.

Several health status indicators are defined below, mostly according to definitions set by the CIHI (4, 6). Some of them are defined in Chapters 4 and 5.

Well-being

Well-being covers the broad measures of the physical, mental, and social state of individuals. Indicators of well-being include subjective assessments, such as self-rated health, a useful measure by which people gauge their health from their own perspective. Studies have shown that functional status is one of the main criteria used by individuals to rate their health, but that self-rated health is also influenced by a person's judgement about the severity of current illness, personal resource to maintain well-being, health behaviour, and family health history (11). Self-rated health is strongly predictive of future health, including the likelihood of dying (12, 13).

Human Biology

Although not listed in the framework, human biology is an important determinant of health and includes age and gender. Women, men, children, and the elderly have different potentials for health and disease (see Chapter 4). Because of their interaction with social and economic conditions, age and gender are incorporated into community and health system characteristics. Genetic inheritance is currently the best example of this human biology indicator. The Human Genome Project offers the potential for complete knowledge of the human gene and the identification of an individual's genetic make-up. A mass screening program for phenylketonuria which is a genetically inherited disease is well established. Genetic screening for diseases raises ethical issues, as it may stigmatize the individuals for a number of reasons e.g., insurability of individual, choice as marriage partner (14). The implications of mass genetic screening will likely emerge as a public health concern.

Health Conditions

Health conditions include alterations or attributes of the health status of an individual that may lead to distress, interference with daily activities, or contact with health services; such a condition may be a disease (acute or chronic), disorder, injury, or trauma, or may reflect other health-related states such as pregnancy, aging, stress, congenital anomaly, or genetic predisposition (10).

There are several subjective and objective indicators of health conditions:

- Body mass index (BMI-Canadian standard), which relates weight to height, is a common method of determining if an individual's weight is in a healthy range. BMI is calculated by dividing weight in kilograms by height in metres squared. The index is as follows: under 20 (underweight), 20 to 24.9 (acceptable weight), 25 to 27.0 (some excess weight), and greater than 27 (overweight). The index is calculated for those aged 20 to 64 excluding pregnant women and anyone under 0.914 metres tall or taller than 2.108 metres.

- Incidence and prevalence of relevant health conditions such as arthritis and rheumatism, diabetes, hypertension, depression, cancer, and injury provide information on the burden of morbidity in the community and are obtained through surveys or other administrative data sources described later in this chapter.
- Information on the incidence of chronic pain is obtained from respondents who report having pain or discomfort that prevents or limits certain activities on a continuing basis. The severity of the pain is measured as severe, moderate, or mild.

Human Function

Human function is associated with the ability to function as a consequence of disease, disorder, injury, or other health conditions. Levels of functionality are considered in terms of functional health (as in impairments related to function and structure), activity limitations, and ability to participate in activities (see Chapter 1) (10).

Information on **functional health** is obtained from population surveys and by determining the proportion of the population aged 12 and older that reports moderate or severe functional problems, according to the Comprehensive Health Status Measurement System, based on eight dimensions of functioning (hearing, seeing, communicating, mobility, dexterity, pain, cognition, and emotion) (15).

Information on **activity limitation** is obtained from the National Population Health Survey, which surveys the population aged 4 and over and also aged 12 and over and asks about disability or handicap or limitations in certain activities because of a physical condition, mental condition, or health problem.

Participation refers to the ability to interact in society and includes aspects such as participation in work, school, or leisure activities. Currently, there are a limited number of indicators of participation in Canada's national health surveys. Other surveys, such as the General Social Survey, are often useful sources of information for indicators on participation and other broader measures of quality of life.

Summary Measures of Population Health

Summary measures of population health combine measures of death and HRQOL into a single summary measure. There are two main classes of summary measures of population health: positive measures of health expectancy (16), such as disability-free life expectancy or health-adjusted life expectancy, and measures of health gaps such as healthy life years (17) or disability-adjusted life years (DALYs) (18).

Life expectancy is the number of years a person is expected to live, starting from birth (for life expectancy at birth) or at age 65 (for life expectancy at age 65), if current mortality rates continue to apply (7). **Disability-free life expectancy** is used to distinguish between years of life free of any activity limitation and years experienced with at least one activity limitation. To that end, disability-free life expectancy establishes a threshold based on the nature of such limitations. Years of life lived in conditions above these thresholds are counted in full. Those lived in conditions below the thresholds are not counted. Thus, the emphasis is not exclusively on the length of life, as is the case for life expectancy, but also on the HRQOL.

Table 3.3   Derivations of Commonly Used Health Status Indicators

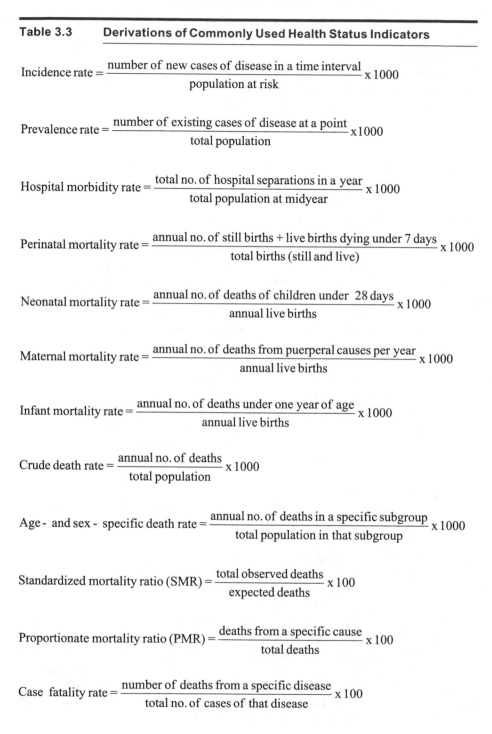

$$\text{Incidence rate} = \frac{\text{number of new cases of disease in a time interval}}{\text{population at risk}} \times 1000$$

$$\text{Prevalence rate} = \frac{\text{number of existing cases of disease at a point}}{\text{total population}} \times 1000$$

$$\text{Hospital morbidity rate} = \frac{\text{total no. of hospital separations in a year}}{\text{total population at midyear}} \times 1000$$

$$\text{Perinatal mortality rate} = \frac{\text{annual no. of still births} + \text{live births dying under 7 days}}{\text{total births (still and live)}} \times 1000$$

$$\text{Neonatal mortality rate} = \frac{\text{annual no. of deaths of children under 28 days}}{\text{annual live births}} \times 1000$$

$$\text{Maternal mortality rate} = \frac{\text{annual no. of deaths from puerperal causes per year}}{\text{annual live births}} \times 1000$$

$$\text{Infant mortality rate} = \frac{\text{annual no. of deaths under one year of age}}{\text{annual live births}} \times 1000$$

$$\text{Crude death rate} = \frac{\text{annual no. of deaths}}{\text{total population}} \times 1000$$

$$\text{Age- and sex- specific death rate} = \frac{\text{annual no. of deaths in a specific subgroup}}{\text{total population in that subgroup}} \times 1000$$

$$\text{Standardized mortality ratio (SMR)} = \frac{\text{total observed deaths}}{\text{expected deaths}} \times 100$$

$$\text{Proportionate mortality ratio (PMR)} = \frac{\text{deaths from a specific cause}}{\text{total deaths}} \times 100$$

$$\text{Case fatality rate} = \frac{\text{number of deaths from a specific disease}}{\text{total no. of cases of that disease}} \times 100$$

DALYs build on the mortality indicators of **potential years of life lost (PYLL)** (discussed in the next section), similar to the way that disability-free life expectancy is an adaptation of life expectancy. DALYs and PYLLs are referred to as **health gap** indicators because they measure the difference (or gap) between death or HRQOL at a specific age compared to a reference age (often 75 years for PYLL or the life expectancy of Japan — the country with the highest life expectancy) for the World Health Organization's calculation of DALYs (18). DALYs consider the mortality gap as well as the gap in disability.

Death

Death includes a range of age-specific mortality rates (e.g., infant mortality) and condition-specific mortality rates (e.g., AIDS), as well as derived indicators (e.g., life expectancy and PYLLs).

Commonly used health indicators in the category of deaths are listed here and their derivations are summarized in Table 3.3.

- **Infant Mortality Rate:** The annual number of deaths in children less than one year of age per 1,000 live births in the same year. The infant mortality rate is commonly used for comparing health among different countries.
- **Perinatal Mortality Rate:** The annual number of stillbirths (gestation of 20 weeks or more) and early neonatal deaths (within the first seven days of life) per 1,000 stillbirths and live births. Perinatal mortality usually reflects standards of perinatal care, maternal nutrition, and obstetric and pediatric care. Stillbirth is defined as a product of conception of 20 or more weeks gestation or fetal weight of 500 grams or more, which did not breathe or show other signs of life at delivery. Death may occur before or during delivery. At what gestational age a miscarriage becomes a stillbirth depends on the policy or law of each province or country and varies from 20–28 weeks.
- **Crude Death Rate:** The annual number of deaths per 1,000 population.
- **Neonatal Mortality Rate:** The annual number of deaths in a year of children under 28 days of age per 1,000 live births in the same year.
- **Maternal Mortality Rate:** The annual number of maternal deaths occuring during pregnancy and from puerperal causes (i.e., deaths occurring during and/or due to deliveries, complications of pregnancy, childbirth, and the puerperium) per 1,000 live births in the same year. According to the WHO, a maternal death is defined as the death of a woman while pregnant or within 42 days of termination of pregnancy, irrespective of the duration and the site of pregnancy (e.g., uterine or extrauterine pregnancy), from any cause related to or aggravated by the pregnancy or its management but not from accidental or incidental causes (7).
- **Age- and Sex-Specific Death Rate:** The annual number of deaths in a particular age and gender group per 1,000 population in that sub-group.
- **Potential Years of Life Lost (PYLL):** The total years of life lost before age 70 or 75 years for people who become deceased between birth and the 70th or 75th year of life. There is no standard cut-off age. It shows the burden of premature deaths by different causes and the cost in terms of person-years lost to society.

- **Proportionate Mortality Ratio (PMR):** The ratio of deaths from a specific cause to the total number of deaths in a given period.
- **Case-Fatality Rate:** The number of deaths from a specific disease per total number of cases of that disease in a given period.
- **Age-Standardized Mortality Rate:** Indicates the overall health of the population and is similar to what is measured by life expectancy. Age-standardization (as opposed to crude rates) allows for comparisons between health regions, provinces, and countries (see Chapter 2).

1.2.   NON-MEDICAL DETERMINANTS

Health Behaviours

Health behaviours include aspects of personal behaviour and risk factors that epidemiological studies have shown to influence health status. Survey data is a rich source of health behaviour and risk-factor indicators, which are discussed in detail in the next chapters. Indicators such as the proportion of high-risk drinkers, the proportion of smokers by age and sex, leisure-time physical activity, and dietary practices all give valuable insight into the patterns of health in the community.

Living and Working Conditions

These indicators are related to the socioeconomic characteristics and working conditions of the population, which epidemiological studies have shown to be related to health (see Chapter 1). Data on living and working conditions are usually obtained through survey and incorporate education, unemployment and income level, housing affordability, youth crime rates, and decision latitude at work.

Decision latitude at work is defined as degree of control that employed workers aged 15 to 74 have over their work circumstances. It has an impact on health of worker. Information about it is obtained by specific survey questions.

Personal Resources

Indicators of personal resources measure the prevalence of factors, such as social support and life stress, which epidemiological studies have shown to be related to health. These are discussed in Chapter 1.

Social support is determined by survey questions that ask about level of perceived social support reported by individuals aged 12 and over, based on responses to four questions about having someone to confide in, someone they can count on in a crisis, someone they can count on for advice, and someone who makes them feel loved and cared for.

Life stress is determined by survey questionnaire determining level of chronic stress reported by the population aged 18 and over based on responses to questions about personal situation.

Environmental Factors

Environmental factors include physical aspects with the potential to influence human health and are discussed in detail in Chapter 9. These indicators are an integral component of monitoring progress toward a safe and clean physical environment. An example of an environmental health indicator is the Air Quality Index (AQI), which is a composite of six continuously measured air pollutants that have evidence of adverse human health effects, namely carbon monoxide, total suspended particulate, ozone, sulphur dioxide, nitrogen dioxide, and total reduced sulphur compounds. When the AQI exceeds certain thresholds, health warnings are issued so that people in vulnerable groups can avoid inhaling outdoor air.

Other indicators of environmental health include water quality measurements of drinking water and recreational water. The number of days that beaches are closed to swimmers because of elevated bacterial counts can also serve as an indicator of recreational water quality. Exposure to secondhand smoke is also considered. The Quebec City Consensus Conference on Environment Health Indicators in 2000 provided a comprehensive picture of the types of environmental indicators needed for surveillance (19).

1.3. INDICATORS OF HEALTH SYSTEM PERFORMANCE

Health system performance indicators fall into several categories: acceptability, accessibility, appropriateness, competence, continuity, effectiveness, efficiency, and safety. At present, there are no agreed-upon indicators developed for acceptability, competence, and continuity. There are few indicators for the other categories.

Acceptability

All care and service provided must meet the expectations of the client, community, providers, and paying organizations, recognizing that there may be conflicting, competing interests among stakeholders and that the needs of the patients are paramount. Patient satisfaction surveys are often used to provide data on acceptability.

Accessibility

Accessibility is defined as the ability of patients to obtain care and service at the right place and the right time, based on needs. Indicators are the proportion of population that receives influenza immunization (65 years and over), Pap smear (women aged 18 to 69 years), and childhood immunization. Waiting times to access specialty or diagnostic care or elective surgery are also used to measure access.

Appropriateness

The care or service provided must be relevant to the patients' needs and based on established standards. The proxy indicator for appropriateness is vaginal birth after Caesarean section, because there is considerable evidence that vaginal birth is safe for many women who have previously delivered in this manner.

Competence

Competence is defined as an individual's knowledge and skills appropriate to the care or service provided. CIHI has begun to report on the volume of procedures done in an institution (for example pancreatic or heart surgery) as a measure of competence.

Continuity

Continuity is defined as the ability to provide uninterrupted, coordinated care or service across programs, practitioners, organizations, and levels of care and service over time. No indicators for this category have been developed.

Effectiveness

Effectiveness is defined as whether or not the intervention or action related to the care or service achieved the desired results. It is measured by a number of indicators. For example, if there are successful programs for immunization, there should be no cases of the related diseases and conditions, such as pertussis, measles, or influenza. Hence, the indicators for effectiveness of immunization programs are the number of cases of pertussis, measles, chlamydia, etc.

Efficiency

Efficiency refers to achieving the desired results with the most cost-effective use of resources. Proposed indicators relate to whether a person requires hospitalization and the expected length of stay versus the actual length of stay in hospital. For example, the level of efficiency can be measured by the percentage of patients hospitalized in acute care facilities for conditions or procedures that can be treated in outpatient facilities and do not require admission. Such hospitalizations are classified as "may not require hospitalization" and are derived from the Case Mix Group (CMG) methodology.

Safety

Safety refers to the minimization of potential risks of an intervention or the environment. Hip fracture is used as an indicator, because it may be the result of intervention, such as when sedatives are given to seniors, or it may be related to the environment, such as loose rugs or poor lighting in dwellings, or it may be related to an interaction of both. The issue of patient safety has become a major focus of interest since the publication of a study by the U.S. Institute of Medicine. There is now considerable work underway to both measure adverse events in health care and improve patient safety (20).

1.4.   COMMUNITY AND HEALTH SYSTEM CHARACTERISTICS

Characteristics of the community or the health system are often referred to as demographic, resource, or utilization indicators. While not indicators of health status or health system performance in themselves, they provide useful contextual information.

Community Characteristics

Examples of these indicators include the age and gender of the population, the population growth rate, ethnicity, language, family size, proportion of single-parent families, and proportion of elderly persons and Aboriginal people (the health of Aboriginal people and the elderly is discussed in Chapter 6). There are a few definitions worth noting.

- **Crude birth rate:** The annual number of live births per 1,000 population.
- **General fertility rate:** The annual number of live births per 1,000 women between ages 15 and 49. This is a more refined measure of fertility, as it includes only those likely to give birth.
- **Total fertility rate:** The average number of children who would be born alive to a woman during her lifetime if she were to pass through all her childbearing years conforming to the age-specific fertility rates of a given year.

Health System Characteristics Inflow/Outflow Ratio

The ratio of inflow to outflow of the health system reflects the balance between the quantity of hospital stays provided to both residents and non-residents by all acute care hospitals in a given region and the extent of acute care use by residents of that region, whether they receive care within or out of the region. A ratio less than one indicates that hospital stays used by residents of a region exceeded hospital care provided within that region, suggesting an outflow effect. A ratio greater than one indicates hospital stays provided by a region exceeded the quantity of stays used by its residents, suggesting an inflow effect. A ratio of one indicates that the volume of hospital discharges in the region is equivalent to that generated by its residents, suggesting that inflow and outflow activity, if it exists at all, is balanced.

Two common measures of hospital use are described below:

- **Hospital separation rate.** The number of hospital separations (discharges and deaths) recorded in the year per 1,000 population. It reflects the frequency at which hospital care is sought, and is influenced by a number of factors such as the availability of care.
- **Hospital days of care.** The total number of days of care for all hospitals per 1,000 population in a year. This rate may also be expressed for certain diseases to allow comparisons.

Other indicators such as hip replacement, knee replacement, and contact with various healthcare professionals indicate availability of services, provider practice patterns, and patient preferences.

Health Expenditures

The proportions of the gross national product (GNP) or the gross domestic product (GDP) spent on health and the per capita expenditure (the average amount spent per person) on health by government and private sector are both indicators of the burden of disease. GNP measures all the goods and services produced by a country in a given year and is a measure of productivity. GDP includes all resources available to the country, irrespective of whether they are earned through local production or foreign investment in the country; it is useful for international comparisons (see Chapter 14). The per capita measure is limited by what costs are included and the scope of adjustment for demographic characteristics of the population.

Health Human Resources

Health care is influenced by the availability of nurses, physicians, and other health professionals and is generally measured as the ratio of healthcare profession to population (see Chapter 14). The mix of healthcare professionals and accessibility to needed professionals determines whether there is an adequate number of human health resources in a particular region or province.

1.5.   ECONOMIC EVALUATION OF HEALTH PROGRAMS

Health programs may be evaluated in terms of their effects on morbidity and mortality (health outcomes), in terms of changes in behaviour (impact), and from an economic perspective (i.e., utilization of resources). An important economic concept is that of efficiency: a program is efficient if it achieves desired results with a minimum of inputs. Different types of economic analysis are used to gauge the cost of a health program in terms of health outcomes. These analyses are often used when evaluating competing programs. The differences in the analyses lie in how the effects of a program are conceptualized and measured.

Cost-Effectiveness Analysis

Cost-effectiveness analysis can be used when the outcomes of procedures or programs vary, but the outcomes can be expressed by a common natural unit such as life years gained (21). The effectiveness of the interventions can then be compared and expressed in dollar figures per natural unit of that outcome. For example, one could calculate the cost of an intervention per year of life gained, or per millimetre of mercury of blood pressure reduction.

Cost-Benefit Analysis

The effects of programs are expressed in health-related terms and then converted to dollar terms. For example, years of life gained are translated to dollars that could be earned during this period by a person of working age. The ratios of benefits to costs are compared for different programs.

Cost-Utility Analysis

Cost-utility analysis refers to the subjective level of well-being experienced by people in differing states of health. Such an analysis uses a variety of techniques such as time trade-offs and the standard gamble. Cost-utility analysis seeks to incorporate the utility of quantity and quality of life in a summary measure such as a quality-adjusted life year (QALY). Interventions can then be compared in terms of the QALYs gained or lost; however there are limitations to this method (22).

1.6.   COMMUNITY EFFECTIVENESS

Efficacy is defined by desired outcomes that are achieved by an intervention in ideal conditions, such as in a randomized control trial. However, the efficacy of an intervention is only one component of its usefulness as it applies in the community. Community effectiveness also depends on coverage and compliance. **Coverage** is the proportion of the target or at-risk population reached by the program: Is it directed at, accessible to, and available to those who would maximally benefit? **Compliance** deals with provider and consumer compliance. Provider compliance indicates the degree to which healthcare providers cooperate with providing the program and all its elements. Consumer compliance indicates the degree to which those who need the intervention use it. This can be expressed in the following relationship:

$$\frac{\text{Community}}{\text{Effectiveness}} = \text{efficacy} \times \text{coverage} \times \frac{\text{provider}}{\text{compliance}} \times \frac{\text{consumer}}{\text{compliance}}$$

1.7.   ECONOMIC BURDEN OF DISEASE

The economic burden of disease is different from economic evaluation of health programs in that it relates to the use of society's resources for broad areas of disease, as opposed to the resources for specific health programs. Resources used for one purpose are unavailable for another, a concept known as opportunity cost. The economic burden of disease has become increasingly prominent in recent years.

The costs of disease are measured in terms of direct and indirect costs. Direct costs measure the expenditure for prevention and treatment of disease. They include publicly funded healthcare costs, education, and research, as well as personal health care, which consists of institutional costs, non-hospital medical care costs, and other costs, such as dental care and prescribed drugs.

Indirect costs measure the loss of productive services due to morbidity and mortality. They include financial loss due to premature death or loss of workdays due to temporary or permanent disability. For example, the number of person-years of productive work lost because of automobile collisions is an indirect cost, or indirect burden, of disease. Usually, data limitations and conceptual problems limit the scope and accuracy of these estimates.

2.   SOURCES OF HEALTH DATA

There is a large volume of Canadian health data available for interpretation. The abundance of health-related data, from a variety of disparate sources, poses problems for comparability. As well, the need to share information across a variety of jurisdictions creates challenges for developing compatible information systems. The challenges are not merely technical. The advent of powerful computers and algorithms for linking databases has also caused significant ethical and social problems. Consequently, Health

Canada in conjunction with Statistics Canada established the Canadian Institute for Health Information in 1994. The CIHI is a federally chartered, independent, not-for-profit organization that consolidated the programs, functions, and activities of the Hospital Medical Research Institute, the Management and Information System Research Group (MIS Group), the Health Information Division of Health Canada, and elements of the Health Statistics Division of Statistics Canada into one body (23). Its primary functions are to collect, process, and maintain a comprehensive number of databases and registries that cover health-related human resources, services, and expenditures, and to set national standards for financial, statistical, and clinical data as well as for health information technology. The CIHI's website, along with Statistics Canada's, is a repository of a wealth of information on different aspects of Canadian health and healthcare system.

2.1.   CENSUS DATA

Statistics Canada conducts a national census every five years in June. All citizens are required by law to participate and complete the short census form (form 2A); a sample of 20% complete a more detailed form (form 2B, the long form). The census is the major source of information on population and demographic information, and of numerator and denominator information for calculating rates. Census undercounting is usually about 3%. Data are collected on many variables, including age, sex, language spoken at home, place of birth, education, and economic status, and are aggregated on a geographical basis according to census tracts.

2.2.   SURVEYS

A health survey is either a cross-sectional (administered to respondents once) or longitudinal study (a survey that is repeated to the same respondents over different periods); it is conducted by interview or examination, or both, of a sample of the population. It can also be conducted with a self-administered questionnaire, by telephone, mail, or personal interview. It can be done regularly and repeatedly (to analyze trends), or as needed to investigate a specific problem (e.g., blood lead levels of children living near lead smelters in Toronto). Longitudinal health surveys directed at a selected or representative sample of the population follow people over time to examine how health determinants, HRQOL, and consequences change among individuals. With proper consent and ethics approval, cross-sectional surveys may be linked to other sources of vital statistics or health administration data. This linkage allows long-term follow-up of the health consequences. For example, the 1978 Canada Health Survey was used to examine the long-term effect of folic acid and heart disease (24). Most commonly, health surveys are used for surveillance of health behaviour, levels of illness, and health consequences. Because health surveys are often representative samples of entire populations, they can examine many related social factors in people who do not necessarily contact the healthcare system.

Although simple in theory, surveys pose many methodological problems. Respondents have been shown to forget even major events. If the questionnaire is neither designed properly nor presented conscientiously, it may give ambiguous or misleading results. If interviewers are not adequately trained, they can easily influence the quality of responses. There is also a problem with missing data.

The federal government established the National Health Information Council (NHIC) to formulate plans on the need for data for the health sector (25). In 1991, the NHIC recommended that an ongoing national survey of population health be conducted. This recommendation was based on the knowledge of the economic and fiscal pressures on the healthcare system and on the requirement for information to improve the quality of health in Canada as well as the effectiveness and efficiency of healthcare services. The survey was first done by Statistics Canada in 1994 and is repeated every two years. The objectives of this National Population Health Survey (NPHS) are to

- aid in the development of public policies by providing measures of the health status of the population;
- provide data that assist in understanding the determinants of health;
- collect data on the economic, social, demographic, occupational, and environmental correlates of health;
- increase the understanding of the relationship between health status and the use of health care resources, including alternative as well as traditional services;
- follow a selected group of people over time to provide information on the dynamic process of health and illness;
- provide the provinces and territories and other clients with a template for a health survey;
- allow the possibility of linking survey data to routinely collected administrative data such as vital statistics, environmental measures, community variables, and health care service utilization (26).

One component of the NPHS is longitudinal and has been following the same group of Canadians since 1994. In 2000–01, the cross-sectional component of the NPHS was expanded into the Canadian Community Health Survey (CCHS), which interviewed more than 120,000 Canadians. The CCHS allowed, for the first time, a close examination of health determinants, HRQOL, and consequences for all 132 health regions in Canada (27).

A number of national and provincial surveys of importance have been conducted in the last five decades (28). General health-related surveys in the past two decades include:

- Canada Health Survey (1978);
- General Social Surveys (1985, 1991);
- Health Promotion Surveys (1985, 1990);
- Ontario Health Surveys (1990, 1997);
- Quebec Health Surveys (1987, 1993).

The following surveys include physical measures of respondents such as blood pressure or cholesterol levels (29).

- Canadian Health Survey (1985);

- Canadian Heart Health Surveys (1986–90);
- Nova Scotia Health Survey (1995).

Surveys devoted to health determinants, special populations, and lifestyles include:

- Canada Alcohol and Other Drugs Survey (1994);
- Surveys of smoking in Canada;
- Youth Smoking Survey (1994);
- Violence against Women Survey (1993);
- Aboriginal Peoples Survey (1991);
- National Longitudinal Survey of Children (1994);
- Labour force surveys.

Several *Health Indicators Reports* describe Canadian and provincial populations (1999–2001) (5).

In 1991 and 1997, Statistics Canada and Health Canada produced an overview of the major population-based surveys in Canada (28, 30). Recently, the CIHI also published a resource guide for data sharing that contains an appendix with an excellent description of the major health-related surveys ongoing or proposed in Canada (31).

2.3. ADMINISTRATIVE DATA

Perhaps the most uniformly recorded and reliable health data are administrative (e.g., rates of hospital admission, treatments, and discharge diagnoses). Administrative and professional bodies require this information for planning and evaluating medical care. Administrative data for hospitalization in most provinces are summarized yearly and entered into a central provincial file, such as those maintained by the CIHI. One of the CIHI's main functions is to prepare easily auditable reports for hospitals to use in quality control and planning, but the data are also suitable for research. Data are also gathered by all provincial health insurance plans, workers' compensation boards, drug utilization plans, and dental health plans. Usually, administrative data are more useful in studying health care rather than the distribution and causes of disease.

The broad utility of administrative data for an understanding of health services has been shown by research institutions in Manitoba and Ontario. The Manitoba Centre for Health Policy and the Institute for Clinical Evaluative Sciences in Ontario (ICES) make extensive use of administrative data to document variations in the delivery of healthcare services and examples of excellence. ICES publishes atlases of healthcare services, which are indispensable for understanding the role of the healthcare system in the broad determinants of health (32, 33). Similarly, the Manitoba Centre for Health Policy, the University of British Columbia, the Centre for Health Services and Policy Research, the Centre for Health, Economics, and Health Policy Analysis at McMaster University, and the Population Health Research Unit of Dalhousie University produce regular reports on different aspects of health services utilization.

2.4.   SURVEILLANCE SYSTEMS

2.4.1.   Health Surveillance

The Network for Health Surveillance in Canada (34) defines health surveillance as: "the tracking and forecasting of any health event or health determinant through the collection of data, and its integration, analysis and interpretation into surveillance products, and the dissemination of those surveillance products to those who need to know." Thus it is the continuous, systematic use of routinely collected, non-identifiable health data used to guide public health action.

Surveillance has the following characteristics:

- it is population based;
- it tends to be prospective and purposeful;
- it usually involves the collection of data in a continuous fashion;
- it goes beyond collecting data to produce surveillance products; and
- it results in information and analytical products that are made available quickly to public health decision makers.

Surveillance of disease or risk factors comes in many different forms, including both the passive and active collection of data. In some situations, surveillance can be a formal or informal network of medical officers of health, physicians, and other healthcare professionals who report unusual occurrences or apparent increases in disease rates to provincial or federal agencies responsible for surveillance. The WHO continuously monitors the Web sites to identify potential emerging health outbreaks or other emergencies that otherwise are difficult to identify.

Many diseases, risk factors, or other determinants of health are targeted for surveillance. Data sources for these may exist as part of health surveys or health administrative databases or they can be specially designed if data sources are otherwise not available. The following are several examples of these special situations.

Many infectious diseases (e.g., measles, chickenpox) and sexually transmitted diseases are reportable — that is, the law requires that they be reported to the local health authority. This reporting provides the data for incidence rates of infectious diseases. The list of reportable diseases in a province is available from the provincial health department or ministry. In Canada, there are 48 reportable diseases. These include diseases ranging from AIDS to yellow fever. This list of national notifiable diseases is agreed upon by consensus among provincial and federal health authorities through the Advisory Committee on Epidemiology (ACE) (see Table 3.4). ACE meets approximately twice a year to update the list (35). Surveillance data for cancer, cardiovascular diseases, notifiable diseases, and injuries for Canada and provinces are available on line at the Health Canada site (35).

Another source of surveillance is the provincial workers' compensation board. In each province, notification of industrial injuries and diseases is required to facilitate claim processing and preventive activities. The Association of Workers' Compensation Boards of Canada (AWCBC) collects information from the provincial and territorial workers' compensation boards (WCBs). These data can provide incidence information on industrial injuries and diseases (36).

Table 3.4   List of Nationally Notifiable Diseases in Canada, 2003

Disease	Disease	Disease
Acute Flaccid Paralysis	Hepatitis B	Rubella, Congenital*
AIDS	Hepatitis C	Salmonellosis
Anthrax*	Human Immunodeficiency Virus	Severe Acute Respiratory Syndrome**
Botulism*	Influenza, laboratory confirmed	Shigellosis
Brucellosis*	Invasive Haemophilus influenzae type b Disease	Smallpox*
Campylobacteriosis	Invasive Group A Streptococcal Disease	Syphilis, Congenital*
Chickenpox	Invasive Meningococcal Disease	Infectious Syphilis
Chlamydia, Genital	Invasive Pneumococcal Disease	Syphilis, Other
Cholera*	Legionellosis	Tetanus*
Creutzfeld-Jakob Disease	Leprosy*	Tuberculosis
Cryptosporidiosis	Malaria	Tularemia*
Cyclosporiasis	Measles	Typhoid
Diphtheria*	Mumps	Verotoxigenic E. coli
Giardiasis	Pertussis	Viral Hemorrhagic Fever* (Crimean Congo, Ebola, Lassa, Marburg)
Gonorrhea	Plague*	West Nile Virus**
Group B Streptococcal Disease of the Newborn	Poliomyelitis*	Yellow Fever*
Hantavirus Pulmonary Syndrome	Rabies*	* Indicates list of notifiable diseases that have few or no cases reported ** Listing pending
Hepatitis A	Rubella	

Disease registries for chronic diseases, especially cancer, are another important source of data, particularly if they are population based. In all provinces, cancer reports are sent by private practitioners, clinics, and pathology departments, and each patient's name and clinical information are entered in a central registry. The completeness of the registry is checked by searching for notations of cancer on death certificates. If the registry is complete, the name of any person who died of cancer should already be entered in the registry records, as cancer is usually detected before death. A 95% agreement between death certificates and registry is the goal in most provinces. Well-kept registries can provide incidence and prevalence data.

There are other registries, including one for children with disabilities in British Columbia and the Canadian National Institute for the Blind. The other examples of disease registries (37, 38) are the Canadian Organ Replacement Register, the Canadian Tuberculosis Reporting System and the Therapeutic Abortion Database.

While many disease registries are active systems of disease identification, others are passive, relying on data collected for other purposes that are then reviewed to ascertain people with specific conditions. One example is the Canadian Congenital Anomaly Surveillance System, which identifies children who have major congenital defects through hospital discharge records from CIHI's discharge abstract databases (a health administrative database). The practice for creating disease registries or surveillance systems using health administrative databases or other sources of information not specially designed for surveillance is increasing in Canada. Recent examples are diabetes registries that are created by identifying people from physician billing or hospital discharge data.

2.5. VITAL STATISTICS

The record of the basic events of the human life cycle — birth, marriage, and death — is appropriately called vital statistics. Throughout history, governments have kept some kind of register of their citizens. As early as 1608, an "Ordinance" in Quebec required the clergy to register births, marriages, and deaths in each parish. By 1667, this registration was required in duplicate, and one copy was forwarded to the "Judge Royal." In late 17th-century England, John Graunt systematized record-keeping, and since then, vital statistics have been the most reliable and consistently recorded data source in the health field.

2.5.1. Birth Certificate
Figure 3.1 is an abridged facsimile of a Statement of Live Birth in Ontario. In Canada, the parents are responsible for filing the certificate with the municipal clerk. It contains relatively limited health information, and there is neither medical history of the mother nor a description of the birth itself. Another form, the Notice of Live Birth or Stillbirth, must be filled out by the attending physician and filed with the provincial registrar. This form provides no information about the father, and records the length of the gestation period and the presence of congenital deformities obvious at birth.

Figure 3.1:   Birth Certificate, Province of Ontario

Province of Ontario (Canada) Office of the Registrar-General *(Abridged)*

Child	1.	2. Sex of Child
Last Name		
Given Names		

Date of Birth	3. Month (by name) day year of birth	4. Please state if mother is: Married, widowed, divorced or single (the term "common law" or "separated" not to be used)
Place of Birth	5. Name of hospital (If not in hospital give exact location where birth occurred.)	
	Borough, city, town, village, township (by name). Regional municipality, county or district	

PARENTS	FATHER		MOTHER	
Name	6. Surname of child's father		10. Maiden name (before marriage)	
	All given names		All given names	
Birthplace	7. City, town, or other place of birth (by name)		11. City, town, or other place of birth (by name)	
	Province (or country if outside Canada)		Province (or country if outside Canada)	
Birthdate	8. Month (by name), day, year of birth	Age (at time of this birth)	12. Month (by name), day, year of birth	Age (at time of this birth)
Usual Residence of Mother	14. Complete street address. If rural, give exact location and Post Office or Rural Route address.			
	Borough, city, town, village, township (by name); Regional Municipality, county or district; Province (or Country)			
Mailing Address of Mother	15. Complete mailing address (if different from 14). If rural give Post Office or rural route address.			

OTHER	16. Duration of pregnancy (in completed weeks)	17. Number of children ever born to this mother (including this birth)	Number liveborn	Number stillborn (after 20 weeks pregnancy)
BIRTH PARTICULARS	18. Weight of child at birth ____ ____ or ____ lbs oz grams	19. Kind of birth State whether single, twin, or triplet	20. If twin or triplet, whether this child was born 1st, 2nd, or 3rd.	

ATTENDANT	21. Name of attending physician (or other attendant)	☐ Physician
	Complete mailing address	☐ Nurse
		☐ Other

Figure 3.2   Death Certificate

CAUSE OF DEATH

Part One

Immediate cause of death   (a) _____

due to, or as a consequence of

Antecedent causes, if any,   (b) _____
giving rise to the immediate   due to, or as a consequence of
cause (a) above, stating the
underlying cause last

(c) _____

Part Two

Other significant conditions   _____
contributing to the death but not
causally related to the immediate
cause (a) above   _____

2.5.2.   Death Certificate

A death certificate must be signed by a licensed physician and includes cause of death, person's name, birth date, sex, and place of residence and death. Figure 3.2 illustrates the part that lists the causes of death. There are three distinct sections for the cause of death. The immediate cause of death is recorded on the first line; for example, a certificate for an elderly person dying of pneumonia with no other fatal health conditions has pneumonia recorded there. The second entry is called "antecedent causes," which means that there may be a condition or disease that gave rise to the immediate cause of death. For example, an immediate cause of death in a woman could be metastatic or secondary cancer of the lung; if the condition that led to this was cancer of the breast, then cancer of the breast would appear on the second line. The third section is "any other significant conditions" that contributed to the death but did not directly cause it. For example, on the death certificate of a person who has chronic bronchitis and dies of uremia as a result of chronic nephritis, uremia would be listed as the immediate cause of death (line a), chronic nephritis would be listed as the antecedent cause of death (line b), and chronic bronchitis would be listed in the second part as another significant condition. When both the immediate cause of death and the antecedent cause are recorded on the death certificate, then the antecedent cause is the one used for data analysis for cause-specific mortality. Other significant conditions may also be recorded separately.

The current system for recording cause of death information has been described as unreliable. There are problems with the ambiguity of the instructions and disease definitions set out by the WHO for use by the physician or coroner when filling out a death certificate. A recent critique suggests the need for greater validity in recording cause of death data (39, 40).

Some causes of death require notification of death to the coroner (or medical examiner). In such cases, a physician must not sign the death certificate. These include situations where there is reason to suspect that the person died by violent means or undue negligence or in an unexplained manner, death in a correctional institution, in police custody, in maternally related situations (e.g., abortion), after anesthesia, in seniors' homes and in work places, and associated with involuntary residence in an institution. Each province has its own statute governing the causes to be notified to the coroner.

Birth and death data usually provide the fertility rate, infant mortality rate, crude death rate, life expectancy at birth, potential years of life lost, and all other mortality rates described earlier.

2.6.   CONSUMPTION DATA

Various production and consumption data can be related to health. The most obvious of these is food. The figures for tonnage of food produced or imported each year are adjusted according to current levels of supplies to produce a "disappearance" figure: the amount of foodstuffs that need to be replaced each year. In general, it is possible to determine the proportion of various foodstuffs actually eaten by humans, so the average per capita consumption of meat, for example, can be calculated for any year. Although this information is useful for following long-term historical trends (compared with dietary inventories of the type collected in surveys carried out by Nutrition Canada), such data are not very reliable, as they tell us little about the habits of any individual.

In the same way, annual production of cigarettes or litres of alcohol can be related to long-term trends in health. More indirectly, data on industrial processes involving hazardous substances, such as asbestos or substances emitting pollutants (e.g., sulphur dioxide from the pulp and paper industry), may be related to levels of health.

3.   RECORD LINKAGE

A wide variety of health data (vital statistics, registries, surveys and reports) is collected about each individual and recorded in many places. Many people feel that if these data were linked, a very useful profile of social, biological, and personal data could be constructed. Relationships between possible causes of disease (industrial exposure, levels of pollution, social conditions, family history) and the individual's history of disease would yield much more precise information than the other sources of data already described. Furthermore, the Canadian system of "geocoding" social and demographic information according to the postal code, and the existence of a centralized agency (Statistics Canada, the ultimate collector and publisher of a great volume and variety of data) set the stage for this record linkage. The 1991 Task Force on Health Information advised that the capacity for linkage of different data elements was critical to fulfilling the potential of the development of systems for health data (25).

Approaches to record linkage include integrating health records at the level of the individual patient from different sources and over time. Record linkage can be achieved by the allocation of personal identifiers, possibly on a lifetime basis, a strategy that has been considered at the provincial level. However, these are not likely to be portable between provinces. Linkage can also be achieved, with varying degrees of accuracy, by matching based on probabilities of linking personal identifying data in two or more data banks. These include the surname, surname at birth (if applicable), first name, date of birth, place of birth, and any other identifiers such as the social insurance number. A record is strongly matched when a high percentage of similarities is obtained. If matched, records for individuals in the two data banks may be merged; however, these data must be of good quality and be sufficiently detailed for the information to be useful.

Record linkage can be employed for both the purposes of administration and research. Health records contain sensitive information about individuals. Linkage and data sharing must be carried out under conditions of strict confidentiality. Confidentiality requirements and consent procedures differ in research and administrative contexts. Data used for administrative purposes can have a direct impact on an individual, whereas research data rarely target individuals, but deal with unlinked aggregate data. In general, it is customary for data collected for administrative purposes to be used for research; the converse is never the case unless explicit consent for such use has been obtained.

Several provinces and the federal government have legislation that protects personal health information. The legislation usually outlines sanctions and punishments that can be brought to bear for violations of confidentiality. Other safeguards for data confidentiality include a mechanism to obtain consent if administrative data are intended for research purposes, a means of informing data subjects on the possible uses of their information, a means of scrambling personal identifiers so that individuals are not identifiable, and adequate legal and physical security controls so that data is secure and access granted only to those with justified access (31).

4. INTERNET AND INFORMATICS

The Internet has made possible both rapid access to databases and the global transfer of information. Most of the data sources listed above, as well as most major scientific journals, are now accessible electronically and can be easily found through search engines. These databases may contain their own powerful search engines that facilitate ease of access. They also contain extensive links to other related sites.

Informatics is the discipline that studies the application of computer technology to the retrieval and analysis of health information. Informatics is likely to become a critical knowledge skill for healthcare workers, and linked computer databases and the Internet will likely become a central and indispensable part of the provision of health care in the 21st century. The CIHI and Statistics Canada are excellent sources for health data.

4.1.   ELECTRONIC HEALTH RECORD

There has been great interest in the personal electronic health record (EHR) and there are a number of joint federal and provincial initiatives (41). The EHR will collect personal health information such as visits to physicians, hospital stays, prescription drugs, laboratory tests, etc. In addition to facilitating the care process, it will be useful in quality control, research, and monitoring of the healthcare system. The issues of privacy, confidentiality, and protection of personal health information in the context of the EHR system are perhaps the most sensitive aspects and need to be addressed (42, 43). While it is the way of the future, a cautious and judicious approach is warranted.

5.   SUMMARY

This chapter dealt with health indicators and sources of health data. **Health indicators** are qualitative and quantitative measures that indicate the health of a population, and are examined on four dimensions, namely health status, non-medical determinants of health, health system performance, and community and health system characteristics.

Health status indicators include indicators of well-being, health conditions of human function and deaths.

Non-medical determinants are factors that are not actual health problems but are believed to be related to the development of disease. The determinants of health include the environment, health behaviour, living and working conditions, personal resources, and environmental factors. Health behaviours include lifestyle-related factors such as drinking and smoking. Living and working conditions include factors such as unemployment rate, education, poverty rate, child poverty rate, and decision latitude at work. Person resources include social support and life stress. With respect to the physical environment, Canadians may be exposed to toxic substances or other environmental hazards from a variety of sources, including food, water, air, soil, and consumer products.

The determinants of human biology include age and sex. Men, women, children, and the elderly have different potential for health and ill health. Another indicator is genetic inheritance.

Health system performance is monitored for different healthcare sectors including hospital care, physician services, and community services such as public health. To date, the main focus of performance monitoring is hospital care. The major categories of health system performance indicators are: acceptability, accessibility, appropriateness, competence, continuity, effectiveness, efficiency and safety.

Community and health system characteristics relate to the psychosocial environment and are commonly described using demographic indicators, such as the age and sex of the population and population growth rate. Indicators of the social environment also include sociodemographic variables (such as ethnicity, language, and family size) and socioeconomic variables (which include education level, literacy, unemployment rates, and income distribution).

There are several **data sources** in Canada. These consist of surveys, administrative data, registries, reports, vital statistics, consumption data, and record linkage. Surveys usually provide prevalence rates for risk factors, disease, disability, and utilization of health services, and can also be used to explore relationships among these factors. Recent surveys of interest include the Canada Community Health Survey, the National Population Health Survey, and the Canadian Heart Health Survey. The most uniformly recorded and reliable health data are administrative. Administrative and professional bodies demand this information for use in planning and evaluation of medical care, and it is more useful in studying health care than the distribution and cause of disease. Disease registries for certain chronic diseases also provide occurrence and prevalence data.

6.   REFERENCES

1.   Health Canada, Canadian Institute for Health Information, Statistics Canada. *Health information needs in Canada.* Ottawa: Canadian Institute for Health Information, 1998.
2.   Canadian Institute for Health Information. 1999. *National Consensus Conference on Population Health Indicators final report.* <secure.cihi.ca/cihiweb/products/phi.pdf> (January 2003).
3.   Roberge R, Berthelot J, Wolfson M. The health utility index: Measuring health differences in Ontario by socio-economic status. *Health Reports* 1995; 7(2):25-32.
4.   Canadian Institute for Health Information. 2002. *Health indicators 2000: Selected health indicators — definitions and data source and technical notes.* <secure.cihi.ca/cihiweb/dispPage.jsp?cw_page=indicators_online_definitions_e> (January 2003).
5.   Canadian Institute for Health Information. 2002. *Health indicators: Related products.* <secure.cihi.ca/indicators/en/related.shtml> (January 2003).
6.   Canadian Institute for Health Information. 2002. *Health indicators: Definitions and data sources.* <secure.cihi.ca/indicators/en/definitions.shtml> (January 2003).
7.   Last J. *A dictionary of epidemiology*, 3rd ed. New York: Oxford University Press, 1995.
8.   Manuel D, Schultz S. *Adding life to years and years to life: Life and health expectancy in Ontario.* Toronto: Institute for Clinical Evaluative Sciences, 2001.
9.   Patrick D, Bergner M. Measurement of health status in the 1990s. *Annual Review of Public Health* 1990; 11:165-83.
10. World Health Organization. 2002. *International classification of functioning, disability, and health.* <www.who.int/icidh> (January 2003).
11. Farmer MM, Ferraro KF. Distress and perceived health: Mechanisms of health decline. *Journal of Health and Social Behavior* 1997; 38(3):298-311.
12. Gold M, Franks P, Erickson P. The predictive validity of a preference-based measure and self-rated health. *Medical Care* 1996; 34(2):163-77.
13. Idler EL, Benyamini Y. Self-rated health and mortality: A review of twenty-seven community studies. *Journal of Health and Social Behavior* 1997; 38(1):21-37.
14. Markel H. The stigma of disease: Implications of genetic screening. *American Journal of Medicine* 1992; 93(2):209-15.
15. Statistics Canada. 2002. *Participation and Activity Limitation Survey: A profile of disability in Canada, 2001—Tables.* <www.statcan.ca/english/IPS/Data/89-579-XIE.htm> (January 2003).
16. Mathers CD, Robine J-M. Health expectancy indicators: A review of the work of REVES to date. In Mathers C, Robine J-M, editors. *Calculation of health expectancies: harmonization, consensus achieved and future perspectives.* London: John Libbey and Company Ltd.; 1993. p. 1-21.

17.   Hyder AA, Rotlant G, Morrow RH. Measuring the burden of disease: Healthy life-years. *American Journal of Public Health* 1998; 88(2):196-202.
18.   Murray CJ, Lopez AD. *The global burden of disease: a comprehensive assessment of mortality and disability from diseases, injuries, and risk factors in 1990 and projected to 2020.* Washington DC: Harvard School of Public Health on behalf of the World Health Organization and the World Bank, 1996.
19.   Quebec City Consensus Conference on Environmental Health Indicators. Selected papers. *Canadian Journal of Public Health* 2002; 93(Suppl 1):S1-S70.
20.   Kohn L, Corrigan J, Donaldson M, editors. *To err is human: Building a safer health system.* Washington DC: National Academy Press, 1999. <www.nap.edu/html/to_err_is_human> (February 2003).
21.   Robinson R. Economic evaluation and health care: What does it mean? *British Medical Journal* 1993; 1993(307):670-3.
22.   McGregor M. Cost-utility analysis: Use QALYs only with great caution. *Canadian Medical Association Journal* 2003; 168(4):433-4.
23.   Canadian Institute for Health Information. 2002. *CIHI profile.* Ottawa. <secure.cihi.ca/cihiweb/dispPage.jsp?cw_page=profile_e> (November 2002).
24.   Morrison HI, Schaubel D, Desmeules M, *et al.* Serum folate and risk of fatal coronary heart disease. *Journal of the American Medical Association* 1996; 275(24):1893-6.
25.   National Health Information Council. *Health information for Canada 1991: Report of the Task Force on Health Information.* Ottawa: Health and Welfare Canada, 1991.
26.   Tambay J, Catlin G. Sample design of the National Population Health Survey. *Health Reports* 1995; 7(1):29-39.
27.   Statistics Canada. 2002. *The Canadian Community Health Survey (CCHS): Extending the wealth of health data in Canada.* <www.statcan.ca/english/concepts/health/cchsinfo.htm> (January 2003).
28.   Kendall O, Lipskie T, MacEachern S. Canadian Health Surveys,1950-1997. *Chronic Diseases in Canada* 1997; 18(2):70-90.
29.   Manuel D. *Population-based health surveys: Measures and methods.* Toronto: Institute for Clinical Evaluative Sciences, 1999.
30.   Adams O, Ramsay T, Millar W. Overview of selected health surveys in Canada, 1985 to 1991. *Health Reports* 1992; 4(1):25-52.
31.   Canadian Institute for Health Information. *Health data sharing in Canada: A resource guide.* Ottawa: Canadian Institute for Health Information, 1995.
32.   Naylor CD, Anderson G, Goel V. *Patterns of health care in Ontario: The ICES practice atlas.* Ottawa: Canadian Medical Association, 1994.
33.   Goel V, Williams J, Anderson G. *Patterns of health care in Ontario: The ICES practice atlas.* Ottawa: Canadian Medical Association, 1996.
34.   Health Canada. 2002. *Network of health surveillance in Canada.* <www.hc-sc.gc.ca/pphb-dgspsp/csc-ccs/network_e.html> (November 2002).
35.   Health Canada. 2002. *Notifiable diseases on-line.* <cythera.ic.gc.ca/dsol/ndis/c_time_e.html> (January 2003).
36.   Association of Workers' Compensation Boards of Canada. 2003. *National work injuries statistics program statistics.* <www.awcbc.org> (January 2003).
37.   Health and Welfare Canada. Special diseases registries issue, Part B. *Chronic Disease in Canada* 1988; 9(4):66-76.
38.   Health and Welfare Canada. Special diseases registries issue, Part A. *Chronic Disease in Canada* 1988; 9(3):50-63.
39.   Myers K, Farquhar D. Improving the accuracy of death certification. *Canadian Medical Association Journal* 1998; 158(10):1317-23.
40.   Lindahl BI, Glattre E, Lahti R, *et al.* The WHO principles for registering causes of death: Suggestions for improvement. *Journal of Clinical Epidemiology* 1990; 43(5):467-74.

41.   Health Canada. 1998. *National Conference on Health Info-Structure: Final report.* <www.hc-sc.gc.ca/ohih-bsi/pubs/1998_nchis/nchis_e.html> (February 2003).

42.   Romanow R. *Building on values: The future of health care in Canada — final report.* Ottawa: Commission on the Future of Health Care in Canada, 2002.

43.   Kirby M, LeBreton M. *The health of Canadians — The federal role; Volume six: Recommendations for reform.* Standing Senate Committee on Social Affairs, Science and Technology, 2002. <www.parl.gc.ca/37/2/parlbus/commbus/senate/com-e/soci-e/rep-e/repoct02vol6-e.htm>.

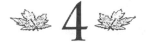

4

DETERMINANTS OF HEALTH AND DISEASE

The non-medical determinants and human biology described in this chapter have a profound direct or indirect effect on health of populations. This chapter describes Canadian demography and socioeconomic factors, as well as Canadians' lifestyle habits and preventive health practices. It includes many statistics in order to describe the characteristics of the population and to indicate the different aspects of their lifestyle and health behaviour that affect their health and utilization of the healthcare system. The next chapters describe the measurable outcomes of the interaction of these determinants of health. Chapters 7 and 8 deal in detail with the effects of these determinants on chronic and communicable diseases. The utilization of the healthcare system, which contributes significantly to health, is also discussed in Part III. Strategies for modifying many of these determinants either at the level of the individual or of society are discussed in Chapters 1, 7, and 11, using the concepts of disease prevention, health protection, health promotion, and healthy public policy.

1. HUMAN BIOLOGY

An individual's genetic make-up affects that person's health in many complex ways, many of which are poorly understood. Genes are generally thought to predispose an individual to certain health conditions, which may manifest themselves when the individual is exposed to certain socioeconomic or environmental factors (1). Within specific populations in Canada, the clustering of certain gene mutations can lead to an increased incidence of specific genetic disorders. For example, in Canadian (Old Colony) Mennonites, due to familial aggregations of autosomal recessive and dominant conditions, diseases that occur more frequently are insulin-dependent diabetes mellitus, autoimmune diseases, Tourette's syndrome, some malformations, inborn errors of metabolism, and other inherited disorders (1). In Quebec, there is a high prevalence of the gene for Tay-Sachs disease among the French Canadian population and a high incidence of sickle cell hemoglobinopathy (HbS) among the black population and those of Central American ancestry (2). Nova Scotia has an indigenous black population that is genetically predisposed to carrying or expressing the gene for sickle cell anemia. The genes for sickle cell anemia and Tay-Sachs are thought to be more prevalent in certain populations because of the protective advantage they may confer under certain environmental conditions. For example, in carriers, the sickle cell mutation may protect against malaria (1).

With the recent advances in molecular genetics, the genes for many inherited, developmental, and psychiatric disorders may eventually be identified. Such medical breakthroughs will raise controversial issues about family planning, disability insurance, confidentiality, and genetic stigmatization. Policies need to be developed to deal with these important ethical questions based on sound empirical research (3). Moreover, with the revolution currently underway in molecular biology, the identification of genetic variants responsible for many conditions that affect health will likely lead to important advances in drug treatment and possibly even to gene therapy (see Chapter 18) (4).

2.   THE DEMOGRAPHY OF CANADIAN POPULATION

Demography is the study of populations, especially with reference to size, density, fertility, mortality, growth, age distribution, migration, and vital statistics. Sociodemographic and socioeconomic indicators represent the interaction of these factors with social and economic conditions. On May 15, 2001, Canada's population was 30,007,095, of whom 49% were male. Of that total, 19.1%, 68.0%, and 12.9% were in the age groups 0 to 14 years, 15 to 64 years, and 65 years and over, respectively. Among those aged 65 and over, 58.1% of the population was female. The Canadian population is projected to be 32.2 million people in 2006; 49.5% will be male, and the population of people aged 65 and older will constitute 13.3% of the total population (see Figure 4.1). In 2001, there were a total of 11.5 million private households of which 8.4 million were families with children aged 24 and under or families without children at home; 70.5% of the families were married couples, 13.7% were common-law families, and 15.7% were lone-parent families. Almost 3 million were one-person households. The average household has 2.6 persons.

The distribution of the population by age and sex between 1901 and 2001 indicates that the population has more than doubled since 1941 (see Figure 4.1). The ratio of males to females has remained roughly constant, but there has been a definite change in the age distribution. In 1901, there were proportionately more children under age 14 compared with 1996, because of early age at marriage and large family size, as is the case in most developing countries. These factors are reflected in the **total fertility rate** (TFR), expressed as number of children a woman can expect to have in her lifetime based on the age-specific fertility rates of a given year. In 1941, compared with earlier years, there were proportionately fewer children under age 14. This was largely due to postponed childbirth during the Great Depression and World War II, which is reflected in low fertility rates during this period. In the late 1940s, the number of births increased during the postwar baby boom, and by 1961, there were proportionately more children under age 14. Generally, birth and fertility rates have

Figure 4.1.   Population Pyramids, 1901–2006

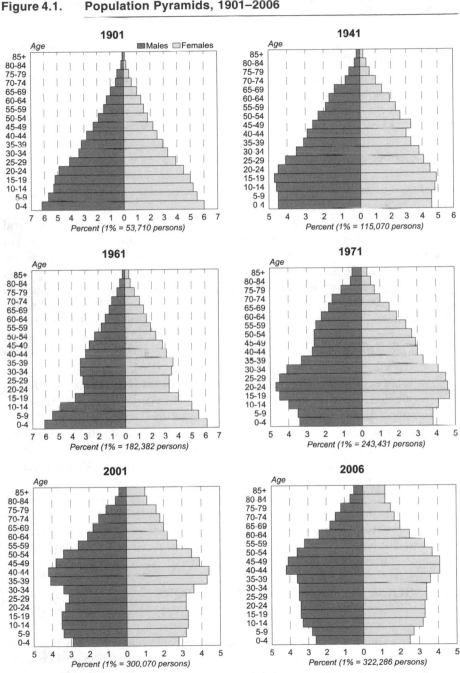

Source: Statistics Canada.

been declining since the baby boom, and the effect on the population's age distribution may be traced in Figure 4.1. Since 1974, the TFR has remained below the level of 2.1, which is the replacement level needed for maintenance of the population at a steady state (5). Total fertility rate for the year 1999 was 1.52 per woman. In Canada, fertility rates are falling for a number of reasons, including the tendency to delay starting families because of economic difficulties experienced by young households or growing fragility of conjugal relationships, increased participation of women in the workforce, increased level of education, more liberal abortion laws, and the availability of contraception. The proportion of children under age 14 decreased in 1971, and the proportion between ages 15 and 29 increased. The decrease in the proportion of young children in the population is reflected in the decreased demand for pediatricians and pediatric units in general hospitals. A temporary increase in this proportion was predicted to occur when the baby boomers grew up and produced families, but it has not happened.

Population growth is the sum of natural increase and net migration. **Natural increase** is the difference between the number of births and number of deaths. For example, for the period of 1991 to 2000, there were a total of 3,716,465 births and 2,088,188 deaths. Thus, the natural increase was 1,628,277 people. **Net migration** is the difference between immigration and emigration. Immigration has always been an important source of population growth in Canada. Between 1991 and 2000, the number of immigrants coming to the country was 2,196,252 whereas 366,081 people emigrated from Canada. Thus, the net migration was 1,830,171 persons. In essence, Canada's population increased by 3.45 million people between 1991 and 2000; the natural increase contributed 47.0% and net migration 53.0%.

Canada has experienced one of the world's smallest census-to-census growth rates in its population. From 1996 to 2001, the nation's population increased only 4.0%. Canada's population five-year growth from 1996 to 2001 was lower than that of United States (5.4%) and Australia (5.9%), but higher than that of Italy (0.4%), Germany (0.4%), Japan (1.3%), the United Kingdom (1.4), and France (1.9%). Only three provinces and one territory had growth rates above national average: Alberta (10.3%), Ontario (6.3%), British Columbia (4.9%), and Nunavut (8.1%).

Geographic distribution also affects the health status of a population. Approximately three quarters of the Canadian population live within 320 km of the border between Canada and the United States, and the remaining population is spread over a vast land mass. Historically, providing healthcare services to a widely dispersed population in northern Canada has been a challenge.

2.1.   SOCIODEMOGRAPHIC INDICATORS

Aging

One important demographic change with far-reaching implications is the rise in the proportion of the population over age 65. Canada's population will continue growing in the next quarter century, but it will age considerably and the proportion of young people will shrink significantly, according to new population projections (6).

An enormous increase in the number of seniors, attributable to the aging of the baby boomers combined with continuing low fertility levels and increasing longevity, will age the population rapidly. In the medium growth scenario, half the population will be over the age of 43.6 by 2026, up substantially from 36.8 in 2000. By 2051, the projected median age will be 46.2.

The baby boomers — those born in the two decades after World War II — will have the most profound impact on the nation's demographics over the next 25 years. In 2000, about one out of every eight people in the population was aged 65 and older. By 2026, one out of every five people will be a senior. By 2016 at the latest, Canada will have far more seniors than children aged 14 and under, a phenomenon never before recorded. Because older Canadians are far more likely than younger Canadians to have physical health problems, seniors have been found to account for a disproportionately larger percentage of patient days spent in general hospitals, allied special hospitals, and even mental hospitals (6). Thus, the growing proportion of seniors in our population will have significant implications for the planning of healthcare services. The health of the elderly is discussed in more detail in Chapter 6.

Immigrant Population

The composition of the Canadian population is changing in relation to ethnicity, and is expected to continue to change as immigrants migrate into Canada from diverse areas of the world. The impact of immigration policies has offset the decreasing Canadian fertility rate. The number of immigrants coming into Canada has been in the range of 200,000 to 225,000 in the last decade.

The 2001 census showed that Canada was home to 5.4 million immigrants, including the more then 2 million who had arrived between 1991 and 2001 (7). The total number of immigrants represented 18.4% of the population in 2001, the largest share since 1932. This share had remained at around 15% to 17% in the latter half of the twentieth century.

The sources of immigration to Canada have also changed greatly. Of those who immigrated in the 1990s, 58% were born in Asia, including the Middle East; 20% in Europe; 11% in the Caribbean, and Central and South America; 8% in Africa; and 3% in the United States. In 2001, European-born immigrants continued to account for the largest proportion (47%) of all immigrants living in Canada, but this figure has declined steadily since 1965. Immigrants born in Asia and the Middle East (31%) were the second largest component and the remainder (22%) were from other parts of the world. Seven of ten of the most frequently reported countries of birth for recent immigrants were the Asian countries of Hong Kong, China, India, the Philippines, Sri Lanka, and Taiwan.

The impact of recent immigration is most clearly seen in big cities. In 2001, Toronto had the largest immigrant population of all Canada's 25 census metropolitan areas, with 43.7% of its population being immigrants, followed by Vancouver (37.5%) and Hamilton (23.6%)

Ethnicity

Ethnic origin, as defined in the 2001 Census, refers to the ethnic or cultural group(s) to which the respondent's ancestors belong. An ancestor is someone from whom a person is descended, and is usually more distant than a grandparent. Ethnic origin pertains to the ancestral roots or background of the population, and should not be confused with citizenship or nationality (8). In 2001, the top 10 ethnic origins reported by Canadians were as follows: approximately 11.7 million (39.4%) people reported their ethnic origin as Canadian; 6.0 million (20.2%) English; 4.7 million (15.8%) French; 4.1 million (14.0%) Scottish; 3.8 million (12.9%) Irish; 2.7 million (9.3%) German; 1.3 million (4.3%) Italian; and approximately 1.0 million each Chinese (3.7%), Ukrainian (3.6%) and North American Indians (3.4%) (7). This number represents total responses to the question of ethnic origin; some respondents had reported more than one ethnic origin. Most people listed as Canadian were born in Canada and had English or French as their first language. This suggests that many of these respondents come from families that have been in Canada for several generations.

Visible Minorities

In the 2001 census, the definition of a visible minority was taken from the *Employment Equity Act:* "persons, other than Aboriginal peoples, who are non-Caucasian in race or non-white in colour." The regulations of the Act specify the following groups as visible minorities: Chinese, South Asians, blacks, Arabs, West Asians, Filipinos, Southeast Asians, Latin Americans, Japanese, Koreans, and Pacific Islanders.

In 2001, Canada was home to almost 4 million people who identified themselves as members of a visible minority (7). They represented 13.4% of the total population in Canada. This proportion has increased steadily over the past 20 years. In 1981, 1.1 million visible minorities accounted for 4.7% of the total population; by 1996, 3.2 million accounted for 11.2%. Three out of every 10 individuals who were visible minorities were born in Canada. A total of 1,029,400 or 3.5% of total population, identified themselves as Chinese in the 2001 census, constituting the largest visible minority population. The next largest groups were South Asians (917,100 or 3.1%) and blacks (662,200 or 2.2%). Together, Chinese, South Asians, and blacks represented two thirds of the visible minority population in Canada. In British Columbia, 22% of the population was a visible minority; in Ontario, the figure was 19%. Seven out every ten people who are members of a visible minority lived in metropolitan Toronto, Vancouver, or Montreal. Toronto was home to 1.7 million of the visible minority population in Canada, and 725,700 lived in Vancouver, representing 37% of the total population of each city; whereas 458,300 lived in Montreal, representing 14% of the total population of Montreal.

Language

Given the ethnic diversity described above, it is not surprising that in 2001, 5.3 million (18.0%) people reported a first language other than French or English. This is defined as the first language learned at home in childhood and still understood by the individual at the time of the census. The most common languages spoken at home were English (67.5%), French (22.0%), and non-official languages (10.5%) (neither French nor English). The non-official languages most frequently listed as a first language were Chinese, Italian, German, Punjabi, and Spanish.

Religion

In 1991, the majority of Canadians were Christians (Catholic, 45.7%, and Protestant, 36.3%) followed by Eastern Orthodox, (1.4%), Jewish (1.2%), Islam (0.9%), Hindu (0.6%), and Sikh (0.5%); 12.5% listed no religious affiliation. The remainder belonged to other religious faiths.

Family Environments

Over the past 20 years, it has been recognized that family abuse and violence affect the health of individual family members. There are three principal types of family violence: spousal violence or abuse, child abuse, and elder abuse (see also Chapter 7). Abuse is threatening or intolerable behaviour that may involve physical violence and threats.

3. SOCIOECONOMIC INDICATORS

Literacy and educational attainment, income, employment and working conditions, and other living conditions are important determinants of the health of a population. This section will describe how these determinants are distributed in the Canadian population.

Literacy and Educational Attainment

Educational attainment is positively associated with health and health behaviour. In the 1996–97 National Population Health Survey (NPHS), 30% of university graduates rated their health as excellent compared with 19% of those with less than a high school education (9). From 1951 to 2001, the levels of schooling continued to increase for all population groups in Canada. Education levels reported here are for aged 25 to 64 i.e., the working-aged population — people who are old enough to have completed their education, but still young enough to work.

Each year the Organization of Economic Cooperation and Development (OECD) conducts an international comparison of education levels in the working-age population of 30 countries. In 2000, Canada ranked fourth among OECD countries with 20% of its population aged 25 to 64 having university education; USA ranked first at 28%, Norway second at 26%, and the Netherlands third at 21%. According to Census 2001, the proportion of Canadians aged 25 and over who had university education was 20.2%; college education 16.0%; trade education 12.1%; 22.7% had completed high school; and 29% less than high school education (10). Canadians with a high school education or below represented more than one-half the working age population in only three provinces and a territory: New Brunswick (53%), Manitoba (51%), Newfoundland

and Labrador (51%) and Nunavut (58%). Between 1991 and 2001, the proportion of female aged 25 to 64 with trade, college or university education increased from 41% to 53%. In 1990s, the immigrants coming to Canada were better educated: 61% of immigrants of working age held trade, college or university credentials reflecting the change in Canadian immigration policy. The level of education attained by Aboriginal peoples aged 25-64 indicated that 38% had less than high school education, 23% had high school diploma, 16% with trade certificate, 15% with college diploma and 8% with the university degree. While educational levels are somewhat lower among Aboriginals than the rest of population, there is considerable improvement over the previous decades.

There are three types of literacy which the 1997 International Adult Literacy Survey explored: prose literacy, or the ability to read and comprehend a passage of text; document literacy, or the ability to complete standard forms such as job applications; and quantitative literacy (sometimes called numeracy), or basic computation skills. In 1994–95, about 17% of Canadians aged 16 to 65 were found to be at the lowest level of prose literacy and another 26% achieved the second lowest level, meaning that 43% of Canadians were able to read at or below the level of only simple material that does not contain complex instructions (9). These limitations may affect health directly in terms of the inappropriate use of medication, inability to communicate effectively with healthcare workers, or difficulty in following instructions including safety instructions at work (see Chapter 18).

The ability to access information for the purposes of maintaining or improving health has been termed "health literacy." Access to and use of information communication technology may have an impact on this (11). Information from the 2000 General Social Survey demonstrates that Canadians with less education and less household income use the Internet less (30%) than those who are more educated and have a greater household income (80%). There is also a difference in Internet use among rural dwellers (45%) versus urban dwellers (55%) and in non-English speaking users (40%) versus English speaking users (59%).

Income

Income is another major socioeconomic indicator. According to the Census 2001, average earnings among the more than 16.4 million people aged 15 and over who had an employment income in 2000 amounted to $31,757, up from $29,596 in 1990 and $29,229 in 1980 (12). Of the total 16.4 million people, slightly fewer than 447,000 (2.7%) individuals earned more than $100,000; and an estimated 6.7 million (41.0%) earned less than $20,000. Higher education was associated with higher income. Recent immigrants earn substantially less than their Canadian-born counterparts even after 10 years in the country. This is true for both those immigrants with low levels of education, as well as those with a university degree.

Statistics Canada has determined low-income cut-off (LICO) points based on a survey of family expenditures. A family that spends more than 54.7% of income on the basic needs of accommodation, food, and clothing is considered to live under strained circumstances and thus falls below the LICO. These levels are adjusted for family size and location. Because there is no accepted definition of poverty, the LICO is used by many to study the characteristics of relatively deprived groups in Canada (9). The average family income in Canada in 1998 was $49,626 (12). This was down from $56,629 in 1996, and represents a lower average than the average family incomes seen since 1978 (9). In 2000, there were 1.1 million Canadian children living in poverty in Canada (13). Certain groups of children are more affected by poverty than others: single-parent families, particularly those headed by a female, Aboriginal children, visible minority children, and children of immigrants and refugees.

Welfare recipients are those who cannot adequately meet their own needs or those of their dependents because of their inability to find work, or because of the loss of a spouse who is the main support of the family, or because of illness, disability, or other reasons. Welfare payments typically fall substantially below the previously described LICOs set by Statistics Canada (14). As of March 2001, there were 1.9 million recipients of social assistance. These included adults who were actual recipients and children living in those households.

Low-income Canadians are more likely to die earlier and to suffer more illnesses than Canadians with higher incomes, regardless of age, sex, race, and place of residence. Even though the gap is narrowing from 1971 to 1996, at each rung up the income ladder, Canadians have less sickness, longer life expectancies, and improved health (15). The effects of poverty on health of children are described in detail in Chapter 6.

Employment and Working Conditions

The social environment includes the working environment. The significance of safety in the work environment is illustrated by the fact that in Canada there are hundreds of work-related fatalities every year (882 in 2000 alone) (16). The number and characteristics of work-related health problems are changing as working environments change. Since World War II, the labour force has shifted gradually from goods-producing jobs in manufacturing, construction, and primary industries to less physically hazardous service-producing jobs, for example in financial, amusement, and business services. Thus the nature of the hazards has changed from those that are physical to those that are psychosocial. The increased participation of women in the work force, generally in the service sector, has led to new concerns about the safety of the working environment for the pregnant mother and fetus. The effect of the physical working environment on health is described in Chapter 10.

Labour markets have also changed dramatically in the last decade due in part to a response to globalization, trade competition, and technological innovation. Many workers in advanced economies now face limited employment prospects and poor working conditions (17). Adverse labour conditions are related to either the availability of work (e.g., unemployment, job insecurity, and overwork) or to the nature of work (e.g., increasing job demands, low job position within a firm, and contingent employment). Unemployment rates in Canada increased from 7.4% in 1981 to over 11.0% in early 1990s, then fell to 7.4% in January 2003. There has recently been a shift to longer standard working hours in some provinces, including Ontario.

Globally, there has been a move toward lean production models (input of fewer resources to do the same job) leading to job strain (18).

All these changes can have profound health consequences. For example, unemployed adults have been found to have gains of over 10% in body mass index (BMI), earlier deaths, and other health problems compared to employed adults (19-21). Two sources of work stress are job strain (a combination of high job demands and low job control) and effort-reward imbalance (the imbalance between the effort put into a job and the rewards of a job in terms of pay, status, recognition, and job security), which have both been found to be associated with diseases such as coronary heart disease and hypertension (see Chapter 1).

The Interaction of Multiple Socioeconomic Conditions

There is a large income penalty for Canadians with low literacy scores. In 1994, among Canadians with the lowest levels of prose literacy, 47% lived in low-income households, compared with 8% of Canadians with the highest levels of prose literacy. Unemployed people were three times more likely than employed people to have a Level 1 category literacy level, and those with higher literacy skills were employed for more weeks of the year than those with low literacy skills (9).

Homelessness

The causes of homelessness are complex. They include poverty, changes in the housing market, reductions in social assistance, family violence, substance abuse, and changing mental health services. As a result, the composition of this group now includes increasing numbers of women and children and other groups in special circumstances, such as adolescents, individuals with mental illness, and Aboriginal people.

Although homeless men and women do not have illnesses that differ from the general population, homelessness is associated with increased health risks. In a Toronto study, mortality rates among men in shelters were higher from 1995 to 1997 than those in the general population(22, 23). There is also evidence that homelessness may add to poor health by posing barriers to the management of health conditions such as diabetes (24). Additionally, many homeless persons are ex-patients of mental health institutions, runaway teenagers, women and children escaping from domestic violence, seniors, alcoholics, and Aboriginal peoples. Estimates for the number of homeless vary because it is difficult to count them; however, the various estimates put the number in the range of 130,000 to 250,000 (25).

Other Living Conditions

Living alone may be associated with social isolation and possibly with lower socioeconomic status and a higher incidence of suicide. In 2001 in Canada, about 3 million individuals (12.1% of the population aged 15 and over) lived alone. Seniors are more likely to live alone: 35% of women and 16% of men in age group 65 and over lived alone The extended survival of senior women and the breakdown of families are major contributing causes.

Stress

Chronic stress has a significant impact on the health of Canadians, and how it affects health was described in Chapter 1. In the 1994–95 Population Health Survey, one in four (26%) Canadians reported experiencing high chronic stress, the remaining equally divided between moderate stress (38%) and low stress (36%). Women are more likely than men to report high stress (29% versus 23% respectively) (26). This is true for all ages except the youngest (age 18–19). The least educated group is more than twice as likely as university graduates to report high stress (31% versus 14% respectively). Men and women between the ages of 35 and 44 reported the highest rates of stress. It is also worth noting that stress is particularly predominant among working parents (75%) and that as stress increases, so too does the rate of family dysfunction (27). Smoking is related to stress: in 1994, 46% of men who reported high levels of chronic stress smoked, compared to 27% of men who experienced low levels of stress. The association is even more pronounced in women, ranging from 45% for those with high stress levels to 21% among women with low stress levels (see Chapter 7).

Clearly, demographic and socioeconomic determinants and chronic stress strongly affect the overall health status of the population, particularly health problems concentrated in certain gender, age, ethnic, or income subgroups (see Chapter 7). It follows then that these determinants in the psychosocial environment are essential considerations for the effective planning of health care and of improvements in health status.

4.   THE PHYSICAL ENVIRONMENT

The physical environment includes physical, biological, chemical, and radiological factors found in food, water, soil, indoor and outdoor air, the built environment, and animal and insect vectors. It is described in detail in Chapter 9. Research carried out in 1993 revealed that most Canadians believed that levels of environmental contaminants were unacceptable and posed a risk to their health (28). Public interest in and knowledge of environmental issues generally has increased over the last 50 years, and concomitantly so has public support for more extensive and strict control of environmental agents. In recent years, the emphasis on chemical and radiological contaminants has changed from mere protection against substances that cause cancer or structural defects to attention to chemicals that can disrupt reproductive, developmental, neurobehavioural, immune system, endocrine, and metabolic processes (28).

Although the negative impact of the environment on health has been widely publicized, the positive impact of the environment must not be forgotten; the environment can have beneficial effects on health, such as the protection of 38% of Canadians against dental caries by fluoridation of municipal drinking water supplies. It should be noted that not all municipal drinking water is fluoridated, since communities decide whether or not to do so. Information on specific physical environmental contaminants is presented in Chapter 9, which deals with environmental health.

Agricultural Exposure

At least 2 million Canadians are involved in activities related to agriculture or livestock on family farms. There are concerns about health and safety issues in modern, competitive agriculture, which depends heavily on mechanization and the use of pesticides, herbicides, fertilizers, fungicides, and efficient feeding techniques (29). Recent widely publicized concerns include the use of genetic technology to produce genetically modified food crops; the widespread use of antibiotics as growth factors in animal agriculture; the suspected relationship of a new variant of Creutzfeld-Jacob disease (CJD) in humans to bovine spongiform encephalophathy (BSE) in beef-industry cows fed animal-containing products; the fecal contamination of drinking water supplies by run-offs from nearby farms; and the adequacy of drinking water regulations and legislation in safeguarding the drinking water supply.

Occupational hazards also exist for those working within agricultural industries. Grain workers and swine and poultry producers are at significant risk for respiratory disorders as a result of intensive feeding techniques and of confinement of poultry. Disabling injuries from accidents also occur. Finally, there is continued concern and research on the links between occupational exposures to different chemicals and neurodegenerative disease, respiratory disease, and cancer (see Chapter 10).

Outdoor Air Quality

Over the past 20 years, Canada has made significant gains in improving outdoor air quality. There has been a decline in the concentration of hazardous air pollutants such as sulphur dioxide, nitrogen dioxide, lead, dust, and smoke. Ground-level ozone (ozone within 11 km of the Earth's surface) creates smog and is one of the most serious air pollution problems in Canadian cities, with significant associations to both respiratory hospital admissions and respiratory mortality. However, the ozone layer (located 11 to 47 km above the Earth's surface in the stratosphere) acts as a barrier to ultraviolet B radiation. The discovery of the depletion of this ozone layer has led to concerns about the increased risks of skin cancer. There has also been concern about global warming, a phenomenon of rising temperatures on Earth that are thought to result from increases in the concentrations of certain greenhouse gases, which is described in detail in Chapter 9.

5.   LIFESTYLE AND BEHAVIOURAL RISK FACTORS

The Lalonde report (see Chapter 1) placed great emphasis on lifestyle elements and the personal behaviour of Canadians as a major factor in determining their health. Emphasis continues to be placed on modifying these risk factors in disease prevention and health promotion, although there is increasing recognition that the social and economic environment in which individuals live and work affects their ability and motivation to change their behaviour and lifestyle. In Canada today, the most common causes of mortality, potential years of life lost (PYLL), hospitalizations, and disability are cardiovascular diseases, cancer, and behaviour- and lifestyle-related injuries (9, 30, 31). The impacts of lifestyle and behavioural risk factors on chronic diseases, injuries, and communicable diseases and their prevention are described in Chapters 1, 7, 8, and 11.

5.1. SUBSTANCE ABUSE

Substance abuse can occur with both controlled (i.e., use is legal under certain circumstances) and uncontrolled (i.e., illegal) substances. For controlled substances, substance abuse is defined as any use in a non-prescribed manner (e.g., non-prescribed use of prescription or other medications, alcohol use by minors). For uncontrolled substances and for the legal use of non-medication controlled substances (e.g., alcohol use by adults), substance use is distinguished from abuse; **substance abuse** is defined as continued use despite recurrent, adverse consequences. Drug dependence has been defined as "a state of psychic or physical dependence, or both, on a drug, arising in a person following administration of that drug on a periodic or continuous basis" (27).

This section will focus on the use of alcohol, tobacco, and illicit drugs. The health effects of excessive use of alcohol and tobacco are described in detail in Chapter 7.

Tobacco

In 2001, 5.4 million or 22% Canadians 15 years and over were smokers — 20% were women and 24% men. This represented the lowest overall level since regular monitoring of smoking began in 1965 (32). For the first time in a decade, smoking prevalence in Quebec was not ranked highest in the country. British Columbia reported the lowest prevalence for current smokers 15 years and older, at 17%; Manitoba, Prince Edward Island, and Newfoundland and Labrador reported the highest prevalence at 26% (32).

In 2001, young adults aged 20 to 24 still had the highest smoking rate of any age group, at 32%. The smoking rate for age group 20 to 24 year for males was 35% and for females 29%. Over the last 15-year period, current smoking prevalence of Canadians aged 45 to 64 dropped from 30% to 20%. However, of the 5.5 million adult daily smokers in the NPHS in 1994–95, 86% still smoked daily in 1996–97. Sex differences were not as apparent after age 45. In the 65–74 age group, 16% of men and 14% of women smoked (33).

There was a significant and large increase in smoking prevalence for 15- to 19-year olds between 1991 and 1994. Since 1994, there has been no significant change in current smoking prevalence of youth (34). The rate of smoking among girls 12 to 14 is 10% compared with 6% in boys the same age (35). The 1998–99 NPHS reported that 25% of females aged 15 to 19 smoked daily compared with 18% of males of the same age.

The First Nations and Inuit Regional Health Surveys (1997) documented that Aboriginal peoples report the highest rates of smoking in Canada, at 62% among the First Nations and 72% among the Inuit. This is almost three times the rate of the Canadian population as a whole. The average age for smoking uptake is also younger (at 10 years) for these populations.

Smoking is closely related to unemployment, income, and education. Smoking rates are twice as high among those who did not complete secondary school as among those who completed university (32.7% versus 15.0%). Smoking rates increase as income decreases — 42% of those in the lowest income group currently smoke, compared with 20% in the highest income group. The unemployed have the highest rate of smoking (46%) (36).

The percentage of ex-smokers continues to grow. In 2001, 24% of the population 15 and older, or about 5.9 million people, reported that they had quit. Smokers find it difficult to quit. Of those who have quit, 54% said it took them one attempt, another 27% took two to three attempts, and 19% took more than four attempts. Most people who quit (82%) claimed that they used their will power only, 8% used nicotine patch, 4% used nicotine gum, 4% reduced daily consumption as a strategy, and 3% used the drug bupropion to help them quit (32).

Alcohol

Liquor authorities, wineries, and breweries sold 2.5 billion litres of alcoholic beverages in 1998–99, up 2.6% from the previous year (37). Beer accounted for the vast majority of sales, 83%, while wine accounted for 11% and spirits 6%. The value of spirits, wine, and beer sales amounted to $12.4 billion in 1998–99, up 5.6% from the previous year. Beer accounted for 53% of this total. Sales of alcoholic beverages by volume should not be equated with data on consumption, because consumption of alcoholic beverages also includes homemade wine and beer, wine and beer manufactured by brew-on-premise operations, and all sales to Canadian residents in duty-free shops.

Per capita sales of alcoholic beverages for people aged 15 and over have decreased from 134 litres in 1976 to 102.6 litres in 1998–99 (37). In 1998–99, each person 15 or older bought an average 6.1 litres of spirits, 11.2 litres of wine, and 85.3 litres of beer. There were noticeable regional differences in sales of the three types of alcoholic beverages. Quebec consumers bought 41% of all the red wine sold in Canada, which represented 7.2 litres per person. Quebec consumers also recorded the highest per-capita sales of white wine, 5.8 litres. Yukon has the highest per-capita sales for domestic beer at 140.7 litres and for spirits at 12.8 litres.

Approximately three of every four Canadians aged 15 or older consumes alcoholic beverages. From the 1998–99 NPHS, about one third of Canadians aged 18 or older consume alcohol at least once a week (33). Men are almost twice as likely as women to consume alcohol weekly. The proportion of people consuming alcohol rises with household income, perhaps reflecting differences in disposable income. People in the highest income group (44%) were more than twice as likely as those at the lowest level (21%) to consume alcohol weekly. However, the level of alcohol consumption among the unemployed is 58% higher than the overall average (36). Overall levels of drinking and rates of heavy drinking are also associated with social isolation and low employment status. Those who have never been married report 24% higher consumption levels than married Canadians.

In 1998–99, 55% of Canadians over age 12 are regular drinkers (someone who consumes one or more drinks per month), 21% drink occasionally, 13% are former drinkers, and 12% of Canadians abstain from alcohol (33). The number of drinks consumed by drinkers aged 12 and over in the week preceding the survey was as follows: fewer than one drink for 27% of drinkers, 1 to 6 drinks for 44%, 7 to 13 drinks for 18%, 14 or more drinks for 18%.

Drinking five or more drinks on one occasion is considered to be heavy drinking; drinking heavily at least 12 times in the previous 12 months is considered regular heavy drinking. In 1998–99, 29% of males who were current drinkers drank heavily in the previous year, compared with 10% of females; 20% of current drinkers were engaged in regular heavy drinking. Regular heavy drinking is most prevalent among young Canadian drinkers and less so with successive age groups. In 1998–99, 33% of drinkers aged 15 to 19 were regular heavy drinkers, as were 38% of drinkers aged 20 to 24 and 23% of drinkers aged 25 to 34, as well as 6% of drinkers aged 65 to 74. Men were more likely to be regular heavy drinkers than women.

An ongoing survey of drug use among adolescents in Ontario found that between 1993 and 1999 the proportion of students reporting use of alcohol increased significantly from 56.5% to 65.7%. The burden of illness due to abuse of alcohol is described in Chapter 7.

Drugs

Although rates of heroin and cocaine use are lower in Canada than in the U.S., many Canadians use illicit drugs and Canada ranks among the countries with the highest rates of illicit drug use (36). In 1994, approximately one in four Canadians (24%) reported the use of an illicit drug at least once in their lifetime. Cannabis is the most widely used illicit drug on a lifetime basis: 23% of Canadians (representing 97% of illicit drug users) reported using cannabis more than once during their lifetime. The proportion reporting the use of LSD, speed, or heroin at least once in their lives is 5.9%, and 3.8% of Canadians reported using cocaine at some point in their lives.

Injection drug use is of great concern because it is a major risk factor for infection with HIV, hepatitis B and C, and other blood-borne diseases (see Chapter 8). Approximately one fifth of recent AIDS cases are attributable to injection drug use (36). Studies have consistently shown higher rates of illicit drug use among Native Canadians and street youth (38, 39). There is no clear pattern regarding the relationship of illicit drug use to income and to education, but illicit drug use is somewhat more common among the unemployed. One distinct characteristic of illicit drug users is that they tend to have a lower degree of social integration — that is, they tend to be more socially isolated and have less investment in social values (36).

According to the Ontario Student Drug Survey, the longest ongoing study of adolescent drug use in Canada, there was a resurgence in adolescent drug use in the 1990s, after a lengthy period of decline during the previous decade. Since 1993, the following have increased steadily in the 1997–99 cycle of the survey: alcohol use (56.5% to 65.7%), heavy drinking episodes (17.7% to 28.2%), cigarette use (23.8% to 28.3%), cannabis use (12.7% to 29.2%), Ecstasy use (0.6% to 4.8%), use of hallucinogens (from 3.1% to 13.6%), and cocaine use (1.5% to 4.1%). Ontario's high school students are also using a greater number of different drugs: 17.4% use four or more drugs, up from 8% in 1993. Conversely, the number of students choosing to remain drug free has dropped from 36.3% to 26.8% (40). Correlating with this increase in drug use is a weakening in the perceptions of risk of harm in drug use, a decrease in moral disapproval of drug use, and an increase in the perceived availability of drugs. About one third of students in 1999 reported exposure to drug selling in their neighbourhood during the 12 months before the survey. Nova Scotia and New Brunswick are also experiencing a trend toward increased use of other illicit drugs. Between 1991 and 1996, cannabis use among students nearly doubled.

Problem Gambling

Legalized gambling increased dramatically in Canada in the 1990s primarily because of the government's desire to increase revenue without additional taxation. Across Canada, there are now more than 50 permanent casinos, 21,000 slot machines, 38,000 video lottery terminals, 20,000 annual bingo events, and 44 permanent race tracks (41). In 2001, Canadians wagered $10.7 billion on some form of government-run gambling activity, four times the amount in 1992. On average, every individual aged 18 and over in Canada spent $424 gambling in 2000, compared with $130 in 1992 (42).

Problem gambling is defined as "a progressive disorder characterized by a continuous or periodic loss of control over gambling; a preoccupation with gambling and with obtaining money with which to gamble; irrational thinking; and a continuation of the behaviour despite adverse consequences" (43). The Canadian Problem Gambling Index is a new survey instrument that places an emphasis on measuring the social impacts of gambling on family, co-workers, and the community at large (44). The cost to families can be great in terms of dysfunctional relationships, violence and abuse, financial pressure, and disruption of growth and development of children.

The estimated lifetime prevalence in the general adult population for problem and pathological gambling combined was reported to be 5.5%. A similar combined prevalence estimate for the adolescent study population was 13.3%. There were no significant differences in prevalence rates between the United States and Canada. Male, youth, Aboriginal ethnic origin, and concurrent substance abuse or mental illness placed people at greater risk of a gambling-related problem (42, 45). In general, participation in gambling rates increase with household income. Bingo is the only gambling activity studied for which there was an inverse correlation with income. High-income households spent more than low-income households on gaming activities other than bingo. However, lower income households spent proportionately more than high income households. Given that gambling revenue goes to the government, this statistic suggests that gambling expenditures may be regarded as a voluntary regressive tax that has proportionately greater impact on people with lower incomes.

5.2.   DIET AND NUTRITION

Food Consumption

Good nutrition is vital to maintaining good health, preventing disease, and reducing the severity of disease all throughout the life cycle. Canada's Food Guide to Healthy Eating recommends the following number of servings per day for the four main food groups: 5 to 12 servings of grain products, 5 to 10 of fruits and vegetables, 2 to 4 of milk products, and 2 to 3 of meat and alternatives (46). The impact of nutrition on health is discussed in Chapter 7.

Food consumption data represents food that is available for consumption (and therefore consumption trends and patterns) but not actual quantities of food consumed in Canada since they do not allow for losses in stores, households, private institutions or restaurants (47, 48). According to 1999–2000 figures on per-capita food consumption, Canadians are eating more fruits and vegetables. Each Canadian had available for consumption just over 124 kg of fruit in 1999, up from 111 kg 10 years ago. Canadians prefer fresh fruit, with bananas, apples, and oranges topping the list. Tropical fruits such as mangoes, kiwis, and papayas have become increasingly popular. Consumption of fresh vegetables (excluding potatoes) in 1999 was 69.5 kg per person, up more than 7% from 1990. Lettuce, carrots, onions, tomatoes, and cabbage have remained popular choices. Consumers also appear to be eating more pasta, specialty and multi-grain breads, and cereal-based snacks. Consumption of cereal products increased to almost 89 kg per person in 2000, up from 74 kg in 1990. The figures in 2000 show that lower fat milk (1% and skim) is being consumed at twice the level of the early 1990s. While the consumption of beef and other red meat is decreasing, beef consumption still represents almost 50% of all red meat consumed. Consumption of pork and chicken, however, is increasing slowly. Fish consumption is up to 10 kg per person, up from 9 kg in 1990. Despite an increase in fruits, vegetables, lean meats, and fish, each Canadian consumes just over 45% more oils and fats than at the beginning of the 1990s. Much of this growth can be attributed to the increasing use of canola, soybean, olive, and other specialty oils for use by households and food service outlets in salad dressings, deep-fried products, and commercially prepared baked goods.

A national survey of adult Canadians was undertaken in 1997–98 to monitor changes in dietary intake, since the previous dietary survey in 1970 showed that the mean dietary percentage of energy derived from protein was 16–18%; from carbohydrate it was 50–56% and from fat it was 29–31%. These are close to recommended levels for different age-sex groups. Fat intake and total calories consumed were down from the previous survey. However, the intakes of dairy products and fruits and vegetables were still lower than recommended levels (49).

The 2001 Tracking Nutrition Trends Survey found that Canadians' interest in nutrition is strikingly divided along gender lines. Men's level of concern about nutrition has waned considerably since 1994, while women's interest in nutrition has remained high: 59% of women consider nutrition to be extremely or very important, compared with less than half (47%) of men. Men are also less likely to rate their eating habits as excellent or very good or to consider themselves knowledgeable about nutrition (50). Congruent with this survey, the 2000–2001 Canadian Community Health Survey (CCHS) found that women consume fruits and vegetables more often than men (51).

Low-income Canadians were more likely to express concerns about the cost of low-fat foods than were high-income Canadians. Among Canadians in the lowest bracket, 40% stated that low-fat products were expensive, compared with 32% of Canadians with the highest incomes; 20% of low-income Canadians stated that grain products were expensive, compared with only 8% of Canadians with high incomes (9). There is evidence that a healthy and nutritious diet may not be affordable to those with low incomes. A Toronto study showed that welfare payment would not allow those on it to afford the costs required to regularly purchase and consume a healthy and nutritious diet (14).

According to the 2000–2001 CCHS, there appeared to be a clustering of health risk factors in both men and women. Those who consumed fruits and vegetables more frequently were also more physically active, less likely to smoke, and less likely to be overweight (51).

Folic Acid

A woman's folic acid intake before conception and during early pregnancy plays an important role in the prevention of neural tube defects and other congenital abnormalities (see Chapter 7). Some evidence also exists that folic acid may reduce the risk of cardiovascular disease and the risks of some cancers. It has been recommended that all women of childbearing age take a daily supplement of folic acid since 50% of pregnancies in North America are unplanned or ill timed, and it is doubtful that even an optimal non-fortified diet can provide adequate folic acid (0.4 mg) to reduce the risk of birth defects (52, 53). A recent study done in women attending a genetics clinic at an Ottawa pediatric hospital showed that while 81% of the women were aware of folic acid and 78% were taking 0.4 mg per day of the vitamin, only 26% had begun the supplementation early enough to reduce the risk of neural tube defects (52).

Food Insecurity

The vast majority of Canadians are food secure— that is, they had access to enough food at all times for an active healthy life; however, some groups of people may be more at risk to food insecurity than others, as shown in a number of studies on food bank use, poverty, and dietary intake. Poverty is one of several factors that impede access to sufficient, safe, and nutritious foods. There are vulnerable people with low incomes who cannot meet their food requirements without compromising other basic needs, such as shelter. Groups most likely to be affected by low incomes in Canada include Aboriginal people, single mothers and their children, people with disabilities, recent immigrants, and those who have not completed high school (54).

One Toronto study that assessed the affordability of a nutritious diet for Toronto households supported by welfare compared welfare incomes to the monthly costs for food, shelter, and other essential expenditures, and indicated that average monthly incomes were insufficient to cover expenses for the families considered in the study. Therefore, discrepancies between welfare incomes and costs of basic needs may explain the vulnerability of welfare recipients to hunger and food insecurity (14).

In 1981, Canadian charities began setting up food banks as a temporary measure to help people deal with emergencies. From 1989 to 1997, the use of food banks in Canada doubled. The pressure on food banks to deliver other kinds of social services has also increased well beyond their capacity to deal with it. Other services, run mainly by civil society organizations, occasionally with support from provincial/ territorial or municipal governments, include community kitchens and gardens, food-buying clubs, and school-based breakfast and lunch programs. These services were also never intended to be long-term solutions, and food banks and other community-based initiatives are now looking to the larger environment for answers (55).

A recent study investigating the food security and nutritional vulnerability of women with children using food banks found that the household incomes of 90% of the women participating in the study, were less than two thirds of Statistics Canada's LICO (56). More than 93% of respondents reported some degree of food insecurity over the previous year, despite their efforts to supplement their food supplies by occasional use of food banks or to increase their disposable income by discontinuing telephone services or delaying bill payments. In addition to their own hunger, more than 25% of the women also reported that their children had gone hungry during the previous month. Furthermore, a significant proportion of the women appeared to have low dietary intakes of iron, magnesium, vitamin A, or folate (57).

Genetically Modified Foods

Rapid growth in the field of genetic engineering, specifically in the development of genetically modified foods, has been the source of a highly contentious debate in the past few years. Genetic engineering began in 1983 with a tobacco plant that was given transgenic characteristics, which made it resistant to an antibiotic. Canada has given approval to 42 genetically modified products including crops such as canola, soy, corn, tomatoes, and potatoes. Plants are only one of five categories of agricultural products derived from biotechnology. Livestock, livestock feeds, fertilizers, and veterinary biologics are also being tested and used throughout the world. Canada is responsible for 10% of the world's genetically modified cropland (compared to the U.S., which is responsible for 75%) and by 2010 worldwide revenues from genetically modified crops are expected to top $25 billion (58).

The risks posed by genetically modified foods include herbicide resistance, causing "superweed"; insecticide resistance — crops with this trait may harm beneficial insects such as the caterpillar of the Monarch butterfly; allergen transfer — the transfer of genetic materials from allergenic materials such as nuts may also transfer the threat to sensitive individuals; antibiotic resistance; and impact on farmers in the developing world, because seeds are available only from multinational corporations. The benefits of genetically modified food include increased food availability, lower food prices, improved nutritional value and other nutritional enhancements (such as the potential to reduce allergenicity, fats, etc.), drought resistance, and reduced need for herbicides and pesticides. No long-term studies are yet available on the impact of genetically modified foods on health.

5.3.   PHYSICAL ACTIVITY AND FITNESS

Physical activity is important for health and well-being. Canada's Physical Activity Guide to Healthy Active Living recommends that Canadians engage in endurance activities four to seven days per week, flexibility activities four to seven days per week, and strength activities two to four days per week (59). More generally, the guide recommends an hour of low-intensity activity every day or 30 to 60 minutes of moderate-intensity activity or 20 to 30 minutes of vigorous intensity activity four to seven days a week.

In 2000–01, 21% of Canadians in the household population aged 12 or older engaged in vigorous physical activity during their leisure time; another 21.6% were moderately active, 49.1% were inactive, and 8.9% did not state their activity level (60). In general, males are more likely than females to engage in vigorous activity. The top five leisure time physical activities for the Canadian population aged 12 and older in 1998–99 were walking, home exercise, gardening, swimming, bicycling, and weight training. Leisure-time physical activity varied with age. Canadians most likely to engage in daily exercise in their leisure time are men and women aged 12 to 19. Daily physical activity decreases for each age group thereafter. Activity levels also varied with income. People in the highest household income group were most likely to be vigorously active.

Leisure-time accounts for only part of an individual's total energy output. Paid work or household chores can also be physically demanding. However, almost a quarter of people aged 12 or older reported that "sitting" best described their usual daily non-leisure activity.

5.4.   BODY MASS INDEX AND OBESITY

The most important factors in maintaining the optimum body weight are dietary practices and active living, with other factors such as genetics and household income playing a role.. The body mass index (BMI) is commonly used to determine if an individual is in a healthy weight range (see Chapter 3). The Canadian standards for BMI are under 20 (underweight), 20 to 24.9 (acceptable weight), 25.0 to 27 (some excess weight), and higher than 27 (overweight). In the 2000–01 CCHS among those 20 to 64 years of age, 8.1% were underweight, 42.9% were an acceptable weight, 15.6% had some excess weight, 31.9% were overweight, and 1.6% did not indicate their weight (60). Since 1985, the proportion of the Canadian population in that age group who are definitely overweight (BMI greater than 27) has increased steadily for both men and women.

An analysis of BMI in relation to household income revealed that a significantly higher proportion of men than women were overweight or obese at all income levels (9). The proportion of women who were overweight fell as household income level increased; however, the opposite was true for men. Therefore, the male-female gap among those who were overweight was greatest in the highest income group (61).

Although BMI is not the best indicator for determining healthy body weight for children, trends indicate that progressively more Canadian children aged 7 to 13 years are overweight and obese. The prevalence of overweight boys has increased from 15% in 1981 to 29% in 1996 and among girls from 15% to 24%. Childhood obesity among Canadian children nearly doubled between 1981 and 1996: in 1981, 5% of boys and girls were obese; in 1996, 13.8% of boys and 11.8% of girls were obese (61). Health Canada has published guidelines for children and youth to increase activity levels (62).

Obesity is a risk factor for multiple health problems including type 2 diabetes and cardiovascular diseases. Adult diet and obesity together have been estimated to account for 30% of cancer deaths (30). NPHS data demonstrate a link between the onset of numerous diseases in Canadians and being overweight or obese. Even when age, education, household income, smoking, alcohol consumption, physical activity level, and personal stress were taken into account, men who classified as overweight or obese in 1994–95 had 1.6 times the odds of being diagnosed with arthritis sometime in the next four years, compared with men in the acceptable weight range. In comparison with women of acceptable weight, those who were overweight or obese had approximately 5.2 times the odds of being diagnosed with diabetes (33).

In Canada, fat and total energy intake has decreased over the last three decades. It is widely believed that energy expenditure has decreased substantially in the last three decades due to physical inactivity, and that the latter is responsible for the increase in obesity (49).

5.5. PLASMA LIPIDS AND LIPOPROTEINS

Abnormally elevated cholesterol, low density lipoproteins (LDL) and triglycerides, and low levels of high density lipoproteins (HDL) are important risk factors for the development of vascular disease, particularly for coronary artery disease (31). At the population level, there is a strong relationship between habitual diet, blood cholesterol levels, and the incidence of coronary heart disease. Serum total and LDL cholesterol levels increase as consumption of saturated fatty acids and dietary cholesterol increases. However, consumption of polyunsaturated fatty acids appears to lower serum cholesterol (63).

According to the 1986–90 Heart Health Surveys, 45% of men and 43% of women had a total plasma cholesterol level above the desirable level of 5.2 mmol/L. Thirty percent of men and 27% of women were in the moderately elevated risk group (5.2-6.1 mmol/L) and 18% and 17% respectively were in the highest risk group (>6.2 mmol/L). The proportion of men and women with a high cholesterol level (>5.2 mmol/L) increased with age, almost doubling from the 25 to 34 age group to the 35 to 44 age group among men and from the 35 to 44 age group to the 45 to 54 age group among women.

5.6.   USE OF PROTECTIVE DEVICES

Seatbelts

Motor vehicle collisions are a leading cause of death and injury in Canada, especially in young adults. The established role of seatbelts in reducing fatalities has been well publicized.

Eighty-eight percent of Canada's 18.7 million motorists aged 16 and older reported that they always insist that all passengers be safely fastened with seatbelts, and only 4% of Canadian motorists rarely or never insisted on such precautions. However, only 60% of men aged 20 to 24 always insisted on their passengers wearing seatbelts, the lowest level of all age and sex groups. There were very few differences among education levels for insistence that passengers wear seatbelts. The proportion of motorists who always insist that passengers wear seatbelts ranged from lows of 77% in Manitoba and Alberta to highs of 89% in Newfoundland and Labrador, New Brunswick, and British Columbia (9).

Bicycle Helmets

Head injuries from mishaps on bicycles affect both adults and children and can be prevented or reduced in severity by the consistent use of a helmet. The provinces of Ontario, British Columbia, and Nova Scotia have legislation involving the use of bicycle helmets (9).

About 29% of Canada's 6 million cyclists claim to always wear a helmet when riding a bike. If those who often wear a helmet are included, this figure rises to only 36%. However, the number of cyclists wearing helmets is up significantly from 1994–95, when only 19% wore a helmet and only 23% always or almost always wore a helmet when riding. The largest proportion (59%) reported that they never wear a bicycle helmet, but this is down from 73% who never wore helmets in 1994–95 (9). When asked why they did not wear a helmet, individuals replied that they did not have a helmet (47%), helmets were uncomfortable (14%), helmets were unnecessary (9%), or they were subject to ridicule as a result of wearing a helmet (4%). Differences in helmet use are strongly associated with education level. There is almost a 2.5-fold difference between the least and most educated groups in helmet use. In terms of education level, 36% of university graduates always wore a helmet, compared with 16% of those with less than a high school degree (64).

5.7.   CELL PHONE USE WHILE DRIVING

In Canada, the number of cellular telephone users has increased from fewer than 100,000 in 1987 to more than 9.5 million by the end of 2001 (65). The availability of cells phones offers some benefit to drivers, such as allowing them to make emergency calls quickly. However, use during driving appears to increase the risk of a motor vehicle collision. In a study of 700 drivers who had cellular telephones and were involved in motor vehicle collisions resulting in substantial property damage but no personal injury, the risk of a collision when using a cellular telephone was four times higher than the risk when a cellular telephone was not used (66). This relative risk is similar to the hazard associated with driving with a blood alcohol level at the legal limit. The risk of a collision was similar for drivers of different ages and driving experience, and was about the same during the day and night, winter and summer (67). Units that allowed the hands to be free offered no safety advantage over hand-held units. Thus, these vehicle collisions may have been the result of a decrease in the driver's attention rather than dexterity. The study suggests that regulations against using a cellular telephone while driving may be justified and more cost-effective than education. As of March 2003, forty one countries such as Brazil, Israel, and Australia have laws against using a cellular telephone while driving. In December 2002, Newfoundland and Labrador was the first Canadian province to pass legislation banning cellular phones while driving.

5.8. SEXUAL PRACTICES

In addition to unplanned pregnancies, unsafe sexual behaviour can lead to serious conditions such as sexually transmitted diseases, infertility, and HIV and other infections. In the 1994–95 NPHS, among people who were sexually active and had more than one partner, 51% of females and 29% of males aged 15 to 19 years reported having had sex without a condom in the previous year. Among youth aged 20 to 24, 53% of sexually active females and 44% of sexually active males reported having had sex without a condom during that period.

Findings from the four-province Atlantic Student Drug Use Survey (1998) found that 26% of Grade 9 students, 37% of Grade 10 students, and 58% of Grade 12 students had sexual intercourse during the previous year. Among sexually active students, 40% had more than one sexual partner, and 50% had unplanned intercourse on at least one occasion when under the influence of alcohol or another drug. Condoms were not consistently used, particularly among older students (9).

6. PREVENTIVE HEALTH PRACTICES

Recent Measures to Improve Health

Almost half the Canadian population aged 12 and older reported changing some behaviour to improve their health in the year before the 1996–97 NPHS. Women and men who recognized the need to change were most likely to say that more exercise was the personal health practice that was most needed. A lack of time and will were cited as the main barriers to making lifestyle changes. Behaviour changes were reported most often in Ontario (50%) and least often in Saskatchewan (39%).

According to the 1998–99 NPHS, women are more likely than men to consider overall health, body weight, and specific diseases or conditions when making food choices: 80% of women versus 63% of men were concerned about maintaining or improving health through food choice. Men seem to become as motivated as women to consider the implications of their food choices only after they have been diagnosed with a major health problem such as heart disease, cancer, or diabetes (60). Despite the substantially higher proportion of overweight men in Canada, women (40%) were still more likely than men (23%) to report recent attempts at weight loss (9). Many Canadians take vitamins with the hope of preventing illness and disease or ensuring good health. The use of supplements is fairly common, especially among women and 45- to 64-year-old men and women.

Immunization

The routine use of vaccines has led to significant reductions in vaccine preventable diseases. Vaccination programs are considered to be the most cost-beneficial health intervention, leading to far more dollar benefits than costs. Routine immunization programs for children are among the most cost-effective interventions, with cost per year of life saved for measles, mumps, and rubella (MMR) immunization for children estimated to be much below $1 (68).

There have been recent successes seen with the introduction of new vaccines. Prior to 1988 in Canada, **Haemophilus influenzae** type b (Hib) was the most common cause of bacterial meningitis and a leading cause of other serious invasive infections in young children. Prior to 1988, there were about 2,000 cases of Hib disease annually. Since the introduction of routine vaccination with Hib conjugate vaccines in 1988, the overall incidence in Canada has decreased more than 90%. In 2000, there were only four cases of Hib disease in children under 5 years of age.

Routine vaccination against many common infectious diseases has made these diseases uncommon (see Table 5.3 in Chapter 5). Consequently, the mortality and morbidity seen with many of such diseases have been forgotten. It can thus be easy for the public to forget the importance of these diseases and become complacent about immunizing against them. The importance of continued vigilance about immunization, however, cannot be underemphasized. When complacency occurs and immunization rates drop, a resurgence of vaccine-preventable diseases occurs. For example, in several developed countries (Britain, Sweden, and Japan) when immunization levels for pertussis dropped due to parental fears of adverse reaction to the vaccine, a dramatic and immediate resurgence in that disease was seen. In Japan, a drop in vaccination rates from 70% to 20-40% led to a rise in pertussis cases from 393 cases and no deaths in 1974 to 13,000 cases and 41 deaths in 1979 (68). Once immunization programs were reinstituted, the numbers began to fall again. The Romanow Commission identified a need for a national immunization strategy as many provinces do not publicly fund four new vaccines (varicella, pneumococcal, meningococcal, and combined pertussis and tetanus vaccine) (69).

At present, across Canada children are routinely immunized against several communicable diseases (see Chapter 8 for details). The recommended vaccines are provided free of charge by provinces to the age groups in which the vaccines are indicated, except those new vaccines listed above.

Jurisdictions assess vaccination coverage at different ages, so a direct comparison of coverage levels is not possible. Reported levels range from 81.0% for four doses at 24 months of age to 97.9% for three or more doses by school entry (4 to 6 years of age) for diphtheria, tetanus, and pertussis (DPT) vaccine; from 80.4% to 93.6% for three or more doses of polio by school entry; from 93.5% to 97.9% for one dose of MMR vaccine by school entry; and from 67.0% for four doses of Hib to 93.4% for three or more doses at school entry. An increase of 5% was found for pertussis coverage between the 1990–91 and 1993–94 cohorts, which likely reflects the 1993 recommendation by the National Advisory Committee on Immunization that certain conditions are no longer considered contraindications to pertussis vaccination. Overall, no statistically significant differences were documented between the coverage levels for children in families with different income levels (70).

A national survey of vaccine coverage in the Canadian population aged 18 and over showed the following selected coverage rates: in 2000–01, 25.8% for influenza (ranging from 13% in those aged 18 to 24 years to 63% in those aged 65 years and over), 0.25% for pneumococcal infections (1% in those aged 65 years and over), and 6% for tetanus and diphtheria (60). The low rates of appropriate immunization among adults are thought to occur because of the targeting of immunization programs, including education about recommendations for immunization and evaluation of coverage, mainly for children. Thus, special efforts are still needed to improve knowledge about recommendations for adult immunizations and to ensure the delivery of vaccines to the right target groups (70).

Dental Hygiene

The vast majority of Canadians (97%) brush their teeth at least once a day and 79% brush their teeth twice a day. This preventive practice is more widespread among women, younger Canadians, and those with a higher education and income.

7.   THE USE OF HEALTHCARE SERVICES

Healthcare organization is also a major determinant of health (and is discussed in Part III of this book). The major feature is the availability of universal health insurance for all Canadians, which has significantly contributed to reducing the inequities in access to health care within the population.

Contact with Healthcare Professionals. According to the 1998–99 National Health Survey, most Canadians visit their doctor at least once a year: 88.5% of females 12 and older reported having had contact with a general practitioner within the last year, compared to 72% of men (71). Contacts were about equally likely for Canadians of all income levels, but older adults were more likely to have visited a general practitioner. Visits to doctors were more common for patients with chronic conditions such as diabetes, asthma, and hypertension than for the population as a whole.

With each step up the income ladder, Canadians were more likely to have visited a dentist. Only 40% of low-income Canadians reported receiving dental services, compared to just fewer than 80% of the most affluent in the 1998–99 NPHS.

Adherence to Recommended Preventive Health Practices. The Canadian Task Force on Preventive Health Care weighs the evidence and makes recommendations on what should — and should not — be included in the periodic health examination (regular check-ups) of Canadians of different ages (see Chapter 11). These recommendations are found in Appendix A.

Screening for Blood Pressure. The task force recommends that all adults over the age of 20 have blood pressure assessments done every two years. High blood pressure (defined as a systolic blood pressure 140 mmHg or higher, or a diastolic blood pressure 90 mmHg or higher) is a major risk factor for coronary artery disease, stroke, peripheral vascular disease, and congestive heart failure. It increases overall cardiovascular risk by two- to three-fold (31).

The Heart Health Surveys of 1986–90 found that 22% of adult Canadians (26% of men and 18% of women) had high blood pressure. However, only 13% of the population had been diagnosed with high blood pressure. In other words, 42% of those who had high blood pressure were unaware that they had high blood pressure. According to the 1996–97 NPHS, 84% of the population had had their blood pressure assessed in the last two years (31).

Research evidence strongly supports the benefits of treating high blood pressure to reduce the incidence of stroke, myocardial infarction, ischemic heart disease, vascular disease, renal disease, and overall death rate. Individuals who have excess weight, are physically inactive, use alcohol heavily, or have excessive salt intake are more likely to develop high blood pressure. High blood pressure is commonly associated with other metabolic cardiovascular risk factors such as insulin resistance, obesity, hyperuricemia, and dyslipidemia.

The 1998–99 NPHS of people aged 12 and over found that 10% of the population was taking blood pressure medication. According to the 1996–97 NPHS, 84% of those diagnosed with high blood pressure were receiving treatment (medication or lifestyle change) for high blood pressure. Many individuals with high blood pressure are treated with medication alone rather than a combination of medication and lifestyle changes, which has been identified as a problem by the National High Blood Pressure Prevention and Control Strategy expert working group (72). This group has also recommended that all hypertensive patients should be assessed for sodium consumption and stress levels. To reduce blood pressure in the population at large, it is recommended that Canadians attain and maintain a healthy BMI, limit their alcohol intake to two or fewer standard drinks per day, and exercise regularly. The DASH diet (Dietary Approach to Stop Hypertension) clinical trials have demonstrated that a diet that emphasizes fruits, vegetables, and low-fat dairy products in addition to restricting dietary sodium, can be highly effective in lowering blood pressure (73).

There is also evidence to suggest that other aspects of blood pressure treatment tend to be inadequate in Canada and elsewhere. Studies done have shown that only a minority of those prescribed treatment achieve target levels of treatment. Even among those with well-controlled hypertension, the rate of cardiovascular events is higher than in age-matched controls because of the undertreatment of their other atherosclerotic risk factors (especially hyperlipidemia) (74).

Screening for Cervical Cancer. The Canadian Task Force on Preventive Health Care recommends that women receive regular Pap smears upon becoming sexually active (or at age 18) until age 69. The frequency can be reduced to every three years after two consecutive normal test results. Seventy-seven percent of women aged 18 to 69 surveyed in the 1998–99 NPHS reported having had a Pap smear in the last three years (75). Those least likely to have had a Pap smear within the last three years are younger women (18 to 19), women without a regular doctor, women with lower levels of education, and women with low incomes. Other factors shown to affect the use of cervical cancer screening include access to screening, awareness of benefits of screening, and anxiety over the procedure.

Screening for Breast Cancer. Clinical examinations and mammography can help detect breast cancer early, when treatment may be more successful. The Canadian Task Force on Preventive Health Care recommends annual screening with clinical breast exam and mammography every two years for women aged 50 to 69. The 1998–99 NPHS found that 66% of women aged 50 to 69 said that they had had a mammogram within the last two years, up slightly from two years before (75). Women with low levels of income and education and those without a doctor were less likely to be screened. Older women, women living in a rural area, women born in Asia, women who were current smokers, women who had infrequent physical activity, and women who were not on hormone replacement therapy were also less likely to have had a mammogram (76).

Recent study has shown that there is sufficient evidence to exclude the routine teaching of breast self-examination (BSE) from the periodic health examination of women in the 40- to 69-year age group. There is not enough evidence to evaluate its effectiveness in women younger than 40 and older than 70 (77).

Alternative Medicine. Alternative medicine refers to a range of services offered outside of the traditional healthcare system. For the purposes of this section, chiropractors are included among alternative healthcare providers.

A survey conducted by the Fraser Institute revealed that 73% of Canadians had used at least one alternative therapy at some point in their life. In this survey, chiropractic was the most common therapy used (36%), followed by relaxation techniques and massage at 23%, and prayer by 21% (78).

The 1998–99 NPHS found that an estimated 16% of Canadians 12 or older said that they had consulted a chiropractor or another type of complementary or alternative healthcare provider in the previous year. This is up from 14% in 1994–95. On average, women, people between the age of 25 and 54, and those with chronic conditions were more likely to use complementary services.

8.   SUMMARY

This chapter dealt with the non-medical determinants and human biology, which has an impact on health and disease in the Canadian population. The determinants of health include human biology, demography, socioeconomics, physical environment, lifestyle and behavioural and risk factors, and healthcare organizations (which are discussed elsewhere in this book).

The genetic potential of the individual is a major aspect of human biology and has an effect on health.

Demographic and socioeconomic indicators represent the interaction of demography with social and economic conditions. In May 2001, Canada's population was 30 million, which has more than doubled since 1941. The ratio of males to females has remained roughly constant, but there has been a definite change in the age distribution. With the availability of better contraception, more liberal abortion laws, and more women participating in the labour force, the proportion of children under age 14 decreased since 1971, while at the same time there has been an increase among those aged 65 and over.

Geographic distributions also affect the health status of a population. Three quarters of the population live within 320 km of the border between Canada and the United States, with the remaining population spread across a vast land mass. This creates a substantial challenge to providing healthcare services, particularly with regard to the northern areas of Canada.

Sociodemographic indicators include aging, immigration, language, and family environments. An important demographic change is the rise in the proportion of the population over age 65. In 2001, seniors represented 12.9% of the population. The composition of the Canadian population is also changing in relation to ethnicity and is expected to continue changing as more immigrants from non-European countries are migrating to Canada. As an example of Canada's ethnic diversity, 5.3 million people reported a first language other than French or English.

The composition of the population in terms of literacy, education, income, and employment influences health. In 1994–95, about 43% of Canadians were able to read at or below the level of only simple material that does not contain complex instructions. These limitations may affect health directly in terms of the inappropriate use of medicines, difficulty communicating with healthcare workers, and difficulty in following instructions.

Income is another major socioeconomic indicator. A family that spends more than 54.7% of income on the basic needs of accommodation, food, and clothing is considered to live under strained circumstances and thus falls below the low-income cut-off (LICO). In 2001, an estimated 1.1 million children under the age of 15 years were living in low-income households. Welfare payments typically fall substantially below the previously described LICOs set by Statistics Canada. Average family incomes have also been decreasing in Canada. The average family income in Canada in 1998 was $49,626, down from $56,629 in 1996, and was lower than the average family incomes seen since 1978.

Labour markets have also changed dramatically in the last decade due in part to a response to globalization, trade competition, and technological innovation. Many workers in advanced economies now face limited employment prospects and poor working conditions related to either the availability of work (e.g., unemployment, job insecurity, and overwork) or to the nature of work (e.g., increasing job demands, low job position within a firm, and contingent employment).

Homelessness is associated with many health risks. The composition of this group now includes increasing numbers of women and children and other groups in special circumstances, such as adolescents, persons with mental illness, and Aboriginal people.

Chronic stress has a significant impact on Canadians. Longitudinal data show that feeling personal stress was predictive of developing chronic conditions.

The physical environment includes physical, biological, chemical, and radiological factors found in food, water, soil, indoor and outdoor air, the built environment, and animal and insect vectors. Public interest and knowledge in environmental issues have increased over the last 50 years, and concomitantly so has public support for more extensive and strict control of environmental agents.

The lifestyle of Canadians is also a major factor in determining their health. The most common causes of mortality, potential years of life lost, hospitalizations, and disability are cardiovascular diseases, cancer, and injuries and are attributable to behaviour and lifestyle such as, misuse of alcohol, tobacco, and illicit drugs. The rate of smoking among Canadian adults in 2001 was 22%. Among youth 15 to 19 years of age, however, there was a significant and large increase in smoking prevalence between 1991 and 1994, and there has been no significant change since 1994. With respect to alcohol, the largest number of alcohol-related deaths stemmed from impaired driving in motor vehicle collisions. Approximately three of every four Canadians aged 15 or older consumes alcoholic beverages, with one half of adults consuming alcohol at least once a month. Approximately one in four Canadians (24%) reported the use of an illicit drug at least once in their lifetime, with cannabis being the most widely used illicit drug.

Over the past few years, gambling has become common in Canadian society. Major public health issues include gambling addiction, family dysfunction, and gambling by youth. Of particular concern is the high prevalence of gambling and gambling-related problems among youth, the poor, and Aboriginal people.

Good nutrition is fundamental to good health and to the prevention of or reduction in severity of disease. Food consumption data in Canada in 1999–2000 suggest that fruit and vegetable consumption have been increasing and red meat consumption has been decreasing since 1990. Although fat and caloric intakes appear to be decreasing over the last decade, obesity is a growing problem among both adults and children in Canada. Nearly half of adult Canadians have a body mass index (BMI) above the target range and one quarter to nearly one third of children are overweight. In 1998-99, only 22% of Canadians in the household population aged 12 or older engaged in vigorous physical activity during their leisure time; almost a quarter of people aged 12 or older reported that "sitting" best described their usual daily non-leisure activity.

Seatbelts and bicycle helmets are examples of protective devices. Eighty-eight percent of Canada's motorists aged 16 and older reported that they always insist that all passengers are safely fastened with seatbelts; however, only 29% of Canadians say they always wear a helmet when riding a bicycle. In Canada, the number of cellular telephone users has increased, and use during driving appears to increase the risk of a motor vehicle collision.

In the 1994–95 NPHS, among sexually active (with more than one partner) 15- to 19-year-olds, 51% of females and 29% of males reported having had sex without a condom in the previous year. Among youth aged 20 to 24, 53% of sexually active females and 44% of sexually active males reported having had sex without a condom during the same period.

Preventive health practices such as immunization, screening, and treatment for high blood pressure, and screening for cervical and breast cancer in women, are measures that can help to improve the health of individuals and the population. High immunization rates in children are important in the prevention of infectious diseases that resurge when immunization rates decrease. Rates of recommended immunizations in adults and seniors are low and require more attention. There is evidence that hypertension may be underdiagnosed in Canadians and that there needs to be improvement in the optimal treatment of hypertensive patients, including treatment that emphasizes lifestyle changes rather than medications alone. In cancer screening, the 1998–99 NPHS found that 77% of women aged 18 to 69 reported having had a Pap smear in the last three years, and 66% of women aged 50 to 69 said that they had had a mammogram within the last two years, up slightly from two years before.

Healthcare organization is also a determinant of health (and is discussed elsewhere in this book). The major feature is the availability of universal health insurance for all Canadians, which has significantly contributed to reducing the inequities in access to health care within the population. In 1998–99, while the majority of Canadians visited their doctors in the past year, 16% of Canadians 12 or older said that they had consulted a chiropractor or another type of complementary or alternative healthcare provider in the previous year, up from 14% in 1994–95.

9.   REFERENCES

1.   Baird P, Scriver C. Genetics and the public health. In Wallace R, editor. *Maxey-Rosenau-Last public health and preventive medicine*. 14th ed. Stamford, CT: Appleton & Lange; 1998.
2.   Yorke D, Mitchell J, Clow C, *et al.* Newborn screening for sickle cell and other haemoglobinopathies. *Clinical and Investigative Medicine* 1992; 15(4):376-83.
3.   Dickson D. Panel urges caution on genetic testing for mental disorders. *Nature* 1998; 395:309.
4.   Health Canada. 1999. *Healthy development of children and youth: The role of determinants of health*. <www.hc-sc.gc.ca/hppb/childhood-youth/spsc/pdf/healthy_dev/partb_8.pdf> (January 2003).
5.   Ford D, Nault F. Changing fertility patterns, 1974 to 1994. *Health Reports* 1996; 8(3):39-45.

6. Statistics Canada. Population projections, 2000–2006. *The Daily* 2001; March 13. <www.statcan.ca/Daily/English/010313/d010313a.htm> (January 2003).

7. Statistics Canada. *2001 census: Canada's ethnocultural portrait — The changing mosaic.* Ottawa: Statistics Canada, 2003. Cat no. 96F0030XIE2001008.

8. Statistics Canada. 2001 Census: definition <www12.statcan.ca/english/census01/products/analytic/companion/etoimm/def.cfm> (February 2003) <www.statcan.ca/english/freepub/82-003-XIE/free.htm> (January 2003).

9. Federal, Provincial and Territorial Advisory Committee on Population Health. *Towards a healthy future: Second report on the health of Canadians.* Ottawa: Health Canada, 1999.

10. Statistics Canada. 2001 Census. *Education in Canada: Raising the standard.* Catlogue no. 96F0030XIE2001012. <www12.statcan.ca/english/census01/Products/Analytic/companion/educ/pdf/96F0030XIE2001012.pdf> (March 2003).

11. Statistics Canada. *Overview: Access to and use of information communications technology.* Ottawa, 2001. Cat. no. 56-505-XIE. <www.statcan.ca/english/IPS/Data/56-505-XIE.htm> (January 2003).

12. Statistics Canada. 2003. *Census: Earning of Canadians: Making a living in the new economy.* <www12.statcan.ca/english/census01/Products/Analytic/companion/earn/pdf/96F0030XIE2001013.pdf> (March 2003).

13. Campaign 2000. 2002. *A report on a decade of child and family poverty in Canada.* <www.campaign2000.ca/rc/unsscMAY02/MAY02statusreport.pdf> (November 2002).

14. Vozoris N, Davis B, Tarasuk V. The affordability of nutritious diet for households on welfare in Toronto. *Canadian Journal of Public Health* 2002; 93(1):36-46.

15. Wilkins R, Berthelot J, Ng E. Trends in mortality by neighbourhood income in urban Canada from 1971 to 1996. *Health Reports* 2002; 13(Suppl):1-28.

16. Association of Workers' Compensation Boards of Canada. 2002. *Key statistical measures, 2000.* Mississauga. <www.awcbc.org/english/board_pdfs/key_2000.pdf> (September 2002).

17. Lavis J, Stoddart G. *Social cohesion and health*: McMaster University Center for Health Economics and Policy Analysis Working Paper Series, 1999.

18. Landsbergis P, Cahill J, Schnall P. The impact of lean production and related new systems of work organization on worker health. *Journal of Occupational Psychology* 1999; 4(2):108-30.

19. Morris J, Cook D, Shaper A. Non-employment and changes in smoking, drinking, and body weight. *British Medical Journal* 1992; 304:536-41.

20. Morris J, Cook D, Shaper A. Loss of employment and mortality. *British Medical Journal* 1994; 308:1135-9.

21. Jin R, Shah C, Svaboda T. The impact of unemployment on health: A review and the evidence. *Canadian Medical Association Journal* 1995; 153(5):529-40.

22. Hwang S. Mortality among men using homeless shelters in Toronto, Ontario. *Journal of American Medical Association* 2000; 283:2152-7.

23. Plumb J. Homelessness: Reducing health disparities. *Canadian Medical Association Journal* 2000; 163(2):172-3.

24. Hwang S, Bugeja A. Barriers to appropriate diabetes management among homeless people in Toronto. *Canadian Medical Association Journal* 2000; 163(2):161-5.

25. Canadian Public Health Association. *Homelessness and health.* Ottawa: Canadian Public Health Association, 1997.

26. Statistics Canada. How healthy are Canadians? *Health Reports* 1999; 11(3):1-119.

27. Schuster C, Kilbey M. Prevention of drug abuse. In Wallace R, editor. *Maxey-Rosenau-Last public health and preventive medicine.* 14th ed. Stamford, CT: Appleton & Lange; 1998.

28.   Health Canada. 1998. *The health and environment handbook for health professionals.* <www.hc-sc.gc.ca/ehp/ehd/catalogue/bch_pubs/98ehd211/98ehd211.htm> (January 2003).

29.   Zedja J, Semchuk K, McDuffie H, *et al.* A need for population-based studies of health and safety risks in Canadian agriculture. *Canadian Medical Association Journal* 1991; 145(7):773-5.

30.   Colditz G, DeJong H, Hunter D, *et al. Human causes of cancer: Cancer causes and control.* Boston: Harvard Center for Cancer Prevention, 1996.

31.   Heart and Stroke Foundation of Canada. *The changing face of heart disease and stroke in Canada.* Ottawa: Heart and Stroke Foundation of Canada, 1999.

32.   Canadian Tobacco Use Monitoring Survey, Health Canada. 2002. *Annual results, 2001.* <www.hc-sc.gc.ca/hecs-sesc/tobacco/research/ctums/2001/summary.html> (January 2003).

33.   Statistics Canada. *Health indicators.* Ottawa, 2001. Catalogue No. 82-221-XIE. <www.statcan.ca/english/IPS/Data/82-221-XIE.htm> (January 2003).

34.   Gilmore J. *Report on smoking prevalence in Canada: 1985–1999.* Ottawa: Statistics Canada, 2000. Cat. no. 82F-0077-XIE. <www.statcan.ca/english/research/82F0077XIE/82F0077XIE.htm> (January 2003).

35.   Steering Committee of the National Strategy to Reduce Tobacco Use in Canada in Partnership with Advisory Committee on Population Health. 1999. *New directions for tobacco control in Canada: A national strategy.* <www.hc-sc.gc.ca/hecs-sesc/tobacco/policy/new_directions/index.html> (November 2002).

36.   Single E. *Substance abuse and population health.* Edmonton, Alberta, June, 1999. <www.ccsa.ca/ADH/single.htm> (January 2003).

37.   Statistics Canada. Control and sale of alcoholic beverages. *The Daily* 2000, June 22. <www.statcan.ca/Daily/English/000622/d000622b.htm> (January 2003).

38.   Gfellner B, Hundelby H. Patterns of drug use among native and white adolescents, 1990-1993. *Canadian Journal of Public Health* 1995; 86:95-7.

39.   Radford J, King A, Warren W. *Street youth and AIDS.* Kingston: Health and Welfare Canada, 1989.

40.   Centre for Addiction and Mental Health. 2001. *Ontario Student Drug Use Survey: Executive summary.* <www.camh.net/addiction/ont_study_drug_use.html> (January 2003).

41.   Korn D. Expansion of gambling in Canada: Implications for health and social policy. *Canadian Medical Association* 2000; 163(1):61-4.

42.   Statistics Canada. Fact sheet on gambling. *Perspectives on Labour and Income* 2002; 3(7). <www.statcan.ca/english/indepth/75-001/online/00702/fs-fi_200207_01_a.pdf> (January 2003).

43.   Topp J, Sawka E, Room R, *et al. Policy discussion paper on problem gambling.* Ottawa: Canadian Centre on Substance Abuse, 1998.

44.   Crockford D, el-Guebaly N. Psychiatric comorbidity in pathological gambling: a critical review. *Canadian Journal of Psychiatry* 1998; 43:43-50.

45.   Health Canada. *A second diagnostic on the health of First Nations and Inuit people in Canada.* Ottawa: Health Canada, 1999. <www.hc-sc.gc.ca/fnihb/cp/publications/second_diagnostic_fni.pdf> (January 2003).

46.   Health Canada. 2002. *Canada's food guide to healthy eating.* <www.hc-sc.gc.ca/hpfb-dgpsa/onpp-bppn/food_guide_rainbow_e.html> (November 2002).

47.   Statistics Canada. Per-capita food consumption, 1999. *The Daily* 2000, November 29. <www.statcan.ca/Daily/English/001019/d001019d.htm> (January 2003).

48.   Statistics Canada. Per-capita food consumption 2000. *The Daily* 2001, October 18. <www.statcan.ca/Daily/English/011018/d011018h.htm> (January 2003).

49.   Gray-Donald K, Jacobs-Starkey L, Johnson-Down L. Food habits of Canadians: Reductions in fat intake over generation. *Canadian Journal of Public Health* 2000; 91(5):381-5.

50. National Institute of Nutrition. 2002. *Tracking nutrition trends 1989-1994-1997-2001.* <www.nin.ca/public_html/Publications/New/rap-vol17-1.pdf> (January 2003).

51. Perez C. Fruit and vegetable consumption. *Health Reports* 2002; 13(3):23-31.

52. Dawson L, Hunter A. Low rate of adequate folic acid supplementation in well-educated women of high socioeconomic status attending a genetic clinic. *Canadian Medical Association Journal* 2001; 164(8):1149-50.

53. Hall J. Folic acid: The opportunity that still exists. *Canadian Medical Association Journal* 2000; 162(11):1571-2.

54. Agriculture and Agri-Food Canada. 1998. *Canada's action plan for food security.* <www.agr.gc.ca/misb/fsb/fsap/fsape.html> (November 2002).

55. Food Security Bureau. 2001. *Canada's action plan for food security.* <www.agr.ca/misb/fsb/fsap/part2e.html> (November 2002).

56. Tarasuk V, Beaton G. Household food insecurity and hunger among families using food banks. *Canadian Journal of Public Health* 1999; 90(2):109-13.

57. Tarasuk V, Beaton G. Women's dietary intakes in the context of household food insecurity. *Journal of Nutrition* 1999; 129(3):672-9.

58. Health Canada. 2001. *Frequently asked questions on genetically modified foods.* <www.hc-sc.gc.ca/english/media/releases/2001/2001_13ebk3.htm> (January 2003).

59. Health Canada. 2000. *Canada's physical activity guide to healthy active living.* <www.hc-sc.gc.ca/hppb/paguide/main.html> (November 2002).

60. Statistics Canada. 2002. *Data tables.* Health Indicators, 2002, no. 1. <www.statcan.ca/english/freepub/82-221-XIE/00502/tables.htm> (January 2003).

61. Tremblay M, Willms J. Secular trends in the body mass index of Canadian children. *Canadian Medical Association Journal* 2000; 163(11):1429-33.

62. Health Canada. 2002. *Activity guidelines for children and youth.* <www.hc-sc.gc.ca/hppb/paguide/guides/en/children/guidelines.html> (February 2003).

63. Luepker R. Heart disease. In Wallace R, editor. *Maxey-Rosenau-Last public health and preventive medicine.* 14th ed. Stamford, CT: Appleton & Lange; 1998.

64. Federal, Provincial, and Territorial Advisory Committee on Population Health. 1999. *Statistical report on the health of Canadians.* Ottawa. <www.statcan.ca/english/freepub/82-570-XIE/free.htm> (November 2002).

65. Health Canada. 2002. *Safety and safe use of cellular phones.* <www.hc-sc.gc.ca/english/iyh/products/cellphones.htm> (January 2003).

66. Redelmeier D, Tibshirani R. Association between cellular-telephone calls and motor vehicle collisions. *New England Journal of Medicine* 1997; 336(7):453-8.

67. Redelmeier D, Tibshirani R. Car phones and car crashes: Some popular misconceptions. *Canadian Medical Association Journal* 2001; 164(11):1581-2.

68. National Advisory Committee on Immunization. *Canadian immunization guide.* Ottawa: Minister of Supply and Services Canada, 2002. 6th edition. <www.hc-sc.gc.ca/pphb-dgspsp/publicat/cig-gci> (January 2003).

69. Romanow R. *Building on values: The future of health care in Canada.* Ottawa: Commission on the Future of Health Care in Canada; Government of Canada, 2002.

70. Health Canada. Canadian national report on immunization, 1996. *Canada Communicable Disease Report* 1997; 23S4(May 1997). <www.hc-sc.gc.ca/pphb-dgspsp/publicat/ccdr-rmtc/97vol23/23s4/index.html> (January 2003).

71. Canadian Institute for Health Information. *Health care in Canada 2001.* Ottawa: Canadian Institute for Health Information, 2001.

72. Health Canada, Canadian Coalition for High Blood Pressure Prevention and Control. *National High Blood Pressure Prevention and Control Strategy: Summary report of the Expert Working Group.* Ottawa, 2000. <www.hc-sc.gc.ca/pphb-dgspsp/ccdpc-cpcmc/cvd-mcv/publications/nhbppcs_e.html> (January 2003).

73. Kosala K. Dietary Approaches to Stop Hypertension (DASH) in clinical practice: A primary care experience. *Clinical Cardiology* 1999; 22(7 Suppl):16-22.

74.   McAlister F, Campbell N, Zarnke K, *et al.* The management of hypertension in Canada: A review of current guidelines, their shortcomings, and implications for the future. *Canadian Medical Association Journal* 2001; 164(4):517-22.

75.   Canadian Institute for Health Information. *Health care in Canada, 2000: A first annual report.* Ottawa: Canadian Institute for Health Information, 2000. <www.cihi.ca> (November 2002).

76.   Maxwell C, Bancej C, Snider J. Predictors of mammography use among Canadian women aged 50–69: Findings from the 1996/97 National Population Health Survey. 2001.

77.   Baxter N. Preventive health care, 2001 update: Should women be routinely taught breast self-examination to screen for breast cancer? *Canadian Medical Association Journal* 2001; 164(13):1837-46.

78.   Buske L. Looking for an alternative. *Canadian Medical Association Journal* 1999; 161(4):363.

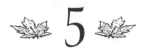

5

HEALTH STATUS AND CONSEQUENCES

The previous chapter examined aspects of Canadian life that affect health. But how does one identify health status and assess its relative significance (1)? As seen in Chapter 3, categories of health status namely, sense of well-being, morbidity, mortality and the ensuing disability and economic burden are the most commonly used measures of health in Canada. Much information is available on death in Canada, but data on morbidity, which to a degree relates to disease outcomes, are more difficult to assess. Several different approaches to assess morbidity are outlined in this chapter. Other outcomes, such as human suffering or quality of life, are no less important but because the methodologies for their measurement are complex and evolving, they are not used as extensively in assessment of health and planning of health care.

1. HEALTH STATUS

1.1. SELF-ASSESSED HEALTH

Perception of Health
The most fundamental health outcome is the individual's perception of well-being. This is frequently associated with other outcomes such as limitation of usual activities, consultation with a healthcare professional, hospitalization, or death. Self-rated health is known to be a good predictor of more objectively measured health problems. The 1996–97 National Population Health Survey (NPHS) asked individuals aged 12 and over to rate their own health as excellent, very good, good, fair, or poor (2). Below are some of the highlights of the survey results.

- Nine out of ten Canadians (90%) assessed their health to be good (27%), very good (38%), or excellent (25%).
- Fewer than one in ten people (9%) reported either fair or poor health.
- For Canadians aged 15 and older, self-rated health has remained approximately the same since 1985, except for a slight decrease in the percentage of people rating their health as fair or poor.

- Older Canadians were more likely to report poorer health. Among those between the ages of 65 and 74, 20% reported that they were in fair or poor health; this number reaches 27% among those aged 75 and over. The percentage of older Canadians reporting fair or poor health appears to be slightly lower in the 1996–97 NPHS than in the 1994–95 NPHS, where 24% of 65- to 74-year-olds and 31% of those age 75 and over reported poorer health.

- Almost all (95%) Canadians with the highest incomes assessed their health to be good, very good, or excellent, compared with 79% of those who were in the lowest income quintile.

Although comparisons between countries must always be made with some degree of caution, among a group of reasonably comparable countries that belong to the Organisation for Economic Co-operation and Development (OECD), in 1995 Canada ranked second along with the United States in the percentage of people who rated their health as good or better. The country with the best rate (92%) was Norway.

Perception of Ill Health

Few data are available on this subject, but the NPHS affords us a look at Canadian perceptions. It inquires into all health problems at the time of the survey, and more than half of the respondents in 1994–95 identified one or more health problems. However, fewer than half of those reporting problems induced the individuals to limit their activity, visit a healthcare professional, or treat themselves with a commercial remedy. The survey identified people with chronic health problems as a proportion of the total population. Of all adults surveyed in 1994–95, 35% (12.5 million) had at least one chronic condition: approximately 28% reported one, 13% reported two, and another 13% three or more. The leading health problems were skin diseases and allergies, reported by 20% of adults, followed by back problems (15%), arthritis and rheumatism (13%), and high blood pressure (9%). It was also observed that chronic health problems were more prevalent among women and that women were also more likely to report multiple chronic conditions. Almost similar findings were obtained in NPHS 1998-99 survey. One of the most common psychiatric disorders is depression.

In 1994, 5.7% of the population aged 15 and over reported having had a depressive episode in the year preceding the survey. Twice as many women reported depression as men (7.6% and 3.7% respectively). High levels of chronic stress and relatively lower incomes were also associated with depression. Although some of this subjective morbidity may be minor in nature, it is worthy of examination to learn more about the relationship between perceived ill health and the pursuit of health care, and the potential role of health education in this process.

In 1967, Robert Kohn estimated the health of a standardized population of 100,000 Canadians based on the following outcomes: the number of individuals who perceive themselves to have at least one health problem or disability, the number of individuals who consulted health professionals or were admitted to hospital for these problems, and the number of deaths (3). It is possible to create similar estimates based on information from the NPHS and other recent sources. Figure 5.1 illustrates these estimates, which give a glimpse of the health of an average group of Canadians on an

Figure 5.1.   **Health of a Population Sample of 100,000 Canadians on an Average Day**

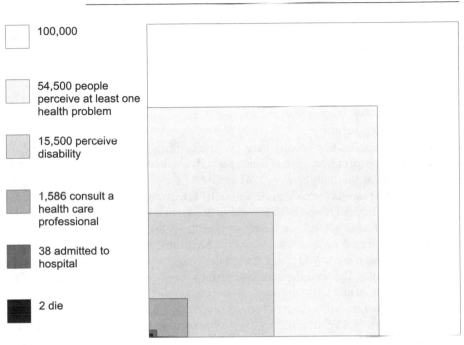

100,000

54,500 people perceive at least one health problem

15,500 perceive disability

1,586 consult a health care professional

38 admitted to hospital

2 die

Source: Adapted from R Kohn. *Royal Commission on Health Services: The health of the Canadian people.* Ottawa: Queen's Printer, 1967.

average day. It is notable that the recent statistics do not differ significantly from those of Kohn 40 years earlier. With the exception of death, these outcomes do not necessarily reflect disease; healthy people may feel ill, see a doctor, and even be admitted to hospital. All these outcomes, however, have consequences for health care and its planning.

Positive Mental Health

One limitation often found in measures of health status is their failure to capture the positive states of health beyond the absence of illness or infirmity. Well-being consists of physical, mental, and social attributes that help individuals to cope successfully with health and functioning. The psychological dimension of well-being fits closely with three measures: sense of coherence, self-esteem, and mastery. **Sense of coherence** is a view of the world that sees events as comprehensible, challenges as manageable, and life as meaningful. **Self-esteem** is the general sense of self-worth a person has, and **mastery** is the extent to which individuals feel their life chances are under their control (2).

The 1994–95 NPHS was the first national Canadian survey to use these measures. Psychological well-being is, on average, lowest among those in the youngest age groups. The most pronounced increases with age occur with sense of coherence. Those aged 75 and older are three times more likely than 18- to 19-year-olds to score high on this measure. These age-related patterns are consistent with measures that capture psychological illness. The prevalence of depression, for example, declines with age. There is little or no relationship found between coherence and education after age standardization. However, self-esteem and mastery are both positively related to education (2).

1.2.   OBJECTIVE INDICATORS

1.2.1.   Life Expectancy

Life expectancy has traditionally been the index of health most commonly used for international comparisons, as relevant data are readily available. Life expectancy at birth in Canada increased significantly between 1941 and 1998 from 63.0 to 75.9 years for males, and from 66.3 to 81.5 years for females; in 1998 overall life expectancy for both sexes combined was 78.6 years. The chief reason is the significant decline in infant mortality, from 61 deaths per 1,000 live births in 1941 to 5.3 in 1998. Life expectancy has increased significantly more for females than for males, such that the gap has broadened from 3.3 years in 1941 to 5.6 years in 1998. This is due to a decline in death rates among women at all ages over a longer period than for males. The sex differential in death rates may be partly attributed to differences in lifestyle, such as smoking, drinking, and occupation (6). Males have traditionally experienced higher mortality from ischemic heart disease, respiratory diseases, and lung cancer, as well as motor vehicle collisions and other unintentional injuries, all of which are related to lifestyle. This increasing difference between the sexes appears to be narrowing and will continue to narrow as lung cancer, injury, and cardiovascular mortality diminish in men (5). Japan had the highest life expectancy at birth in 1998 — 84 for females and 77.2 for males. Life expectancies in other developed countries are listed in Chapter 12 (see Table 12.5). In 1998, Canada's life expectancy ranked third among member countries of the Organisation for Economic Co-operation and Development (OECD), behind Japan and Switzerland (6).

1.2.2.   Mortality

The overall age-standardized mortality rate in Canada was 6.5 deaths per 1,000 people in 1996. In 1994, Canada ranked fifth behind South Korea, Japan, Iceland, and Switzerland. The lowest rate, in South Korea, was 5.5 per 1,000 (2). The overall mortality rate is important, but much more information is gained by examining mortality in more detail. Mortality may be expressed in terms of life expectancy, age- and sex-specific death rates, causes of death by age and sex, and potential years of life lost (PYLL). Most of these terms are explained in Chapter 3. Each yields different useful information about Canadian health.

Trends and Causes in Age- and Sex-Specific Death Rates (1951–1998)

Age-standardized overall mortality rates declined steadily between 1950 and 1998 for both men and women (7). Figure 5.2 illustrates age-specific mortality rates for both

Figure 5.2.   Trends in Age- and Sex-Specific Mortality Rates per 1,000 Population in Canada, 1951–1998

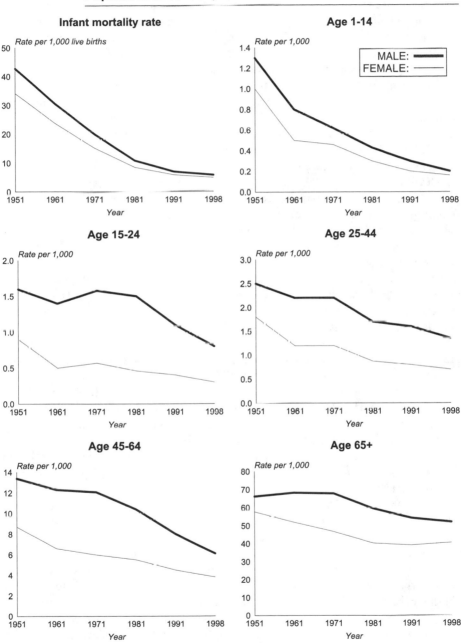

Source: Adapted from Health Field Indicators, Health and Welfare Canada, 1986, and Statistics Canada.

sexes from 1951 to 1998. Figure 5.3 provides an overview of the prevailing causes of death by sex and age group in Canada in 1998. Among those under the age of one year, there has been a steady decline in mortality rates throughout this period and it appears to be continuing. Infant mortality refers to the deaths of children under one year of age (8). There has been a steady decline in infant mortality rates in Canada throughout this period, falling below six deaths per 1,000 for the first time in 1998. In 1998, the rate was 5.6 deaths per 1,000 births. Infant mortality rates in males (6.7 per 1,000) have always been and continue to be higher than those in females (5.5 per 1,000). In 1996, Canada ranked 12th among 17 OECD countries compared. The lowest infant mortality rates found internationally occur in Japan (3.8 per 1,000), Finland, Sweden, and Norway (4.0 per 1,000 in the latter three countries). The highest rates are found in Greece (7.3 per 1,000), New Zealand (7.4 per 1,000), and the United States (7.8 per 1,000) (2). In 1998, infant mortality rates appear to have dropped further for both males (5.7 per 1,000) and females (4.8 per 1,000). In 1998, the most important cause of infant mortality and perinatal deaths (combination of stillbirths and early neonatal deaths) was perinatal complications. Also important were congenital anomalies and sudden infant death syndrome (SIDS) (9). Although perinatal complications and congenital anomalies are still the two most important causes of death among infants, there has been great progress in preventing death due to these factors (8).

From 1 to 14 years of age, mortality rates continue to decline slowly to very low levels. In 1998, the number-one cause of death in this age group is injuries, particularly from motor vehicle collisions and accidental drowning in those under 10, and motor vehicle collisions and suicides in those 10 to 14 (9). Such injuries are preventable. Although deaths due to most external causes and diseases have declined considerably, the mortality rate from suicide has increased. Between 1971 and 1996, the rate of suicide among those aged 10 to 14 has nearly tripled (8).

More recently, however, there has been a significant drop in the death rate of those aged 15-24, especially for males. This is due mainly to a decrease in mortality from motor vehicle collisions, which may be a result of the introduction of lower speed limits, highway safety design, installations of air bags, increased seat belt usage, and better trauma care for injured individuals. In spite of this favourable trend, most of the deaths in this age group must be regarded as preventable, and there is much room for improvement (10).

Among those aged 25 to 44, mortality rates were relatively stable throughout the 1960s and early 1970s, with a decline starting in the 1970s and continuing today. In this age group, male rates are about double the female rates, and the leading causes of death for males are suicides and motor vehicle collisions. In females, the leading causes of death are suicides and motor vehicle collisions in those under 35, and cancers of the breast and then lung in those 35 to 44. Excess male mortality is due largely to the much higher numbers of deaths from suicides, motor vehicle collisions, and ischemic heart disease. Lung cancer mortality rates are higher among women than men in this age group (9).

Among those aged 45 to 64, female mortality rates have been slowly declining for several decades. Male rates on the other hand were relatively stable until the mid 1970s but have fallen since. Male rates are now just over 1.5 times those of females. This is, in part, due

Figure 5.3.   Causes of Death by Age and Sex, Canada, 1997

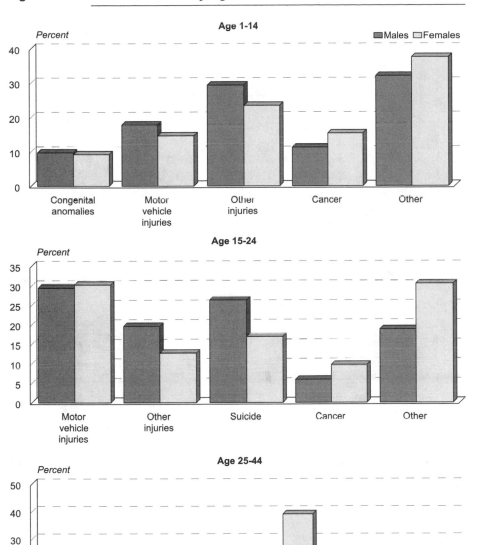

Continued

Figure 5.3.   Causes of Death by Age and Sex, Canada, 1997 (continued)

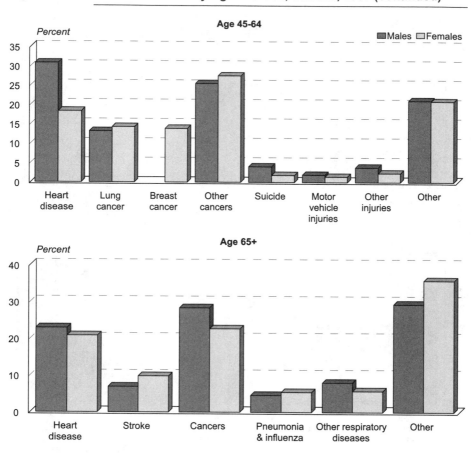

Source: Statistics Canada. *Deaths.* Ottawa, 1997. Catalogue No. 84F0209XIB.

to the decline in mortality from ischemic heart disease, the leading cause of death in men at these ages. In this age group, cancer is the leading cause of death in both men and women, followed by diseases of the circulatory system. In men, the leading causes of cancer deaths are lung followed by colorectal cancer. In women under age 55, breast cancer is the leading cause of cancer death followed by lung cancer; for women aged 55 to 64, lung cancer is the leading cause followed by breast cancer. Lung cancer mortality rates for men start to exceed those for women after age 50 (9).

Beyond age 65, there remains a wide gap between male and female death rates, with male rates remaining much higher than female rates. Male rates continue to decline but female rates appear to be stable since the mid 1980s. In this age group, the main causes of death in women under age 75 are cancer, particularly lung and breast, followed by diseases of the circulatory system, particularly ischemic heart disease and stroke. For women over age 75, circulatory diseases become the leading cause of death. In men under age 75, the leading cause of death is cancer, particularly lung and colorectal cancer, followed by diseases of circulatory system, particularly ischemic heart disease and stroke. In men over age 75, circulatory diseases are the number-one cause of death. As men age, prostate cancer becomes an important cause of mortality, becoming the second leading cause of cancer death between 75 and 84, and then the leading cause of cancer death after age 85. Respiratory illness is the third leading cause of death in men and women aged 65 to 89, but becomes the second leading cause of death after age 90 (9).

Overall Causes of Death

As listed in Table 5.1, the overall leading causes of death ranked by number of deaths for men are diseases of the circulatory system (particularly ischemic heart disease and stroke), cancer (particularly lung and prostate cancers), respiratory diseases (particularly chronic obstructive pulmonary diseases and pneumonia or influenza), injuries (particularly suicides and motor vehicle collisions), and diseases of the digestive system (particularly chronic liver disease or cirrhosis and gastrointestinal hemorrhage). For women, the five leading causes of death are diseases of the circulatory system (particularly ischemic heart disease and stroke), cancer (particularly lung and breast cancers), respiratory diseases (particularly pneumonia or influenza and chronic obstructive pulmonary diseases), injuries (particularly accidental falls and motor vehicle collisions), and diseases of the digestive system (particularly chronic liver disease or cirrhosis and non-infective enteritis and colitis) (9,10). Based on current knowledge of the etiology of these health problems, many of these deaths could be prevented or delayed by lifestyle modifications, attention to social and environmental conditions, and vaccinations. Diabetes is also important as a cause of death, as are the diseases associated with aging such as Alzheimer's disease, senile and presenile dementia, and Parkinson's disease.

Potential Years of Life Lost

For any cause of death, the PYLL is calculated by totalling the years of life remaining until a defined age (typically 70 or 75) for each person who dies of that cause between birth and that defined age. Thus, for PYLL before age 75, a person who dies at age 21 would contribute 54 years to the total. This indicator has the main effect of assessing premature mortality, which may be useful for setting priorities for prevention.

Figure 5.4 lists the main causes of PYLL before age 70 in Canada. Immediately apparent is the importance of cancer, heart diseases, suicide, and injuries. PYLL due to heart disease, suicides, and injuries are much higher for men than women, with rates for males three times, four times, and two times, respectively, as high as rates for females (2). Cancers have been the leading cause of PYLL since 1984. Suicides are the only major cause of PYLL that have increased since 1970. PYLL from heart disease, unintentional injuries, respiratory diseases, and strokes have been decreasing over the last two decades. If suicide is excluded, Canada ranked second lowest in PYLL before age 70 per 100,000 when compared to other OECD countries in 1995 (2).

Table 5.1.   Leading Causes of Death and Death Rate by Sex, Canada, 1998

Cause	Number	Percent	Rate per 100,000		
			Total	Males	Females
Cancer	60,597	27.8	200.3	216.2	184.8
Heart disease	43,029	19.7	142.3	158.1	126.7
Stroke	15,634	7.2	51.7	43.3	59.9
Other circulatory diseases	20,726	9.5	68.5	65.2	71.8
Respiratory diseases	21,833	10	72.2	76	68.5
Injuries	13,262	6.1	43.8	59.3	28.7
Diabetes mellitus	5,756	2.6	19	19.3	18.8
Alzheimer's disease	2,810	1.3	9.3	6	12.5
Dementia	2,791	1.3	9.2	6	12.4
Chronic liver disease and cirrhosis	2,166	1	7.2	9.6	4.8
Parkinson's disease	1,286	0.6	4.3	4.8	3.7
Other causes	28,199	12.9	93.2	90.6	95.8
All causes	218,089	100	721	754.4	688.4

Source: Statistics Canada. 1998. *Leading causes of death at different ages, 1998.* <www.statcan.ca/english/IPS/Data/84F0503XPB.htm> (January 2003).

1.2.3.   Morbidity

Mortality indicators, although very important, are clearly only one measure of the health status of a population. Morbidity, which is related to disease outcomes other than death, is difficult to quantify due to a relative paucity of accurate information. No single source of information reflects all morbidity, but by looking at several sources, one can gain an appreciation of the nature and extent of morbidity and detect trends. It is also important to remember that in examining a particular health problem, some aspects of morbidity may be more relevant than others. For example, time off work may

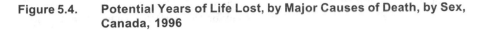

Figure 5.4. **Potential Years of Life Lost, by Major Causes of Death, by Sex, Canada, 1996**

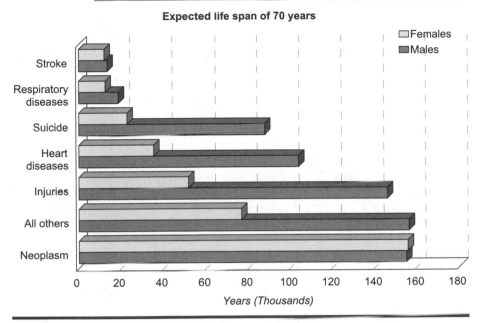

Source: Statistics Canada. *Health indicators.* Ottawa, 1999. Catalogue No. 82-221-XIE.

be a better reflection of morbidity associated with the common cold than hospital admission rates, which might more appropriately be used to assess the morbidity of bleeding duodenal ulcer; similarly, the incidence of disease is a better measure for disease with shorter duration such as streptococcal infection, whereas the prevalence of disease provides a measure of chronic diseases, such as diabetes. Each of the sources described in this section is valuable in assessing some aspect of morbidity.

Quality of Life

The concept of measuring quality of life is increasingly popular in the healthcare sector as an outcome measure of a procedure, drug, or service provided, reflecting the importance of quality not merely quantity of life and was described in Chapter 3.

Health-adjusted life expectancy (HALE) is a population health indicator that modifies life expectancy by a value-weighted index such as the Health Utility Index (see Chapter 3 for a detailed explanation of terminology and concepts). Monitoring HALE answers whether Canada is achieving the goal of the World Health Organization's Healthy People 2000, namely "to add life to years and years to life." In 1996–97, Canada's HALEs for men and women were 69.8 and 73.9 years respectively, whereas life expectancy at birth for men was 75.7 and women 81.3 years. Disability-free life expectancy at birth for both men and women combined was 68.6 years, and for men 66.9 years and women 70.2; from this one can conclude that non-institutionalized Canadians could expect to live over 90% of their lives in good health in 2000–01(11). Disability-free life expectancy at age 65 years for both sexes was 11.7 years and for men 10.9 years and for women 12.4 years in 2000–01. Although women live longer than men, they live a smaller proportion of it in good health as a result of higher prevalence of conditions such as arthritis and mental disorders (12). People living in large metropolitan areas and urban centres have the longest life expectancies and disability-free life expectancies in Canada. Each province can be divided into several regions and when data are examined at the health region level, high obesity rates, high daily smoking rates, and high rates of depression are associated with shorter disability-free life expectancies (4).

Survey results from 1996–97 indicate that other health measures related to quality of life may be improving over time. Two such measures, long-term activity limitation and disability days, appear to be better in recent cohorts than previous cohorts. In 1996–97, those aged 50 to 85 reported a significantly lower prevalence of activity limitation compared with those of the same age in 1978–79. Similarly, for disability days, both men and women aged 50 to 67 in 1996–97 reported a significantly lower number of bed-days compared to those the same age in 1978–79. Women aged 68 to 85 in 1996–97 also reported a significantly lower number of bed days compared to those the same age in 1978–79 (13).

Cancer

Although reporting cancer cases to provincial cancer registries is voluntary in some provinces, the provincial cancer agency maintains a database of potential causes of malignancies through case-control studies that allows the long-term evaluation of the effect of new therapies, early detection programs, and changes in environmental and lifestyle factors. Cancer registries are also able to give information on other health outcomes including incidence. In 2001, there were an estimated 134,000 new cases of cancer (excluding 70,000 new cases of non-melanoma skin cancer) diagnosed in Canada (see Table 5.2). Deaths from cancer in 2001 were estimated at 65,300. The leading causes of cancer mortality in men were lung, prostate, and colorectal. In women, the leading causes of cancer mortality were lung, breast, and colorectal (14). In men, prostate cancer had the highest incidence rates, followed by lung and colorectal cancers; in women, breast cancer had the highest incidence, followed by lung and colorectal cancers.

Communicable Diseases

As described in Chapter 3, selected diseases in Canada are reported to central authorities on a voluntary or mandatory basis. These centralized reports constitute an important source of information on morbidity. The disease-specific case definitions set out in the Canadian Communicable Disease Surveillance System are used for federal surveillance (15, 16). Most provinces provide annual summaries of reportable communicable diseases incorporating time trends. Most of the communicable diseases for which reporting is mandatory are reasonably well controlled, and appear in the population with low frequency (see Table 5.3). Cases of vaccine-preventable diseases, however, continue to occur, and vigilance about continued vaccination remains a requirement if rates of these diseases are to remain low. Some major sexually transmitted

Table 5.2. **Distribution of Estimated New Cases and Deaths for Major Cancer Sites, Canada, 2001**

Site	Male		Female	
	Incidence n=68,600	Mortality n=34,600	Incidence n-65,300	Mortality n=30,700
Lung	17.6	30.8	14	24
Breast	–	–	29.8	17.8
Prostate	26	12.4	–	–
Colorectal	13.5	10	12.1	9.7
Leukemias and lymphomas	8.4	7.8	7.2	7.4
Oral, larynx, esophagus	6	6.4	2.5	2.6
Pancreas	2.2	4.3	2.5	5.4
Ovary	–	–	3.9	4.9
Uterus and cervix	–	–	7.5	3.6
Stomach	2.6	3.4	1.6	2.5
Bladder	5.1	3	1.9	1.5
Kidney	3.5	2.6	2.3	1.8
Melanoma	2.9	1.4	2.8	1.1
All others	12.2	17.9	11.9	17.7

Source: National Cancer Institute of Canada. *Canadian cancer statistics 2001*. <www.ncic.ca/english/e_news/e4_news.html> (February 2003).

diseases (STDs), such as chlamydia, continue to show high incidence rates. HIV infections in Canada have shifted from occurring primarily among men who have sex with men (MSM) to injection drug users (IDUs). Between 1985–94 and 1997, new HIV diagnoses attributed to MSM decreased from 75% to 38%, while those attributed to IDUs increased from 8% to 33%. New diagnoses attributed to heterosexual transmission have also increased in this period from 7% to 22%. Cumulatively from January 1985 up to December 2001, there were 50,277 positive HIV tests, 18,034 AIDS cases, and 12,619 AIDS deaths in Canada (17).

After decades of declining rates, the incidence rates of tuberculosis (TB) in Canada have remained stable since 1987. The epidemiology in Canada has been changing due to new patterns of travel, immigration, and trade and also related to emergence of multi-drug resistance mycobacteria and comorbidity with HIV; most TB cases are now diagnosed among those born outside Canada, although TB rates are also very high in the Aboriginal population (2). The tragedy in Walkerton, Ontario, in 2000, due to a

Table 5.3.   Incidence Rate per 100,000 People of Vaccine Preventable Diseases and Notifiable Diseases in Canada, 1999

Disease category	Cases per 100,000 persons
Selected vaccine-preventable diseases	
Chicken pox	135.7
Diphtheria	0
Haemophilus influenzae type b	0.10
Measles	0.10
Mumps	0.30
Meningococcal infection	0.7
Rubella	0.08
Congenital rubella syndrome	0
Pertussis	20.0
Paralytic poliomyelitis	0
Tetanus	0
Selected notifiable diseases	
Chlamydia	138.2
Gonorrhea (1998)	17.7
Syphillis (2000)	0.3
Tuberculosis (1998)	5.9
Campylobacter	37.7
Salmonella	18.4
Giardia	17.2
Hepatitis A (1996)	2.9
Hepatitis B (1999)	4.2
Hepatitis C	63.6
Shigella	3.6
E. coli 0157	4.9
HIV/AIDS	1.4

Source: Health Canada. 2002. *Notifiable Diseases On-Line*. <cythera.ic.gc.ca/dsol/ndis/c_time_e.html> (January 2003).

water-borne outbreak of *Escherichia Coli* related to failure of a community water treatment system, once again raised the profile of enteric food-borne and water-borne diseases, and has been an important reminder of the need for continued vigilance in maintaining the environmental and public health measures necessary in the control of infectious diseases. Table 5.3 shows data from Health Canada indicating the 1999 incidence of several notifiable diseases in Canada.

Occupational Injuries and Illness

Since the advent of widespread financial compensation for injuries and illness in the working environment, the Association of Workers' Compensation Boards of Canada (AWCBC) maintains a reporting system. In 2000, there were 392,502 work injuries involving time lost from work. This amounted to a rate of 25 injuries per 1,000 workers (18). The number of reported injuries in 2000 was at an all-time low after increases were seen in the 1980s when it peaked at 48.5 injuries per 1,000 workers in 1987. The work-injury rates of men are generally higher than those of women. Young workers have higher injury rates than older workers. Forestry and logging had the highest rates of compensated injuries, but transportation, wholesale trade, manufacturing, and construction also had compensated work injury rates above average. Among the white collar sector, government and health had the highest rates of work injuries (2). According to data collected in 1994, the most common injuries were strains and sprains (which accounted for about half), contusions, and wounds. Occupational diseases are infrequent compared with injuries (see also Chapter 10) (19).

Statistics Canada has also attempted to assess workplace illness and disability through the 1996–97 NPHS and the 1997 Labour Force Survey. According to the 1996–97 NPHS, 8.9% of those aged 16 or older who had been working in 1994–95 had developed chronic back problems two years later. This was equivalent to 1 million new cases (20). The 1997 Labour Force Survey attempted to determine the absence rates for full-time paid workers in Canada, including the reasons for absence. In this 1997 survey, 3.4% of full-time employed men and 5.1% of full-time employed women (excluding women on maternity leave) were absent each week due to illness or disability, compared to 1.2% and 1.7% respectively due to personal or family responsibilities (21).

Causes of Hospitalization

General Hospitals. Hospitalization rates may vary according to availability of beds and local medical practice. However, although hospitalization data omit important information about morbidity in outpatients, they reflect the magnitude of serious illness and use of vital resources. Figure 5.5 indicates the pattern of major causes of hospitalization in general hospitals in Canada (in 1998–99) in ascending order of importance. Expressing hospitalization in terms of separations is useful for looking at the burden caused by conditions affected by frequency rather than length of stays, such as obstetrical admissions. In 1998–99, there were a total of 3 million hospital separations (22). Delivery without complication is not true morbidity but must be considered in planning for hospital services. Apart from pregnancy and childbirth, the five leading causes of hospital separations except for cancers listed as benign tumours

Figure 5.5.   Leading Causes of Discharges and Number of Days in General Hospitals, Canada, 1998–99

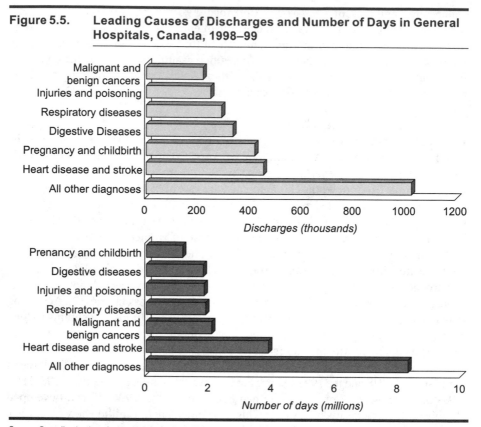

Source: Canadian Institute for Health Information. 1999. *Hospital morbidity database.* <secure.cihi.ca/cihiweb/dispPage.jsp?cw_page=services_hmdb_e> (January 2003).

are also the five leading causes of death. While not shown in the figure, mental illness is one of the leading causes of hospitalization for males accounting for 6% of total 1.2 million discharges from hospital and 11.2% of total 9.3 million days used by males (see Chapter 7).

In terms of overall hospital separations, women were more likely than men to be hospitalized. Women were more likely to be hospitalized for pregnancy and childbirth, cancer, heart disease and stroke, digestive and respiratory diseases. Men were more likely to be hospitalized for heart diseases and stroke, digestive and respiratory diseases, injury and poisoning, malignant and benign tumours, and mental disorders. Hospitalizations for respiratory diseases are highest for those under 12 and in those over 65; for injury and poisoning, hospitalizations are most common in youth 15 to 24 years old and those over age 65. Between 1990–91 and 1995–96, there was a decrease in the number and rate of hospital separations (2).

Another way of expressing hospitalization is in terms of patient days, which is useful for looking at the burden of illnesses requiring longer hospital stays. In 1998–99, Canadians spent 20.9 million days in general and allied hospitals. This represents a

Table 5.4. **Separations, Days of Care, and Average Length of Stay in Psychiatry and General Hospitals by Diagnosis, 1999–2000**

Type of mental disorder	Separations (%) n=199,308	Days of care (%) n=9,022,382	Average length of stay (days)
Senile and presenile organic conditions	4.8	13.4	126.9
Alcoholic psychosis	2.9	1.5	24.2
Schizophrenic psychosis	15.6	29.3	85
Affective psychosis	25.1	13.6	24.5
Other psychosis	10.4	10.1	44
Neurotic and personality disorders	10.2	3.1	13.7
Alcoholic dependence syndrome	5.5	1.2	9.6
Drug dependence	2.2	0.5	10.5
Mental retardation	0.3	7.0	977.5
Others/unclassified	23.0	20.3	40
Total	**100**	**100**	**45.3**

Source: Canadian Institute for Health Information. February 26, 2002

decrease from the 41.4 million patient days in hospital in 1990–91. The average length of hospital stay for 1998–99 was seven days, down from 11.5 days in 1990–91. In 1995–96, circulatory system diseases accounted for 18% of patient days, the highest number of days spent in hospital (see Figure 5.6). Most age groups had lengths of stays that were less than the average, while elderly Canadians typically had hospitalizations that lasted longer than average (23 days) (2).

Mental Hospitals. Table 5.4 illustrates the mental health problems treated in general and psychiatric hospitals in Canada (see Chapter 7). In 1995–96, affective psychoses including bipolar disorder accounted for 23% of psychiatric admissions while schizophrenia and alcohol–drug dependence accounted for 15% and 12% respectively. Across all ages, females are hospitalized more frequently than males for depressive disorders, affective psychoses, and adjustment reactions. Males are more likely than females to be hospitalized for schizophrenia and alcohol or drug dependence. Affective psychoses and alcohol or drug dependence have the highest rates of hospitalization among those aged 35 to 44, schizophrenia among those aged 25 to 44, and depressive disorders among seniors. The latter contrasts with the prevalence of outpatient depression, which declines with age (2).

Dental Morbidity

Dental illness is considered separately in this chapter in order to emphasize its significance. Dental diseases are associated with a great deal of morbidity. Dental health is important to an individual's overall health status since it can affect the functional, psychological, and social aspects of life. Dental problems are also associated with time lost from work and school (2).

The Health Promotion Survey in 1990 indicated that overall, 84% of Canadian adults reported having one or more of their natural teeth (23). This proportion was fairly consistent throughout all provinces, with the exception of Quebec, where 73% of the population were dentate. The proportion of toothless persons increased with age; 35% of those aged 55 to 64 and 50% of those over age 65 are toothless. This measure may be said to reflect dental disability and is useful in planning dental care. In 1994, 10.3% of Ontarians aged 12 years and over reported being edentulous (toothless). Gender differences were very small in each age group, with slightly more women than men living with this condition (24).

As there is no large-scale reporting by dental health professionals and hospitalization is infrequent, the only information on dental morbidity comes from studies and surveys (25-27). Dental caries and periodontal disease were assessed by means of indices based on a dental examination. The index for caries, for example, was the score for DMFT (decayed, missing, or filled teeth) or score for DEFT (decayed, extracted, or filled teeth), which identifies the number of teeth involved with caries. The rate of dental caries in elementary school children in Canada, particularly in Ontario, shows a steady long-term decline, which appears to be continuing (28). From previous studies, the Canadian average of DMFT at age 13 was 3.1. Ontario had the lowest (1.7); British Columbia (2.9) and Alberta (3.1) were in the middle; Quebec (4.2) and the Atlantic provinces (5.5) had the highest DMFT index in 13-year-old children. When Canadian DMFT rates were compared to those of other developed nations, Canadian children rated favourably. It must also be noted that the prevalence of dental morbidity was unevenly distributed, with immigrant children having the highest levels of caries: 52.4% of Canadian-born children had a DEFT/DMFT score of 0 compared to 37.6% of those born outside of Canada (28).

2.   CONSEQUENCES

The consequences of illness are personal disability, impairment, or handicap, as well as the utilization of healthcare resources in the management of the condition. There is also an economic burden that illness poses to the community. Certain aspects of the utilization of hospitals data were presented above; the utilization of health resources is described in Chapter 14.

2.1. DISABILITY

Disability as a measure of morbidity (see Chapters 1 and 3) has been defined in various ways. All definitions include the notion of the inability to carry on usual functions of living and working. All attempts subdivide disability by degree of severity. Sources of disability information include surveys, disability pension plans, and records of time lost from work due to ill health. As previously discussed, the 1997 Labour Force Survey showed that 3.4% of full-time employed men and 5.1% of full-time employed women (excluding women on maternity leave) were absent each week due to illness or disability and that days lost per worker due to illness or disability were 5.3 and 7.6 days per year for males and females respectively (29). The NPHS in 1996–97 examined short-term and long-term disability, as well as functional health status. Short-term disability was based on the individual's experience during the previous two weeks; disability days were recorded if the individual was unable to do things he or she would normally do for all or most of the day. One or more disability days were reported by 13% of Canadians in 1996–97, down from 15% of Canadians in 1994–95. However, the mean number of days in the last two weeks where disability was experienced was slightly higher than in 1994–95. Since the 1978–79 Canada Health Survey, there has been an 18% increase in the mean disability days. Since these values are not age standardized, they likely reflect the disability experienced by an aging population. Females aged 15 and older reported more disability days than males, and were somewhat more likely to report one or more days. With increasing years beyond the teens, there is also a steady increase in two-week disability days, reaching a maximum of 1.65 days for Canadians aged 75 and older. There is an inverse relation between education and income and the number of two-week disability days experienced: those with the highest income and education had the lowest disability days, while those with the lowest income and education had the highest average number of disability days (2).

Statistics Canada's 2001 Participation and Activity Limitation Survey (30) uses the World Health Organization's framework of disability provided by the International Classification of Functioning and described in Chapters 1 and 3. This framework defines disability as the relationship between body structures and functions, daily activities, and social participation, and recognizes the role of environmental factors. It considers overall functional health based on nine dimensions of functioning (vision, hearing, speech, mobility, dexterity, feelings, cognition, memory, and pain). Data described below are derived from this survey.

One out of every seven (14.6%) Canadians aged 15 and over — an estimated 3.4 million people — reported some level of disability in 2001. Disability rates increased with age; they were lowest in age group 0 to 14 years at 3.3%, 9.9% in age group 15–64, 40.5% in age group 65 and over, and highest in age group 75 and over, in which just over half of the individuals reported disabilities. In general, the disability rate was higher among women. About 1.9 million women aged 15 and over, or 15.7%, reported having a disability, compared with just over 1.5 million men (13.4%). As noted, the highest rates occurred in the group aged 65 and over, with more than one half of both men and women reporting a disability. The severity and type of disabilities individuals suffer are described in Chapter 6.

Activity limitations were reported for almost 181,000 (3.3%) children aged 14 and under. Of these, 26,000 were younger than five and about 155,000 were school aged. Almost 43% of children with disabilities had severe or very severe disabilities. Although children aged 14 and under had the lowest rates of disability, they had their own unique conditions. The most widespread disability, reported for 118,000 youngsters, was related to chronic health conditions such as asthma that reduced their activities. Learning disabilities were reported for an estimated 100,000 school-aged children (5 to 14). These children accounted for almost two-thirds of all school-aged children who reported disabilities.

2.2. PHYSICIANS' SERVICES

Since the advent of government health insurance in Canada, it has been possible to acquire information about the kinds and numbers of illnesses treated by physicians outside hospitals. National data on reasons for visits are unavailable, and provincial comparisons are difficult due to differences in reporting, but an example of data from the Saskatchewan Health Care Commission for 2001–02 is shown in Table 5.5. These data indicate that the largest numbers of services were related to health check-ups, respiratory conditions, cardiovascular and urinary conditions, rheumatic diseases, and diabetes (31). For all physicians' services, whether inside hospitals or in the community, these services accounted for approximately 45% of all visits to Saskatchewan physicians.

The 1996–97 NPHS assessed the distribution of visits to different healthcare professionals, as well as the frequency of physician visits in the preceding 12 months. Among Canadians aged 12 and over, 93% visited a healthcare professional in that period. Of these, 81% visited a general practitioner or family physician, 60% a dentist, 34% an eye specialist, 22% a specialist physician, and the remainder other professionals including chiropractors, nurses, physiotherapists, social workers, psychologists, and speech therapists (2). In terms of billed physician services, Saskatchewan data for 2001–02 showed that of the total 10.9 million services provided and billed to the health insurance plan, 65.2% of services were billed by general practitioners, followed by 6.7% by internists, 5.4% by anesthetists, 3.2% by ophthalmologists, 2.5% by pediatricians, 2.4% by obstetricians, 2.0% by general surgeons, and 1.7% each by cardiologists, psychiatrists, and otolaryngologists; the remaining 7.5% was billed by all other specialists (31).

In 1996–97, 75% of those who saw a physician made two or more visits. Most saw the family physician or general practitioner within the physician's office. In 1996–97 and 1998–99, women were more likely than men to see a physician and the proportion of Canadians who made physician visits increased with age (2, 32). Those with higher incomes were more likely to visit a health professional than those with lower incomes.

2.3. MEDICATION USE

In the 1996–97 NPHS, almost two thirds of Canadians aged 12 and over reported taking some type of medication, with 30% of Canadians overall taking three or more

Table 5.5. Utilization of Physicians' Services by Common Medical Conditions, Saskatchewan, 2001–02

Conditions	Number of services (thousands)
General medical examination	480
Acute upper respiratory infection (except influenza)	471
Hypertension	350
Diseases of genitourinary tract	317
Ischemic heart disease	236
Chronic sinusitis and other respiratory symptoms	200
Rheumatic disease	181
Diabetes mellitus	171
Arthritis	160
Otitis media	150
Psychosis	148
Asthma	145
Bronchitis	142
Neurosis	128
Eczema	122
All others	4,212
Total	7,613

Source: Saskatchewan Health, Medical Services Branch. *Annual Statistical Report 2001-02*, Government of Saskatchewan.

different types of medication at the same time This represents a large increase from 1978–79, when 48% of Canadians aged 15 and older reported using medication and only 7% reported taking three or more medications. In 1996–97, the most common form of medications taken were pain killers, followed by cough and cold remedies, then stomach remedies, and blood pressure medications. In 1998–99, 65% reported taking pain killers, 20% cough and cold medications, 10% stomach remedies, and 10% blood pressure medications. Nine percent had taken allergy medication and 8% had been on antibiotics. Women were more likely than men to be on one or two drugs but less likely to be on three or more at the same time; they were also more likely to be on antidepressant medications. Medication use increased noticeably after age 45. Among Canadians 75 and older, 46% were taking three or more drugs at the same time. Antidepressant medication and stomach remedies are used increasingly with increasing age; asthma and allergy medications were more common among the younger ages. Antidepressants, stomach remedies, and asthma medications were more commonly used among low-income than among high-income persons (2, 32).

With the advent of provincial drug plans in a number of provinces, large-scale data describing the prevalence of drug use have now become available (33). Saskatchewan's drug plan covers most of the province's population and includes annual deductibles and co-payments for benefits under the prescription drug plan. Certain classes of individuals, such as those on social assistance or residing in special care homes, are exempted from the deductible program; others pay the deductible and co-payment depending upon income, whether they are receiving seniors benefits or other benefits, or whether they need very high cost drugs. The highlights of the Drug Plan in Saskatchewan are as follows (33).

- At June 30, 2000, a total of 930,965 individuals, representing approximately 515,029 family units were eligible to receive Drug Plan benefits.
- A total of 633, 698 individual beneficiaries representing 434,591 family units purchased eligible prescriptions (those prescribed by physicians and those classified as drugs on the beneficiary list). This represents 68% of eligible individuals.
- There were 7.5 million prescriptions processed during the fiscal 12-month period.
- An average of 11.9 prescriptions were dispensed to each active beneficiary exempted from the deductible program. An average of 9.1 prescriptions were dispensed to each active beneficiary under the deductible and co-payment program.
- An average of 16.3 prescriptions were dispensed to each family unit exempt from the deductible program. An average of 13.5 prescriptions were dispensed to each family unit under the deductible program.
- Individuals who were on a special support program (69% were senior families), such as paraplegics, people with chronic renal disease, or people with cystic fibrosis, received 37.3 prescriptions to each active beneficiary and 51.0 prescriptions to each family unit.
- Four categories — central nervous system drugs, anti-infectives, cardiovascular drugs, and hormones and substitutes — accounted for 69.3% of all prescriptions and 61.2% of all Drug Plan payments.
- The average number of prescriptions per active beneficiary was 11.9 and it increased with age: there were 3.3 prescriptions for people aged 0 to 4 years and 33.4 for people aged 85 and over.
- The average drug cost of a prescription was $22.36.

2.4.   USE OF DENTAL CARE SERVICES

Oral diseases and dental problems are largely preventable, and regular check-ups (one visit in a one- to two-year period) are important for dental health. Dental visits, however, are largely determined by the ability to pay for services. Visits to the dentist tend to increase with increased household income. Dental insurance coverage was strongly associated with household income, with 70% of those at the highest income level having dental insurance compared to 23% of those at the lowest incomes (34). According to the 1998–99 NPHS, 56% of Canadians aged 15 or older had dental insurance. However, only 25% of those aged 65 and older had dental insurance coverage (16).

In 1998–99, 60% of Canadians 12 year of age and older had visited a dentist or orthodontist in the year before the survey. The rates of contact with dental care professionals were highest among the young (84% of 12 to 14 year olds) and decreased with age (40% of those aged 65 and older). Except for those over 65, females had higher contact rates than males. Contact with a dentist was also higher among urban residents (61%) compared to rural residents (54%). The proportion of the population aged 15 and older who have contact with a dentist has increased from 48% in 1978–79 to 61% in 1998–99 (16).

The reasons that people seek dental care varied with household income. In 1996–97, only 36% of those with the lowest incomes cited cleaning and fluoride treatment as a reason for visiting the dentist, compared to 48% in the highest income group. In contrast, 25% of those in the lowest income group went to a dentist for a filling or tooth extraction, compared to 13% of those with the highest incomes. Overall, the following reasons were cited for visiting a dentist: for cleaning, fluoride, or maintenance (43%), to ensure there are no problems (36%), to take care of teeth, gums, or dentures (20%), for a filling or extraction (17%), to maintain good dental health (12%), because the check-up is insured (9%), or to catch problems early (5%) (the total does not add up to 100% as some individuals gave multiple responses)(34).

The reasons for not seeking dental care varied with income and dental insurance coverage. Among those with the lowest incomes, 20% mentioned cost, compared to 10% of those with the highest incomes; 22% of the uninsured mentioned cost, compared to 6% of those with dental insurance. Pain and embarrassment were more commonly cited as reasons for avoiding a dental visit among those with high incomes and dental insurance compared with those of low income or without dental coverage (34).

2.5. ECONOMIC BURDEN

The total economic burden of ill health is associated with both direct costs related to health expenditures and indirect costs such as disability, time lost from work, and costs related to premature death. Health expenditures, or direct health-related spending, refer to expenditures for which the primary objective is to improve or prevent the deterioration of health status. They include public and private sector spending on personal health care, and public spending for public health and administration of the healthcare system. Health expenditures over time are related to population growth, utilization per capita, and increased prices associated with health goods and services. Health expenditures can be grouped into seven major uses: hospitals, physicians, drugs, other professionals, other institutions, capital, and other health spending. Per capita expenditure is useful for comparisons over time because it removes the effect of population growth on total costs.

Figure 5.6.   Cost of Illness by Major Disease by Category, Canada, 1998

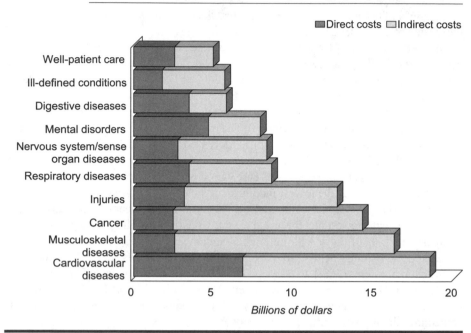

Source: Health Canada. 2002. *Economic burden of illness in Canada, 1998.* <www.hc-sc.gc.ca/pphb-dgspsp/publicat/ebic-femc98/index.html> (November 2002).

In terms of total economic burden of ill health that takes into account direct as well as indirect costs, estimates for Canada in 1998 were $159.4 billion (compared to $97 billion in 1986 and $156.9 billion for 1993), of which 52.7% or $83.9 billion were direct costs and 47.3% or $75.5 billion were indirect (Figure 5.6) (35). Of the total expenditures in 1998, the leading causes in the category of direct expenditure were hospital care costs (17.3%) and professional services (13.3%); professional services include medical (7.3%) and other healthcare practitioner services (5.0%). Drug costs accounted for 7.8% of total costs. Expenditures for care in other institutions accounted for 5.0% and additional direct health expenditures, which include other professionals, capital expenses, public health, health research, etc., accounted for 15.2%. In the category of indirect costs, premature mortality accounted for 21.0% of the total cost and morbidity costs due to long-term disability 20.2%. The remainder of the indirect costs covered short-term disability (6.2%).

The top five most costly diseases in Canada in 1998 were cardiovascular disease, musculoskeletal diseases, cancer, injuries, and respiratory diseases (see Figure 5.6). These conditions accounted collectively for more than half (55.8%) of the total costs. Cardiovascular disease was the leading cause of both direct ($6.8 billion) and indirect costs ($11.7 billion), making it the most expensive category overall. Musculoskeletal disorders and cancer ranked next (total cost of $16.4 and $14.2 billion respectively), followed by injuries (total cost of $12.7 billion). Overall, chronic conditions were responsible for the major economic burden.

3. SUMMARY

The health status indicators related to sense of well-being, mortality and morbidity and ensuing disability and economic burden are the most commonly used measures of health in Canada.

Overall age-standardized mortality rates declined steadily between 1950 and 1997 for both males and females. The trend in age- and sex-specific death rates between 1951 and 1998 indicates that over this period death rates have been declining at different rates for different age groups. Among those under 1 year of age, there has been a steady decline in mortality rates. In 1998, the infant mortality rate per 1,000 live births fell for the first time below 6 to 5.6 per 1,000 live births. The main causes of these deaths were perinatal complications, followed by congenital anomalies and sudden infant death syndrome. Between 1 and 14 years of age, mortality rates continue to decline slowly. In 1998, the leading cause of death in this age group was injuries, which are largely preventable. While deaths due to most external causes and diseases have declined considerably, between 1971 and 1996, the rate of suicide among those aged 10 to 14 has nearly tripled. Among those aged 15 to 24, the most significant causes of death are injuries due to motor vehicle collisions and suicide. Recently, there has been a significant drop in the death rate for this age group, particularly for males.

Among those aged 25 to 44, the decline in mortality rates that began in the 1970s has continued. Male mortality rates in this age group are about double the female rates. In males, the leading causes of death are suicides and motor vehicle collisions throughout this age group. In females, the leading causes of death are suicides and motor vehicle collisions in those under 35 and cancers of the breast and then lung in those 35 to 44. Excess male mortality is due largely to the much higher numbers of deaths from suicides, motor vehicle collisions, and ischemic heart disease.

Female and male mortality rates have been declining among those aged 45 to 64. Male rates are now just over 1.5 times those of females. In this age group, cancer is the leading cause of death in both men and women, followed by diseases of the circulatory system.

Beyond age 65, there remains a wide gap between male and female death rates, with male rates remaining much higher than female rates. Male rates continue to decline but female rates appear to be stable since the mid 1980s. The major causes of death for both men and women are circulatory system diseases (including ischemic heart disease and strokes), cancers, and respiratory illnesses.

The overall leading causes of death ranked by number of deaths for both men and women are diseases of the circulatory system, cancer, respiratory diseases, injuries, and diseases of the digestive system. Based on current knowledge of the etiology of these health problems, many of these deaths could be prevented or delayed by lifestyle modifications, attention to social and environmental conditions, and vaccinations. Lung cancer is the most frequent cause of cancer death in both males and females; lung cancer exceeded breast cancer as the leading cause of cancer death in women in 1997. Diabetes is also important as a cause of death, as are the diseases associated with aging such as Alzheimer's disease, senile and presenile dementia, and Parkinson's disease.

No single source of information reflects all morbidity. There are several useful sources of information for assessing different aspects of overall morbidity. For example, communicable disease information is obtained through mandatory reporting of disease to public health authorities. Most of these communicable diseases are reasonably well controlled; however, vigilance about continued vaccination remains a requirement if rates of vaccine-preventable diseases are to remain low. Continued vigilance is required to maintain the environmental and public health measures necessary in the control of enteric food-borne and water-borne infectious diseases. Some of the major sexually transmitted diseases, such as chlamydia, continue to show high incidence rates. The epidemiology of tuberculosis in Canada has been changing due to new patterns of travel, immigration, and trade. With regard to occupational injuries, data collected from workers' compensation for such injuries provide important information related to their morbidity. Forestry and logging had the highest rates of compensated injuries, but transportation, wholesale trade, manufacturing, and construction also had above-average compensated work injury rates. Another aspect of morbidity that has been documented is hospitalization. Excluding pregnancy and childbirth, the five leading causes of hospital separations are also the five leading causes of death overall. Although mental illness is not a leading cause of mortality, it is one of the leading causes of hospitalization, both in terms of numbers of separations but also, more importantly, in terms of patient days spent in hospital. In 1998-99, circulatory system diseases accounted for the highest number of days spent in hospital, followed by cancer. Morbidity is also associated with dental disease. Dental caries in elementary school children has been declining steadily.

The consequences of illness are disability, impairment, or handicap, as well as the utilization of healthcare resources and economic burden to the community. Since 1978–79, there has been an increase in the mean short-term disability days, likely reflecting the disability experienced by an aging population. In 2001, 3.6 million Canadians (12.4%) aged 12 and older reported a long-term disability or handicap or limitation due to a health problem. The main causes of long-term disability were musculoskeletal disorders (particularly back muscle problems) and nervous system conditions (including vision and hearing difficulties). Increased short- and long-term disability rates were associated with being female, increased age, and lower education and income.

The total economic burden of ill health is associated with both direct costs (related to health expenditures) and indirect costs (such as disability, time lost from work, and costs related to premature death). Hospitals and physicians are associated with the highest health expenditures in terms of total economic burden of ill health that takes into account direct as well as indirect costs. Estimates for Canada from 1998 were $159.4 billion, of which $83.9 billion were direct and $75.4 billion were indirect costs. Premature mortality, chronic disability, and short-term disability accounted for much of the indirect costs. Cardiovascular disease was the leading cause of both direct and indirect costs.

4.   REFERENCES

1.   Canadian Centre for Health Information. *Health Indicators*. Ottawa: Statistics Canada, 1991.
2.   Federal, Provincial, and Territorial Advisory Committee on Population Health. 1999. *Statistical report on the health of Canadians*. Ottawa. <www.statcan.ca/english/freepub/82-570-XIE/free.htm> (November 2002).
3.   Kohn R. *Royal Commission on Health Services: The health of the Canadian people*. Ottawa: Queen's Printer, 1967.
4.   Statistics Canada. How healthy are Canadians? 2002 annual report. *Health Reports* 2002; 13(supplement). <www.statcan.ca/english/IPS/Data/82-003-SIE2002001.htm> (January 2003).
5.   Nault F, Wilkins K. Deaths 1993. *Health Reports* 1995; 7(1):51-60.
6.   Statistics Canada. How healthy are Canadians? *Health Reports* 1999; 11(3):1-119.
7.   Statistics Canada. Death: Shifting trends in how healthy are Canadians. *Health Reports* 2000; 12(3):41-6.
8.   Statistics Canada. How healthy are Canadians? Annual report 2002. *Health Reports* 2000; 12(3):1-110. <www.statcan.ca/english/freepub/82-003-SIE/free.htm> (January 2003).
9.   Statistics Canada. 1998. *Leading causes of death at different ages, 1998*. <www.statcan.ca/english/IPS/Data/84F0503XPB.htm> (January 2003).
10.   D'Cunha C. 2002. *2002 Chief Medical Officer of Health Report—Injury: Predictable and preventable*. <www.gov.on.ca/health/english/pub/ministry/injury_rep02/injury_mn.html> (November 2002).
11.   Statistics Canada. 2002. *Data tables*. Health Indicators, vol. 2002, no. 1. <www.statcan.ca/english/freepub/82-221-XIE/00502/tables.htm> (January 2003).
12.   Manuel D, Schultz S. *Adding life to years and years to life: Life and health expectancy in Ontario*. Toronto: Institute for Clinical Evaluative Sciences, 2001.
13.   Chen J, Millar W. Are recent cohort healthier than their predecessors? *Health Reports* 2000; 11(4):9-24.
14.   Canadian Cancer Society. 2001. *Canadian cancer statistics 2001*. <www.ncic.cancer.ca/pubse.htm> (November 2002).
15.   Health and Welfare Canada. Canadian Communicable Disease Surveillance System: Disease-specific case definitions and surveillance methods. *Canadian Disease Weekly Report* 1991; 17(Supplement 13):35-6.
16.   Statistics Canada. Health care services: recent trends. *Health Reports* 1999; 11(3):91-109.
17.   Health Canada. 2002. *HIV and AIDS in Canada*. <www.hc-sc.gc.ca/pphb-dgspsp/publicat/aids-sida/haic-vsac0602/pdf/haic-vsac0602.pdf> (February 2003).
18.   Association of Workers' Compensation Boards of Canada. *Work injuries and diseases, 1998-2000*. Mississauga: Association of Workers' Compensation Boards of Canada, 2001.
19.   Statistics Canada. *Work injuries, 1992-1994*. Ottawa: Government of Canada, 1995.
20.   Perez C. Chronic back problems among workers. *Health Reports* 2000; 12(1):41-55.
21.   Akyeampong E. Work absence: new date, new insights. *Perspectives on Labour and Income* 1998; 10(1):16-21.
22.   Canadian Institute for Health Information. 1999. *Hospital morbidity database*. <secure.cihi.ca/cihiweb/dispPage.jsp?cw_page=services_hmdb_e> (January 2003).
23.   Statistics Canada. *Health Promotion Survey, 1990*. Ottawa: Minister of Supply and Services, 1993.
24.   Jokovic A, Locker D. *Oral health status of Ontarians aged twelve years and over*. North York, ON: North York Public Health Department, 1995.
25.   Public Health Branch. *Dental health indices, 1987/88 survey*. Toronto: Ontario Ministry of Health, 1991.

26.   Payette M, Brodeur JM, Lepage Y, *et al. Enquête Santé Dentaire Québec, 1989-90.* Montreal: Département de la Santé commautaire, Hôpital Saint-Luc, 1991.

27.   Gray H, Gunther D. *A comprehensive review of dental caries experience shown by grade 7 students in the provincial health units of British Columbia.* Victoria: Dental Health Branch, Minister of Health, Government of British Columbia, 1987.

28.   Mair P. Preliminary findings from the 1994 Ontario Children's Dental Health Survey. *Canadian Journal of Community Dentistry* 1995; 10(2):38-43.

29.   Statistics Canada. 2003. *Days lost per worker due to illness or disability by sex, Canada and provinces.* <www.statcan.ca/english/Pgdb/health47c.htm> (January 2003).

30.   Statistics Canada. 2002. *A profile of disability in Canada, 2001: Tables.* <www.statcan.ca/english/IPS/Data/89-579-XIE.htm> (January 2003).

31.   Saskatchewan Health, Medical Services Branch. 2002. *Annual Statistical Report 2001-2002.* <www.health.gov.sk.ca/Report.pdf> (January 2003).

32.   Statistics Canada. Health care/self care. *Health Reports* 2001; 12(3):33-8. <www.statcan.ca/english/freepub/82-003-XIE/art3.pdf> (January 2003).

33.   Saskatchewan Health, Drug Plan and Extended Benefits Branch. 2002. *Annual Statistical Report 2000-01.* <formulary.drugplan.health.gov.sk.ca/publications/2000-2001%20Annual%20Report.pdf> (January 2003).

34.   Millar W, Locker D. Dental insurance and use of dental services. *Health Reports* 1999; 11(1):55-65.

35.   Health Canada. 2002. *Economic burden of illness in Canada, 1998.* <www.hc-sc.gc.ca/pphb-dgspsp/publicat/ebic-femc98/index.html> (November 2002).

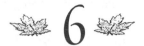

6

THE HEALTH OF
VULNERABLE GROUPS

The previous two chapters outlined the determinants of health, health status, and consequences in the Canadian population as a whole. This chapter examines the health of certain vulnerable groups in Canadian society: Aboriginal peoples, seniors, poor children, and people with disabilities. The health of each of these groups reflects the influence of the determinants of health. For the first three groups, the determinants are race and age as well as physical, psychosocial, socioeconomic, and environmental factors. The fourth group, people with disabilities, has been chosen as an example of how the determinants of health frequently interact and compound further the inequities in health relative to the rest of the population.

1.   THE HEALTH OF ABORIGINAL PEOPLES

According to the census, Aboriginal peoples, also known as the First Nations peoples or Native Canadians, fall into four groups; Status Indians, non-Status Indians, Métis, and Inuit. "Status Indian" has specific legal connotations and is defined as Aboriginal peoples registered under the *Indian Act* (1). This group has signed treaties with the federal government that accord them certain privileges to be compensated for having relinquished certain land rights. Four centuries of colonization — being subjugated and stripped of their land, religion, culture, language, and autonomy — have taken their toll on the physical, mental, emotional, spiritual, and cultural health of the Aboriginal communities. Today's determinants of health reflect these injustices.

Aboriginal people define health and illness in terms of balance, harmony, holism, and spirituality rather than in terms of the western concepts of physical dysfunction and disease within the individual (2). Some First Nations refer to this concept as the "medicine wheel," a holistic wheel consisting of the four quadrants or components of health: physical, mental, emotional, and spiritual. For achieving health, there must be harmony among all these components.

Unless otherwise indicated, the information in this section comes from *A Second Diagnostic on the Health of First Nations and Inuit People in Canada* (3). Interested readers are advised to read other publications listed in the end notes (2, 4-6).

Because of limitations related to health determinants and status information on the Métis and non-Status Indian populations, this section will focus primarily on the health information available for those registered as First Nations and Inuit. There is generally less information available about off-reserve Aboriginal people except for recent publications by Statistics Canada and others, which indicate the health and health determinants of these populations to be poor compared with other Canadian populations (7-10).

1.1.   DEMOGRAPHY

The beginning of the 20th century represents the lowest point in the size of the population of Aboriginal people in Canada, with subsequent steady recovery since then, so that today it is at its highest level post-Confederation. (11). The 2001 census, which asked respondents to specify whether they were North American Indian, Métis, or Inuit, found that 976,305 or 3.3% of Canadians reported that they were Aboriginal compared with 2.8% or 799,010 five years ago (12). Of these, 608,850 (62%) people were North American Indian, 292,310 (30%) were Métis, and 45,070 (5%) were Inuit, and the remainder 3% identified themselves with more than one Aboriginal group.

This population growth is due to a natural increase. The crude birth rate per 1,000 population declined from 44.3 in 1965 to 27.3 in 1993, but in 2000 the fertility rate among the Aboriginal population was still 50% higher than the general Canadian population. Similarly, Aboriginal death rates remain higher than the rates for other Canadians. In 1996–97, First Nations and Inuit people throughout Canada had mortality rates at about 1.5 times the national mortality rate. Although life expectancy increased about 10 years between 1975 and 2000, life expectancy at birth was 68.9 years in 2000 for Registered Indian males and 76.3 years for females, substantially lower than the life expectancy of 76.3 years for Canadian males and 81.5 years for females. The high birth rate of Aboriginal people, coupled with a consistently lower life expectancy, ensures a relatively young population compared to the general population. In 2001, the median age of the Aboriginal population was 24.7 years compared with 37.7 years in the general population: 33.2% were aged 0 to 14 years and 4.1% were aged 65 years and over, compared to 19.1% and 12.9%, respectively, for the general Canadian population. Although the Aboriginal population accounted for only 3.3% of Canada's total population, Aboriginal children represented 5.6% of all children in Canada. The gender distribution (a ratio of 49 men to 51 females) is approximately the same as for all Canadians.

Of the total Aboriginal population in 2001, 19.3% lived in Ontario, 8.1% in Quebec, 5.4% in the Atlantic region, and 67.3% lived in the four western provinces. Ontario had the highest absolute number (188,315) of Aboriginal people accounting for less than 2% of its total population, followed by British Columbia with 170,025 people or 4.4% of its population. However, when viewed as a percentage of the total provincial or territorial population, Aboriginal peoples constituted 85% of Nunavut, 51% of the Northwest Territories, and 23.0% in the Yukon Territory. Ontario had more North American Indians than any other province. Alberta had the largest Métis population, while Nunavut had the largest Inuit population. In 2001, almost half (49.0%) of the Aboriginal people lived in urban areas; 31% lived on Indian reserves and settlements and the remainder (20%)

lived in rural non-reserve areas. There are approximately 2,284 reserves in Canada. In 2001, 25% of all Aboriginal people lived in 10 of the nation's 27 census metropolitan areas; Winnipeg had the greatest number (55,755), followed by Edmonton, Vancouver, Calgary, Toronto, Saskatoon, Regina, Ottawa-Hull, Montreal, and Victoria.

1.2. DETERMINANTS

1.2.1. Psychosocial and Socioeconomic Environment

Family violence is an important psychosocial issue faced by many Aboriginal communities. Results of four studies show that at least 75% of Aboriginal women have been victims compared with 7% of Canadian women. Up to 40% of children in some northern First Nations communities have been abused by a family member, and elder abuse has also been identified as a serious problem in some First Nations communities.

The socioeconomic environment, indicated by education, employment, and income, is an important predictor of the health status of a population. In 1996, 54% of the Aboriginal population, compared with 35% of the non-Aboriginal population, had not completed high school. Compared to 16% of the non-Aboriginal population, only 4.5% of the Aboriginal population had a university degree. However, there has been some improvement among those at younger ages: for those in their 20s, an increased percentage of people have completed a non-university post-secondary diploma or degree (from 19% in 1981 to 23% in 1996); for on-reserve students, there has been an increase in the number remaining until Grade 12 for consecutive years of schooling (from 37% in 1987–88 to 74% in 1997–98).

Among First Nations people living on reserves, the unemployment rate was 29% in 1997–98, triple the national unemployment rate at the time. Forty-six percent of First Nations people on reserves rely on social assistance, a rate four times higher than the general Canadian population. As has been discussed elsewhere in this chapter, incomes on social assistance typically fall far below the low-income cut-off (LICO) set by Statistics Canada. **LICO** is defined by Statistics Canada as those whose family spends 54.7% or more of its gross income on food, shelter, and clothing creating economic hardship and strained living circumstances.

In addition to high unemployment rates, in 1995 one third of employed Aboriginal people 15 and older (compared to 25% of non-Aboriginal Canadians) worked in some of the lowest paying occupations, and the percentage of those employed in management positions was 1.5 times lower than those who were non-Aboriginal. In 1995, the mean income of employed Aboriginal people was 50% lower than the national average. Average earnings of Aboriginal people on reserves were lower than those of Aboriginal people not living on reserves. Forty-four percent of Aboriginal people have incomes falling below the LICO, compared with 20% of the total Canadian population. Twice as many Aboriginal children live in single-parent or low-income families as other Canadian children (32%). Although they constitute only 3% of the Canadian population, Aboriginal people account for 16% of the sentences to correctional facilities.

On and off reserves, relative homelessness has been well documented by both government and other sources including the Royal Commission on Aboriginal Peoples

(13). With high prevalence of the risk factors for homelessness — high unemployment, welfare dependency, poverty, substance abuse, physical and mental health problems, and domestic and sexual abuse — Aboriginal people have been identified to be the group perhaps most at risk for becoming homeless in Canada. Many Aboriginal people alternate between living on the reserve in the summer and in the city in the winter, leading to problems associated with consistent housing in the city.

1.2.2.   Physical Environment

Crowded living conditions are associated with increased risks of transmission of a number of infectious diseases including tuberculosis, hepatitis A, and shigellosis. In 1991, the average number of people per occupied private dwelling for on-reserve Registered Indians was 4.1, compared to 2.7 for the total Canadian population. Only 1% of Canadian dwellings had more than one person per room compared with 22% of on-reserve dwellings.

Housing condition is also an important determinant of health. Inefficient ventilation systems and high humidity can promote the growth of moulds, which has recently been identified in Aboriginal housing as a problem , that can induce respiratory and immune system illnesses. The availability of adequate water supplies and sewage disposal is important in the control of infectious diseases. Housing on reserves appears to be improving (from 46% in 1991–92 to 54% in 1997–98); however, nearly half the houses are still inadequate in terms of needing major repairs, having poor ventilation, and being overcrowded.

Environmental contaminants such as polychlorinated biphenyls (PCBs) and mercury can accumulate in fish and marine mammals, and ingestion of high levels of these compounds within such food sources can pose health risks to children (particularly the developing fetus and newborns). First Nations and Inuit people are considered at higher risk for exposure because of their traditional diets (see Chapter 9). In studies on Inuit from Quebec and Nunavut and on the Montagnais in Quebec, the amount of PCBs and mercury in infants' bodies has been found to be much higher than in other infants from similar areas and to be above the thresholds for cognitive and neurological impairments. In another study amongst the Cree in James Bay, mercury levels were high in a much smaller proportion of the population in 1993 (2.7%) than in 1988 (14.2%). The issue of environmental contaminant exposure through traditional food sources is complex because game meat and fish are important sources of nutrients, are a healthier diet (compared to processed non-traditional foods), and contribute to cultural and spiritual bonds for the Aboriginal people.

1.2.3.   Lifestyle and Behavioural Risk Factors

Smoking

In 1997, First Nations and Labrador Inuit people 15 years old and over smoked at a rate of 62%, more than double the general smoking rate of the Canadian population (29%). First Nations and Labrador Inuit smokers begin smoking very early in life (at six to eight years of age) and show a rapid increase in initiation at ages 11 and 12.

Alcohol and Substance Abuse

Alcohol and substance abuse, including the abuse of solvents, is considered a major problem within many Aboriginal communities. Information from addiction treatment centres, hospitalizations for alcohol-related causes, and violent deaths (e.g., suicides) have shown that alcohol is the abused drug of choice among Aboriginal Canadians. There are also more severe consequences of alcohol and substance abuse. Risks for alcohol-related problems are two to six times higher in Aboriginal youth than non-Aboriginal youth. Binge and chronic drinking are a problem among Aboriginal people and lead to risks of fetal alcohol syndrome (FAS) or fetal alcohol effects (FAE) in pregnancy. The incidence of FAS and FAE are variously reported in range of 100 cases per 1,000 births in Aboriginal communities, compared with 0.33 for FAS in western countries. Aboriginal men may be more likely to abuse alcohol; Aboriginal women may be more likely to abuse other drugs alone.

Drug abuse also constitutes an important problem. In the Northwest Territories, Aboriginal people 15 and older were 3 to 3.5 times more likely than non-Aboriginal people to have used illicit drugs such as marijuana, hashish, LSD, speed, cocaine, crack, or heroin. Use of solvents and non-beverage alcohol (such as rubbing alcohol) is also a major problem among Aboriginal youths, with 20% having used solvents and with one third of users under 15 years of age. In the Northwest Territories, Aboriginal people 15 and older had 11 times the risk of having used solvents compared to the non-Aboriginal population and 24 times the risk compared to the general Canadian population.

Problem Gambling

Problem gambling may be an increasing problem among Aboriginal youth and adults. In Alberta, almost half of the Aboriginal students in grades 5 to 12 who participated in a study were either problem gamblers or at risk of becoming one. Another Alberta study in 1994 found that 22% of Aboriginal people aged 15 and older were problem gamblers, 40% were moderate pathological gamblers, and 15% were severe pathological gamblers.

Nutrition

Many Aboriginal people in Canada, particularly in remote communities, experience all or most aspects of food insecurity due to low incomes, safety risks due to pollutants in the traditional food supply, quality problems associated with inappropriate shipping, handling, and home preparation of commercial foods, and disruptions to access caused by interruptions in shipping or changes in animal migratory patterns. More and more Aboriginal people are turning to commercial foods, which are more expensive and not always as nutrient-dense as traditional foods. The cost of commercial food is high, as is the cost of supplies for fishing and hunting (14).

Physical Activity

With the reduction in fishing, hunting, and trapping that has accompanied acculturation and the loss of traditional ways of life, Aboriginal people now lead much more sedentary lives. According to the 1994–95 National Population Health Survey, 20% of Aboriginal residents in Northern Canada had active leisure time activities, compared to about 28% of non-Aboriginal northern residents (15).

Body Mass Index

The combination of genetic factors, changes in diet, and physical inactivity has led to a high prevalence of overweight among First Nations people. In a study of Northern Ontario residents, 29% of youth aged 5 to 19 and 60% of adult women were obese. Another study of adult Cree and Ojibwa in Northern Canada found a higher prevalence of overweight in the Aboriginal compared to the non-Aboriginal population; almost 90% of women aged 45 to 54 had a body mass index of 26 or over. Fat distribution in Aboriginal peoples tends to occur primarily in the abdominal area, which is associated with increased risks for a number of chronic diseases including hypertension, coronary heart disease, stroke, premature death, breast cancer, and type 2 diabetes and its complications such as renal failure and blindness (16).

Sexual Practices

According to the Ontario First Nations Healthy Lifestyle Survey in 1993 (17), two out of every five males and one out of every five females reported multiple sexual partners in the 12 months prior to the survey; 15% of respondents reported having sexual partners both within and outside the community; 60% of respondents reported having unprotected sexual intercourse at least some of the time, and only 13% of respondents reported protected intercourse only. About two thirds of Aboriginal women surveyed by the Aboriginal Nurses Association of Canada indicated that they did not use condoms (18). Condom use and the consistency of use were associated with learning about sex from family and through health services (17).

1.2.4.   Healthcare Organizations

The federal government is responsible for the health care of Aboriginal peoples on reserves, and the provincial government for those off the reserves (see Chapter 13 for details). Different legislative acts, federal reports, and Supreme Court decisions have shaped the federal health policy for Aboriginal people and are well outlined in the Kirby report (2). Two thirds of Aboriginal peoples live in rural or remote areas, where healthcare services are often provided by nurses or community health workers supplemented by visits from physicians. In the 1994–95 NPHS, only 50% of those from the Northwest Territories and the Yukon had seen a general practitioner, compared with 77% from the provinces. Aboriginal northerners were much more likely to have seen a nurse (41% versus 18%). Aboriginal northerners were less likely to have seen a dentist than non-Aboriginal northerners (15).

Admission rates for general and mental hospitals, usually located at great distances from the communities themselves, are high compared with other Canadian rates. In 1996–97, data from the Prairies indicated that First Nations people had a hospitalization rate 2.5 times that of the general Canadian population.

Immunization

First Nations 2-year-olds living on reserves were found to have lower vaccination coverage than the 2-year-olds in the rest of Canada in 1997. Immunization rates in 2- and 6-year-old Aboriginal children have also been found to be well below the national immunization target rates of coverage. This is an important issue, especially when combined with some of the issues related to housing and living conditions (e.g., crowding) on reserves that facilitate infectious disease transmission.

Geographic isolation also makes it difficult to provide appropriate services to northern communities. The priorities set by Aboriginal people are frequently at variance with those developed by the government, and many strategies for delivering health programs are inappropriate. However, in recent years, many Aboriginal communities have assumed the administration and management of health care in their own communities.

1.3.   HEALTH STATUS AND CONSEQUENCES

1.3.1.   Mortality

Despite a decline in Aboriginal mortality, the gap in mortality between the Aboriginal and the general Canadian population remains wide. In 1996–97, mortality rates among First Nations and Inuit people from Eastern and Western Canada and the Prairie provinces were almost 1.5 times higher than the national rate (3).

Infant Mortality

In 1995–97, infant mortality rates among First Nations people in Eastern and Central Canada, the Prairie provinces, and British Columbia were up to 3.5 times the national infant mortality rates. Neonatal death rates were up to double the general Canadian rates, while post-neonatal mortality rates were up to almost four times higher, contributing high infant mortality rates. The common post-neonatal mortality causes are infectious diseases, respiratory diseases, sudden infant death syndrome (SIDS), and injuries. The relative risk of Indian children dying of SIDS is approximately three times higher than for non-Indian children (6).

Causes of Death

In 1996, for Canada as a whole, the four leading causes of death were circulatory diseases, neoplasm, respiratory diseases, and injuries (19). The leading causes vary among different Aboriginal populations in Canada: in the Atlantic provinces and Quebec, the leading causes were circulatory system diseases followed by cancer, then injuries and poisonings. In the Prairies and British Columbia, the leading causes were injuries and poisonings, followed by circulatory system diseases and then cancer. Overall, among all Aboriginal peoples in Canada, between 1979 and 1993, the four leading causes of death in order of decreasing frequency were unchanged: injury and poisoning, diseases of the circulatory system, cancer, and diseases of the respiratory system.

Although there has been an overall improvement in mortality rates from injury and poisoning, in 1996–97 First Nations and Inuit people were 6.5 times more likely to die of injuries and poisoning than the total Canadian population. The suicide risk among Registered Indians also varies by age and community, but is generally 2.5 times that of the general Canadian population (19). In 1994, the suicide rate for Aboriginal people aged 15 to 24 was up to eight times higher than that of other Canadian youth (20).

Potential-Years-of-Life-Lost

In 1996, the main causes of potential years of life lost (PYLL) among the Canadian population were cancer followed by injuries and then cardiovascular diseases (20). In 1997, data from Western Canada show injuries and poisonings to be the leading causes of PYLL among the Aboriginal population. In 1993, Aboriginal PYLL was two times higher than that of the general Canadian population. In addition to injuries and poisonings, sudden infant death syndrome, congenital anomalies, and perinatal conditions were important causes of PYLL among Aboriginal people in 1993.

1.3.2.   Morbidity

Infectious Diseases

A variety of infectious diseases are found at higher incidence and prevalence in the Aboriginal population. Botulism, sometimes fatal, occurs in Aboriginal (and more frequently, Inuit) communities due to ingestion of fermented marine mammal meat, raw or parboiled fish, or salmon eggs. Since 1994, AIDS cases have been declining in the general Canadian population; in the Aboriginal Canadian population, however, the number of AIDS cases has risen dramatically. In 1997, the prevalence of AIDS in Aboriginal Canadians (33.2 per 100,000) was 11 times the national rate of 3.1 per 100,000. Injection drug use was responsible for 19% of AIDS cases in Aboriginal men and 50% in Aboriginal women.

Tuberculosis (TB) is also an important issue in the Aboriginal population. Although incidence rates have decreased between 1991 and 1996, with an average decline of 7% per year, the age-standardized incidence rate in Status Indians (35.8 per 100,000) greatly exceeds that of Canadian-born non-Aboriginal persons (2 per 100,000) (21). In 1996, the incidence rate of TB among persons living on reserves was 40 per 100,000. In 1996, the highest provincial TB incidence rate in the Aboriginal population was in Saskatchewan (105 per 100,000).

The increase in AIDS cases seen among Aboriginal persons has important implications for TB because infection with HIV is a risk factor for active TB. Crowded living conditions, which are prevalent on reserves or in homeless shelters, aid the transmission of infectious diseases including TB. Data from Western Canada show that 42% of TB cases in Aboriginal people are due to recent infection compared to 12% of cases in the general Canadian population (with the remainder of active cases due to reactivation of old infection). The movement of many Aboriginal people between reserves and inner city locations adds to the challenges of control in terms of spread of disease geographically and because such movement has been identified as a risk factor for defaulting on treatment (21).

Table 6.1.   **Comparison of Age-Adjusted Prevalence of Chronic Conditions in First Nations and Inuit and the General Canadian Population**

| Chronic condition | Gender | Age-Adjusted Prevalence (%) | | Ratio of First Nations and Labrador Inuit to Canadian population |
		First Nations and Labrador Inuit	General Canadian population	
Heart problems	Male	13	4	3.3
	Female	10	4	2.5
Hypertension	Male	22	8	2.8
	Female	25	10	2.5
Diabetes	Male	11	3	3.7
	Female	16	3	5.3
Arthritis and rheumatisim	Male	18	10	1.8
	Female	27	18	1.5

Source: *A second diagnostic on the health of First Nations and Inuit people in Canada*, p7. Health Canada ©. Reproduced with the permission of the Minister of Public Works and Government Services Canada, 2003.

Chronic Conditions

Table 6.1 shows the prevalence of a number of self-reported chronic diseases and conditions in Aboriginal people compared to the non-Aboriginal Canadian population. In 1997, those chronic diseases and conditions at higher prevalence in the Aboriginal population included heart problems and hypertension (about 2.5 to 3 times more likely to be reported than the general Canadian population), diabetes (almost four times more likely to be reported in Aboriginal men and more than five times more likely to be reported in Aboriginal women compared to the general Canadian population), and arthritis and rheumatism (about 1.5 to 2 times more likely to be reported than the general Canadian population) (21).

Before 1940, there was no evidence of diabetes among Aboriginal Canadians (22). Today, however, the age-standardized prevalence of type 2 diabetes among Aboriginal peoples is at least three times that of the general population. Approximately two thirds of the First Nations people with a diagnosis of diabetes are women. The incidence of type 2 adult-onset diabetes in children as young as six years old appears to be increasing at a rapid rate (23). The combination of genetic predisposition with a high prevalence of obesity (particularly central obesity) and physical inactivity contribute to the increased risks of diabetes. Although dietary acculturation has occurred in many Aboriginal communities, the association between diabetes and dietary factors has not been demonstrated consistently (24).

Disability

Studies from the late 1990s indicate that disability rates among Aboriginal people aged 15 and over were high compared with the total Canadian population. According to the 1999 First Nations and Inuit Regional Health Survey (FNIRHS) (25), one quarter of those aged 55 and older had activity limitation in the home and one third had hearing problems. Overall, 15% of the Aboriginal population surveyed had hearing problems, a rate twice as high as the general Canadian population. The National Advisory Council on Aging has reported that the length of disability experienced by Aboriginal Canadians is about twice that of non-Aboriginal Canadians. According to the FNIRHS, chronic conditions were associated with activity limitations. As indicated above, incidence of FAS and FAE is higher among aboriginal communities, leading to physical, mental and emotional disabilities among children.

1.4.   FUTURE DIRECTIONS

The continued improvement of Aboriginal health will require attention to be paid to the determinants of health. The poor psychosocial, socioeconomic, and physical environments within which many Aboriginal people live contribute greatly to the difficulty in achieving healthy lifestyles and to the much poorer health status in the Aboriginal population. Cultural insensitivity has often led to the paternalistic imposition of ineffective interventions. Five basic areas must be addressed to improve Aboriginal health, namely health research, a greater sensitivity to Aboriginal culture, a continuing process of control of health service and other aspects of local government services transfer to the communities, increased opportunities for the success of Aboriginal peoples in various healthcare professions, and an overall improvement in the socioeconomic status of Aboriginal Canadians (5). To achieve these ends, several efforts have been put in place to establish areas of Aboriginal self-government, and the federal government is transferring control of healthcare services to the local level of Aboriginal government or band councils (see Chapter 13). Ultimately, self-determination remains one of the hopes for improving the health of Aboriginal people.

In 1996, the Royal Commission on Aboriginal Peoples delivered a comprehensive report on all aspects of Aboriginal peoples' life, including their health, and made a number of recommendations related specifically to Aboriginal health (13). The Royal Commission recommended that the Aboriginal health and healing system should embody the following characteristics: equity in access to health and healing services and in health status outcome; holism in its approach to problems and their treatment and prevention; Aboriginal authority over health systems and, where feasible, community control over services; and diversity in the design of systems and services to accommodate differences in culture and community realities. The federal government responded in 1998 by stating four objectives: to renew partnerships, strengthen Aboriginal governance, develop a new fiscal relationship, and support strong communities, people, and economies (26). It pledged $350 million to support the development of community-based healing for the legacy of psychological and physical abuse endured in the residential schools to which Aboriginal children were sent until 1969. Also in 1998, the Aboriginal Healing Foundation, an independent non-profit corporation, was established to address the healing needs of all Aboriginal peoples. A number of health sciences programs now have programs to recruit Aboriginal students, and many regional health authorities seek Aboriginal participation in their governance. Professional organizations provide their members with cross-cultural awareness, and the Society for Obstetrics and Gynecologists has published *The Guide for Health Professionals Working with Aboriginal Peoples* (27). Models of traditional healing practices along with western medicine are being developed in a number of provinces. The federal government has allocated almost two billion dollars in its 2003 budget for improvements in health and well-being of Aboriginal people. The Aboriginal Canada Portal is a useful site with links to national Aboriginal organizations, 12 federal government departments with Aboriginal mandates, all provincial governments, and organizations with Aboriginal responsibilities, as well as related Aboriginal community information (28).

2.   THE HEALTH OF SENIORS

This section identifies some characteristics relevant to the health of seniors. Seniors are a heterogeneous group, each generation having a different social history. However, for the purpose of comparison, seniors as a group are divided into three sub-groups, the young elderly (65 to 74 years), the middle elderly (75 to 84), and the old elderly (85 and over). The number of seniors and their proportion in the population of Canada continue to grow, particularly the number of the old elderly.

Aging is a lifelong process, encompassing a series of transitions from birth to death. Reaching the age of 65 does not therefore herald old age. Even though disability increases with age, aging and poor health are not synonymous. It is not clear how much functional disability is intrinsic to the aging process or whether death is always the result of a disease process, which is the prevalent biomedical model. The degree of handicap also depends on society's response. **Successful aging** has been defined in terms of retaining the ability to function independently, remaining mobile, and undertaking all the activities of daily living (e.g., dressing, bathing, using stairs, getting in and out of bed, eating). In addition to age itself and measures of physical and mental health status, two major social predictors of successful aging have been identified: not having one's spouse die and not entering a nursing home. These indicate the interaction of biological and psychosocial factors (29).

There is controversy about the biological process of aging. The organism can be viewed as having a preprogrammed life span (natural limit) after which natural death occurs (due possibly to a general decline in withstanding external stressors); the life span in humans is approximately 120 years based on a woman who survived from 1875 to 1997 (30). As increasing proportions of the population age to the natural limit, survival tends to "rectangularize" the mortality curve. The onset of chronic disease may be postponed, thus compressing the period of disability, a concept known as "compression of morbidity" (31, 32). However, life expectancies, currently around 80 years, have a long way to go to achieve the natural limit. Some studies suggest that the average period of decreased vigour will probably increase if life expectancy increases to the natural limit, and that chronic diseases will occupy a large proportion of the life span (33, 34). There may be a biological basis for the female health advantage related to the genes in the X chromosome that surpasses lifestyle and environmental influences (35).

2.1.   DEMOGRAPHY

In 2001, there were 3.8 million Canadians over the age of 65 years, constituting approximately 12.9% of the population. It is estimated that by 2021, there will be 6.7 million seniors, more than 18% of the population. This increase is attributed to an increase in average life expectancy, the aging of the baby boomers, and the projected decline in fertility (36).

Another striking trend is the expanding population of senior women, particularly among those aged 80 and over. There were 932,000 people in that age group in 2001, an 11.8% increase from the 1996 census and over four times the level in 1971. In 2001, two thirds of people aged 80 years and over were women. The female proportion of the population over age 65 has increased from 49% in 1951 to 57% in 2001 and will likely be approximately 60% in 2001, due to the increased longevity of women on average and the gain in female life expectancy relative to males. Widows constitute 45.7% of the senior female population, whereas widowers are only 13.6% of senior men.

2.2.   DETERMINANTS

2.2.1.   Psychosocial and Socioeconomic Environment

Income

Seniors' incomes have increased substantially since the early 1980s, narrowing the gap between seniors and the rest of the population. In contrast to the slower decline in percentage of Canadian adults and children with low incomes, the proportion of seniors with low incomes has decreased significantly. In 1980, 34% of seniors met the criteria for living under the LICO, compared to 21% in 1992 (37). By 1997, 19% of Canadian seniors lived in a low-income situation. In 1997, the inflation-adjusted average income of those aged 65 and older was 18% higher than it was in 1981, compared with a decline in income seen in those aged 15 to 64. However, seniors still have lower average incomes compared to those under 65. Men aged 65 and older have higher incomes than females of this age group. Senior women are twice as likely as men to have incomes below the LICO (38).

The primary government transfer programs for seniors are the Old Age Security (OAS) program and the Canada or Quebec Pension Plan (CPP/QPP). All Canadian citizens or legal residents over aged 65 and older are eligible for OAS benefits, while those with little or no other income may also be eligible for additional benefits in the form of the Guaranteed Income Supplement (GIS) (39). Currently, seniors depend heavily on public pensions and income security plans, which comprise their single largest source of income. However, because 64% of seniors own their own home, and are frequently mortgage-free, income is not the only relevant indicator of socioeconomic status for the elderly. In 1998, 6% of seniors were still a part of the paid workforce (38).

Living Situation

Seniors may be stereotyped as being passive and dependent; however, the majority are "well elderly" who remain healthy into their 80s or even 90s, needing only minimal assistance. In 1996, 93% of Canadian seniors lived at home in a private household, although this proportion declines with increasing age. Ninety-eight percent of seniors aged 65 to 74 lived at home, compared with 91% of those aged 75 to 84 and 66% of those aged 85 and over. Among those living at home, 69% of seniors lived with family members. Fifty-seven percent lived with a spouse, while 7% lived with members of their extended family. In 1996, 29% of seniors were living on their own (38).

Although many seniors are largely able to take care of themselves and live independently, in 1996, 84% of those aged 65 and older reported getting some help with household or personal chores. Sixty-seven percent had help with housework or household maintenance; 51% with transportation, grocery shopping, banking, and bill paying; 39% had someone checking on them by phone; 23% had some kind of emotional support; and 12% received help related to personal care. Although men and women were approximately equally likely to receive help for household or personal tasks, senior men were more likely than women to get help with housework, while senior women were more likely to get emotional support, have someone check on them, and to get help with transportation, shopping, banking, bill paying, and personal care (38).

According to the 1994–95 NPHS, more than 50% of those reporting that they need assistance with personal care such as washing, dressing, or eating received no formal home care. Among those in need of help with the instrumental activities of daily living such as preparing meals, grocery shopping, housework, and heavy household chores, the percentages not getting home care was even larger (40).

In 1996, 7% of seniors lived in an institution, down from 10% in 1971. People aged 65 and over, however, still represent the majority (75%) of Canadians living in an institution. In 1996, 34% of those aged 85 and older, 9% of those aged 75 to 84, and 2% of those aged 65 to 74 lived in an institution (38). The factors associated with living in an institution include health status, particularly with a diagnosis of dementia, the absence of a spouse, low income, low education, and advanced age (41, 42).

Elder Abuse

Elder abuse (see also Chapter 7) includes physical/emotional/financial abuse, physical neglect, and maltreatment, including questionable institutionalization. Approximately 7% of elderly Canadians experienced some form of emotional or financial abuse by an adult child, caregiver, or spouse in a five-year period (43).

Emotional abuse was reported most frequently (7%) followed by financial abuse (1%). Very little physical or sexual violence was reported (43).

Accurate estimates of the prevalence of elder abuse within institutions are not available. Abuse within institutions can include the inappropriate or excessive use of physical or chemical restraints, such as restrictive "gerrichairs," bed railings, or sedatives. Ontario's *Patient Restraints Minimization Act* (2001) stipulates that a physician must specifically order a restraint and document the indication for its use, that the physician must obtain consent from either the patient or proxy, and that all acute care hospitals must have "least restraint" policies in place (44). Strategies to combat elder abuse are aimed at increasing public awareness, enhancing the training and working conditions of those employed at institutions, providing support services for abusers, conducting further research, and encouraging prevention by fostering independence for seniors through adequate housing and income.

2.2.2. Physical Environment

With advancing age, there is less ability to tolerate hazards in the physical environment, which may be exacerbated by wandering and forgetfulness associated with dementia. There is also increasing prevalence of visual, auditory, and locomotive disability, predisposing seniors to possibly serious falls; gait disorders may also result in falls and subsequent injury. In fact, falls in the elderly are a threat to health. In 1995, more than 2,100 deaths among Canadians aged 65 and over listed accidental fall as the underlying cause. Hip fractures are the second leading cause for senior women and the fifth leading cause for senior men of admission to hospitals in 1995–96; 90% of hip fractures are caused by falls (45). While many falls are due to intrinsic changes such as decreasing visual acuity and mobility, they are also caused by preventable extrinsic factors such as poor lighting, loose rugs, and medications (46).

Motor vehicle collisions are another cause of mortality and morbidity among seniors. A recent study concluded that impaired visual processing and glaucoma may play a role in crashes involving older drivers (47). There are many other conditions (e.g., musculoskeletal, neurodegenerative) that affect seniors that can have an impact on their ability to drive. Many provinces require mandatory vision and written tests every one to two years for all drivers aged 80 and over, and physicians and optometrists are required to report people with conditions that may make driving dangerous. It may be very difficult to assess the fitness to drive in many elderly drivers who do not have gross deficits. The Canadian Medical Association has produced guidelines that address the responsibilities of physicians in determining medical fitness to drive (48). Additionally, concerns about road safety must be weighed against the desire to maintain the mobility of seniors: driving provides a sense of personal control, can allow timely access to care, and can reduce social isolation in municipalities with limited public transit systems.

2.2.3. Lifestyle and Behavioural Risk Factors

Alcohol, Smoking, and Drug Use

Seniors are less likely to smoke than those in younger age groups and smoking among seniors also decreases with age. In 1996–97, 15% of men and 10% of women aged 65 and older who were living at home smoked, compared to 21% of 55- to 64-year-olds and 28% of 25- to 54-year-olds (38).

The pattern was similar for alcohol use. In 1996–97, whereas more than 50% of those under age 65 had at least one drink a month, only 49% of senior men and 29% of senior women did so. Forty-two percent of seniors aged 65 to 74 were drinking at least once a month, but only 30% of those over age 75 did so. Compared with 4% to 5% of those under age 65 who have five or more drinks on any one occasion at least once a week, only 1% of seniors reported doing so (38).

In contrast, seniors are more likely than younger Canadians to take prescription or over-the-counter medication. In 1996–97, while two thirds of Canadians took some type of medication, 84% of seniors living at home took some form of medication within two days (19, 49). Fifty-six percent took more than one medication in the same period. Use of multiple medications increased with age. In 1996–97, 52% of those aged 65–74, 61% of those aged 75–84, and 65% of those aged 85 and over took two or more medications in a two-day period (38).

Nutrition

A review of Canadian surveys concluded that 10–28% of elderly Canadians were at risk for deficiencies of calcium, beta-carotene, and vitamins A, C, and D (50). Protein, zinc, iron, and vitamin B6 were also frequently deficient. In a 1990 Quebec survey, senior females consumed only 77% of predicted energy requirements, while senior males consumed 92%; 55% of senior males, and 53% of senior females consumed more than 30% of their energy requirements as fat, exceeding the fat level recommended by Canada's Food Guide to Healthy Eating (51). Both senior men and women were deficient in calcium, and senior women were also mildly deficient in folate.

Exercise and Other Activities

Television viewing accounted for the largest proportion of leisure time activity among seniors, with those over age 60 watching about 4.9 hours per day of television in 1997. However, 50% of people aged 65 and older reported being regularly physically active, with an additional 12% reporting occasional physical activity. This compares to 66% of 15- to 24-year-olds and 55% of 25- to 64-year-olds who regularly took part in physical activity in 1997. A significant proportion of seniors attend a place of worship or religious function at least once a week (37%) and seniors are also travelling (an average of 0.7 trips per person internationally and three domestic trips per person in 1997) (38).

2.3.   HEALTH STATUS AND CONSEQUENCES

2.3.1   Mortality

There have been gains in life expectancy among Canadian seniors over the course of the last century. This has resulted from long-term declines in death rates in this age group. Between 1921 and 1981, the average life expectancy of a woman at age 65 increased by five years while that of a man of the same age increased by two years. Between 1991 and 1996, men have made more gains than women with the average life expectancy of a 65-year-old man increasing 0.5 years compared to 0.2 years in women. From 1980 to 1996, the age-standardized mortality rate among those aged 65 and older decreased by 12%. In 1996, death rates for men aged 65 and older (5,600 deaths per 100,000) were higher than those for women (3,600 per 100,000) (38). Common causes of death among seniors are shown in Figure 5.3, in Chapter 5.

2.3.2.   Morbidity

In 1996–97, most seniors (78%) living at home stated that their health was good, very good, or excellent; 16% reported their health as fair and only 6% reported that their health was poor. The percentage of seniors who described their health as fair or poor increased with increasing age, with negative self-reported health being more likely to occur in women than men: 85% of women and 78% of men aged 65 and over reported in 1996–97 that they had been diagnosed with at least one chronic health condition. Arthritis and rheumatism were the chronic health problems most commonly reported among seniors (42%), followed by high blood pressure (33%), allergies (22%), back problems (17%), chronic heart problems (16%), cataracts (15%), diabetes (10%), chronic bronchitis or emphysema (6%), asthma (6%), sinusitis (5%), ulcers (5%), cataracts (5%), migraine headaches (4%), and the effects of a stroke (4%) (38).

Among conditions that cannot be self-reported because they render the person cognitively impaired, dementia is an important cause of morbidity among seniors. In 1991, the Canadian Study of Health and Aging identified a prevalence of dementia of 8.0% — approximately a quarter of a million Canadians (252,500) (52, 53). The prevalence increased sharply with age: 2.4% of those aged 65 to 74 had dementia, 11.1% of those aged 75 to 84, and 34.5% of those aged 85 and over. About half of these people lived in institutions, and approximately two thirds of these cases were due to Alzheimer's disease. Alzheimer's disease caused dementia in more women (69%) than men (53%); dementia in men was more likely to have a vascular cause (30% versus 14% for women). Women with dementia were also more likely to be institutionalized, attributable to the fact that they are less likely to have a spouse to care for them at home. In 1995, 78% of those with Alzheimer's or other dementia lived in an institution (38).

The annual net cost of dementia in Canada has been estimated at more than $3.9 billion, $2.18 billion of which goes toward long-term institutionalization (54). Of those with dementia living in the community, 92% have either a family member, relative, or friend as an unpaid caregiver (52). These caregivers rarely have access to community support services, and are more vulnerable to chronic health problems and depressive symptoms than are those caring for the non-demented elderly.

2.3.3. Consequence

Disability

In 2001, 40.5% of Canadians aged 65 and over had a long-term disability or handicap. The proportion increases with age: 31.2% of those aged 65 to 74, 53.3% of those aged 75 and over had a long-term disability or handicap (see Section 4) (55).

Several health conditions are associated with activity limitations and disability in seniors. Chronic pain can affect activities in seniors. In 1996–97, 25% of seniors living at home reported experiencing chronic pain or discomfort, and 20% said that chronic pain prevented them from being able to carry out at least some activities. Although injuries serious enough to impair normal activities are less likely to occur in seniors than in younger age groups, 7% of women and 4% of men aged 65 and over had injuries severe enough to limit their normal activities in 1996–97 (38).

Dental Health

Approximately half of Canadians aged 65 and over retain none of their natural teeth (37), and in 1990 approximately 77% of seniors had not seen a dentist in the preceding year (56). In Ontario, 48% of the edentulous (toothless) and 15% of those with teeth reported a limited ability to chew. The dental health of seniors living in institutions was poorer: 25% of those in collective living centres required dental treatment urgently and 75% required preventive dental services. Almost 30% of seniors (the proportion increasing with age) reported that because of dental problems they avoided eating with other people, avoided laughing or smiling, were embarrassed by the appearance of their teeth or condition of their mouth, or avoided conversation with others (57). Low income was associated with edentulousness and with decreased likelihood of having visited a dentist within the previous year.

2.4.   HEALTHCARE UTILIZATION

Hospitalization

Hospital use rises dramatically with age. In 1996–97, the rate of hospitalization among those aged 65 and over was three times that of those aged 45 to 64. Among seniors, this rate also increased with increasing age; the number of hospital separations/ discharges per 100,000 people aged 75 and older was 70% higher than the number per 100,000 people aged 65 to 74. The average length of stay in a person aged 65 and over was 17 days compared with nine days for those aged 45 to 64, seven days for those aged 35 to 44, and less than seven days for those under age 35. Older seniors tend to have longer hospital stays than younger seniors and senior women have longer stays than men (38).

Home Care

In 1997, 10% of those aged 65 and older received support from a homecare service (38). By comparison, in 1994/95, only 1–2% of those under 65 used homecare services (37). The percentage of senior men and women receiving homecare service support increased with increasing age. Women were more likely than men in the same age group to receive home care (40).

2.5.   FUTURE DIRECTIONS

Longer life expectancy combined with decreased fertility has led to a growing proportion of seniors in the population. Most jurisdictions in Canada have recognized the need for increased and improved geriatric services. Many have planned for the expected increase in the number of seniors by increasing funding for gerontology programs, and some are considering a one-stop service delivery model in which a case manager organizes necessary service delivery at appropriate locale. Health promotion for seniors is an important approach to the development and maintenance of optimum levels of functioning as aging occurs. These approaches may incorporate physical activity, social support, awareness of adverse drug response, nutrition counselling, and programs to prevent falls. Increasingly, need for the end of life program including palliative care for seniors has been recognized, and universal home care programs dealing with the situation have been recommended by both Kirby and Romanow commissions (58, 59).

3.   THE HEALTH OF CHILDREN LIVING IN POVERTY

Over the last three decades, the number of Canadian youth who live in poverty has increased steadily until the early 1990s, and then levelled off; since 1997, it has been declining. Canada has no official poverty line. However, Statistics Canada uses the LICO to identify those who are considered to be living under economic hardship and strained circumstances because the family spends 54.7% or more of its gross income on food, shelter, and clothing (19).

3.1.   DETERMINANTS

3.1.1   Psychosocial and Socioeconomic Environment

With regards to child poverty in Canada, the following trends emerged between 1989 and 1999 (unless specified), indicating the importance of social variables on levels of poverty (60, 61):

- the number and percentage of poor children increased from 936,000 (14.4%) in 1989 to 1.5 million in 1996 (21.1%) and then declined to 1.1 million (16.5%) in 2000;
- the number of poor children in families with full-time employment increased by 15%;
- the number of poor children in two-parent families increased by 33%;
- the number of poor children in single-parent families led by a female increased by 44%;
- the number of children in families with incomes less than $20,000 increased by 32%;
- the number of children living in unaffordable rental housing (1989–96) increased by 91%; and
- social assistance benefits (1990–2000) decreased by 19%.

Some groups of children are more affected by poverty than others: in 1996 when average child poverty levels were 23.4%, poverty rates for Aboriginal children were 52.3%, rates for visible minority children were 42.7%, and rates for children with disabilities were 37.0%.

The most recent UNICEF report, "Child Poverty in Rich Nations," ranked the 23 rich nations belonging to the Organisation for Economic Co-operation and Development. Sweden ranked first for having the lowest level of poverty (2.6%); Canada ranked 17th at 15.5%; U.S. 22nd at 22.4%, and Mexico at 23rd with highest level of poverty (26.2%). Child poverty rates in Canada vary considerably among the provinces. In 1999, the prevalence of child poverty ranged from 16.3% in Alberta to 25.7% in Newfoundland with an average of 18.5% for Canada overall (60). The provinces vary in terms of their poverty levels and their social structure (62). The size of the community's population affects child poverty rates, with larger communities having higher rates of child poverty; for example, the child poverty rate in the city of Toronto in 1999 was 32.2% (63).

Parental depression and family dysfunction have important effects on the development of children. When parents have difficulty coping with life, work, family, or parenting, they may be unable to provide their children with the necessary emotional, social, and physical support. A poorly functioning family deprives children of a supportive home atmosphere and positive relationships. Data from the 1994–95 National Longitudinal Survey of Children and Youth (NLSCY) show that children from low-income families were two times more likely to live in poorly functioning families compared to children in high-income families (64). Nearly 20% of children in low-income families lived with a parent who had depressive tendencies, compared with less than 5% of children in high-income families (65).

3.1.2. Physical Environment

Meeting the physical needs of children, as well as the physical safety of the environment in which they live, are important issues related to poverty. Being able to meet the physical needs for food and shelter is a challenge increasingly faced by poor children and their families in Canada. Because of decreased government support for subsidized housing in recent years, many cities now have long waiting lists for assisted housing. In 1998, Toronto had 21,557 families with children on such waiting lists (64). In 1996, 30% of couples with children, 58% of single-parent families, and 76% of single parents under 30 years of age who rent had a problem with the affordability of rent (19).

Food security is also an important issue. In 1998–99, children were the age group most likely to live in food-insecure households (66, 67). Although 10% of Canadians lived in food-insecure households, 14% of Canadian children lived in such households (68). In 1998, although children made up 27% of the Canadian population, 31% to 54% of food bank users in Canada were children. Furthermore, hunger has become an important issue in Canada, with 206 of 16,639 families in the 1996–97 NLSCY reporting the experience of hunger (defined as "the inability to obtain sufficient nutritious, personally acceptable food through normal food channels or the uncertainty that one will be able to do so"). Although children from families that depend on social assistance were more likely to go hungry than children of employed parents, more than half the families that had hungry children reported having a wage or salary. Thus, food security problems in Canada are being experienced by working poor families as well as those on social assistance (see Chapter 7) (19).

In addition to concerns about availability of food and housing, the condition and location of housing can also expose children to environmental contaminants and unsafe conditions. Housing conditions, for example, can affect mould growth, which can have adverse health effects on children. Housing conditions can also affect exposure to toxic substances such as lead. The risk of physical harm to children is increased when they live in unsafe or problem neighbourhoods where drug use, drug dealing, excessive public drinking, or the threat of violence occurs. Low-income families often live downwind or downstream from sources of environmental contaminants, and adults are often employed in dangerous occupations. In addition, children are at an increased risk of exposure to hazardous substances if their parent or parents work in a dangerous occupation(64).

Additional adverse effects on the physical and mental health of children can occur as a result of the lack of suitable play and recreational spaces for children living in poor neighbourhoods. In 1994–95, 60% of very poor children almost never participated in supervised sports, compared with 27% of well-off children and 45% of not-poor children. Similarly, the rate of almost never participating in unsupervised sports also increased as income levels decreased (64).

3.1.3.   Lifestyle and Behavioural Risk Factors

As discussed above, supervised and unsupervised sports participation in children decreased with income levels. Additionally, parents who rely on food banks to help feed their children have limited ability to make decisions over their children's nutrition. Thus, the capacity for healthy behaviour as it relates to physical activity and nutrition can be greatly undermined by being in poverty.

Studies have shown that risk behaviour may be more prevalent among poor children. In 1990 in Ontario, among children under age 15, 48.9% of poor children smoked, compared to 20.7% of well-off children, and 46% of sexually active adolescents from low-income families reported never using a condom, versus 32% of those of high-income families (69).

3.1.4.   Healthcare Utilization

Lower consumption of medical care may also contribute to the negative impact of poverty on health. Canadian studies have shown conflicting results on this issue because of differing definitions of benefits and services, differing population units (families compared with per capita), and lack of controls for confounding factors such as age and sex (70). Per capita costs of medical services in Ontario did not vary significantly with income. Low-income families had a greater number of physician visits, but less costly services were provided per visit, and a greater proportion of visits were hospital-based rather than office-based. With regard to children, except for the lowest income group, benefits and average cost of services increased with increasing income. Rates of healthcare system utilization are higher among poor children than those who are better off. In Ontario in 1990, 14% of children up to age 19 on family benefits had been admitted to hospital in the preceding year, compared to 8% of those not on family benefits. In the preceeding year 35% of those on family benefits had visited an emergency department (versus 27% of children without benefits), and 33% had at least one chronic health problem (versus 26% of children without benefits) (69). Poor children also had less access to dental care than children from more affluent families; according to the NLSCY, 56% of poor children under age 12 did not visit a dentist in 1993, compared to 37% of children in non-poor families.

3.2. HEALTH STATUS AND CONSEQUENCES

3.2.1. Mortality

As in the case of adult poverty, the association between childhood poverty and increased disease and death has been well documented. Socioeconomic differences in children's health are seen from a very early age (71).

Infant Mortality

In Canada, the lower the income of a neighbourhood, the higher the rates of infant mortality and low birth weight. Since 1971, despite tremendous improvements in the infant mortality rates, Canadian infant mortality rates are still highest in the poorest neighbourhoods and lowest in the wealthiest neighbourhoods. In 1996, the infant mortality rate in the poorest neighbourhoods in Canada was 6.5 per 1,000 live births compared to 3.9 per 1,000 in the richest neighbourhoods. The rate was thus almost 70% higher in the poorest neighbourhoods compared to the richest neighbourhoods in Canada. Furthermore, although the income-related disparity in infant mortality rates had been decreasing between 1971 and 1991, there has been little decrease in this disparity since 1991 (71).

Low birth weight (LBW) is one of the major risk factors for infant and perinatal mortality, and childhood disability as well as other health problems. In recent years, income-related disparities in LBW have shown an increase in Canada. In 1986, the LBW rate for the richest urban neighbourhoods was 4.9% while it was 6.9% in the poorest neighbourhoods. In 1996, the rate had stayed the same in the richest neighbourhoods but had declined in almost all other income quintiles. There was an increase of 13% in the disparity between the richest and poorest neighbourhoods (71).

Child Mortality

Deaths are higher in poor children compared to children from higher socioeconomic strata. Overall mortality was higher in 1971 and 1986 for poor children than for those who are not poor. Total mortality in boys aged 1 to 14 years was 2.0 times higher in the lowest income level than in the highest. The mortality rate for girls who were poor was 1.5 times higher in both 1971 and 1986.

Injury is the number-one cause of death in children beyond infancy (see Chapter 7). In 1991, overall rates of injury-related deaths in Canada were highest in the poorest children. The inverse injury-related mortality gradients by socioeconomic status were seen mostly in boys and may be attributable to unsafe housing, close proximity of housing to high traffic areas, a lack of safe play spaces, and limited access to supervised recreation and sports. Additionally, income plays a clear role in injury-related deaths due to fire and homicide. The poorest 20% of children are at the highest risk of dying from fires or homicides. While the rate of dying in a fire is 1.7 per 100,000 and from homicide is 2.5 per 100,000 in these children, these rates respectively in children from other income quintiles are 0.4 or less per 100,000 and 1.1 or less per 100,000 respectively (64).

3.2.2. Morbidity

General measures of health status are usually directly related to socioeconomic status: the higher the socioeconomic status of children, the better their health is. Socioeconomic status, particularly the education level of the parents, has been found to be an important determinant of perceived health among Canadian children. According to the 1996–97 NLSCY, children under age 12 whose parents did not graduate from high school were almost three times more likely to have poorer health compared to children of university graduates. Likewise, the former children were also more likely to perceive a decline in their health between the 1994–95 and 1996–97 NLSCY (71). Studies done previously in the U.S. have found that low-income children had lower parental ratings of general health and slightly more restricted activity days, more bed disability days, and a higher rate of school absenteeism (72). The Ontario Child Health Study found that the prevalence rates of chronic health problems per 1,000 children who were below the poverty line was 237, compared with 183 per 1,000 children above the poverty line (73).

Mental Health

The 1994–95 NLSCY assessed the impacts of household income on children's behaviour and frequency of psychosocial problems. Although children with hyperactivity symptoms and delinquent behaviour can be found across all income groups, the poorest group of children (those who lived in households with incomes of less than $20,000 per year) were at the highest risk. Hyperactivity and delinquency have been found to be associated with poorer school performance, higher illiteracy, lower school attendance, and increased problems in getting along with others. In the NLSCY, differences in hyperactivity and delinquency problems were less significant in children from households across income groups over $30,000 (which is the approximate LICO for a two-parent, two-child family) (64).

Very poor children (who live in households with a family income below 75% of the LICO) are at particularly elevated risks for psychosocial problems including repeating a grade in school, impairment in social relationships, and having one or more emotional or behavioural disorders. Among children who were poor (living in households with family incomes 75% to 100% of the LICO), 3% had impairments in social relationships, 8% had to repeat a grade, and 23% had one or more emotional or behavioural disorders. Among children who were very poor, 7% had impairments in social relationships, 11% had repeated a grade, and 29% had one or more emotional or behavioural disorders. This was compared to 2% with impairments in social relationships, 4% who repeated a grade and 19% who had one or more emotional or behavioural disorders among children who were well-off (64).

Nutrition

Low-income children are at greater risk for nutritional disorders. Previous studies have shown that poor children are more likely to develop iron-deficiency anemia. Iron-deficiency anemia was found in 25% of 218 infants aged 10 to 14 months whose mothers lived in the five poorest districts of Montreal (74). Low-income mothers tend to discontinue breastfeeding early and switch to using cow's milk (which is known to cause occult intestinal bleeding and possibly contribute to iron-deficiency anemia in infants). A follow-up evaluation of infants whose iron status and treatment were known demonstrated lowered scores on mental and developmental tests at five years of age, raising the issue of whether iron-deficiency anemia, even if treated, causes irreversible defects (75).

Food security, discussed above, is also an important issue related to nutrition. The use of food banks limits the ability of parents to make decisions about their children's nutrition. Furthermore, food insufficiency and hunger among poor children and families have become important issues in Canada (19).

Dental Health

Two surveys of randomly selected 13- and 14-year-olds in Alberta and Quebec found that dental caries, as measured by the decayed/missing/filled teeth (DMFT) index, varied inversely with social class (76, 77). The ratio of filled teeth to the DMFT index, which reflects the amount of dental care received, was directly related to social class. The social class gradient was largest in Quebec, with an F/DMFT ratio of 65.1% for the highest socioeconomic group and only 17.4% for the lowest.

3.2.3. Disability

The rate of childhood disability in 1986 was more than twice as high among children from poor families compared with affluent ones. Seven percent of children from the poorest quintile had some degree of disability, compared with 3.5% from the richest. The differences between income quintiles were even more pronounced when only severe disability was considered, in which case the rate was 2.7 times higher among the poor compared with the rich.

An important issue related to children with disabilities and child poverty is due to the effects of children's disability on family income. Currently, existing employment programs are not flexible enough to give parents sufficient time off to establish skills and supports needed to support a child with disabilities. Furthermore, the lack of satisfactory childcare arrangements for children with disabilities is an important crisis faced by many families with children with disabilities. As a result, many parents of children with disabilities are forced to leave the workforce and end up subsisting on social assistance. In 1996–97, 79% of households with children under 11 years of age with activity limitation had employment income compared to 87% of households with children of the same age without activity limitation (64).

3.2.4.   Illness and Well-being in Later Life

Some researchers have proposed the idea that an impoverished early childhood results in developmental changes that can determine one's health and well-being throughout life. "Programming" and "latency" are terms that have been used to describe this concept (78-80). In essence, those who experience inadequate nurturing and stimulation in the earliest years of life (up to six years of age, and under three years in particular) will suffer higher rates of ill health and poor intellectual, social, and economic performance through their entire lives. This effect is proposed as being independent of their socioeconomic status in later life.

Birth weight, as already indicated, is closely linked with socioeconomic status. A number of ecological studies from the Environmental Epidemiology Unit at Southampton, England, suggest that fetal and early childhood growth (reflected by birth weight and weight at 1 year of age) correlate with such adult conditions as coronary heart disease, stroke, hypertension, diabetes mellitus, chronic obstructive lung disease, ovarian cancer, suicide, autoimmune thyroiditis, abdominal obesity, atopy, and renal failure; metabolic or physiological programming are thought to occur at critical periods of early development (78).

Recent studies have shown that health outcomes later in life, including cardiovascular disease risks and cognitive function in adulthood, are affected by socioeconomic conditions during childhood. In a case-control study of Swedish women, although the effects on cardiovascular disease risks were stronger for later life disadvantage, early-life socioeconomic disadvantage was also an independent risk factor (81). In another study of Finnish men, socioeconomic conditions in childhood were found to influence adult cognitive functioning, independent of adult educational attainment. Maternal education and paternal occupation appeared to be critical determinants (82).

3.3.   FUTURE DIRECTIONS

Decreasing child poverty is needed to decrease the adverse child and later adult life health and social problems associated with child poverty. Government programs, as well as appropriate income and taxation legislation, are an essential means of preventing child poverty in Canada.

Governments at the federal and provincial levels have pledged to address the issue of child poverty directly even though many critics consider the government's financial commitment inadequate. Any such programs to improve the well-being of children must be part of a greater societal approach that includes strategies to promote economic growth in all areas of the country, reductions in unemployment, wage increases, increases in the rates of social assistance, accessible and affordable high-quality child care, and the removal of other barriers that prevent economically disadvantaged, vulnerable groups from gaining employment. Early childhood education and care are viewed by many as central in strategy to reduce poverty (61). One study showed that adults born in poverty who participated in a high-quality, active-learning preschool program at ages 3 and 4 have half as many criminal arrests, higher earnings and property wealth, and greater commitment to marriage. It also showed that over participants' lifetimes, the public is receiving an estimated $7.16 for every dollar originally invested (83). In 2000, the federal government announced $2.2 billion over five years toward early childhood education — indeed a step in the right direction.

4. THE HEALTH OF PEOPLE WITH DISABILITIES

People with disabilities face many difficulties in both their daily activities and their meaningful participation in society; physical and social environment influences a great deal in their functioning. In this section, instead of focusing on how determinants of health influence health, focus is on how the determinants of health frequently interact and compound further the inequities in health relative to the rest of the population. The Word Health Organization's framework of disability provided by the International Classification of Functioning defines disability as the relationship between body structures and functions, daily activities, and social participation, and recognizes the role of environmental factors. It considers overall functional health based on nine dimensions of functioning (vision, hearing, speech, mobility, dexterity, feelings, cognition, memory, and pain). Statistics Canada's 2001 Participation and Activity Limitation Survey (PALS) used this framework in its recent survey (84). This framework is described in Chapters 1 and 3.

4.1. EXTENT AND TYPES OF DISABILITIES

According to the 2001 PALS, there were 3.4 million (14.6%) Canadians aged 15 and over and 180,930 children who reported disabilities (see Chapter 5). Disabilities increase with age, the lowest rate being in children at 3.3% and highest (53.3%) among people over 75. In general, the disability rate was higher among women. About 1.9 million women aged 15 and over (15.7%) reported having a disability, compared with just over 1.5 million men (13.4%). The highest rates occurred in the age group 75 and over, with more than one half of both men and women reporting a disability. Of the 3.4 million adults reporting disabilities, about one-third (34.1%) reported mild levels of disability, one quarter reported moderate levels, and 41% reported severe or very severe levels (see Table 6.2). The type of disability reported most often involved mobility (see Table 6.3). Slightly fewer than 2.5 million people aged 15 and over had difficulty walking, climbing stairs, or moving from one room to another. More than 1 million adults reported having hearing difficulties and some 600,000 had a problem with their vision. More than half a million adults reported limitations that were the result of emotional, psychological, or psychiatric conditions. Among seniors aged 65 and over, mobility problems affected an estimated 1.1 million individuals. In addition, more than 887,000 (69.5%) seniors reported they were disabled because of pain.

Activity limitations were reported for almost 181,000 (3.3%) children aged 14 and under. Of these, 26,000 were younger than five and about 155,000 were school aged. Almost 43% of children with disabilities had severe or very severe disabilities. Although children aged 14 and under had the lowest rates of disability, they had their own unique

Table 6.2.   Severity of Disability among Adults Aged 15 Years and Over
               with Disabilities, by Sex, 2001

Severity of disability	Both sexes		Men		Women	
	Number	%	Number	%	Number	%
Total	3,420,340	100.0	1,526,900	100.0	1,893,440	100.0
Mild	1,165,470	34.1	555,110	36.4	610,360	32.2
Moderate	855,330	25.0	375,380	24.6	479,950	25.3
Severe	919,310	26.9	383,570	25.1	535,740	28.3
Very severe	480,220	14.0	212,830	13.9	267,390	14.1

Note: Data exclude Yukon, Northwest Territories, and Nunavut. Data may not add
to total because of rounding.

Source: Statistics Canada, Participation and Activity Limitation Survey: A profile of disability in Canada. *The Daily*, December 3, 2002.

conditions. The most widespread disability, reported for 118,000 youngsters, was related
to chronic health conditions that reduced activities, such as asthma. Learning disabilities
were reported for an estimated 100,000 school-aged children (5 to 14). These children
accounted for almost two thirds of all school-aged children who reported disabilities.

4.2.   DETERMINANTS

4.2.1.   Psychosocial and Socioeconomic Environment

Unless otherwise indicated, the information in this and suqsequent sections comes
from *A Portrait of Persons with Disabilities* (85).

Education

According to the 1991 Health and Activity Limitation Survey (HALS), on average
people with disabilities have lower levels of educational attainment compared with
those without disabilities. Among those aged 35 to 54 in 1991, persons with disabilities
were twice as likely to have less than a Grade 9 education and were only half as likely
to have a university degree. Similar disparities in educational attainment were seen for
those aged 15 to 34 and 55 to 64. As with people without disabilities, those at younger
ages generally had higher levels of educational attainment than those who were older.
There were few differences in the educational attainment of women and men with
disabilities.

Among those aged 15 to 34, women with disabilities tended to have higher educational
levels than men; among those aged 35 or older, men were more likely than women to

Table 6.3.   Types of Disability

Type of Disability	%
Mobility	71.7
Pain	69.5
Agility	66.6
Hearing	30.4
Seeing	17.4
Psychological	15.3
Learning	13.2
Memory	12.3
Speech	10.6
Developmental	3.5

Note: Data exclude Yukon, Northwest Territories, and Nunavut.

Source: Statistics Canada, Participation and Activity Limitation Survey, 2001. *The Daily*, December 3, 2002.

have university degrees but also were more likely than women to have fewer than nine years of education. Those with mild disabilities had higher educational levels than those with more severe disabilities. Barriers to education included prolonged interruptions to education, enrolment in fewer courses, and beginning school later as a result of a disability.

The majority of children with disabilities were in some type of formal educational program. Ninety percent attended regular school, and another 7% were being tutored. Children with mild disabilities were more likely to attend regular school compared to children with more severe disabilities. Only 3% of those with mild disabilities were in special education schools, compared to 18% of those with moderate or severe disabilities. Barriers to education increased with severity of disabilities: in 1991, 77% of children with severe disabilities, 61% of those with moderate disabilities, and 25% of those with mild disabilities took longer to achieve the same level of schooling as their classmates without disabilities; 36%, 13%, and 6% respectively started school late because of their disabilities; and 29%, 18%, and 6% respectively had school interruptions because of their disabilities.

Income

Although the proportion of people with disabilities who are employed is smaller than the proportion of people without disabilities, 65% of those aged 35 to 54 and 58%

of those aged 15 to 34 were part of the paid work force in 1991. Those with mild disabilities were more likely to be employed than those with more severe disabilities. The majority (76%) of employed persons aged 15 to 64 with disabilities worked at least 30 hours a week. The higher the educational attainment of persons with disabilities, the more likely they were to be employed.

Earnings from employment are the major source of income of people aged 15 to 64 with disabilities. According to the 1991 HALS, income from employment represented 73% of all income of people aged 15 to 64 with disabilities. In 1990, 30% of those aged 15 to 64 and 13% of those aged 65 and over with disabilities received disability-related income from one or more of the following sources: social assistance (12% of those aged 15 to 64), Canada or Quebec Pension Plan (10%), workers' compensation, employer-sponsored disability insurance plan (3%), or employment insurance sickness benefits or private disability insurance (1%).

In all age groups, the income of people with disabilities is below that of people without disabilities. In 1990, the incomes of men aged 55 to 64 were 60% those of men the same age without disabilities; the incomes of men and women aged 35 to 54 were 70% those of people the same age without disabilities; the incomes of men and women aged 15 to 34 and men aged 65 and over were 80% those of their counterparts without disabilities; and the incomes of women aged 65 and over were 90% those of women the same age without disabilities. People with severe disabilities tended to have lower incomes than those with mild or moderate disabilities.

4.2.2.   Physical Environment

According to the 1991 HALS, most people with disabilities live in private households (93%); only 7% aged 15 and over lived in health-related institutions. Twenty-two percent of those with severe disabilities lived in institutions. Seniors with disabilities (15%) are more likely than their younger counterparts (aged 15 to 64) to live in a health-related institution (2%) (88). Among those living at home, a number encountered difficulties with using basic household facilities. Among those aged 15 and older in 1991, 12% reported some difficulty using the bathtub or shower, 5% accessing cabinets, 4% with laundry equipment, 4% operating the stove, and 3% using sinks and counters. The percentage of people with disabilities reporting the above difficulties exceeded the percentage reporting modifications in the home to accommodate their difficulties. In 1991, 5% of those aged 15 and over with disabilities reported needed special features, such as ramps or widened hallways, to enter or leave their homes.

In 1991, 39% of those aged 15 and over with disabilities living at home received help with doing heavy housework, 21% with shopping, 20% with everyday housework, 13% each with meal preparation and personal finances. Family members were the most common source of help with household tasks. However, 9% also received assistance with heavy housework from private organizations and 6% from friends and neighbours. Volunteer organizations played little role in helping with household tasks.

Another important aspect of the physical environment for people with disabilities is transportation. Although most are able to get around without assistance, 6% of those aged 15 and over with disabilities are housebound, and 13% require help with travelling short distances. Those who are more likely to require help with getting around their communities include seniors, particularly senior women, and people who have severe disabilities. Although only 3% of those with disabilities use specialized transportation to move around locally, 5% of seniors and 9% of those with severe disabilities use such services (85).

4.2.3. Lifestyle and Behavioural Risk Factors

Substance Abuse

Adults with severe physical disabilities are sometimes assumed to be susceptible to alcohol and drug abuse due to potential low self-esteem, social isolation, and other problems caused by their physical conditions. However, a survey of college students in wheelchairs found that the rate of alcohol and illicit drug use was similar to the general college population. Approximately 20% of students with disabilities are considered problem users of drugs and alcohol. Another survey administered to university students with disabilities found 40% drinking alcohol one or more times a week and 14% smoking marijuana one or more times a week. Again, however, these rates are similar to the general college population (86). As with young adults in general, drug usage among students with disabilities is correlated with a previous history of drug usage.

Among adults with disabilities, the percentage who drink and smoke decreased between 1986 and 1991. In 1991, 40% of adults with disabilities drank alcohol compared to 43% in 1986. The percentage who drank alcohol every day remained the same at 5%. The percentage of adults with disabilities who smoked cigarettes dropped from 33% in 1986 to 28% in 1991 (87).

Nutrition

Children with disabilities are at increased risk for malnutrition, attributable either directly or indirectly to several factors: physical disability, cognitive delay, altered nutrient requirements caused by their medical condition, and drugs used to treat their medical condition. Children with severe developmental disabilities are significantly below their expected weight. One third of children with disabilities have been found to be below the third percentile for weight, primarily the result of eating dysfunction, which affects a notable portion(88).

Physical Activity and Other Activities

Among adults with disabilities in 1991, 61% reported participating in physical activity each week. Thirty percent attended religious services or related activities each week and 15% participated in volunteer work each month. Among children with disabilities in 1991, 93% participated in physical activities, 51% participated in community physical recreation programs, and 34% in community competitive sports programs. Twenty-three percent of children with disabilities were not able to participate in some physical activities (88).

4.3.   FUTURE DIRECTIONS

As indicated in Chapter 1, the impairments and handicaps related to disability are mediated by the social context of the person. Societal attitudes toward people with disabilities, and the degree of modification of the physical, psychosocial, and socioeconomic environments to integrate them and allow their maximal participation, have a great impact on their quality of life and their ability to participate fully in and contribute to the community. As has been shown, the majority of people with disabilities are able to live independent lives and participate in the paid labour force. However, barriers are still encountered. Thus, the major social policy issues to be addressed in the 21st century for the people with disabilities in Canada are integration of Canadians with disabilities into mainstream society, and ensuring services are available to accommodate the increasing number of people with disabilities resulting from an aging population.

5.   SUMMARY

This chapter examined the health of certain vulnerable groups in the Canadian population in terms of the determinants of their health, health status, and consequences. The groups considered were Aboriginal peoples, seniors, poor children, and people with disabilities.

Aboriginal peoples, also known as the First Nations peoples or Native Canadians, fall into four groups: Status Indians, non-Status Indians, Métis, and Inuit. "Status Indian" has specific legal connotations and is defined as Aboriginal peoples registered under the *Indian Act*. In 2001, there were 976,305 Aboriginal people in Canada, of which 33.2% were under age 14 years, 62.7% between ages of 15 and 64, and 4.1% aged 65 and over. In 1996–97, First Nations and Inuit people throughout Canada had mortality rates that were about 1.5 times the national mortality rate.

In 2001, almost half (49.0%) of the Aboriginal people lived in urban areas; 31% lived on Indian reserves and settlements and the remainder (20%) lived in rural non-reserve areas. Forty-four percent of Aboriginal people have incomes falling below Statistics Canada's low-income cut-off. Twice as many Aboriginal children live in single-parent and low-income families (32%) as other Canadian children. Aboriginal people have been identified as the group perhaps most at risk for becoming homeless in Canada.

In 1997, First Nations and Labrador Inuit people 15 years old and over smoked at a rate of 62%. Alcohol and substance abuse, including the abuse of solvents, are considered major problems within many Aboriginal communities. The combination of genetic factors, changes in diet, and physical inactivity has led to a high prevalence of overweight among First Nations people. This in turn has led to a high incidence of chronic diseases and their predisposing conditions, including heart problems, hypertension, and type 2 diabetes. As a result of poverty and poor living conditions, certain infectious diseases such as tuberculosis also occur at a much higher incidence in the Aboriginal population compared to the general Canadian population. The prevalence of AIDS in Aboriginal people was eleven times the national rate. The increased AIDS cases are important, since HIV is a risk factor for active tuberculosis.

The federal government is responsible for the health care of Aboriginal peoples on reserves, and the provincial government for those off the reserves.

One of the major solutions proposed by Aboriginal people to improve their health status is to have self-government and gain control over their health, social, and educational programs.

The conventional definition of a **senior** is someone aged 65 years or over. The number and proportion of seniors in the population continues to grow with a tendency toward an increasing proportion of the old elderly (over age 85). In June 2001, seniors accounted for 12.9% of the population. In 2001 two thirds of people aged 80 years and over were women. Seniors' incomes have increased substantially since the early 1980s; however, seniors still have lower average incomes compared to those under 65. Many seniors are at risk of falls and injuries due to increased rates of visual, auditory, and locomotive disabilities. As well, they have low tolerance levels to the presence of hazards in the physical environment and are often on medications that may increase the risk of falls.

In 1996, 93% of Canadian seniors lived at home in a private household, although this proportion declines with increasing age. Seniors are less likely to smoke than those in younger age groups and smoking among seniors also decreases with age. The pattern was similar for alcohol use. Seniors are more likely than younger Canadians to take prescription or over-the-counter medication.

In 1996, death rates for men aged 65 and older were higher than those for women. In 1996–97, most seniors living at home stated that their health was good, very good or excellent. Arthritis and rheumatism were the chronic health problems most commonly reported among seniors, followed by high blood pressure, allergies, back problems, chronic heart problems, and cataracts. Among conditions that cannot be self-reported because they render the person cognitively impaired, dementia is an important cause of morbidity among seniors. Hospital usage, both in terms of admission rates and lengths of stay, rises dramatically with age.

There is a recognized need for improved geriatric services. Health promotion for seniors is important to the development and maintenance of optimum levels of functioning as aging occurs. These approaches include physical activity, social support, nutrition counselling, and programs to prevent falls.

Over the last three decades, the number of Canadian children living in poverty has increased steadily until the early 1990s when it levelled off; since 1997, it has been declining. In 2000, there were 1.1 million (16.5%) children living in poverty. Several groups are at particular risk for poverty, particularly single mothers, immigrants, and Aboriginal people. Children living in poverty face issues in their socioeconomic, psychosocial, and physical environments that can lead to short- and long-term social, educational, and health disadvantages. It is well documented that poor children have poorer health, although the exact mechanisms of how poverty affects health are still being elucidated.

Meeting the physical and psychosocial needs of children, as well as the physical safety of the environment in which they live, are important issues related to poverty. Parental depression and family dysfunction have important effects on the development of children. Data from the 1994–95 National Longitudinal Survey of Children and Youth show that children from low-income families were two times more likely to live in poorly functioning families compared to children in high-income families. Food security is also an important issue.

Poor children are at higher risk for a range of poor health and social outcomes. Injury is the number-one cause of death in children beyond infancy. Although children with hyperactivity symptoms and delinquent behaviours can be found across all income groups, the poorest group of children were at the highest risks. Very poor children, who live in households with a family income below 75% of the LICO, are at particularly elevated risks for psychosocial problems including repeating a grade in school, impairment in social relationships, and having one or more emotional or behavioural disorders.

Government programs, as well as appropriate income and taxation legislation, are an essential means of preventing child poverty in Canada.

According to the 2001 Participation and Activity Limitation Survey, there were 3.4 million (14.6%) Canadians aged 15 and over and 180,930 (3.3%) children who reported disabilities. Disabilities increase with age. Of the 3.4 million adults reporting disabilities, one third reported mild levels of disability, one quarter reported moderate levels, and the remaining 41% reported severe or very severe levels. The type of disability reported most often involved mobility.

Individuals with disabilities tended to have less formal education than those without disabilities, as disabilities can interfere with education. In all age groups, the income of people with disabilities is below that of people without disabilities.

Societal attitudes toward people with disabilities, and the degree of modification of the physical, psychosocial, and socioeconomic environments to integrate them and allow their maximal participation, have a great impact on their quality of life and their ability to participate fully in and contribute to the community. Two of the major social policy issues identified for the 21st century for people with disabilities in Canada are their integration into mainstream society, and ensuring services are available to accommodate the increasing number of people with disabilities resulting from an aging population.

6.   REFERENCES

1.   Government of Canada. 1995. *Indian Act.* <www.solon.org/Statutes/Canada/English/I/I-5.html> (November 2002).
2.   Kirby M, LeBreton M. 2002. *The health of Canadians: The federal role. Volume 2: Recommendations for reform.* Standing Senate Committee on Social Affairs, Science and Technology. <www.parl.gc.ca/37/1/parlbus/commbus/senate/com-e/SOCI-E/rep-e/repjan01vol2-e.htm> (November 2002).

3. Health Canada. *A second diagnostic on the health of First Nations and Inuit people in Canada.* Ottawa: Health Canada, 1999. <www.hc-sc.gc.ca/fnihb/cp/publications/second_diagnostic_fni.pdf> (January 2003).

4. Manitoba Centre for Health Policy. 2002. *The health and health care use of Registered First Nations people living in Manitoba: A population-based study.* <umanitoba.ca/centres/mchp/reports/rfn_pdfs.htm> (November 2002).

5. Waldram JB, Herring DA, Young TK. *Aboriginal health in Canada: Historical, cultural, and epidemiological perspectives.* Toronto: University of Toronto Press, 1995.

6. MacMillan H, MacMillan A, Offord DR, *et al.* Aboriginal health. *Canadian Medical Association Journal* 1996; 155(11):1569–978.

7. Richards J. *Neighbors matter: Poor neighborhoods and urban Aboriginal policy.* Toronto: C.D. Howe Institute, 2001.

8. Hanselmann C. *Urban Aboriginal people in Western Canada: Realities and policies.* Calgary: Canada West Foundation, 2001.

9. Tjepkema M. 2002. *The health of the off-reserve Aboriginal population.* <www.statcan.ca/english/freepub/82-003-SIE/82-003-SIE2002003.pdf> (November 2002).

10. Shah CP, Dubeski G. First Nations peoples in urban settings: Health issues. In Masi R, Mensah L, McLeod KA, Oakville K, editors. *Health and Cultures: Exploring the Relationships.* Oakville: Mosaic Press, 1993.

11. Siggner AJ. The socio-demographic conditions of Registered Indians. *Statistics Canada: Canadian Social Trends* 1986; 1(1):1-9.

12. Statistics Canada. 2003. *Aboriginal peoples of Canada: A demographic profile.* <www12.statcan.ca/english/census01/products/analytic/companion/abor/pdf/96F0030XIE2001007.pdf> (January 2003).

13. Royal Commission on Aboriginal Peoples. *Gathering strength: Report of the Royal Commission on Aboriginal Peoples — Volume 3.* Ottawa: Canada Communication Group, 1996.

14. Food Security Bureau. 2001. *Canada's action plan for food security.* <www.agr.ca/misb/fsb/fsap/part2e.html> (November 2002).

15. Diverty B, Perez C. The health of northern residents. *Health Reports* 1998; 9(4):49-55.

16. Luepker R. Heart disease. In Wallace R, editor. *Maxey-Rosenau-Last public health and preventive medicine.* 14th ed. Stamford, CT: Appleton & Lange; 1998.

17. Myers T, Calzavara LM, Cockerill R, *et al. Ontario First Nations AIDS and Healthy Lifestyle Survey.* Toronto: LB Publishing Services, 1993.

18. Aboriginal Nurses Association of Canada. *HIV/AIDS and the impact on Aboriginal women in Canada.* Ottawa: Aboriginal Nurses Association of Canada, 1996.

19. Federal, Provincial, and Territorial Advisory Committee on Population Health. 1999. *Statistical report on the health of Canadians.* Ottawa. <www.statcan.ca/english/freepub/82-570-XIE/free.htm> (November 2002).

20. Task Force on Suicide in Canada. *Suicide in Canada.* Ottawa: Minister of National Health and Welfare, 1994.

21. FitzGerald J, Wang L, Elwood R. Tuberculosis: 13. Control of the disease among Aboriginal people in Canada. *Canadian Medical Association Journal* 2000; 162(3):351-5.

22. D'Cunha C. *Diabetes: Strategies for prevention.* Toronto: Ontario Ministry of Health and Long-Term Care, 1999.

23. Diabetes Division Bureau of Cardio-Respiratory Diseases and Diabetes. *Diabetes in Canada.* Ottawa: Laboratory Centre for Disease Control, 1999. <www.hc-sc.gc.ca/hpb/lcdc/bcrdd/diabetes/docpub_e.html> (November 2002).

24. Young T, Reading J, Elias B, *et al.* Type 2 diabetes mellitus in Canada's First Nations: Status of epidemic in progress. *Canadian Medical Association Journal* 2000; 163(5):561-6.

25. First Nations and Inuit Regional Health Survey National Steering Committee. *First Nations and Inuit regional health survey: National Report, 1999.* Ottawa: Health Canada, 1999.

26.   Royal Commission on Aboriginal Peoples. *Gathering strength: Canada's Aboriginal action plan*. Ottawa: Government of Canada, 1997.

27.   Society for Obstetricians and Gynecologists of Canada Policy Statement. Guide for health professionals working with Aboriginal peoples. *Journal of Society for Obstetricians and Gynecologists of Canada* 2000; 22(12):1070-81.

28.   Canada. 2002. *Aboriginal Canada portal*. <www.aboriginalcanada.gc.ca> (November 2002).

29.   Roos P, Havens B. Predictors of successful aging: A twelve-year study of Manitoba elderly. *American Journal of Public Health* 1991; 81(1):63-8.

30.   Bradbury R. 1999. *Jeanne Louise Calment*. <avsunxsvr.aeiveos.com/longevity/jlcinfo.html> (Febuary 2003).

31.   Barer ML, Evans RG, Hertzman C, *et al*. Aging and health care utilization: New evidence on old fallacies. *Social Science and Medicine* 1987; 24(10):851-62.

32.   Fries JF. Aging, natural death, and the compression of morbidity. *New England Journal of Medicine* 1980; 303(3):130-5.

33.   Ableson J, Paddon P, Stohmenger C, editors. *Perspectives on health*. Ottawa: Statistics Canada; 1983.

34.   Schneider E, Brody J. Aging, natural death, and the compression of morbidity: Another view. *New England Journal of Medicine* 1983; 309(14):854-6.

35.   Wylie CM. Health-related contrasts between older men and women. In Isaacs B, editor. *Recent Advances in Geriatric Medicine*. Churchill Livingstone: Melbourne; 1985.

36.   Government of Canada. *Canada's seniors: A dynamic force*. Ottawa: Ministry of Supply and Services, 1988.

37.   Federal, Provincial, and Territorial Advisory Committee. *Report on the health of Canadians: Technical appendix*. Ottawa, 1996.

38.   Statistics Canada. *A portrait of seniors in Canada*. Ottawa: Ministry of Supply and Services, 1999.

39.   Human Resources Development Canada. 2002. *Old Age Security and Canada Pension Plan*. <www.hrdc.gc.ca/isp/common/home.shtml> (November 2002).

40.   Wilkins K, Park E. Home care in Canada. *Health Reports* 1998; 10(1):29-37.

41.   Trottier H, Martel L, Houle C, *et al*. Living at home or institution: What makes the difference for seniors? *Health Reports* 2000; 11(4):49-56.

42.   Glazebrook K, Rockwood K, Stolee P, *et al*. A case control study of the risks of institutionalization of elderly people in Nova Scotia. *Canadian Journal of Aging* 1994; 13:104-17.

43.   Statistics Canada. 2002. *Family violence in Canada: A statistical profile*. <www.statcan.ca/english/IPS/Data/85-224-XIE.htm> (November 2002).

44.   Government of Ontario. 2001. *Patient Restraints Minimization Act, 2001*. <192.75.156.68/DBLaws/Statutes/English/01p16_e.htm> (February 2003).

45.   Wilkins K. Medications and fall-related fractures in the elderly. *Health Reports* 1999; 11(1):45-53.

46.   Tinettie M, Speechley M, Ginter S. Risk factors for falls among elderly persons living in the community. *New England Journal of Medicine* 1988; 319(26):1701-7.

47.   Millar WJ. Older drivers - a complex public health issue. *Health Reports* 1999; 11(2):59-71.

48.   Canadian Medical Association. *Determining medical fitness to drive: A guide for physicians*. 6th ed. Ottawa: Canadian Medical Association, 2002.

49.   Health care/self care. *Health Reports* 2001; 12(3):33-8.

50.   Chandra R, Imbach A, Moore C, *et al*. Nutrition of the elderly. *Canadian Medical Association Journal* 1991; 145(11):1475-87.

51.   Santé Québec, Bertrand L, editors. *Les québécoises et les québecois mangent-ils mieux? Rapport de l'Enquête québécoise sur la nutrition, 1990*. Montreal: Ministère de la Santé et des Services sociaux; 1995.

52. Canadian Study of Health and Aging. Patterns of caring for people with dementia in Canada. *Canadian Journal on Aging* 1994; 13(4):470-87.
53. Hill G, Frobes W, Berthelot J, *et al.* Dementia among seniors. *Health Reports* 1996; 8(2):7-10.
54. Ostbye T, Crosse E. Net economic costs of dementia in Canada. *Canadian Medical Association Journal* 1994; 151(10):1457-64.
55. Statistics Canada. 2002. *A profile of disability in Canada, 2001: Tables.* <www.statcan.ca/english/IPS/Data/89-579-XIE.htm> (January 2003).
56. Locker D, Leake JL, Hamilton M, *et al.* Oral health status of older adults in four Ontario communities. *Journal of the Canadian Dental Association* 1991; 57(9):727-32.
57. Locker D, Leake JL, Lee J, *et al.* Utilization of dental services in four Ontario communities. *Journal of the Canadian Dental Association* 1991; 57(9):879-81.
58. Kirby M, LeBreton M. 2002. *The health of Canadians: The federal role. Interim report, volume 3: Health care systems in other countries.* Standing Senate Committee on Social Affairs, Science and Technology. <www.parl.gc.ca/37/1/parlbus/commbus/senate/com-e/SOCI-E/rep-e/repjan01vol3-e.htm> (September 2002).
59. Romanow R. *Building on values: The future of health care in Canada.* Ottawa: Commission on the Future of Health Care in Canada; Government of Canada, 2002.
60. Campaign 2000. 2002. *Putting promises into action: A report on a decade of child and family poverty in Canada.* <www.campaign2000.ca/rc/unsscMAY02/unintro.html> (January 2003).
61. Campaign 2000. 2002. *Poverty amidst prosperity.* <www.campaign2000.ca/rc/rc02/intro.html> (January 2003).
62. Canadian Institute of Child Health. 2002. *Fact sheets.* <www.cich.ca/facts.htm> (November 2002).
63. Canadian Council on Social Development. 2002. *Highlights: The progress of Canada's children 2002.* <www.ccsd.ca/pubs/2002/pcc02/hl.htm> (November 2002).
64. Canadian Institute of Child Health. *The health of Canada's children, 2000.* Ottawa: Canadian Institute of Child Health, 2000.
65. Canadian Council on Social Development. *The progress of Canada's children, 1997.* Ottawa: Canadian Council of Social Development, 1997.
66. McIntyre L, Connor S, Warren J. Child hunger in Canada: Results of the 1994 National Longitudinal Survey of Children and Youth. *Canadian Medical Association Journal* 2000; 163(8):961-5.
67. McIntyre L, Glanville N, Officer S, *et al.* Food insecurity of low-income lone mothers and their children in Atlantic Canada. *Canadian Journal of Public Health* 2002; 93(6):411-5.
68. Che J, Chen J. Food insecurity in Canadian households. *Health Reports* 2002; 12(4):11-21.
69. Canadian Institute of Child Health. *The health of Canada's children: A statistical profile.* 2nd edition. Ottawa: Canadian Institute of Child Health, 1994.
70. Manga P. *Equality in access and inequalities in health status.* Markham: Fitzhenry and Whiteside, 1987.
71. Statistics Canada. Health status of children. *Health Reports* 1999; 11(3):25-34.
72. Kovar MG. Health status of U.S. children and use of medical care. *Public Health Reports* 1982; 97(1):3-15.
73. Cadman D, Boyle MH, Offord DR. Chronic illness, function conditions, and limitations in Ontario children: Findings of the Ontario Child Health Study. *Canadian Medical Association Journal* 1986; 135(7):761-7.
74. Lehmann F, Gray-Donald K, Mongeon M, *et al.* Iron deficiency anemia in 1-year-old children of disadvantaged families in Montreal. *Canadian Medical Association Journal* 1992; 146(9):1571-7.
75. Lozoff B, Jimenez E, Wolf AW. Long-term development outcome of infants with iron deficiency. *New England Journal of Medicine* 1984; 325(10):687-94.

76.   Stamm JW, Dixter CT, Langlair RP. Principal dental health indices for 13-14-year-old Quebec children. *Canadian Dental Association Journal* 1980; 46(2):125-37.

77.   Stamm JW, Lizaire A, Fedori D, *et al.* Dental health status of Alberta school children. *Canadian Dental Association Journal* 1980; 46(2):98-107.

78.   Joseph K, Kramer M. Review of the evidence on fetal and early childhood antecedents of adult chronic disease. *Epidemiologic Reviews* 1996; 18(2):158-74.

79.   Hertzman C, Wiens C. Child development and long-term outcomes: A population health perspective and summary of successful interventions. *Social Science and Medicine* 1996; 43(7):1083-95.

80.   Mustard F. Ideas, collaboration, and healthy children. *Ideas* 1996; 3(1):3-8.

81.   Wamala S, Lynch J, Kaplan G. Women's exposure to early and late life socioeconomic disadvantage and coronary heart disease risk: The Stockholm Female Coronary Risk Study. *International Journal of Epidemiology* 2001; 30:275-84.

82.   Kaplan G, Turrell G, Lynch J, *et al.* Childhood socioeconomic position and cognitive function in adulthood. *International Journal of Epidemiology* 2001; 30(256-63).

83.   Schweinhart L, Barnes H, Weikart D. 2002. *Significant benefits: The high/scope Perry Preschool study through Age 27.* <www.highscope.org/Research/PerryProject/ perryfact.htm> (January 2003).

84.   Statistics Canada. 2001. *Canadians with disabilities.* <www.statcan.ca/english/freepub/ 85F0033MIE/85F0033MIE01002.pdf> (January 2003).

85.   Bergob M. *A portrait of persons with disabilities.* Ottawa: Statistics Canada, 1995.

86.   Substance abuse among the disabled. *Science News* 1989, October 7.

87.   McDowell I, Praught E. *Selected characteristics of persons with disabilities residing in households.* Ottawa: Statistics Canada, 1994.

88.   Evers S, Munoz M, Vanderkooy P, *et al.* Nutritional rehabilitation of developmentally disabled residencies in a long-term care facility. *Journal of the American Dietetic Association* 1991; 91(4):471-3.

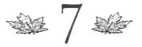

CHRONIC DISEASES AND INJURIES

The major causes of mortality, morbidity, and the burden of illness in the Canadian population are described in Chapter 5. Overall, cardiovascular disease and cancer are the leading contributors to **chronic disease**, which is usually defined as a condition lasting three months or longer. A significant proportion is due to injuries, either unintentional (e.g., motor vehicle collisions) or intentional (e.g., homicide). The economic and personal burden of chronic illness to Canada is substantial. There are a number of risk factors that influence the development of chronic diseases. Some of these are modifiable, such as those related to lifestyles, whereas others such as age, sex, or genetic make-up are not amenable to change. Substance use (predominantly tobacco use and excessive alcohol use), poor nutrition, and physical inactivity are major risk factors for chronic illness and play a part in several diseases; hence they are discussed first to avoid the repetitiveness in terms of preventive strategies.

This chapter presents detailed information on the burden of illness caused by chronic non-communicable diseases, emphasizing current approaches to prevention and control. As many chronic illnesses are preventable, primary and secondary prevention and, more recently, health promotion have emerged as increasingly important. The underlying principles of disease prevention and health promotion that provide the framework are discussed in Chapter 1.

Most of the data presented here come from published studies, government sources, and non-governmental organizations. Data, particularly percentage figures for risk factors and economic estimates of the burden of illness, quickly become out of date. Also, due to differences in methods, definitions, and time of data collection, incidence and cost figures vary slightly from report to report. The methods section of the reports cited explain how their estimates were made. The organizations cited, such as the Heart and Stroke Foundation, Statistics Canada, Health Canada, Canadian Institute for Health Information, and the National Cancer Institute of Canada, produce annual or semi-annual compilations of statistics. Updates can be found on their Web sites.

1.   MAJOR MODIFIABLE LIFESTYLE ISSUES

The major underlying causes of many chronic diseases are substance use and abuse in the form of tobacco use and excessive alcohol use, improper diet, and physical inactivity. As mentioned above, in order to avoid repetitiveness, the strategies for primary prevention of major diseases are described in the sections on substance abuse and diet.

1.1.   SUBSTANCE USE AND ABUSE

Although much media attention focuses on drugs such as cocaine and heroin, the burden of illness caused by tobacco and alcohol, which are readily available, socially sanctioned, and promoted widely, is greater. These substances are each discussed below in the context of that burden, and then discussed together in the context of control and prevention of the consequences of their use and abuse. A risk continuum framework of the spectrum of problems arising from use and abuse of these substances and the appropriate level of response are provided in Chapter 1 (see Figure 1.1).

1.1.1.   Tobacco

Tobacco smoking is the most important preventable cause of death in Canada. The trends and prevalence rate of smoking are described in Chapter 4. In Canada, 45,000 deaths each year are attributable to the use of tobacco products (1). In 1995, tobacco was estimated to cause 15.7% of premature years of life lost (PYLL) and 6.5% of hospital admissions (2). Tobacco smoking is estimated to be responsible for one third of PYLL due to cancer, one quarter of PYLL due to heart disease, and one half of PYLL due to respiratory disease (3).

Smoking is the primary cause of lung cancer and is a major cause of cancers of the larynx, esophagus, mouth, bladder, kidney, and pancreas. The risk of these cancers decreases rapidly after smoking cessation (4). The age-standardized mortality rates for lung cancer per 100,000 persons have increased from 58.7 for males and 10.2 for females in 1972 to an estimated 68.6 for males and 37.0 for females in 2001 (3). The overall cancer death rates of male smokers are double those of non-smokers. Female deaths, while much lower in number than males, have risen proportionately at a greater rate than for males within the last 15 years, paralleling the increase in female smoking. The overall cancer death rate of female smokers is 30% greater (and rising) than that of non-smokers. Maternal smoking is the preventable cause of low birth weight (small-for-gestational age), in Canada. Infants born to women who smoke, on average weigh 150 grams less than those of non-smoking mothers (5). These infants are at increased risk of preterm birth and sudden infant death syndrome, and maternal smoking has been associated with impaired physical and intellectual development (6). Smoking is a major cause of cardiovascular diseases such as heart disease and stroke, and of chronic respiratory diseases; it is the first and third most frequent cause of hospitalization in Canada (1, 7, 8). Women who use oral contraceptives and smoke are also at increased risk of subarachnoid hemorrhage and thromboembolism. The relative risk of dying increases in individuals with asthma and chronic obstructive pulmonary disease (COPD), including bronchitis and emphysema in those who smoke. Smoking also increases the mortality rates of individuals.

In 1995, there were an estimated 193,772 hospitalizations related to tobacco use in Canada. Ischemic heart disease was the largest contributor with 52,297 hospital separations, followed by COPD (37,506), lung cancer (21,212), and stroke (13,671) (2). In terms of economic burden, Health Canada estimates that the societal costs attributable to smoking for 1992 were approximately $11 billion, of which $3 billion was spent on direct healthcare costs such as hospitalization and physician time. The remaining $8 billion was due to lost productivity, including foregone household income (9). Caution should be exercised with these figures as they are old and do not take into account inflation.

Tobacco marketing has traditionally relied on portraying smoking as glamourous and liberating. Despite some evidence of shifting social norms and attitudes toward smoking, the effectiveness of this marketing is evident in the higher rates of smoking among young women. In 2000, smoking prevalence in Canada for people 15 years and older was slightly more than 6 million, or 24% of the population. This represents the lowest overall level since regular monitoring of smoking began in 1965 (10). While this is encouraging, between 1991 and 1994 there was a significant and large increase in smoking prevalence for people between 15 and 19 years, and this rate has stayed high since 1994. For example, the rate of smoking among girls aged 12 to 14 is 10%, compared with 6% in boys the same age, and 29% among girls 15 to 17 compared with 22% in boys the same (1).

Environmental Tobacco Smoke

Smoking is a hazard not only to those who smoke but also to non-smokers exposed to environmental tobacco smoke (ETS). In 1990, the Report of the Working Group on Passive Smoking stated that there is strong evidence of an association between residential and workplace exposure to ETS (also referred to as secondhand smoke), and respiratory illness (11). Six major scientific reviews have identified ETS as the known or suspected cause of 15 diseases or health conditions (12). The relationship between ETS and adverse health effects is now well accepted. ETS is a mixture of exhaled smoke (mainstream) and smoke emitted from the smouldering tobacco (side stream). It contains more than 4,000 chemicals, of which 42 are known carcinogens. Besides ETS being a known mucous membrane irritant, exposure is linked to increases in mortality from lung cancer and cardiovascular disease among non-smokers, and has serious consequences for children.

For children, exposure to ETS is a risk factor for respiratory symptoms, middle ear disease, sudden infant death syndrome, and bronchitis, pneumonia, and other lower respiratory tract infections, and it exacerbates asthma. It is also thought to have adverse impacts on cognition and behaviour, and to decrease lung function, induce asthma, and exacerbate cystic fibrosis. In adults, ETS causes heart disease, lung cancer, and nasal sinus cancer and has also been linked to stroke, breast cancer, cervical cancer, and miscarriages (12). Approximately 1,100 to 7,800 Canadians die each year due to ETS. Effective tobacco control includes bans on smoking in the workplace and public places, including restaurants and bars, both to protect non-smokers and to facilitate quitting by reducing opportunities to smoke (13).

In 2000, 25% of the 2.4 million households with children under the age of 12 reported regular exposure of children to ETS in their homes from cigarettes, cigars, or pipes. This appears to be a substantial improvement from 1996–97, when ETS exposure occurred in 33% of such homes. Nevertheless, approximately 900,000 children under the age of 12 continue to be regularly exposed to ETS in the home. Children in British Columbia, Ontario, and Alberta were much less likely to be exposed to ETS in the home, while children in Saskatchewan and Quebec are much more likely to be exposed (10).

Tobacco Control

A person's decision to use tobacco is the result of a complex interaction of factors that varies from one individual to another. Ninety percent of adult smokers begin smoking before age 18 and youth smoking is strongly influenced by role modelling by parents and other adults (youth whose parents smoke have ready access to tobacco and perceive that smoking is socially normal behaviour) and the price of cigarettes (higher prices reduce initiation). Reducing tobacco use requires a comprehensive, multifaceted approach that targets different groups in different settings and addresses, at a minimum:

- prevention (preventing smoking initiation among non-smokers);
- cessation (assisting smokers to reduce their consumption, quit, and prevent relapse); and
- protection (protecting non-smokers from ETS and other harmful effects of tobacco) (14).

Interventions for Smoking Cessation by Healthcare Professionals

For smokers, the benefits of quitting are significant, including increased exercise tolerance and decreased risks of cardiovascular disease and lung cancer. These health gains occur within a relatively short time after quitting. Most smokers would like to quit, but the relapse rate is very high because of the addictive nature of nicotine and social pressures. In most smoking cessation programs, a quit rate of between 15% and 20% is considered a success. Most smokers attempt to quit several times before they finally succeed.

Smoking cessation counselling is widely recognized as an effective clinical practice. Even a brief intervention by a healthcare professional significantly increases the cessation rate. A smoker's likelihood of quitting increases when he or she hears the message from a number of healthcare providers from a variety of disciplines. Healthcare professionals can tailor their messages to individuals and work with them on an individual basis. Clinical practice guidelines, practice tools, quick reference guides, and other resources are available to healthcare professionals. Pharmacotherapy has been shown to increase the cessation rate significantly and works best when combined with counselling.

However, healthcare professionals encounter barriers, such as doubts about their own effectiveness in motivating behaviour change and finding time during a busy day for counselling. Also, funding mechanisms have traditionally overlooked preventive care except in some jurisdictions, with little or no reimbursement for smoking cessation interventions, follow-up, or support, and there is insufficient public awareness of the smoking cessation services provided by healthcare professionals. Many healthcare professionals may become frustrated by high relapse rates among smokers.

Expanding access to cessation counselling and services (e.g., assessment, counselling, pharmacotherapy, ongoing support, relapse prevention strategies) involving healthcare professionals should be part of a comprehensive national tobacco control strategy that also includes prevention and protection measures such as legislation, tax increases, product regulation, restrictions on tobacco advertising and promotion, restrictions on smoking in public places, and public education campaigns.

Legislation and Community Action

In 1996, Bill C-71 was passed to regulate the manufacture, sale, labelling, and promotion of tobacco products. The legislation further limits youth access to tobacco products, restricts the promotion of tobacco products, increases health information on tobacco packages, and establishes powers to regulate tobacco products. Specifically, there can be no self-service displays, vending machine sales, or mail-order distribution, and photo identification is required for confirmation of minimum age. Advertising of tobacco products is curtailed, and sponsorship links reduced. The logo of the company and other brand elements are limited to the bottom 10% of the display surface; sponsorship items containing brand information are restricted to publications catering to a predominantly adult audience. More detailed reporting on the sales of tobacco products, promotional activities, and distribution and manufacturing practices, as well as information on toxic substances, is required from tobacco manufacturers. There are stringent regulations that require graphic health warning messages to cover 50% of principal display surfaces of all tobacco products sold in Canada (15).

Recently across Canada, many municipal and regional jurisdictions have introduced or are in the process of introducing strengthened bylaws to protect non-smokers and workers from environmental tobacco smoke. Since January 2000, at least 51 Canadian municipalities have bylaws (either already in place or coming into force at a later date) that ban or restrict smoking in restaurants and bars; in Nova Scotia, since January 1, 2003, it is illegal for people under 19 years of age to possess tobacco. The federal *Non-Smokers' Health Act* passed in 1988 restricts smoking to enclosed designated smoking rooms in federally regulated workplaces and protects about 8% of the workforce. All provinces except Prince Edward Island have laws that restrict smoking to some extent. Prince Edward Island, however, uses administrative rules to restrict or ban smoking in provincial government workplaces. In British Columbia, Saskatchewan, Ontario, New Brunswick, Nova Scotia, and Newfoundland and Labrador, policy directives prohibit smoking in provincial government workplaces. All provinces, except Prince Edward Island, Nova Scotia, and Quebec, authorize their municipalities to pass bylaws controlling smoking in workplaces and public places (12). Aside from ETS protection, bylaws that restrict or ban smoking in workplaces and public places have also been found to be effective in decreasing cigarette consumption and increasing smoking cessation among smokers.

In 1999, the National Tobacco Strategy was developed and identified five aspects to control tobacco effectively and comprehensively at the local, provincial/territorial, national, and international levels, as follows (1).

- Policy and legislation includes measures such as increasing taxation for tobacco products across Canada.
- Public education provides relevant information concerning tobacco products, such as ingredients and constituents of smoke.
- Industry accountability and product control establish restrictions on advertising of tobacco products and related sponsorship and encourage legislation to recover the healthcare costs resulting from tobacco product use from tobacco companies.
- Research explores tobacco cessation strategies, the impact of health determinants on tobacco use, monitoring knowledge, attitudes and behaviour about smoking, and ETS among children, youth and adults.
- Building and supporting capacity for community action includes providing training and resources, supporting coalition developments, including those specifically for francophones, Aboriginal peoples, and minority ethnic groups, involving youth as advisors, activists, and peer models, and promoting the implementation of practice guidelines for healthcare professionals to identify, counsel, and monitor patients who use tobacco.

The strategy is based on a population health approach and addresses a range of factors that determine health such as social, economic, and physical environments, personal health practices, individual capacity and coping skills, and health services. Following litigation in the United States, interest in taking legal action directed specifically at the tobacco industry has grown, facilitated in part by access to thousands of tobacco industry documents revealing evidence of industry deception regarding health risks and marketing strategies.

Effectiveness of Tobacco Control Strategies

A report by the Surgeon General in the U.S. has provided the following information about the effectiveness of different modalities in tobacco control (16):

- Educational strategies, in conjunction with community-based and media-based activities, can postpone or prevent smoking onset in 20% to 40% of adolescents.
- Physician advice alone to quit smoking produces cessation rates of 5% to 10%.
- Pharmacological treatment of nicotine addiction, combined with behavioural support, will allow 20% to 25% of smokers to remain abstinent at one year post-treatment.
- Regulation of advertising and promotion, particularly at young people, is very likely to reduce both uptake and prevalence of smoking.
- Smoking bans and restrictions and restriction of minors' access to tobacco contribute to changing social norms and may influence prevalence directly.

The World Health Organization states that one of the most important interventions is price increases (via taxation). Estimates of the subsequent impact vary but the current consensus is a 4–5% reduction in consumption for each 10% increase in price with greater effects among young people (17).

1.1.2. Alcohol

Various diseases and injuries are associated with alcohol consumption, including cirrhosis, suicide, breast cancer, upper respiratory and gastrointestinal tract cancers, and injuries from motor vehicle collisions and work-related incidents. Trend and prevalence rates for drinking are discussed in Chapter 4. A study that examined substance abuse in Canada estimated that 6,507 Canadians died in 1995 because of alcohol consumption. The largest number of alcohol-related deaths stemmed from impaired driving (see below), followed by cirrhosis and then suicide (2). In Canada, in 1995, 172,126 PYLL and 82,014 hospitalizations were attributable to alcohol use (2). For alcohol-related mortality, PYLL, and hospitalizations, men far outnumber women. Alcohol is estimated to account for 2.1% of cancer mortality in Canada (18); this is consistent with the estimates of 3% of cancer mortality attributable to alcohol more globally (4).

Although mortality and PYLL to society are of concern, the impact of alcohol on the health of Canadians is shown more strongly in terms of morbidity and economic burden. The economic costs of alcohol abuse are estimated at $7.5 billion per year. The largest costs are associated with lost productivity due to morbidity and premature mortality ($4.1 billion), law enforcement ($1.4 billion), and direct healthcare costs ($1.3 billion) (19). In addition, excessive alcohol use can fuel family and social problems.

Alcohol has both acute and chronic effects on health. The acute effects of heavy drinking include increases in blood pressure and an increased risk of cardiac arrhythmia. As little as one drink affects cognition, neuromotor function, and judgement, and attenuates performance of skilled tasks. Blood alcohol concentration (BAC) is very closely associated with risk of injury and severity of injury; risk of motor vehicle collisions increases with increasing BAC. Cross-sectional surveys show that drinking as many as five drinks per day is highly correlated with reported social problems (home life, work, legal, financial). Alcohol use may also accompany suicide attempts and criminal activities.

Excessive long-term alcohol use can also lead to chronic health problems. There is no threshold level for many health problems (i.e., risk is lowest for non-drinkers, occurs at all levels, and increases with levels of intake). Chronic alcohol-related problems include diseases of the liver (hepatitis, cirrhosis), pancreas (pancreatitis), and nervous system (neuropathy, dementia); cancer of the upper respiratory and digestive systems, liver, colon, and breast; gastritis and peptic ulcers; cardiomyopathy; and nutritional deficiencies (e.g., thiamine deficiency).

Alcohol use during pregnancy can impair physical and mental development of the fetus and increase the risk of congenital defects. The most severe but uncommon example is fetal alcohol syndrome (FAS), which usually occurs in children of mothers with serious alcohol problems or who are alcohol dependent. However, measurable effects on child growth, development, and behaviour can occur with use below levels associated with dependence. There is no risk-free level for alcohol use in pregnancy (20).

There is some evidence to suggest that alcohol consumption may reduce mortality from cardiovascular disease. Cardiovascular mortality rates are lower in France where wine consumption is high, which has led to the "French paradox." There has been debate about recommending alcohol consumption because of increased rates of cirrhosis found in France (21). The protective effect against coronary artery disease and ischemic stroke occurs over a wide range of intakes (from fewer than 4 drinks/week to 5–6 drinks/day); however, the risk for heart disease does not diminish with increased intake and the risk of other health problems increase with intake. An average of greater than 14 drinks per week is associated with increased risk of premature death in men; an average of greater than 9 drinks per week associated with increased risk of liver cirrhosis and breast cancer in women. The Low-Risk Drinking Guidelines, which are endorsed by several Canadian addiction management organizations, state that if you do not drink alcohol, starting just for these health benefits is not recommended. (22).

There are four categories of alcohol use (23):

1. **Low-Risk Drinking:** A maximum of two drinks a day, with a weekly limit of 14 drinks for men and 9 for women.
2. **Hazardous Drinking:** Alcohol consumption at levels that expose the drinker to a high risk of physical complications. Levels of consumption far below those diagnosed as alcohol dependent are associated with increased risks of adverse health consequences (23).
3. **Alcohol Abuse:** It relates to use that results in physical or psychosocial dysfunction (24).
4. **Alcohol Dependency:** It relates to physical and psychological dependence on alcohol (24).

The Low-Risk Driving Guidelines also state that some people should not use alcohol or should limit its consumption to less than the amount described as low-risk drinking, including those with liver disease, psychiatric illness, gastritis and ulcers, uncontrolled blood pressure, and uncontrolled diabetes. Similarly, alcohol consumption should be avoided or restricted for those taking certain medications, such as sedatives, sleeping pills, pain killers, as well as those with a personal or family history of serious drinking problems. Women who are pregnant or trying to conceive should avoid alcohol, and anyone operating any type of vehicle or working with machinery or dangerous equipment should also avoid or restrict intake, as well as those with any legal or other restriction on drinking,

Men have a greater risk disorders than women of developing alcohol use, with a male-to-female ratio of 2–3:1. Although most common in people under age 45, the prevalence is thought to be underestimated in the elderly due to less satisfactory screening tools. Alcohol use disorders are seen across all levels of socioeconomic status but are somewhat more prevalent with lower socioeconomic status. A family history of serious drinking problems is likely the strongest predictor of alcohol abuse. First-degree offspring of an alcohol-dependent parent are three to four times more likely to develop alcohol dependence than those without such a family history. Adoptee studies show that both genetic and environmental factors play a role in determining risk of alcohol use disorders (23).

Early Detection and Brief Interventions by Healthcare Professionals

Physicians and primary healthcare providers are well positioned to identify problem drinking and alcohol dependence quickly and offer early intervention for patients whose alcohol use is increasing their risks for medical and psychosocial consequences. Short questionnaires, such as the Michigan Alcoholism Screening Test (MAST) (25) or CAGE questionnaires (26), are often used to detect problematic alcohol use. Newer instruments include the Alcohol Use Disorders Identification Test (AUDIT) and the TWEAK instrument (27, 28). For adolescents, the Adolescent Drinking Index (ADi) is useful (29).

For treatment, brief intervention programs such as physician advice to reduce alcohol consumption for those at an early stage of problem drinking have shown to be effective, especially for those with hazardous but non-dependent drinking. For those who are physically dependent on alcohol, efficient approaches include behavioural self-control training (involving goal setting and self-monitoring), controlling the rate of consumption, and learning substitutes for drinking behaviour. For dependent individuals, more intensive treatment is often needed. Groups such as Alcoholics Anonymous can be beneficial in assisting motivated problem drinkers. Persons with stable social situations and with fewer years of problematic drinking have a better prognosis. Most heavy drinkers do not seek treatment (23).

Population-Based Prevention for Alcohol

Increases in overall or per capita consumption are associated with higher rates of heavy drinking and with increased frequencies of alcohol-related problems. Therefore, an important population-based approach to preventing hazardous drinking and alcohol-related problems is to decrease overall alcohol consumption. Comprehensively, this can be done by paying attention to the 4 E's (23):

- **Economic Accessibility.** A study done in Scotland showed that overall consumption and associated adverse effects fell when prices were increased via excise duty. Heavy drinkers reduced consumption as much as light and moderate drinkers and alcohol-dependent persons reduce alcohol consumption as a function of beverage costs. In an experimental study, reductions in price of alcoholic drinks led to significant increased consumption by both casual and heavy drinkers; a subsequent increase in price caused drinking to drop to previous levels. Liver cirrhosis rates have been found to respond directly and fairly quickly to major restrictions on availability, including economic availability, that produce declines in per capita consumption. Prices affect the number of youths drinking beer and the number of heavy beer drinkers among youth. Dramatic effects are seen in the rates of motor vehicle collisions in youth as a result of excise tax policies.
- **Environmental or Physical Availability.** Although the effectiveness of this factor is mixed, taken together there is evidence that physical availability can affect consumption in heavy and moderate drinkers and reduce alcohol-related problems. Prohibition was successful in reducing consumption and health risks. Cirrhosis mortality rates dropped after institution of Prohibition in the U.S. and gradually increased to previous levels after repeal of prohibition. In Paris during periods of rationing in the two world wars, consumption by both heavy and moderate drinkers

was reduced. In Finland, a marked increase in overall consumption occurred after alcohol became available in previously dry areas.

- **Enforcement of Laws Affecting Accessibility and Use by Youth.** There is much evidence that lower drinking ages are correlated with higher consumption of alcohol and incidence of alcohol-related problems, especially among teens.
- **Education.** Public education is essential to increase public knowledge about reducing risks associated with alcohol use and equip people with the skills to implement the actions needed to reduce the risks of their alcohol use to themselves and others. Small, interactive, peer-based education programs in schools have been found to be effective in increasing knowledge about drug use, facilitating anti-drug-use attitudes, and decreasing the use of tobacco, alcohol, marijuana, and illicit drugs.

1.2.   HEALTH PROMOTION IN RELATION TO SUBSTANCE USE

Even though the majority of Canadians have no personal problem with the use of alcohol or other drugs, including tobacco, there remains the enormous economic burden to society in general and the suffering of those close to the people affected. Federal, provincial, and municipal governments have developed policies to reduce this burden and try to achieve an environment free of substance abuse for all citizens. Because a plethora of information has entered the public arena, healthy choices in relation to substance use need to be promoted as easy choices and to be supported by changes in societal norms.

The health promotion approach focuses on enhancing, maintaining, or regaining the physical, psychological, and social dimensions of health. Health promotion action implies policies, services, and programs designed to enhance the healthfulness of individuals and their environments, not just the physical but also the social, cultural, and economic environments. Swarbrick's Model Program for Substance Abuse Prevention gives a good guide to community participation at all levels of planning for a community program to combat substance abuse (30). School-based policies on alcohol, drugs, and smoking can complement integrated education and prevention programs that incorporate smoking cessation programs and drug education curricula. Peer-assisted learning uses the influence of peers in smoking prevention programs. In post-secondary schools, server intervention, designated-driver programs, and education programs should also be implemented along with campus policies. In the home setting, parents should be encouraged to discuss alcohol and smoking issues and values with children. Educational material supporting smoke-free homes and self-help smoking cessation kits can be introduced into the home. Parents can be educated about quitting smoking and alcohol use. Workplaces provide further sites for health promotion policies such as alcohol and smoke-free policies, health programs, smoking cessation programs run by trained staff and drinking driving countermeasure programs. Furthermore, the healthcare setting itself can be a useful role model by adopting smoke-free workplace policies, and providing education and smoking cessation support. Early detection and intervention programs for alcohol abuse are the responsibility of healthcare providers.

As noted in Chapter 1, harm reduction programs are now recognized as important components in the reduction of risk from substance abuse, such as needle exchange programs.

1.3. NUTRITION

Chapter 4, Determinants of Health and Disease, provided information on the nutritional and dietary status of Canadians. Diet, particularly excessive fat intake and insufficient intake of fruits and vegetables, is a major factor in the development of many chronic diseases, including the two leading killers, cardiovascular disease (31) and cancer. A diet high in saturated fatty acids and dietary cholesterol and low in polyunsaturated fatty acids is the most important dietary contribution to high serum total and LDL cholesterol levels, which are important risk factors for cardiovascular diseases (8, 32). Although there is a possible role for total and saturated animal fat intake in some cancers, the scientific evidence regarding diet and cancer is far stronger for the protective effect of increased fruit and vegetable consumption. Scientific evidence that a diet high in fruits and vegetables protects against cancers of the lung, mouth, pharynx, esophagus, stomach, colon, and rectum, and probably protects against cancers of the breast, bladder, and larynx is the basis for recommendations from several groups to eat at least 5 to 10 servings of fresh fruit or vegetables daily (33). Nutrition is also a factor in the prevention of neural tube and other congenital anomalies, osteoporosis, chronic liver disease, and dental health. Obesity is a risk factor for diabetes and synergistic with other risks for cardiovascular disease (CVD).

National guidelines for nutrition have been published by Health Canada in the report called Nutrition Recommendations (34), which recommends that the Canadian diet should provide:

- energy consistent with the maintenance of body weight within the recommended range;
- essential nutrients in amounts recommended;
- no more than 30% of energy as fat (33 g/1,000 kcal or 39 g/5,000 kJ) and no more than 10% as saturated fat (11 g/1,000 kcal or 13 g/5,000 kJ);
- no more than 55% of energy as carbohydrate (138 g/1,000 kcal or 165 g/5,000 kJ) from a variety of sources;
- no more than 5% of total energy as alcohol, or two drinks daily, whichever is less;
- no more caffeine than the equivalent of four regular cups of coffee per day;
- a reduction in the sodium content of the Canadian diet; and
- fluoridation of community water supplies containing less than 1 mg/L fluoride to that level.

On a practical level, Canada's Food Guide to Healthy Eating provides the following key nutrition messages for healthy Canadians over the age of two (35): enjoy a variety of foods; emphasize cereals, breads, other grain products, vegetables, and fruit; choose lower fat dairy products, leaner meats, and foods prepared with little or no fat; and limit salt, alcohol, and caffeine.

1.4.   PHYSICAL INACTIVITY

Physical inactivity creates a significant health and economic burden in Canada. About $2.1 billion, or 2.5% of the total direct healthcare costs, and about 21,000 lost lives were attributable to physical inactivity in 1999. A 10% reduction in the prevalence of physical inactivity could potentially reduce direct healthcare expenditures by $150 million a year (36). Risks of coronary artery disease, stroke, colon cancer, breast cancer, osteoporosis, and type 2 diabetes are all increased with physical inactivity (36, 37). Physical activity is important in maintaining a healthy body weight and improving serum lipids, cholesterol, and blood pressure (8, 32).

People who are overweight may be able to reduce their level of risk of some health consequences by engaging in regular exercise. Overweight or obese men who reported at least a moderate level of leisure-time physical activity in 1994–95 had significantly lower odds (0.5) of being diagnosed with heart disease over the next four years, compared with overweight/obese men with a low level of activity (38). One study in the United States reported that unfit men who were within the acceptable weight range had a higher risk of mortality than did overweight men who were fit (39).

Canada's Physical Activity Guide to Healthy Active Living recommends that Canadians engage in endurance and flexibility activities four to seven days each per week and strength activities two to four days per week (40). More generally, the guide recommends an hour of low-intensity activity every day or 30 to 60 minutes of moderate-intensity activity or 20 to 30 minutes of vigorous intensity activity four to seven days a week. Only 34% of Canadians aged 25 to 55 years are meeting this recommendation (36). About two thirds of Canadians are physically inactive.

1.5.   HEALTH PROMOTION FOR NUTRITION AND PHYSICAL ACTIVITY

The Ottawa Charter for Health Promotion strategies (creating healthy environments, reorienting health services, and increasing prevention, as described in Chapter 1) can be applied to improving diets and physical activity and reducing the burden of illness. In encouraging healthy eating and increased physical activity, for example, action should be directed to the community at large, involving the media and community organizations in promoting healthy eating and physical activity campaigns. Healthy food policies in schools can be introduced by healthy choices among cafeteria items. Policies ensuring that children get regular physical activity through physical education classes and extracurricular activities are examples of appropriate school policies (41). In urban settings, examples of an environment conducive to physical activity are safe walking or biking paths and shopping malls opened early in winter for seniors to walk in. Individuals and families can receive educational material to promote healthy eating habits and physical activity in home environments. Labelling the content of grocery and menu items facilitates healthy choices at the point of purchase in grocery stores and restaurants. Similar strategies can be implemented in workplaces and healthcare settings (34). Affordability of healthy food choices and recreational facilities is also important to ensuring accessibility to healthy and nutritious foods and physical activity for all people, particularly the populations living in poverty who are most vulnerable to a range of chronic diseases related to obesity and physical inactivity. Nutrition action should also include policy and regulatory changes to agricultural, marketing, and trade practices, to facilitate more widely available healthy choices of food.

The importance of the broader determinants of health has been recognized in the development of programs and policies to improve the nutritional status of Canadians and address issues such as food insecurity and genetically modified foods (see Chapter 4). Canada has committed to the World Food Summit to develop an action plan for food security both at home and abroad; the plan deals with issues of production and availability of nutritionally adequate and safe food as well as access or capacity to such food (42). Quebec's ministry of health (Ministère de la santé et des services sociaux), together with the regional boards, plans to implement specific strategies and actions that contribute to the accessibility of sufficient, acceptable, and reasonably priced nutritious food to its population. Financial support is given to each region to encourage the development of pilot projects, such as collective kitchens, food cooperatives, and food-buying groups with farmers and others (43).

Responsibility for genetically modified food is shared by the Canadian Food Inspection Agency, for environmental safety, and Health Canada, for human health and safety issues (see Chapter 12). The Cartagena Protocol on Biosafety of 2000 requires countries exporting crops grown with the aid of biotechnology to state that they "may contain" genetically modified organisms (44). However, labelling at the consumer level is voluntary. The issue of mandatory labelling is contentious, not only as an issue of safety, health, and nutrition, but also as an issue of the "consumers' right to know" (45). Health Canada has passed legislation requiring labelling of food constituents, however labelling for genetically modified food is not required by law.

Nutrition for Health: An Agenda for Action (46), published in 1996, describes a multisectoral collaboration that identifies the priorities for improving nutrition from the perspective of population health. Four strategic directions were identified: reinforce healthy eating practices; support nutritionally vulnerable populations; enhance the availability of foods that support healthy eating; and support nutrition research. The steering committee identified the need to collect data on important core indicators of population nutritional status.

1.6. CHRONIC DISEASE PREVENTION AND CONTROL STRATEGY

As can be seen from this section, the use of tobacco and alcohol, a diet high in saturated and dietary cholesterol and low in vegetables and fruits, and physical inactivity contribute significantly to a number of chronic diseases, including cardiovascular diseases such as coronary heart disease and stroke, a number of cancers, diabetes, and osteoporosis. To date, many initiatives for preventing chronic disease and promoting health have focused on education and on building individual knowledge and skills. Increasingly, however, it is recognized that such initiatives remain limited if they are not accompanied by supportive environments and healthy public policy. It is now becoming widely accepted that the prevention and control of chronic diseases require multilevel and comprehensive approaches (47), much as the control of infectious diseases has required and still requires environmental controls, and the use of policies, regulations, and legislation within and outside the health sector (48). As a result, there has been a growing movement in Canada to develop a single coordinated strategy to address the common risk factors shared by multiple chronic diseases.

2.   SPECIFIC DISEASES

2.1.   CARDIOVASCULAR DISEASE

Trends

Ischemic heart disease (IHD) is the most common form of cardiovascular disease (CVD). Acute myocardial infarction (heart attack) is the most widely recognized form of ischemic heart disease. In terms of prevention, CVD is often grouped with cerebrovascular disease (stroke), because the two diseases share risk factors. Since the first national mortality statistics were published in 1921, CVD has been the leading cause of death in Canada. CVD is currently the cause of death of more than one third of Canadians (8). CVD mortality rates today are almost half those in 1969 and have declined at about 2% per year, but the mortality rates for stroke have not changed significantly in the past 10 years. Statistics Canada projections suggest that although the number of CVD deaths for men will not increase, the numbers for women will have increased by 28% between 1995 and 2016, due in large part to higher rates of tobacco use among women.

Cardiovascular disease is the leading cause of death worldwide, but rates vary considerably among countries. In the mid 1990s, age-standardized mortality rates for all cardiovascular disease in men ranged from a high of 1,051.7 deaths per 100,000 in the Russian Federation, to a low of 232.7 deaths per 100,000 in Japan. In 1996, Canada's rates per 100,000 were 307 for men and 185 for women. Caution must be used in comparing between countries because the statistics are collected and calculated using different methods. Among 22 selected countries, Canada ranks 11th in mortality from ischemic heart disease, at a rate of 186.1 deaths per 100,000 for men and 95 per 100,000 for women. Canada has the lowest stroke mortality rates in men (51 per 100,000) and the second lowest in women (42 per 100,000) after France.

Unfortunately, incidence data for CVD is lacking in Canada, so it is unclear whether incidence is decreasing even though mortality rates are decreasing. There is a recent initiative to expand the Canadian Heart and Stroke Surveillance System. Worldwide there are remarkably few reports of CVD incidence, likely because existing systems do not allow for easy determination. Recently, however, findings of the World Health Organization (WHO) Monica Project involving a multinational prospective assessment of incidence over 10 years found that most western industrialized countries have shown a small but significant decrease in incidence in all age groups and in both sexes (8).

Data in the following sections come from reports published by the Heart and Stroke Foundation and the Federal, Provincial and Territorial Advisory Committee on Population Health unless otherwise specified (7, 8, 49).

Mortality

CVD is the leading cause of death in Canada (79,457 or 36% of deaths in 1997), and the third leading cause of potential years of life lost (164,417 years of life lost to heart disease and strokes). For men of all ages, 36% of deaths are attributable to CVD, while in women the percentage is slightly higher, at 38%. After menopause, the proportion of all female deaths due to CVD increases. In men, the risk of death due to CVD increases steadily from age 35 to 84.

Morbidity

CVD is the leading cause of hospital admissions for men and women excluding pregnancy and childbirth (see Chapter 5). While the hospitalization rates for heart disease and stroke have decreased slightly, the actual number of hospitalizations has increased due to rapid increase in the elderly population (see Chapter 4).

In 1998, approximately 26.4 million (9%) of visits made by Canadians to physicians were for CVD. One half of these visits were for the management of high blood pressure. The number of prescriptions for cardiovascular conditions increased by 6.4% from 1997 to 1998, a figure that represents the largest single increase in the last 55 years. In 1998, an estimated 32.5 million prescriptions, or 12.8% of the total 254.2 million prescriptions dispensed in Canada, were dispensed for the treatment of CVD. The economic impact of CVD is high, accounting for 11.6% ($18.5 billion) of the total cost of illness classified by diagnostic category in 1998 ($6.8 billion in direct costs and $11.7 billion in indirect costs) (50) (see Chapter 5).

Risk Factors

Sociodemographic factors are important risk factors in CVD. Age is the dominant risk factor: the risk increases with age. Sex is also important, with risks being higher in men. There is a 10-year lag for women in development of coronary artery disease. A positive family history for CVD at younger ages is a strong predictor of risk for future generations. CVD risks vary with ethnicity, although the degree to which this is due to genetic factors or sociocultural ones is unclear. Studies on migrating populations suggest a predominance of sociocultural influences, including diet, in the occurrence of coronary heart disease among migrants. Rates and risk factors for coronary heart disease move toward the rates of the population of the destination country within a generation.

In Canada, CVD death rates show a gradient with socioeconomic status; thus, the rate of CVD-related deaths is 35% higher in men and 11% higher in women of the lowest income quartile compared to the highest quartiles. The prevalence of CVD risk factors is also inversely related to socioeconomic status in Canada (51). The relationship of socioeconomic status to risk factor prevalence is stronger and more consistent for education than income, and is particularly strong for smoking and excess weight; persons with higher education tend to smoke less and are less obese.

Tobacco smoking is responsible for more deaths due to heart disease and stroke than deaths due to cancer. Smoking increases the risk of all major forms of heart disease and stroke, and peripheral vascular disease. Women who smoke and use oral contraceptives are at increased risk of subarachnoid hemorrhage. Epidemiological data from multiple countries confirms that individual smokers have higher risks of CVD than non-smokers and that there is a dose-response relationship, meaning that risk increases with amount and duration of smoking. (32).

Dyslipidemias, notably elevated cholesterol, low-density lipoprotein (LDL), and triglyceride levels, and low high-density lipoprotein (HDL) levels, increase risks of coronary artery disease. Elevated total serum cholesterol and LDL increase risk of stroke. The 1986–90 Heart Health Surveys report that 45% of men and 43% of women had total plasma cholesterol greater than 5.2 mmol/L (18% men and 17% women had levels of at least or greater than 6.2 mmol/L) (see Chapter 4). Epidemiological studies comparing populations find a strong relationship between diet, average blood cholesterol levels, and incidence of coronary heart disease. Higher dietary fat consumption raises total and LDL cholesterol levels. The composition of fats is also important since higher saturated fatty acid and dietary cholesterol consumption raise serum cholesterol while polyunsaturated fatty acid consumption appears to reduce serum cholesterol. There is some debate about whether monounsaturated fats have a neutral or cholesterol-lowering effect (32).

Hypertension, or high blood pressure (BP), is defined as systolic blood pressure (SBP) greater or equal to 140 mmHg or diastolic blood pressure (DBP) greater or equal to 90 mmHg. It is a major risk factor for coronary artery disease, stroke, peripheral vascular disease, and congestive heart failure (CHF). Hypertension increases the overall CVD risk by two to three times, with even greater increases in risk of cerebrovascular hemorrhage and CHF more significantly than coronary heart disease and thrombotic stroke. The risk factors for developing high BP include being overweight, physical inactivity, heavy alcohol use, and excessive salt intake. Marked sodium depletion reduces blood pressure in people with severe hypertension. Dietary sodium restriction (i.e., a low- or no-salt diet) enables people with high BP to be controlled with lower doses of antihypertensive medications.

Physical inactivity increases risk of CVD. Level of physical activity is inversely related to risk of mortality from coronary heart disease. A recent review reported that risk of physical inactivity increases the risk of first event of coronary heart disease and there was a significant and graded relationship between physical inactivity and risk of first event. Physical inactivity has an effect on mortality risk of coronary heart disease independent of other risk factors such as serum lipid levels, LDL, hypertension, and diabetes (32).

Overweight is defined as having a body mass index (BMI) above 25 (see Chapters 3 and 4). Excess weight is defined as having a BMI 26 or 27 and obesity as BMI greater than 27 (8). Being overweight is a risk factor for developing high BP and diabetes; it also affects blood lipids. People with greater waist-to-hip circumference ratio (WHR) have higher risks of coronary heart disease, premature death, type 2 diabetes, and cancer in women. Several studies have shown that the fat distribution is better correlated with occurrence of several diseases than general measures of overweight or obesity (32).

Clinical, pathological, and epidemiological evidence all support a causal role for diabetes in coronary heart disease. Type 2 diabetes increases risks of developing high blood pressure, stroke, heart disease, and vascular disease, particularly in women. People with diabetes have not only higher risks of CVD but also more severe disease and higher mortality. Other risk factors (aside from hyperglycemia) — physical inactivity, body weight, blood pressure, blood lipid levels, dietary composition, and smoking — greatly affect the risk of coronary heart disease in diabetics. Diabetes can be prevented by maintenance of healthy weight through healthy nutrition and regular physical activity.

Drinking more than two alcoholic drinks per day increases risks of high BP and CVD. Alcohol abuse increases risk for hemorrhagic stroke and subarachnoid hemorrhage. There is a curvilinear, J-shaped relationship between levels of alcohol consumption and risk of mortality from heart disease; individuals who do not drink alcohol are at higher risk for heart disease than individuals who drink one drink per day (32). The cardioprotective effects of alcohol appear to occur with as little as one drink every other day.

Several psychosocial factors appear to be risk factors for CVD (see Chapter 1). Myocardial ischemia can be precipitated by mental stress (such as anxiety or anger). The impact of stress is mediated by the individuals' ability to cope and by their surrounding support network. There is evidence linking hostility (rather than type A personality) to increased risks of coronary heart disease in men. Several prospective population-based studies have established an association between stronger social support (social connectedness) and reduced risk of death, including mortality from CVD; whether this is causal is unclear (32).

Several external physical factors also appear to be important. Exertion in the cold (e.g., snow shoveling) is associated with myocardial ischemia and infarction. Emergency room visits for acute coronary syndromes and cardiac arrest increase after heavy snowfalls. Half of myocardial infarctions (heart attacks) occur in winter and when temperatures are lowest, with most deaths occurring after brief exposure to cold.

Prevention

Although age, sex, family history, and ethnicity cannot be altered, many other CVD risk factors e.g., hypertension, smoking, physical inactivity and obesity are amenable to preventive health practices. Chapter 11 outlines efficacious manoeuvres to deal with these modifiable risk factors at individual level.

Smoking cessation lowers risk of coronary heart disease. After one year, excess risk is reduced by about half; after 15 years of cessation, the risk is similar to that of a non-smoker. Similarly, prognosis improves in survivors of myocardial infarction who quit smoking compared to those who continue smoking. The MRFIT study showed that the success rate for smoking cessation in the first year and for up to four years in high-risk participants was 40% under ideal supportive circumstances (32).

The Working Group on Hypercholesterolemia and Other Dyslipidemias recently recommended serum lipid screening in women over the age of 50 and men over the age of 40 and in adults with two or more risk factors for coronary artery disease, with clinical evidence of coronary artery disease, peripheral vascular disease, or carotid atherosclerosis, with diabetes mellitus, and with family history of dyslipidemia or coronary artery disease (52).

The cholesterol threshold for initiating treatments depends on a calculation of the overall risk of coronary heart disease based on the other risk factors present in the individual (i.e., the higher the overall risk, the lower the cholesterol value needed to start treatment). Treatments for high and very high cholesterol involve medications as well as lifestyle modifications; treatments for those at medium to low risk start with lifestyle modifications (for three to six months) first. Pharmacological treatment of high blood cholesterol levels reduces acute myocardial infarctions (heart attacks) by 25% over four years in most studies; it also reduces the rate of stroke.

The Canadian Task Force on Preventive Health Care recommends that all adults over age 20 have blood pressure screening done every two years. The 1996–97 National Population Health Survey (NPHS) showed that 84% of Canadians had BP checked in the last two years, the highest rates being found in the over-65 age group and the lowest rates in the 25–44 age group (8).

Small amounts of alcohol appear to be cardioprotective, and for those who choose to drink, moderate consumption should be the goal. Non-drinkers should not start drinking solely for cardioprotective benefit as the adverse health effects of alcohol use overweigh its benefits. Regular alcohol use is often accompanied by enhancement of overeating, underactivity and smoking (32). Effective control of blood sugar, weight, and hypertension in diabetes decreases the risk of heart disease and stroke.

2.1.1.   Community-Wide Approaches to Heart Health

The decline in cardiovascular mortality in Canada has been attributed, in part, to the reduction in the prevalence of smoking, reduced consumption of dietary fat, and improved detection and management of hypertension, as well as to improved surgical and medical approaches to treatment of symptomatic heart disease. The current widespread prevalence of risk factors, however, remains a concern.

From a population perspective, initiatives can be undertaken to shift the distribution of risk factors and protective factors in a population. Epidemiological studies comparing populations find a strong relationship between diet, average blood cholesterol levels. and incidence of coronary heart disease. There is also a consistently strong relationship between high average population blood pressure and increase salt intake. Thus, healthier diets with lower saturated fat, cholesterol, and salt intakes and increased polyunsaturated fat intake can be promoted across the adult population. Likewise, population-based approaches to increasing physical activity and social networks and supports, and decreasing stress are integral to effective community-wide approaches.

Community-based models for primary (and secondary) prevention of heart disease, using many of the health promotion strategies described in Chapter 1, have spread, following demonstration of their effectiveness for reducing cardiovascular disease risk in populations in several studies.

Models used in North Karelia, Finland, and the Stanford Five-City Study (53-55) have provided the basis for the Canadian Heart Health Initiative (CHHI) undertaken by Health Canada in partnership with the provinces and the Heart and Stroke Foundation of Canada (56). This multidisciplinary, intersectoral initiative has five phases: national policy development, surveys of cardiovascular disease risk factors in all ten provinces and the development of a national database on cardiovascular risk factors, the implementation of provincial heart health demonstration programs, evaluation of the demonstration heart health programs, and the diffusion of the findings and interventions to communities across Canada. Such community-based population-wide approaches, backed by research, can be expected to reduce the prevalence of risk factors for cardiovascular disease, and trends in prevalence of some risk factors, such as smoking, are encouraging. Actions to further improve diet and to encourage active lifestyles are important strategies that need more attention.

Promoting heart health equity calls for an approach in which health is seen as a shared responsibility between individuals and the systems that influence their health, and there have been calls to coordinate the CHHI with a broader initiative that includes the prevention of other chronic diseases since multiple chronic diseases often share similar risk factors. Community-based interventions for CVD prevention have traditionally targeted educated, middle class people who are already highly motivated to change their lives, mainly through the dissemination of messages about modifying lifestyle behaviour. These methods have been largely ineffective in reaching people living in disadvantaged circumstances. Inadequate financial resources, limited education and illiteracy, unemployment or underemployment, and isolation make people less easy to reach through conventional health education methods, and their circumstances rarely provide enabling environments for behaviour change (57).

2.2.   CANCER

Trends

After CVD, cancer is the second leading cause of death in the Canadian population (3). The mortality rate for all cancers combined among men has been declining since 1988, mainly due to the decrease in mortality rates for lung and colorectal cancers. When lung cancer is excluded, there has been a steady, significant decline in combined cancer mortality rates in women since the 1970s.

Lung cancer is the number-one cause of cancer mortality among both men and women. In women, its incidence and mortality rates started to level off in 1993 following several decades of rapid increase. This trend reflects a decline in smoking rates that began in the 1970s; however, smoking rates still remain more than four times as high as in 1971.

Colorectal cancer is the third most common cancer for both men and women; both incidence and mortality have been declining steadily over the past 15 years. Mortality rates for Hodgkin's disease and stomach cancer have been decreasing steadily over time. Thyroid cancer, although relatively rare, has the most rapidly increasing incidence for both men and women in the last decade. Mortality rates have decreased for men and stayed stable for women.

The steady increase in breast cancer incidence since the 1960s levelled off in 1993. Mortality rates for breast cancer in women have declined steadily since 1986. The divergent trends in incidence and mortality are consistent with the benefits of screening and treatment.

Prostate cancer incidence started to decline in 1994 following a rapid increase likely secondary to the use of early detection techniques. Prostate cancer mortality rates are stable.

Mortality

In 2001, an estimated 134,100 new cases of cancer and 65,300 deaths from cancer occurred (see Table 5.2 in Chapter 5). One third of all potential years of life lost are due to cancer. Cancer occurs primarily in older Canadians, with 70% of new cancer cases and 81% of deaths due to cancer occurring among those who are at least 60 years old (3).

For men, the three most common cancers are lung, colorectal, and prostate. Based on 2001 estimates, men have a lifetime probability of 1 in 9 of developing prostate cancer, 1 in 11.5 of developing lung cancer, and 1 in 16 of developing colorectal cancer.

The three leading cancers for women are lung, breast, and colorectal. Women have a lifetime probability of 1 in 9.5 of developing breast cancer, 1 in 18 of developing colorectal cancer, and 1 in 19 of developing lung cancer.

Morbidity

Cancer was responsible for 7.3% of the total 3 million hospitalizations in 1998-99 and 9.9% of the total 20.9 million hospital days; the average length of hospitalization (9.5 days) for cancer patients was 2.5 days longer than the overall average length of stay. Cancer was the second most costly component of health care in 1998, with $2.5 billion in direct costs and $11.7 billion in indirect costs (50).

A prognostic indicator for cancer is the ratio of deaths to cases expressed as five-year survival probability or recurrence-free survival duration. Overall, the ratio was 49% from estimated figures for Canada in 2001. Prognosis for individual cancers varies from poor (ratio greater than 50%: lung, adult leukemia, pancreas, stomach, ovary, brain, multiple myeloma, and esophagus) to fairly good (ratio of greater than 30% but less than 50%: colorectal, non-Hodgkin's lymphoma, female bladder, kidney, oral, and larynx) to very good (a ratio of 30% or less: breast, prostate, melanoma, uterus, thyroid, cervix, Hodgkin's disease, testes, and male bladder).

Risk Factors

While a few cancers may be associated with inherited genetic factors (e.g., polyposis of the colon and the inherited form of retinoblastoma), behavioural and environmental factors are considered important determinants. According to one study, two thirds of cancer deaths can be linked to tobacco use, diet, obesity, and lack of exercise, as follows: 30% of total cancer deaths due to tobacco; 30% due to adult diet and obesity; 5% each due to a sedentary lifestyle, occupational factors, viruses and biological agents; 3% alcohol; 2% each exposure to ultraviolet radiation and environmental pollution (58).

Variations in cancer rates among immigrants provide supportive evidence of environmental effects in the development of some neoplasms. Proportional mortality rates for cancers of the stomach and lung in Ontario show a gradient for different generations of immigrants from the same country. The highest rates are for the immigrants themselves, intermediate for the first generation, and lowest for the second generation. Changes in lifestyle, dietary patterns, or other environmental exposure may be responsible for this observed shift.

Workplace and environmental exposures to high concentrations of certain chemicals increase risks of some cancers (see Table 10.2 in Chapter 10). For example, inhalation of asbestos and chromium is associated with cancer of the lung, and benzidine and beta-naphthylamine with bladder cancer.

2.2.1. General Framework for Cancer Control

Miller has devised an excellent planning framework for cancer control strategies, which could be usefully applied to the control of other chronic diseases (59). The steps are the following:

- **Assess the current situation:** Determine the relative importance of cancer to other diseases, determine the relative importance of different cancer sites, identify differences between provinces in the range of indicators, as well as differences between Canada and other countries, and determine the availability of resources for cancer control. Indicators may include the number of cancer cases diagnosed (incidence), number of deaths from cancer, survival, sex ratio, cumulative incidence, premature mortality, and trends.
- **Set objectives for cancer control:** Reduce morbidity from cancer, reduce mortality from cancer, and improve the quality of life of cancer patients.
- **Evaluate possible strategies.**
- **Set priorities using quantitative assessments:** Determine the potential effectiveness of different strategies, determine the potential cost of different strategies, determine the cost effectiveness of all different and competing strategies, modify the priority for action on the basis of other considerations, and monitor trends in disease to evaluate effectiveness of strategies.

2.2.2. Site-Specific Cancer Control

The following sections discuss specific types of cancer. The etiology for different cancers is different and diverse. For some cancers, the risk and protective factors are well known while they are relatively unknown for others. For those with such known factors, primary prevention is important. Smoking, for example, is a risk factor for several cancers and therefore an important target for primary prevention activities. For cancers with less well-defined risk and protective factors, secondary and tertiary prevention — where available and appropriate — should be emphasized.

Lung Cancer

Lung cancer remains the leading cause of cancer death for both sexes. Almost one third of the cancer deaths in men and almost one quarter in women are due to lung cancer alone. In 2001, 7,400 women will die of lung cancer, compared with 5,500 deaths expected for breast cancer. In men, the 10,700 lung cancer deaths far exceed the 4,300 deaths due to prostate cancer (3). Because of its relative frequency among Canadians and poor survival rates, lung cancer is by far the leading cause of death due to cancer.

Effective tobacco control is of utmost importance in lung cancer. Cigarette smoking is the main cause of lung cancer, accounting for at least 80% of all new cases in women and 90% of those in men. Pipe and cigar smoking are also linked to lung cancer. ETS is a risk factor for lung cancer, as carcinogens are present in the tobacco smoke inhaled by bystanders. Environmental contaminants such as asbestos and arsenic are associated with increased risk of lung cancer. Occupational exposure to radon increases lung cancer risk. Air pollution, in particular motor vehicle exhaust and industrial emission releases of polycyclic aromatic hydrocarbons, are known to be carcinogenic (60).

There is convincing evidence that the risk of lung cancer can be decreased through a high intake of fresh fruits and vegetables. The risk for individuals with a high consumption of fresh fruit and vegetables is about one half that of individuals with much lower consumption. According to the Canadian Task Force on Preventive Health Care, there is fair evidence to advise smokers to follow a diet high in green leafy vegetables and fruit; however, it recommends against routine chest x-rays or sputum cytology screening for lung cancer in healthy asymptomatic Canadians (60).

Colorectal Cancer

An estimated 17,200 new cases and 6,400 deaths from colorectal cancer will occur in Canada in 2001 (3). It is the third most common cancer and most frequent cause of death from cancer in both men and women.

The risk of colorectal cancer increases with age. The elderly are more likely to develop colorectal cancer, with the highest probability among those in their 70s. Age-standardized incidence and mortality rates have been declining since 1985. There has been a greater decline in the mortality rates for women than men, perhaps due to changes in exposures to risk factors (e.g., diet, exogenous hormones, physical activity) or prevention programs that have benefited women more than men. Recent research suggests that the non-steroidal anti-inflammatory drugs (NSAIDs) may protect against colorectal cancer, and increased use of these medications in the last two decades may have contributed to the decline.

Early detection and screening for colorectal cancer may also have contributed to the recent decline in rates. Early detection procedures include fecal occult blood test (detects blood in the stool); sigmoidoscopy, colonoscopy, which allow direct visualization of the colon; and an indirect procedure involving x-rays and barium enema. The implementation of large population-based screening programs is controversial and much debated, because of the sensitivity and specificity of the tests, cost-effectiveness, compliance (most large trials are able to achieve 50% compliance at most), ethical issues (lack of informed consent of negative aspects of test), and the capacity of the healthcare system to provide equitable access to facilities for diagnosis and treatment (61, 62). The Expert Panel and Cancer Care Ontario and Canadian Task Force on Preventive Health Care recommend screening for general population aged 50 and over by annual or biennial fecal occult blood (63, 64).

Breast Cancer

In 2001, 19,500 Canadian women were diagnosed with breast cancer, and 5,500 died of the disease. It is the most frequent new cancer among women and the second most common cause of cancer death in women after lung cancer.

Age is the most significant risk factor for breast cancer. Other risk factors are family history, history of benign breast disease, and high levels of radiation exposure to the chest. Risk factors that show definite association but do not contribute to high incidence levels include obesity in postmenopausal women; reproductive factors such as never having had children, being 30 or older at first full-term pregnancy, early onset menstruation, late onset menopause; and sociodemographic risk factors such as living in an urban area, higher socioeconomic status, and having been born in North America or Northern Europe. There is controversy over whether oral contraceptives are a risk factor, and there is a suggested link with postmenopausal estrogen replacement therapy (65).

There is evidence that dietary and lifestyle factors play a role in breast cancer. The risk of breast cancer appears to increase with increasing alcohol consumption, and women who drink alcohol should have no more than 9 drinks per week. There is some evidence that consumption of meat and that higher levels of total and saturated fat intake possibly increase the risk of breast cancer. Higher levels of vegetable and fruit consumption probably decrease the risk, as do higher levels of dietary carotenoids, fibre, and physical activity. The World Cancer Research Fund's expert panel report states that "plant-based diets, together with the maintenance of recommended body mass and regular physical activity, may decrease the incidence of breast cancer by about 33–50%" (33). The report also states "these habits will have the most benefit if established before puberty and maintained throughout life."

Although tamoxifen, an anti-estrogenic compound, has demonstrated effect in decreasing the risk of breast cancer recurrence, it is not currently recommended for the routine prevention of breast cancer in healthy women (in the three trials so far, two showed no benefit and one showed benefit; there were significant side effects including blood clots and uterine cancer in all three trials) (65). The Canadian Task Force on Preventive Health Care recently stated that there is fair evidence to recommend against the use of tamoxifen to reduce the risk of breast cancer in women at low or normal risk of the disease. It recommends that women at high risk be counselled on the potential benefits and harms of breast cancer prevention with tamoxifen (66).

About 5% of cases of breast cancer are due to an autosomal dominant inherited predisposition. It is possible to test some people at high risk for inherited mutations to the BRAC1 and BRAC2 genes. Women with some mutations to the BRAC1 or BRAC2 gene may have a 56% to 85% lifetime risk of acquiring breast cancer (67).

The mainstay of prevention of breast cancer remains early detection and treatment. The Canadian Task Force on Preventive Health Care recommends annual screening with a clinical breast exam and mammography for women aged 50 to 69 (68). The Canadian Task Force on Preventive Health Care now recommends that women aged 40 to 49 be informed of the potential benefits and risk of screening mammography and assisted in deciding at what age they wish to start mammography (69). Recent evidence has shown that there is sufficient evidence to exclude the routine teaching of breast self-examination (BSE) from the periodic health examination of women aged 40 to 69, and there is insufficient evidence to evaluate its effectiveness in women younger than 40 and older than 70 thus precluding recommendation of teaching breast self-examination to women in this age group (70).

Prostate Cancer

As of 2001, prostate cancer is the third most frequently occurring cancer in Canadian men. It is estimated that 17,800 new cases will be diagnosed in 2001, as compared with 12,100 lung cancers. However, the number of men who will die from prostate cancer (4,300) is far less than the number of Canadian men who will die of lung cancer in 2001 (10,700).

The Canadian Task Force on Preventive Health Care does not recommend population screening for prostate cancer and states that there is fair evidence to exclude both the transrectal ultrasound and the prostate-specific antigen (PSA) test. The major issue is the lack of evidence that there is a survival benefit from early detection of prostate cancer. Modeling by several groups suggests no benefit and potential harm if one considers the side effects of treatment, particularly incontinence and impotence after surgery. Also there are low positive predictive values of the PSA test, which range from 8% to 33%; at best 67% of patients identified as having a positive result will undergo unnecessary biopsy (71). There is currently poor evidence either to include or to exclude the digital rectal examination from regular health check-ups, because only the posterior and lateral aspects of the prostate can be palpated, leaving 40% to 50% of cancers beyond reach (71).

The role of nutrition in the primary prevention of prostate cancer is receiving more research attention. Evidence exists that soy isoflavones, lycopenes from tomatoes, vitamin D, and selenium may play a role in the primary prevention of prostate cancer (72). There is a small but significant association of high consumption of total and saturated animal fat which indicates increase in risk. The higher levels of physical activity possibly decrease the risk of prostate cancer (33).

Leukemia

Childhood leukemia is the most common form of childhood cancer. In Canada, approximately 1 in 6,400, or 1,644, children are diagnosed with leukemia before the age of 19 years. The death-to-case ratio was 0.24, which indicates good prognosis for children with leukemia. A Canadian case-control study of childhood leukemia in relation to exposure to power-frequency electric and magnetic fields found little support for a relationship between the two (73). At present there are no primary prevention programs available.

Cancer of the Cervix

Cancer of the cervix is ranked 11th for incidence and deaths from cancer in Canadian women. An estimated 371,000 new cases of invasive cervical cancer are diagnosed worldwide each year, representing nearly 10% or all cancers in women. In 2001, nearly 1,450 new cases of cervical cancer were estimated to have been diagnosed in Canadian women and 420 women died of the disease. The highest incidence rates were found in

Nova Scotia, Newfoundland and Labrador, and Prince Edward Island. Among the Canadian Inuit, cervical cancer accounts for nearly 15% of all cancers among women. The age-standardized rate is six times higher than the national average among Aboriginal Canadian women in Saskatchewan (74).

There has been a decline in the age-standardized incidence and mortality rates in Canada since 1960. Declines in cervical cancer incidence and mortality coincide with increased Papanicolaou smear (Pap) screening, which is interpreted as evidence of the role of Pap smears in decreasing cervical cancer incidence. It is now well established that human papillomavirus (HPV) infection is the central causal factor in cervical cancer. HPV infections are the most common sexually transmitted diseases today. There are more than 100 types of HPV, which are divided into groups according to oncogenic risk. Other factors increasing risk include higher numbers of sexual partners, younger age of first sexual intercourse, tobacco smoking, long-term use of oral contraceptives, and diet (a high intake of fruits and vegetables and foods containing beta carotene and vitamin C possibly reduces the risk of cervical cancer).

The Canadian Task Force on Preventive Health Care recommends that women receive regular Pap smears upon becoming sexually active (or at age 18) until age 69. The frequency can be reduced to every three years after two consecutive normal test results. For women with Pap results of uncertain significance, cytological evidence of HPV infection in the smear will likely play a bigger role in guiding decision making about intervention and frequency of follow-up (74). There is an ongoing and promising research in development of vaccine for HPV to eradicate cervical cancer in future (75).

Stomach Cancer and Helicobacter pylori

In 2001, nearly 2,800 new cases of stomach cancer were estimated to have been diagnosed in Canada and 1,950 died of the disease. Recent findings strongly implicate *Helicobacter pylori (H. pylori)* infection in the development of adenocarcinoma and some lymphomas of the stomach. Studies have supported the role of *H. pylori* infection at young ages in the pathogenesis of stomach cancers (4, 58).

Cancer and the Environment

The incidence of melanoma and non-Hodgkin's lymphoma has been increasing rapidly in recent years. Environmental and occupational exposures as well as genetic factors are causal factors in both these cancers. Exposure to ultraviolet light is an important cause of melanoma. Factors also associated with non-Hodgkin's lymphoma are exposures to phenoxyacetic acid herbicides, solvents, and viruses. Table 10.2 in Chapter 10 lists other occupational and environmental substances that are considered by the International Agency for Research on Cancer (IARC) to cause cancer in humans when exposed for prolonged periods or in very high concentrations (see also Chapters 9) (76).

2.3.   RESPIRATORY DISEASES

Common respiratory diseases include asthma, chronic bronchitis, emphysema, and pneumonia.

Mortality

In 1996, non-cancer respiratory diseases were the third leading cause of death, the fifth leading cause of PYLL, and the third leading cause of hospitalization in Canada (7). There were 10,301 deaths from non-cancer respiratory diseases, accounting for 9.2% of deaths in Canada (77). There is a J-shaped curve for the age-specific mortality rates for both sexes, with mortality higher in the very young and very old age groups.

Morbidity

The total economic cost of respiratory diseases in 1998 was $8.5 billion; direct costs accounted for $3.5 billion and indirect costs for $5 billion (50). For chronic bronchitis, emphysema, and asthma combined, Health Canada estimates that in 1993 the direct costs were $1.3 billion and the indirect costs $3 billion (78). Incidence, prevalence, hospitalization, and mortality rates from asthma, a chronic inflammatory disorder of the airways causing recurrent episodes of wheezing, breathlessness, chest tightness, and cough, are increasing in Canada and many industrialized countries. (79). In Canada, the prevalence and death rates of childhood asthma have risen sharply over the past two decades (80). It is also becoming more prevalent among low-income adults over the age of 35 (78). The causes of these increases remain under study. According to the 1996–97 NPHS, more than 2.2 million Canadians (12.2% of children under age 19 years and 6.3% of adults) have been diagnosed with asthma at some time in their lives (78). The rate of hospital separations/discharge for asthma in children aged 0 to 14 years increased sharply from 311 per 100,000 in 1978–79 to 514 per 100,000 in 1983–84, but decreased to 488 per 100,000 in 1994–95 (80). The persistence of inappropriate asthma management by practitioners and inappropriate use of asthma medications by patients, despite the presence of guidelines, leads to higher risks of fatal asthma attacks and significantly increased use of healthcare resources (81).

Risk Factors

Important factors influencing respiratory disease mortality rates include smoking (active and ETS), respiratory pathogens, and indoor and outdoor air pollution (see Chapter 9). Smoking is considered an important risk factor for frequency and severity of respiratory illness. In children, exposure of the fetus, infants, and young children to tobacco smoke increases the risk of asthma. Except where open combustion of fuel is used for cooking or heating (as with wood fires), ETS is generally the most important source of indoor air pollution. In adults, exposure to work-related agents leading to occupational asthma is estimated to cause 5% to 15% of adult-onset asthma (78).

Higher air pollution levels in a number of Canadian communities also lead to higher rates of hospital admissions for respiratory diseases (82, 83) (see Chapter 9). Specifically, higher levels of ground-level ozone, acid aerosols, and particulate matter are associated with increased hospitalization rates for respiratory disease. Inhaled ozone causes an inflammatory response that can result in decreased pulmonary function, increased cough, and chest tightness. Nitrogen dioxide and sulphur dioxide have also been linked to reduced lung function in people with asthma. In a recent study of six Canadian sites, there was variation in the prevalence rates of asthma, with prevalence higher in highly industrialized cities such as Hamilton and lower in more rural areas such as Prince Edward Island (79).

Prevention

Approaches to prevention and cessation of smoking and prevention of exposure to ETS are discussed in the section on substance abuse. Regarding respiratory infections, some research evidence indicates that children who have been breastfed have lower risks of developing asthma (78). Prevention of occupational disease and protection of worker health are addressed in Chapter 10. Health promotion in relation to air pollution is discussed in Chapter 9. Societal actions such as use of public transit, use of fuel-efficient vehicles, and monitoring for industrial pollution can reduce the sources of air pollution, including the combustion of fossil fuels by vehicles, power plants, and industries that lead to the formation of particulates, nitrogen oxides, and volatile organic compounds (nitrogen oxides and volatile organic compounds interact to form ground-level ozone in the presence of heat and sunlight). In addition, better adherence to clinical management guidelines by both healthcare providers and patients for asthma is needed and likely leads to reduced fatality, hospitalization, and healthcare utilization from asthma.

2.4. DIABETES

Diabetes mellitus is a chronic condition that results from the body's inability to produce sufficient insulin or use it properly, leading to chronically high levels of blood glucose. Long-term complications include cardiovascular disease, kidney disease, blindness, neuropathy, lower limb amputations, dental disease, and complications in pregnancy. There are two types of diabetes: type 1, also known as insulin-dependent diabetes, with onset mainly in childhood or adolescence, and type 2, also known as non-insulin dependent diabetes, which occurs primarily in the older population (typically after age 40). Type 2 diabetes is the most common, accounting for 90 to 95% of diagnosed cases of diabetes. With the aging population, and increases in obesity, diabetes-related mortality and morbidity have become an important public health problem (84).

Mortality

In 1996, there were 5,447 deaths for which diabetes was certified as the underlying cause. The actual number of deaths for which diabetes is a contributing cause is estimated to be five times as high. Diabetes is ranked as the seventh leading cause of death in Canada, and it accounts for approximately 25,000 PYLL prior to age 75.

Projections for diabetes mortality trends up to 2016 show a linear increase among females and an exponential increase among males. Age-standardized mortality rates for diabetes have increased since the early 1980s from 15.0 per 100,000 population, to 16.8 in 1996. Since 1983, the age-standardized PYLL due to diabetes has also increased (85).

Morbidity

Diabetes is diagnosed in an estimated 60,000 Canadians every year. According to the National Diabetes Surveillance System (NDSS), it is estimated that one third of all cases of diabetes are undiagnosed in Canada (86). The NDSS found that 4.8% or just over 1 million Canadians aged 20 and older had diabetes (4.6% of women and 5.0% of men); prevalence rates increase with age. One percent of Canadians aged 20 to 39 had been diagnosed with diabetes, and prevalence increased in each successive age group, to a high of 13.5% for all seniors aged 75 or older. In 1998-99, males were more likely to have diabetes in all age groups. The prevalence of diabetes is very high in aboriginal populations: 8.5% of North American Indian peoples on Indian reserves and settlements; 5.3% each for North American Indians off reserves and Métis and 1.9% of Inuit people.

In 1998, the economic burden of diabetes was estimated to be up to $1.6 billion; $0.4 billion in direct healthcare costs and $1.2 billion in indirect costs (86). A person with diabetes typically has medical costs that are two to five times higher than costs for a person without diabetes (84).

Risk Factors

It is important to distinguish between the risk factors for diabetes and those for diabetes-related complications. The risk factors for complications include poor control of diabetes, as well as smoking and high blood pressure. The risk factors for diabetes differ for type 1 and type 2 diabetes. Race and ethnicity are accepted risk factors for type 1 diabetes. Geographical variations also occur: the World Health Organization has reported the highest rates of type 1 in Scandinavia, intermediate rates in Canada and the United States, and low rates in Japan and Tanzania. Genetic susceptibility is also a factor in type 1 diabetes but does not play as strong a role as in type 2 diabetes. Type 1 diabetes is possibly linked with diet and exposure to viruses. Some evidence exists on the possible protective effect of breastfeeding (85).

For type 2 diabetes, the prevalence increases rapidly with age; usual onset is after age 40. Increased risk of diabetes with a positive family history of diabetes is probably due to genetic and environmental factors. Obesity is a well-recognized risk factor when measured as the level of obesity, the duration of obesity, and the body-fat distribution (i.e., WHR). Compared to those who do not have diabetes, a substantially large proportion of people with diabetes between 35 and 64 years are overweight i.e., BMI greater than 25 (59% versus 32%) (85). Physical inactivity is a known risk factor as it leads to overweight. While levels of physical inactivity are similar for those with and without diabetes in the 35 to 64 age group, those over 65 years with diabetes are less active than those who do not have diabetes. A 1% increase in the number of Canadians who are physically active would result in an expected annual saving of $877,000 in the direct costs of treating type 2 diabetes (87). Ethnicity has been accepted as an independent risk factor for type 2 diabetes. Certain ethnic groups such as Aboriginal, African, Hispanic, and Asian have a higher rate of type 2 diabetes. Before 1940, there was no evidence of diabetes among Aboriginal Canadians. Today, however, the age-standardized prevalence of diabetes among this population is at least three times that of the general population. Approximately two thirds of the First Nations people diagnosed with diabetes are women. The incidence of type 2 diabetes in Aboriginal children as young as 6 to 8 years old appears to be increasing rapidly (85).

Prevention

Prevention for diabetes takes three forms: primary, secondary, and tertiary prevention. At present, because there are no known modifiable risk factors for type 1 diabetes, there are no well-defined strategies for primary prevention. Primary prevention of type 2 diabetes, however, calls for the reduction of obesity and physical inactivity. The 1998 Clinical Practice Guidelines for the Management of Diabetes in Canada recommends a program of weight control through diet and regular exercise to help prevent type 2 diabetes. Canada's Food Guide to Healthy Eating and Canada's Physical Activity Guide to Healthy Active Living provide guidelines on a healthful diet and how to achieve health benefits from physical activity (35, 40).

Secondary prevention involves screening to identify diabetes in asymptomatic people. The Canadian Task Force on Preventive Health Care recommends against such screening for type 2 diabetes, because of a relatively low overall rate of diabetes in the general population and the lack of cost-benefit for mass screening. Screening is not recommended for type 1 diabetes.

Tertiary prevention tries to delay or prevent the complications of diabetes. In type 1 diabetes, tight glycemic control can reduce microvascular complications such as blindness and kidney disease. In type 2 diabetes, tight control of blood sugar and blood pressure levels has been shown to reduce both microvascular and macrovascular complications (heart disease and stroke). In those with diabetes, the treatment of hyperlipidemia and hypertension also reduces risks of heart disease and stroke. For all people with diabetes, regular foot and eye examinations with early treatment can help to prevent limb amputations and progression of retinopathy.

2.5   CONGENITAL DISORDERS

Congenital disorders include congenital anomalies and genetic diseases that may or may not be apparent at the time of birth. A **congenital anomaly** is an abnormality of structure, function, or body metabolism that is present at birth (even if not diagnosed until later in life) and may result in physical or mental disability, or is fatal (88).

Mortality and Morbidity

There are approximately 400,000 children born in Canada each year, of which 2% to 3% are born with a serious congenital anomaly (89). Congenital anomalies are now the second leading cause of death in infants (approximately 30% of all infant deaths in 1996), after perinatal causes. Among those aged 1 to 14 years, anomalies are the third leading cause of death (11% of all deaths in 1996), after unintentional injuries and neoplasms. Among children born in Canada in 1995, there were 13,629 anomalies, giving a rate of 483.5 per 10,000 live births. The most common anomalies were musculoskeletal anomalies (130.6 per 100,000 live births) followed by congenital heart anomalies (78.8 per 100,000). The musculoskeletal anomalies occurring most frequently were congenital dislocation of the hip and clubfoot (7).

Risk Factors

Recognized genetic conditions such as chromosome or single gene defect accounts for 15% to 25% of all congenital anomalies. Environmental factors account for 8% to 12% of etiological factors and include the following (89-91):

- maternal-related conditions such as maternal infection with herpes, syphilis, rubella, toxoplasmosis, or cytomegalovirus and lack of adequate amount of folic acid in diet;
- drug use during pregnancy such as anticonvulsants or teratogenic drugs; or
- chemical exposures such as alcohol or pesticides.

A multifactorial origin is considered when there is a combined influence of genes and environmental factors that interfere with normal embryological development. Multifactorial inheritance is the underlying etiology of most common congenital anomalies and accounts for 20% to 25% of all congenital disorders. The majority, 40%-60% of congenital anomalies have unexplained causes (89).

There are now more than 200 identified genetic and metabolic disorders. Many, but by no means all, can be diagnosed prenatally. Some can cause mental retardation (for example, phenylketonuria). Preconception counselling in susceptible populations may lead to mating patterns that reduce risks of some genetic and metabolic disorders. Prenatal fetal testing may also be offered to inform decision making regarding pregnancy termination. Certain genetic disorders have high frequencies in genetically defined ethnic groups; thalassemia, for example, occurs once in every 25 Italian births, Tay-Sachs disease affects about one in every 1,000 births to Ashkenazi Jews, and phenylketonuria has an incidence of 1 in 10,000 live Caucasian births. Five percent of Caucasians are carriers for cystic fibrosis.

Prevention

With regard to preconception and periconception, a woman's folic acid intake plays an important role in the prevention of neural tube defects and other congenital abnormalities (see Chapter 4, for folic acid intake in Canadian population). In Canada since 1998, white flour, enriched pasta, and cornmeal have been fortified with folic acid on a mandatory basis to improve dietary folate intakes, with the goal of reducing the rate of neural tube defects. The amount of folic acid supplement was kept low because of concerns that higher amounts would create a risk of anemia for individuals with undiagnosed vitamin B12 deficiency. The prevalence of low serum B12 levels has been found to be relatively more prevalent, especially among people over 50 years of age (92). The other examples include excellent glucose control in insulin-dependent diabetic women, changing anticonvulsant therapy in epileptic women and preconception identification and counselling of couples who, by virtue of their ethnic background, are known or suspected carriers of certain genetic disorders (89)

With regard to prenatal diagnosis, a number of prenatal screening methods detect congenital malformations or chromosomal abnormalities (89). These include screening maternal serum for alpha fetoprotein, human chorionic gonadotropin, and unconjugated estriol (the triple screen for Down syndrome and neural tube defects), chorionic villus sampling (CVS), amniocentesis, fetoscopy, and ultrasound examination. CVS provides the earliest available screen for fetal karyotype and molecular prenatal diagnosis at 8 to 12 weeks; however, it requires considerable technical skill. The early detection of abnormalities, however, allows for the termination of pregnancy in the first trimester when the procedure is medically less difficult and safer. Amniocentesis is the most commonly performed screening procedure, usually done at 15 to 16 weeks; it is associated with a less than 1% risk of miscarriage. Fetoscopy can be used to check for fetal malformations at 17 to 18 weeks, during which it is possible to obtain a blood sample. Ultrasonography requires a high level of skill to do well and can only identify structural abnormalities, but offers the dual advantages of being non-invasive and giving immediate results.

In 1996, the Canadian Task Force on Preventive Health Care reviewed the triple screening process for detecting Down syndrome. It stated that there is fair evidence to offer triple-marker screening as part of a comprehensive prenatal program to women under the age of 35. There is fair evidence to offer amniocentesis or CVS to women 35 years or older and to those with a history of a Down's syndrome fetus or of a chromosome 21 abnormality (93).

Research conducted by the Royal Commission on New Reproductive Technologies showed that 5% of prenatal diagnostic tests indicated that the fetus had a serious congenital anomaly or genetic disease. In this subset, 80% of women and couples chose to terminate the pregnancy (94). The Royal Commission recommended that prenatal diagnosis be done only with adequate counselling, and that representatives of people with disabilities be included in the development of appropriate counselling materials to address concerns about eugenics. With the human genome sequence now available, the commission's recommendations are likely to assume greater importance, as prenatal diagnostic tests become available for more and more conditions. (94).

With regard to gene therapy, a variety of genetic technologies may play a role in preventing and treating certain genetic diseases. Aside from prenatal diagnostic and screening tests, there are pre-implantation diagnosis and gene therapy (95). Pre-implantation diagnosis can be used by couples known to be at increased risk of having a child with a serious, single gene, or chromosomal disorder. For those undergoing in vitro fertilization, a zygote cell can be evaluated for chromosomal make-up or particular genes using genetic probes, and only zygotes without an identified abnormality selected for implantation in the uterus (95). Gene therapy involves inserting genetic material into a human being with the intention of correcting a particular disorder or disease. More than 300 clinical trials in human gene therapy are now underway or approved (see Chapter 18).

2.6. ARTHRITIS

The term "arthritis" incorporates a set of diverse but related conditions, including osteoarthritis and rheumatoid arthritis (96). Osteoarthritis is a degenerative disease characterized by degeneration of joint cartilage and leading to pain and stiffness accompanied by a loss of function. The prevalence of osteoarthritis increases with age. Rheumatoid arthritis is a chronic inflammatory joint disease of autoimmune etiology that leads to swelling stiffness and pain in multiple joints (97). It affects 1 in 100 Canadians.

Arthritis causes morbidity, a reduction in the quality of life, and physical disability. In the 1998–99 NPHS, 15% of Canadians aged 12 and older were diagnosed with arthritis or rheumatism. Women are more likely (19%) to have arthritis compared with men (11%) in all age groups; 56% of females aged 75 or older have arthritis, whereas 38% of males in the same age are affected. Residents of Nova Scotia and Saskatchewan were more likely to have arthritis or rheumatism compared with those living in other provinces.

Among people with arthritis, 90% report difficulty with mobility and 66% report having trouble with or being unable to climb stairs; 70% report being moderately to severely disabled, and that they depend on others for care and assistance; 20% of adult Canadians with arthritis are unable to travel long distances because of their condition. In a recent Canadian study, disability caused by arthritis was found to be significantly associated with non-participation in the labour force (98). Arthritic conditions are also a common cause of healthcare utilization and medication use. It is estimated that the number of Canadians diagnosed with arthritis will have increased in 2031 to 6.5 million, or by 124%, from 2.9 million in 1991. About half the increase will be among those aged 45 and older (99).

2.7.   CHRONIC PAIN

Chronic pain can affect not only physical health, but also emotional well-being. It can invade all aspects of an individual's life — at home and at work, in personal and in business relationships. People afflicted with chronic pain spend more time in hospital and see physicians more often than those who are not afflicted (38). In 1998–99, 16% of females aged 12 or older reported that they usually suffer from pain, compared with 12% of males. This may be attributed to the fact that pain-causing conditions such as migraines and arthritis are more prevalent among females. This difference between men and women is not significant after the age of 65.

2.8.   OSTEOPOROSIS

Osteoporosis is a health state predisposing to disease (fracture). The World Health Organization defines osteoporosis as bone mineral-density more than 2.5 standard deviations below the mean for young adults (100). Functionally, bone is also considered osteoporotic if it has sufficiently decreased density that it would be unable to withstand the traumas of normal activities or if there has already been a spontaneous or non-traumatic fracture. Osteoporosis is a major health problem in Canada, causing fractures, disability, pain, and deformity in a growing number of adults, especially women. One in four women over age 50 will be afflicted with osteoporosis. Up to two million Canadians may be at risk of osteoporosis fractures during their lifetime. The rate of fractures may be increasing much faster than can be accounted for by population aging (101).

Osteoporosis increases risk of fracture and death among elderly people. Osteoporosis-related hip fractures result in death in up to 20% of cases. Women's mortality rates from osteoporosis-related fractures are greater than the combined mortality rates from cancers of the breast and ovaries. Osteoporosis in men is also on the rise; one in eight men over the age of 50 is affected. The annual cost of all osteoporosis-related fractures in Canada is more than $1 billion.

Important predictors of osteoporosis are increased age, low body weight, poor muscle strength, and estrogen deficiency (101). The probability of developing osteoporosis is determined largely by the peak bone mass accumulated during growth and the rate of its loss during aging. Risk and protective factors have been identified for each of peak bone mass and rate of loss. Adequate calcium intake during childhood, adolescence, and early adulthood is important in maximizing peak bone mass. Adequate physical activity during childhood and adolescence is also a determinant of peak bone mass. Genetic factors and family history are important risk factors. Long-term use of medications affecting bone density, particularly corticosteroids, also increases risks of osteoporosis.

Once peak bone mass is reached in adulthood, bone loss with aging becomes a critical factor. Estrogen is a major factor preventing bone loss in women. Thus, with reduced estrogen production as women age, and particularly with menopause, osteoporosis risk increases. Estrogen replacement in the form of hormone replacement therapy (HRT) after menopause therefore slows the rate of bone loss and reduces risks of both osteoporosis and osteoporotic fractures. Inadequate calcium and vitamin D intake and physical inactivity accelerate bone loss, increasing risks of osteoporosis. Thin women are at higher risk than women of higher weight because of lower estrogen production, decreased mechanical stress on their bones, and decreased fat padding for protection during a fall. Smoking increases risks of osteoporosis, probably by lowering of estrogen levels. Heavy alcohol use may increase the risk of osteoporosis (97).

Since osteoporosis is difficult to reverse once it is established, the burden of this disease can be minimized only through preventive efforts in health behaviour such as increasing weight-bearing exercise, high calcium intake, and therapeutic approaches. Primary prevention involves interventions to increase peak bone mass development and limit bone loss at later ages. The former requires adequate intakes of calcium, physical activity, and not smoking early in life. Estrogen replacement following menopause limits bone loss, but recent studies indicate that HRT increases the risk of stroke, heart attack, and breast cancer. (102). Bisphosphonates are also used in the treatment of established osteoporosis and are a useful alternative to HRT in postmenopausal women (101). Adequate calcium and vitamin D intakes through diet or a combination of diet and supplementation, physical activity, and not smoking are also recommended for older people to help reduce bone loss (97).

In addition, fall prevention in the elderly is an important step toward reducing injury and improving quality of life. Exercise programs tailored for people at risk for osteoporosis or who have it are aimed at increasing strength, coordination, balance, and flexibility to reduce the risk of falls and fractures. Exercises aimed specifically at balance such as tai chi have been shown to prevent falls.

3.   MENTAL HEALTH

3.1.   BURDEN OF ILLNESS

Most of this section is based on *A Report on Mental Illness in Canada* (103). Mental health is as important to daily living as physical health. In fact, they are intertwined. **Mental health** is a state of well-being in which the individual realizes his or her own abilities, can cope with the normal stresses of life, can work productively and fruitfully, and can contribute to his or her community (104). **Mental illnesses** are characterized by alterations in thinking, mood, or behaviour associated with significant distress and impaired functioning over an extended period. Mental illnesses may occur together; for example, an individual can have depression and anxiety disorder or addiction. In developed countries, mental illness accounts for 4 of the 10 leading causes of disability and affects people of all ages, educational and income levels, and cultures; onset of most mental illness occurs during adolescence and young adulthood. A complex interplay of genetic, biological, personality, and environmental factors causes mental illnesses. Mental illnesses are responsible for a large and measurable burden of illness in the Canadian population: 20% of Canadians will experience a mental illness during their lifetime.

The major mental illnesses in Canada are mood disorders, schizophrenia, anxiety disorders, personality disorders, eating disorders, suicide, and addictions. Eighty-six percent of hospitalizations for mental illness occur in general hospitals and 14% in provincial psychiatric hospitals. In 1999–2000, individuals with mental illnesses used approximately 9 million hospital days; these were equally divided between provincial psychiatric and general hospitals (see Table 5.4 in Chapter 5). The average length of stay was 45 days; because of the severity of disease, patients in psychiatric hospitals have longer stays than those in general hospitals. In 1999–2000, the rate of hospitalization (admission) in general hospitals for all the mental illnesses listed above except addiction was 319 per 100,000 population (273 for men, 388 for women); they accounted for 3.8% of all admissions and consumed 1.5 million hospital days. For the past four decades the rate at which patients were admitted for mental disorders from general and psychiatric hospitals continues to decline. This downward trend is largely due to increased emphasis on treating mental disorders in outpatient and community clinics and the transfer of long-term care patients to residential care facilities.

The economic burden of mental health problems in Canada in 1998 was estimated to be $14.4 billion. This amount includes direct costs of $6.3 billion and indirect costs of $8.1 billion including short-term sick days, long-term disability, and premature death. These costs are higher than those reported in Chapter 5, due to a methodology refined by the author (105).

Risk Factors

Mental illnesses are the result of complex interactions among genetic, biological, personality, and environmental factors; however, the brain is the final common pathway for behaviour, cognition, and mood. Mental illnesses are more common in close family members of a person with mental illness, suggesting a genetic basis to the disorders. For reasons that may be biological, psychosocial, or both, age and sex affect rates of mental illness. Environmental factors such as family situations, workplace pressures, and socioeconomic status can precipitate the onset or recurrence of mental illness, and often determine the severity or chronicity of illness. Health behaviour, such as substance use and learned patterns of thought and behaviour, can influence the onset, course, and outcome of mental illness. Many studies have reported that socioeconomic status is inversely related to the development of mental illness, due in part to the safety net provided through greater income and social connectivity to persons of higher social economic status (103).

3.2. MENTAL HEALTH PROMOTION

Addressing the biopsychosocial determinants of mental illness can promote mental health and perhaps prevent some mental illness. **Mental health promotion** is the process of enhancing the capacity of individuals and communities to take control of their lives and improve their mental health. Mental health promotion is an umbrella term that covers a variety of strategies, all aimed at having a positive effect on mental health. The encouragement of individual resources and skills and improvements in the socioeconomic environment are among them. It uses strategies that foster supportive environments and individual resilience, while showing respect for culture, equity, social justice, interconnections, and personal dignity. The underlying principles include building on participants' and communities' competencies and strengths, demonstrating cultural sensitivity and responsiveness, involving meaningful consumer participation, addressing issues in the everyday life context of individuals, and ensuring the personal dignity of individuals (106).

At the level of the individual, a sense of control, social support, and meaningful participation are important in helping to reduce stress, anxiety, burnout, and frustration. At a systemic level, strategies that create supportive environments, strengthen community action, develop personal skills, and reorient health services can help to ensure that the population has some control over the psychological and social determinants of mental health (107). For example, a stress management training program for low-income women in Quebec proved effective by reducing anxiety and depression. Participants also reported an increased sense of control over their environment that enabled them to act positively, for example by returning to school, changing their living situations, and finding work (106). Thus mental health promotion requires multisectoral action, involving a number of government sectors such as health, employment/industry, education, environment, transport, and social and community services as well as non-governmental or community-based organizations such as health support groups, churches, clubs, and other bodies.

3.3.   COMMON MENTAL ILLNESSES AND PROBLEMS

Common mental illnesses and problems are described in the following section, except for major substance use issues (tobacco and alcohol) already discussed at the beginning of this chapter. Most of the information is derived from *A Report on Mental Illness in Canada* (103), unless otherwise specified.

Mood Disorders

Mood disorders include major depression, bipolar disorders, and dysthymia (depression or irritability for at least two years). Approximately 8% of adults will experience major depression at some time in their lives. During any 12-month period, between 4% and 5% of the population will experience major depression. The onset of mood disorders usually occurs during young adulthood, although it can occur at all ages. Women are twice as likely as men to be diagnosed with depression.

The risk factors for depression are family history of mood disorder, a history of early loss (typically a parent before the age of 11), stress, and chronic and debilitating illness. Individuals with mood disorders are at high risk of suicide.

Schizophrenia

Schizophrenia is one of the most serious mental illnesses in Canada and affects 1% of the Canadian population. Onset is usually in early adulthood. In 1996, the total cost of schizophrenia in Canada was estimated to be $2.3 billion.

A combination of genetic and environmental factors is considered responsible for schizophrenia. Immediate family members of individuals with schizophrenia are 10 times more likely to develop schizophrenia, and children of two parents with schizophrenia have a 40% chance of developing it. Identified contributors to risk of schizophrenia include prenatal or perinatal trauma, and viral infection.

Anxiety Disorders

Anxiety disorders include general anxiety disorder (GAD), specific phobia, post-traumatic stress disorder, social phobia, obsessive-compulsive disorder, and panic disorder. Anxiety disorders affect approximately 12% of Canadians; prevalence is lower in men (9%) compared with women (16%) during a one-year period. As a group, anxiety disorders are the most common mental illness. The one-year prevalence rates for different disorders in Canada are as follows: general anxiety disorder, 1.1%; specific phobias, 6.2% to 8.0%; social phobias, 6.7%; obsessive-compulsive disorder, 1.8%; and panic disorder, 0.7%. Women report and are diagnosed with anxiety disorders more frequently than men.

Personality Disorders

Personality disorders exist in many forms, such as borderline, antisocial, dependent, and paranoid. Estimates of the one-year prevalence rate of antisocial personality disorder is 1.7%; other personality disorders range from 1% to 10%. Based on U.S. data, about 6% to 9% of the population has a personality disorder. Antisocial personality disorder is more common among men (particularly among prison inmates) than women, while borderline personality disorder is more common among women.

Eating Disorders

Eating disorders include anorexia, bulimia, and binge eating disorder. They are more common amongst girls and women (90% of cases) than boys and men (10% of cases). Approximately 3% of women will be affected by an eating disorder during their lifetime.

Factors believed to contribute to eating disorders include: biological, such as gender, and psychosocial, such as poor body image; overvaluation of appearance; societal promotion of the thin body image; and peer-group weight concerns.

Suicide

Mortality. Suicide is an important preventable cause of mortality and PYLL in Canada, especially among Canadian youth (108). Suicide is the third leading cause of PYLL after cancer and unintentional injuries (7). Suicides account for 90% of the deaths from intentional injuries in Canada (109).

In 1996, there were 3,941 suicides in Canada, or 11 deaths from suicide per day. This translated to a rate of 13 per 100,000 population. Suicide rates increased between 1970 and 1978, fluctuating between 13 and 15 per 100,000 in the 1980s, and remaining stable at 13 per 100,000 since 1989. Males are four times more likely than females to complete suicide while females are more likely to attempt suicide; 78% of completed suicides in 1996 were male. The highest male rates of suicide occur among 20- to 24-year-olds and 30- to 44 year olds, while the highest female rates occur among 35- to 54-year-olds (7). Women are more likely to attempt suicide by overdose while men are more likely to use firearms.

Youth suicide is an important issue in Canada. Canada was the only one of 21 western countries where the male suicide rate in 15- to 24-year-olds exceeded the rate for the general male population. Canada's ranks third after Australia and the Russian Federation in suicide among male youth and third after Sweden and the Russian Federation among female youth. Since 1970, teen suicide rates have been on the rise in Canada (7, 38). Rates doubled for 15- to 19-year-olds between 1970 and 1983, entirely accounted for by males (7). Between 1971 and 1996, the rate of suicide among those aged 10 to 14 has nearly tripled. Among this age group, rates of suicide are also much higher in boys than in girls.

Another group with high rates of suicide in Canada is the Aboriginal population. Although it varies according to age and community, the suicide risk among Status Indians is estimated at three to six times that of the general Canadian population (103) (see Chapter 6).

Risk Factors. Many factors contribute directly or indirectly to suicide risk. Among them, the two most important are a recent history of mental disorder and substance abuse. Those who suffer from depression are at high risk of suicide. Alcoholism is the second most commonly reported problem, after major depression, to be associated with suicide. Certain personality disorders, such as borderline and antisocial personality disorders, increase risks of suicide (attempts) (7).

Other high-risk groups include gays and lesbians, who have a suicide rate two to six times that of comparable unmarried heterosexuals (7). Childhood sexual abuse may also increase risk of suicide. There are also situational risk factors for suicide. Suicide clusters among teenagers and young adults suggest that suicides may sometimes be caused by exposure to suicide or suicidal behaviour in others. Stressful life events, such as the death of a loved one or recent job loss, often appear to be precipitants of suicide and may increase the risk of suicide by a factor of 5 to 10. Loss or disruption of normal social support systems, such as occur with divorce, unemployment, or migration, also appear to increase the risk of suicide. A lack of social support networks appears to interact with other risk factors, such as clinical depression and recent stressful life events, to increase the risk of suicide (110).

Prevention and Health Promotion. Strategies for suicide prevention can be categorized into five broad categories (110):

- Improving the identification, referral, and treatment of persons at high risk of suicide by various caretakers and "gatekeepers." Examples include training primary care physicians and healthcare professionals to recognize and refer patients with clinical depression, and school-based screening programs to identify suicidal youth.
- Treating underlying risk factors for suicide. Examples include treating those with mental illness such as clinical depression, and treating alcoholism and drug abuse through rehabilitation programs.
- Decreasing individual vulnerability to suicide through education of the general population. Examples include education to help individuals cope with problems that can lead to suicide and increasing public awareness about the resources available in the community to those who need help for specific problems.
- Improving accessibility of self-referral resources for suicidal people. Examples are hotlines and walk-in crisis centres.
- Limiting access to lethal means of suicide. Examples are legislation to reduce accessibility to firearms, physical restrictions to high places, and limiting amounts of potentially lethal medications dispensed to those who are depressed.

Stress

Stress is a ubiquitous feature of modern life. It is part of a larger set of psychological factors that may contribute to illness. Psychological factors include internal factors, such as personality, attitudes, and reactions to events, and external factors, such as social supports and employment. **Stress** can be broadly defined as the psychic or physiological disequilibrium caused by an event. It has been linked to increased risk for cardiovascular disease, is considered a predisposing factor for depression, and is linked to decreased work performance The level of chronic stress experienced by the Canadian population was described in Chapter 4.

Longitudinal data from the NPHS show that feeling personal stress in 1994–95 was predictive of developing chronic conditions over the next four years, even when age, socioeconomic status, and several health-related behaviours (smoking, drinking, body mass index, leisure-time activity) were taken into account. Men who had experienced high personal stress in 1994–95 had twice the odds of having been diagnosed with migraine, ulcers, or arthritis by 1998–99 compared with those who did not report high stress. Women who were under high personal stress in 1994–95 and had not experienced a major depressive episode in the preceding year had high odds of reporting such an episode in 1996–97 and 1998–99, compared with women who had not been under stress.

There are different sources of chronic stress. Personal stress can arise from trying to do too much at once, from having too much expected by others, from feeling too much pressure to be like others, from people being critical, and from feeling as though one's work is not appreciated. In the 1994–95 NPHS, 45% of women aged 18 and over and 38% of men reported they were trying to do too much at once (38).

Work stress arises from physically demanding labour, low support from co-workers and supervisors, job insecurity, job strain, effort-reward imbalance, and long working hours. Two sources of work stress have been found to be strongly and consistently associated with diseases such as coronary heart disease and hypertension: job strain, which is a combination of high job demands and low job control, and effort-reward imbalance, which is the imbalance between the efforts put into a job and the rewards of a job in terms of pay, status, recognition, and job security (111-113). Job strain has also been shown to be associated with depression, workplace injuries, and sickness absence (114). In 1994–95, 40% of Canadians aged 15 to 64 reported physically demanding jobs, 30% reported low support from co-workers, 15% reported low support from supervisors, 20% reported job strain, and 18% reported their jobs were insecure. Job stressors tended to be most common in low-income households. While men were more likely to report high physical demands, women were more likely to report job strain (38).

Stress management consists of identifying stressors and finding ways to organize life to reduce demands. Positive guided imagery, relaxation tapes, meditation, and exercise have been reported to give benefit in helping to cope with stress. A recent Canadian study showed that those who are moderately and highly active showed significantly lower levels of psychological distress compared with inactive individuals (115). Social support, including affection, social interaction, emotional or informational support, and tangible support (to do specific tasks in times of need), also often help people to cope with stress. In 1998–99, most Canadians aged 12 and older reported having access to these forms of social support (38).

Although individuals need to find ways to manage the stress in their lives, stress prevention needs also to consider sources of stress in life and work that may not be modifiable by the individual. Examples of these include improvements to stressful working conditions and the larger social environment in which we live.

4.   INJURIES

Mortality

Injuries are the leading cause of death during the first half of life, and second to cancer as a cause of PYLL. Potential years of life lost from injuries in those under age 65 accounted for 47% of the total Canadian PYLL in 1996. Although mortality rates due to unintentional injuries in children aged 1 to 14 have been decreasing for the past three decades, injuries remain the leading cause of death of children under age five, school-aged children, and young adults (116).

In 1997, there were 12,791 deaths from injury in Canada, or 35 deaths per day. Two thirds of injury deaths were due to unintentional injuries and one third from intentional injuries. Unintentional injuries include motor vehicle collisions, falls, drowning, burns, and poisonings. Suicides accounted for 90% of the deaths from intentional injuries (109). Among the First Nations people in canada, injury is the number-one cause of death (109). Among registered Indians and Inuit, injuries accounted for 28 and 35 percent, respectively, of all deaths compared with 8% of deaths in the general Canadian population (117). Males have much higher mortality rates from injury than females.

Morbidity

In the 12 months between 1998 and 1999, more than 195,000 Canadians were hospitalized for injuries, which accounted for 1,800,000 hospital days and 7% of all acute care hospitalizations (109). Injuries in people aged 65 years and over accounted for the majority (43%) of admissions. The number of injuries among females peaked at around age 80 and the peaks for males in the late teenaged years, the late 30s and the late 70s (118). Non-fatal injuries also lead to long-term impairment or disability.

In terms of economic burden, injury ranks fourth after cardiovascular, musculoskeletal diseases and cancer. Injury accounts for 8% or $12.7 billion of the economic burden of illness in Canada in 1998. The direct cost was $3.2 billion and induirect cost was $9.5 billion. Falls account for 40% of the cost, motor vehicle collisions for 20%, and the remaining 40% for drowning, poisoning, fires, and other non-intentional injuries (119).

4.1.   UNINTENTIONAL INJURY

Childhood injuries

Mortality. Injury is the leading killer of children in every industrialized country and claims the lives of more than 20,000 children annually in the 26 richest nations of the world (120). The most common cause of death by injury for children is motor vehicle collisions (41%), followed by other unintentional injuries (16%), drowning (15%), intentional harm (14%), fire (7%), falls (4%), poisoning (2%), and firearm accidents (1%). Canada has a poorer than average rate of child deaths caused by fire and other intentional injuries. In 2001, UNICEF reported that Canada's rate of death from injury among children is higher than that of several other industrialized nations (120). Canada's death rate is 9.7 per 100,000 children, almost double that of Sweden (5.2). If Canada had Sweden's rate of child injury death, 1,233 of the 2,665 deaths over the five-year period of 1991–95 might have been prevented. As indicated in Chapter 6, children living in the poorest income areas are at greatest risk of dying from injuries.

Motor Vehicle Injuries

Mortality. The highest percentage of PYLL arises from fatal motor vehicle injuries, since mortality from this cause occurs primarily in the young. Motor vehicle injuries are the number-one cause of injury death among children aged 1 to 14 (116). Mortality rates from motor vehicle injuries are highest in those aged 15 to 24 and in the elderly (77). The mortality rate for motor vehicle injuries has steadily declined since the 1960s. They cost almost $1.7 billion every year and are one of the most significant types of injury causing permanent disability (119).

Risk Factors. Important risk factors for motor vehicle collisions include the mental attitude and condition of the driver, the design and condition of the vehicle, road design and conditions, cell phone usage while driving, and seatbelt usage. Driving while intoxicated is a major factor in collisions: 42% of fatally injured drivers had alcohol in their blood and 35% were over the legal limit of a blood alcohol concentration (BAC) of 0.08% (18).

Prevention of Unintentional Injury

The Canadian Public Health Association (CPHA) drafted a position paper in 2002 on injury prevention and control, which makes the following points and is relevant to non-intentional as well as intentional injuries (109). Most injuries are preventable. Injuries are the result of many complex factors; therefore, any effort to prevent or reduce the severity of injuries must involve multiple sectors, disciplines, jurisdictions, and approaches. The public health approach ideally consists of primary prevention, such as safety promotion, secondary prevention, such as emergency response, and tertiary prevention, such as rehabilitation, in addition to health promotion strategies such as safe working environment and better vehicle design. Current efforts in Canada are still fragmented and require strong and continuing national leadership.

For preventive efforts to be instituted, the population must understand that injuries are not "accidents" or "acts of fate." Injuries are the result of predictable events. The main causes of injury to Canadians at all ages are preventable. Infants and toddlers can be protected from injuries related to motor vehicles, drowning, burns, poisoning, falls, and suffocation. Injuries among school-aged children from motor vehicles, drowning, and fires or burns can be prevented (109). Preventive measures such as redesigning playgrounds and targeting hazards in the home would help decrease the number of needless injuries of children. The net savings could total over $126 million every year (119).

For motor vehicle collisions, primary preventive methods include environmental as well as individual measures. Environmental methods include public education, improved vehicle and roadway design, speed controls, random breath testing for alcohol, decreasing public tolerance for drinking and driving, improved emergency response and trauma care, graduated licensing of new drivers, and other legislative and enforcement measures such as banning use of cellular phones while driving (109). Wearing seatbelts and installing air bags can reduce motor vehicle injuries by 61%. Given that about 40% of all fatal motor vehicle crashes are related to alcohol, mortality could be reduced by 20% through a reduction in drunk driving. Reducing the speed limit by 10 km/hour could lead to a 15% decrease in mortality. Poor road design accounts for 10% of crashes. Implementing a prevention strategy based on buckling seatbelts, driving sober, slowing down, and paying attention on the roads could result in 2,800 fewer hospitalizations and save $500 million annually (119).

Among teens and young adults, traffic-related injuries and suicide are important and preventable, as are sports-related injuries. Among older adults, prevention of falls can help reduce mortality and morbidity. These falls can be averted by recognizing risk factors such as history of falls, impairment related to cognition, balance and gait, low body mass index, the misuse of medications, and hazards in the home. Over $138 million annually could be saved by targeting these risk factors through prevention programs (119).

As described above, multiple prevention methods can reduce the number of fatal injuries. A multisectoral response involving action at the individual level as well as actions by government and non-government sectors involved with education, transportation, urban planning, automobile manufacturing, emergency response, pre-hospital trauma care, and consumer advocacy has been crucial.

Haddon's matrix, a useful framework, conceptualizes unintentional injuries as resulting from interactions between host (person), agent or vector (e.g., a car), and environment (121) (see also Figure 1.3 in Chapter 1). Interventions directed toward the host, agent, or environment may reduce the onset or extent of injury sustained. Injury occurs when forces are applied beyond the capability of the organism to withstand them. In Haddon's matrix, preventive injury interventions are organized in a two-dimensional matrix in which pre-injury, time of impact, and post-injury preventive measures are considered in relation to the person, the agent causing the injury, or the environment. In the pre-injury phase, attention should be directed at eliminating the source of the energy, reducing exposure to it, or increasing the magnitude of resistance to it. Attention directed at the injury should reduce the magnitude and duration of exposure and decrease the host's susceptibility to injury. In the post-injury phase, the environment can be altered to reduce the source of the injury in the future and facilitate the rescue and resuscitation of victims in the short term. For example, in relation to motor vehicle collisions involving children, pre-injury strategies include appropriate use of car seats and seatbelts for all children in cars, teaching children road safety, use of bicycle helmets, reduction of vehicular speed especially in areas with schools and in residential areas, and road design. Protection at the time of injury involves the restraining action of seatbelts and helmets' ability to reduce brain damage. Post-injury prevention involves ready access to trauma centres and a review of injury sites for future precautions.

Preventive measures can be active or passive. Active measures require the host to take some action in order for the intervention to work (e.g., putting on a seatbelt or wearing a helmet). Passive measures are structural interventions that require no action by the host (e.g., antilock brakes and airbags). The most successful public health measures are usually passive ones. In addition to this framework and conceptualizing measures as active or passive, it is also helpful to think of public health strategies in terms of the 4E's: education, environmental modification, enforcement, and engineering (122).

4.2. INTENTIONAL INJURY

Intentional injury includes suicide, which has been addressed in the mental health section, homicides and firearm-related deaths, physical and emotional abuse, and acts of war.

4.2.1. Homicides and Firearm-Related Deaths

Mortality

In the 1990s, the overall homicide rate in Canada averaged 2.0 to 2.7 per 100,000. In Canada, 1,252 firearm-related deaths on average were reported each year between 1989 and 1997. Of these, 80% were suicides, 15% were homicides, and 4% were related to unintentional injuries. In a 1991 Canadian study, the risk of death from a firearm in Canada was found to be comparable to the risk of death from a motor vehicle injury (2.37 deaths per 10,000 firearms versus 2.4 per 10,000 vehicles respectively) (123). A comparison made in 1992 among 26 developed countries found Canada's firearm-related death rate to be the sixth highest. Direct and indirect costs associated with firearm-related deaths in Canada was estimated at $6.6 billion in 1993 (124, 125).

Gun Control

About 1,200 to 1,300 firearm-related deaths occur each year in Canada. Gun control has been highlighted as an important potential strategy in prevention of both suicides and homicides. The number of suicides using firearms has declined since the introduction of gun control legislation in 1978. Case-control studies done in the U.S. have shown that homes with a firearm have an increased risk of firearm-related death in household members and relations compared with households without firearms: the risk is 4.7 times higher for suicide and 2.7 times higher for being the victim of a homicide. Even in homes where the weapon was kept locked up or rendered inoperable, the risk of suicide was three times higher than in homes without firearms (124). Aside from suicides and homicides, firearms also result in unintentional injuries and unintentional firearm deaths (UFDs). There are approximately 50 UFDs each year in Canada (125).

Many experts believe that a crucial factor in reducing the number of firearm-related deaths and injuries is to reduce accessibility to firearms. This can be done by reducing the number of firearms found in homes and by ensuring that household firearms are stored more safely. Both strategies are addressed in the *Firearms Act*. Rules determining firearm storage have been in place under this act since 1993. Firearms must be stored unloaded, rendered inoperable or inaccessible, and preferably stored separately from ammunition (124). All owners of firearms must also obtain a licence that must be renewed every five years and is required for the purchase of ammunition as well as guns. Those with histories of violence are not permitted to get a licence, and ownership is now tied to increased accountability and education on the proper storage and handling of firearms. Firearms are required to be registered since January 1, 2003, in a new system designed to assist in limiting access to firearms by persons who may be more likely to use them inappropriately (126). As well, the registry facilitates more accurate statistics in order to help assess the effectiveness of prevention efforts.

4.2.2.   Domestic Violence

Spousal Abuse

In Canada, 7% of people who were married or living in a common-law relationship reported experiencing some type of violence by a partner during the previous five years (127). There is significant underreporting due to confounding factors, including secrecy surrounding the issue of family violence, economic dependence of the victim on the perpetrator, lack of knowledge about available help, and fear of repercussions for reporting the event. The five-year rate of violence was similar for women (8%) and men (7%). Women were more likely than men to report what could be considered severe forms of violence. Women were more than twice as likely as men to report being beaten (25% vs. 10%), five times more likely to report being choked (20% vs. 4%), almost seven times more likely to report being sexually assaulted (20% vs. 3%) and almost twice as likely to report being threatened by or having a gun or knife used against them. Generally, younger people are at greater risk of experiencing spousal violence than are older people. Men were more likely than women to report being slapped (57% versus 40%), having something thrown at them (56% versus 44%), and being kicked, bitten, or hit (51% versus 33%). Women were three times more likely than men to be injured by spousal violence and five times more likely to require medical attention. During the five-year period almost one quarter (24%) of spousal violence victims feared their lives were in danger. This fear was much more prevalent among women than men: 38% of women compared to 7% of men feared for their lives. In the past 20 years, one third of homicide victims were related to their killers. The rate of spousal homicide, in particular wife killings, has been reduced by half since 1980, from 15 per million couples to 7 per million couples. Approximately half a million children have heard or witnessed a parent being assaulted during the five-year period. The Canadian Task Force on Preventive Health Care has published a useful report on the prevention and treatment of violence against women (128).

Child Abuse and Neglect

Child abuse consists of neglect and physical, emotional, or sexual abuse. A recently published Canadian study found that an estimated 135,573 child maltreatment investigations were carried out in Canada in 1998, with an annual incidence rate of 21.5 investigations per 1,000 children (129). Child maltreatment cases investigated consist of four primary categories: physical abuse (31%), sexual abuse (10%), neglect (40%), and emotional maltreatment (19%). Of the total cases investigated, 45% were substantiated, 22% remained suspected, and 33% were unsubstantiated. Despite the existence of mandatory reporting laws in provinces and territories requiring citizens to report child abuse and neglect, it has been estimated that as many cases are not reported to child welfare agencies. Parents are responsible for 66% of physical assaults and 42% of sexual assaults against children and youth under 18 years of age (130). From 1974 to 1999, 63% of the 1,990 solved homicides of youths up to age 17 were committed by family members.

The effects of violence extend beyond the physical harm endured: stress, poor mental health, lack of social connection, and substance abuse can all occur in victims of violence. Children raised in violence-prone homes suffer from depression, post-traumatic stress disorder, peer conflicts, and conduct disorders as well as a host of other behavioural problems.

Elder Abuse

Elder abuse includes emotional, financial, physical neglect, and maltreatment, including questionable institutionalization. A 1992 survey estimated that approximately 4% of Canadians over age 65 may be victimized annually (131). Two thirds of the violence experienced by older adults was committed by non-family members. Among those victimized by a family member, older adults were most likely to be victimized by adult children. Older adults are more likely to experience emotional and financial abuse than physical or sexual violence. There is no one theory that can adequately account for the abuse of older adults. Theories include spousal abuse grown old and learned abusive behaviour by children; some researchers point to the negative societal attitudes toward the elderly (130).

Risk Factors

A number of factors appear to increase the risk of domestic violence. Women and men from all income levels and all educational backgrounds reported experiencing spousal violence. The victims' level of education also showed no relationship to exposure to spousal violence. Alcohol, however, appears to be a factor related to the rates of spousal violence: heavy drinking is associated with elevated rates of violence, and rates of spousal violence were six times higher for victims whose partners drank heavily compared with those victims whose partners drank moderately or not at all.

There also appears to be a generational cycle of violence. The 1993 Violence Against Women Survey provided evidence to support such a theory (132). According to this survey, men who witnessed violence committed by their fathers were three times more likely than men without these childhood experiences to be violent toward their wives. Children who have heard or seen physical fights between adults or teenagers in their home are more than twice as likely to be physically aggressive as those who have not heard or seen such fights (130).

The 1999 General Social Survey reported that 20% of Aboriginal peoples reported being assaulted by a spouse in the five-year period before the survey, compared with 7% of the non-Aboriginal population. About one half of Aboriginal peoples who were assaulted by a spouse reported that a child had seen the incident (130).

Prevention

The prevention of domestic violence is complex. It is recognized that a multifactor strategy is necessary for violence prevention. While the self-reported rates of partner violence amongst men and women are roughly equivalent, the severity of male-perpetrated violence is greater than that of female-perpetrated violence and hence violence against women receives major attention. Successful prevention requires first that the problem be acknowledged and addressed by communities and governments. In 1995, the federal government released the Federal Plan for Gender Equality, which clearly recognized violence against women as a crucial area. It identified as priorities supporting community-based actions undertaken by women's organizations, such as addressing the root causes of violence, increasing media awareness and involving the media in counteracting violence, supporting shelters for battered women, achieving reform related to criminal justice, addressing violence in Aboriginal on-reserve and Inuit communities, promoting women's safety in the workplace, and undertaking research and analysis on issues related to violence against women. The Canadian Task Force on Preventive Health Care has published a useful report on spousal abuse (128).

Strategies needed to reduce victimization of seniors include: regulation of long-term care and nursing home facilities and education of staff in these facilities; consumer protection laws that would protect the elderly from financial manipulation and accessible, affordable trusteeship can reduce the opportunities for families to financially abuse their elder members (see Chapter 6).

5. SUMMARY

This chapter surveys the current approaches in disease prevention and health promotion in relation to major non-communicable chronic diseases and injuries in Canada. Chronic illnesses are the cause of the major burdens of illness and death in Canada.

These illnesses are preventable, and hence there is increasing emphasis on the role of primary and secondary prevention. Many chronic illnesses have substance abuse (alcohol and tobacco), poor quality diet, and physical inactivity as major underlying causes.

Smoking is the number-one preventable cause of death in Canada. In Canada, 45,000 deaths each year are attributable to the use of tobacco products. It is estimated to be responsible for one third of potential years of life lost (PYLL) due to cancer, one quarter due to heart disease, and one half due to respiratory disease. There is strong evidence of an association between residential and workplace exposure to environmental tobacco smoke (ETS), or secondhand smoke and ill health. For children, exposure to ETS causes respiratory symptoms, middle ear disease, sudden infant death syndrome, and bronchitis, pneumonia, and other lower respiratory tract infections; it also impairs fetal growth, causing low birth weight and babies who are small for their gestational age, and it exacerbates asthma. In adults, ETS causes heart disease, lung cancer, and nasal sinus cancer and has also been linked to stroke, breast cancer, cervical cancer, and miscarriages.

There is good evidence that healthcare providers, including physicians and non-physicians, can be effective in motivating people to quit smoking using brief interventions by incorporating smoking cessation messages that are repeated on multiple occasions and reinforced. Educational strategies, in conjunction with community-based and media-based activities, can postpone or prevent smoking onset in 20% to 40% of adolescents. Regulation of advertising and promotion, particularly aimed at young people, is very likely to reduce both uptake and prevalence of smoking. Clean air regulations (i.e., smoking bans and restrictions) and restriction of minors' access to tobacco contribute to changing social norms and may influence prevalence directly. The most effective intervention on tobacco control is raising the price.

There are various diseases and injuries associated with alcohol consumption, such as cirrhosis, suicide, breast cancer, upper respiratory and gastrointestinal tract cancers, and motor vehicle and other injuries. The largest number of alcohol-related deaths stemmed from motor vehicle collisions due to impaired-driving followed by cirrhosis and then suicide. There are four categories of alcohol use: low-risk drinking, hazardous drinking, alcohol abuse, and alcohol dependency. A family history of serious drinking problems is likely the strongest predictor of risk for problem drinking.

Interventions by healthcare professionals can be categorized into secondary prevention (screening) and tertiary prevention (treatment of an alcohol-use problem). Physicians and primary health care providers are in a good position to quickly identify problem drinking and alcohol dependence using questionnaires such as CAGE or MAST. For treatment, good evidence exists for the effectiveness of brief intervention programs for those at an early stage of problem drinking. Groups such as Alcoholics Anonymous can be beneficial in assisting motivated problem drinkers.

Effective health promotion programs in relation to substance abuse should be comprehensive, coordinated, and participatory. A comprehensive approach should focus on education, environmental controls, economic levers, and enforcement of legislation and regulations.

Diet, particularly excessive caloric intake and insufficient intake of fruits and vegetables, is a major factor in the development of many chronic diseases, including the two leading killers: cardiovascular disease and cancer. Nutrition is also an important factor in the prevention of neural tube and other congenital anomalies, osteoporosis, chronic liver disease, and dental health. National guidelines for nutrition have been published by Health Canada.

Obesity is an increasing problem in Canada among both adults and children. Obesity is a risk factor for multiple diseases including diabetes and cardiovascular disease (CVD). Ideal body mass index is associated with both healthy eating and with physical activity.

Physical inactivity creates a significant public health burden in Canada. Risks of coronary artery disease, stroke, colon cancer, breast cancer, osteoporosis, and type 2 diabetes are all increased with physical inactivity. Physical activity is important in maintaining a healthy body weight, and improving serum lipids and cholesterol and blood pressure. There is evidence that physical activity and body mass index exert independent effects on health. Canada's Food Guide to Healthy Eating and Canada's Physical Activity Guide to Healthy Active Living provide physical activity recommendations for Canadians.

CVD (heart disease and stroke) is the leading cause of death in Canada. It is also the leading cause of hospital admissions for men and women excluding pregnancy and childbirth. The most common forms are ischemic or coronary heart disease (IHD) and cerebrovascular disease (stroke).

CVD has many risk factors that can be targeted for prevention. Modifiable risk factors include smoking; dyslipidemias (elevated cholesterol, LDL and triglycerides, and low HDL levels), which are affected by the quantity and types of fats consumed; hypertension, which is affected by overweight, physical inactivity, heavy alcohol use, and excessive salt intakes; physical inactivity; obesity; and diabetes, which is affected by obesity and physical inactivity. More recently, several other potentially modifiable risk factors have been identified: mental stress, hostility, physical exertion in the cold, air pollution, and infectious agents. Dietary antioxidant intake and social supports appear to protect against CVD.

Cancer ranks second overall as a leading cause of death. It is the number-one cause of PYLL in both men and women. Prognosis for individual cancers varies from poor (lung, adult leukemia, pancreas, stomach, ovary, brain, multiple myeloma, and esophagus) to fairly good (colorectal, non-Hodgkin's lymphoma, female bladder, kidney, oral, and larynx) to very good (breast, prostate, melanoma, body of the uterus, thyroid, cervix, Hodgkin's disease, testis, and male bladder). Although a few cancers may be associated with inherited genetic factors, behavioural and environmental factors such as the use of tobacco and alcohol, exposure to environmental tobacco smoke (ETS), diet, physical inactivity, obesity, exposure to and infection with certain infectious agents, exposure to ultraviolet radiation, occupational carcinogen exposure, and environmental pollution are important determinants.

Lung, colorectal, breast, and prostate are the most common cancers in Canadians. Smoking causes 90% of lung cancer. There is convincing evidence that a diet high in fruits and vegetables protects against lung and colorectal cancers, and also probably against breast cancer. The Canadian Task Force on Preventive Health Care recommends annual screening with clinical breast exam and mammography every two years for women aged 50 to 69.

Respiratory diseases constitute the third leading cause of death, the fifth leading cause of PYLL, and the third leading cause of hospitalization in Canada. Important risk factors include smoking, respiratory pathogens, and air pollution. In Canada and many industrialized countries, increases have been seen in asthma incidence, prevalence, hospitalization, and mortality rates.

Diabetes is ranked as the seventh leading cause of death in Canada. The main risk factors for type 2 diabetes are obesity and physical inactivity. Primary prevention strategies are important in type 2 diabetes. However, for both types, medical and healthcare interventions play important roles in helping to delay or prevent complications.

Congenital anomalies are now the second leading cause of death in infants after perinatal causes. Among those aged 1 to 14 years, anomalies are the third leading cause of death after unintentional injuries and neoplasms. The most common anomalies are musculoskeletal followed by congenital heart anomalies. Etiological factors for malformations include hereditary or familial tendencies, and non-genetic factors such as maternal diabetes mellitus, teratogenic drug use during pregnancy, and maternal infection with herpes, syphilis, rubella, toxoplasmosis, or cytomegalovirus. Other etiological factors are nutritional deficiencies (such as folic acid deficiency), exposure to external environmental agents, and factors related to personal lifestyle choices such as substance abuse during pregnancy. A variety of genetic technologies may have a role in the prevention and treatment of certain genetic diseases, and the advent of new technologies raises many ethical issues.

Arthritis and chronic pain conditions are important causes of morbidity in the Canadian population. Although the mortality for these conditions is low, quality-adjusted life is poorer for those with severe arthritis or chronic pain. These conditions increase in incidence with age and are major causes of health service utilization and medication use.

Osteoporosis is a major health problem in Canada, causing fractures, disability, pain, and deformity in a growing number of adults, especially women. Risk and protective factors for osteoporosis include adequate calcium intake during childhood, adolescence, early adulthood, and later in life; physical activity during childhood, adolescence, and later on; family history; race; medical factors or medications affecting bone density; body weight; smoking and possibly heavy alcohol use. Estrogen is a major factor in preventing bone loss in women. Because osteoporosis is difficult to reverse once it is established, the burden of this disease can be reduced only through preventive efforts focusing on diet, physical activity, and medical therapy where indicated. In addition, fall prevention in the elderly is an important step toward reducing injury and improving quality of life.

The major mental illnesses in Canada are mood disorders, schizophrenia, anxiety disorders, personality disorders, eating disorders, suicide, and addictions. The economic burden of mental health problems in Canada in 1998 was estimated to be $14.4 billion. Mood disorders include major depression, bipolar disorders, and dysthymia. Approximately 8% of adults will experience major depression at some time in their lives. Schizophrenia, which affects 1% of the population, is one of the most serious mental illnesses in Canada. Anxiety disorders affect approximately 12% of Canadians, and personality disorders exist in many forms such as borderline, antisocial, dependent, and paranoid. Estimates of the one-year prevalence of antisocial personality disorder is 1.7% and other personality disorders range from 1% to 10%. Approximately 3% of women will be affected by an eating disorder during their lifetime.

Suicide is an important cause of mortality and PYLL in Canada, especially among Canadian youth, as there is a steady and significant increase in the teen suicide rate. Another group with high rates of suicide in Canada is the Aboriginal population. Suicides account for 90% of the deaths from intentional injuries in Canada. The two most important factors contributing to suicide are a recent history of mental disorder and substance abuse.

Chronic stress, including personal stress and work stress, is associated with the development of both mental and physical health problems.

Injuries are the leading cause of death during the first half of the human life span, and are second to cancer as a leading cause of PYLL. Two thirds of injury deaths are due to unintentional injuries and one third from intentional injuries. Unintentional injuries include motor vehicle collisions, falls, drowning, burns, and poisonings. Among Status Indians and Inuit, injuries account for 28% and 35%, respectively, of all deaths, compared with 8% of deaths in the general Canadian population.

Important risk factors for motor vehicle collisions include the mental attitude and condition of the driver, the design and condition of the vehicle, road design and conditions, and seatbelt usage. Driving while intoxicated is a major factor in collisions. Primary preventive methods must therefore include environmental as well as individual measures.

Most injuries are preventable: they are the result of many complex factors and therefore any effort to prevent and reduce the severity of injuries must involve multiple sectors, disciplines, jurisdictions and approaches; the public health approach is required. Haddon's matrix is a useful framework for analyzing injuries and their prevention.

Violence is an important public health concern. There were, on average, 1,252 firearm-related deaths reported each year between 1989 and 1997. Of these, 80% were suicides, 15% were homicides, and 4% were related to unintentional injuries.

Of those who are married or living in a common-law relationship, 7% have experienced some type of violence by a partner in the last five years. Child abuse consists of neglect and physical, emotional, or sexual abuse; in 1999, children and youth under 18 years of age made up 60% of all sexual assault victims and 20% of all physical assault victims. Parents are responsible for 66% of physical assaults and 42% of sexual assaults against children and youth under 18 years of age. There is significant underreporting of both child abuse and spousal abuse. Elder abuse includes emotional, financial, and physical neglect, and maltreatment, including questionable institutionalization. It is estimated that approximately 4% of elderly Canadians may be abused annually.

6.   REFERENCES

1.   Steering Committee of the National Strategy to Reduce Tobacco Use in Canada in Partnership with Advisory Committee on Population Health. 1999. *New directions for tobacco control in Canada: A national strategy.*<www.hc-sc.gc.ca/hecs-sesc/tobacco/policy/new_directions/index.html> (November 2002).
2.   Single E, Jurgen R, Robson L, *et al.* The relative risks and etiological fractions of different causes of death and disease attributable to alcohol, tobacco, and illicit drugs use in Canada. *Canadian Medical Association Journal* 2002; 162(12):1669-75.
3.   Canadian Cancer Society. 2001. *Canadian cancer statistics 2001.* <www.ncic.cancer.ca/pubse.htm> (November 2002).
4.   Colditz G, DeJong H, Hunter D, *et al. Human causes of cancer: Cancer causes and control.* Boston: Harvard Center for Cancer Prevention, 1996.
5.   U.S. Department of Health and Human Services. *The health consequences of smoking: Nicotine addiction.* Rockville, MD: U.S. Department of Health and Human Services, Public Health Services, Centres for Disease Control, Office of Smoking and Health, 1989.
6.   Health Canada. 2002. *Canadian perinatal health report, 2000.* <www.hc-sc.gc.ca/pphb-dgspsp/publicat/cphr-rspc00/pdf/cphr00e.pdf> (February 2003).

7.   Federal, Provincial and Territorial Advisory Committee on Population Health. 1999. *Statistical report on the health of Canadians*. Cat. 82-570-XIE. <www.statcan.ca/english/freepub/82-570-XIE/free.htm>

8.   Heart and Stroke Foundation of Canada. *The changing face of heart disease and stroke in Canada*. Ottawa: Heart and Stroke Foundation of Canada, 1999.

9.   Health Canada. 1995. *Tobacco control: A blueprint to protect the health of Canadians*. <www.hc-sc.gc.ca/hecs-sesc/tobacco/research/archive/tobac_control.html> (November 2002).

10.   Health Canada. 2000. *You're not the only one smoking this cigarette*. <www.hc-sc.gc.ca/hecs-sesc/tobacco/research/ctums/ETS_factsheet_2000_eng.html>

11.   Spitzer W, Lawrence V, Dales R, *et al*. Links between passive smoking and disease: A best-evidence synthesis. *Clinical and Investigative Medicine* 1990; 13(1):17-42.

12.   Ontario Tobacco Research Unit. 2001. *Protection from second-hand tobacco smoke in Ontario: A review of the evidence regarding best practices*. <www.otru.org/pdf/special_ets_eng.PDF> (November 2002).

13.   Ontario Medical Association. 2003. *The duty to protect: Eliminating second-hand smoke from public places and workplaces in Ontario*. <www.oma.org/phealth/2ndsmoke03.pdf> (February 2003).

14.   Canadian Medical Association, *et al*. Tobacco: The role of health professionals in smoking cessation. 2001. <www.cma.ca/advocacy/news/2001/01-17.htm> (November 2002)

15.   Health Canada. 2001. *New tobacco regulations become law*. <www.hc-sc.gc.ca/english/media/releases/2000/2000_67e.htm> (January 2003).

16.   U.S. Department of Health and Human Services. 2000. *Reducing tobacco use: A report of the Surgeon General*. <www.cdc.gov/tobacco/sgr_tobacco_use.htm> (November 2002).

17.   World Health Organization. 2003. *Tobacco free initiative: Economic interventions*. <tobacco.who.int/page.cfm?sid=52> (February 2003).

18.   Canadian Centre on Substance Abuse. 2000. *Canadian profile 1999: Alcohol*. <www.ccsa.ca> (November 2002).

19.   Single E. 1996. *The concept of harm reduction and its application to alcohol*. <www.ccsa.ca/hr-uk-1.htm> (November 2002).

20.   Health Canada. 1996. *Joint statement: Prevention of fetal alcohol syndrome, fetal alcohol effects in Canada*. <hc-sc.gc.ca/hppb/childhood-youth/cyfh/pdf/english.pdf> (November 2002).

21.   Kahan M. Identifying and managing problem drinkers. *Canadian Family Physician* 1996; 42:661-71.

22.   Centre for Addiction and Mental Health. 2002. *Low-risk drinking guidelines*. <www.camh.net/addiction/pims/low_risk_drinking.html> (November 2002).

23.   Cook B, Abreu J. Alcohol-related health problems. In Wallace R, editor. *Maxey-Rosenau-Last public health and preventive medicine*. 14th ed. Stamford, CT: Appleton & Lange; 1998. p. 847-60.

24.   American Psychiatric Association. *Diagnostic and statistical manual of mental disorders*. DSM-IV. Washington DC: American Psychiatric Association, 2000.

25.   Selzer ML. The Michigan Alcoholism Screening Test: The quest for a new diagnostic instrument. *American Journal of Psychiatry* 1971; 127(12):1653-8.

26.   Ewing JA. Detecting alcoholism: The CAGE questionnaire. *Journal of American Medical Association* 1984; 252(14):1905-7.

27.   National Institute on Alcohol Abuse and Alcoholism. 2000. *Alcohol use disorders identification test (AUDIT)*. <www.niaaa.nih.gov/publications/audit.htm> (February 2003).

28.   National Institute on Alcohol Abuse and Alcoholism. 2000. *TWEAK*. <www.niaaa.nih.gov/publications/tweak.htm> (February 2003).

29.   National Institute on Alcohol Abuse and Alcoholism. 2000. *Adolescent drinking index (ADi)*. <www.niaaa.nih.gov/publications/adi2.htm> (February 2003).

30.   Swarbrick M. Model program for substance abuse prevention. *Public Health and Epidemiology Reports Ontario* 1991; 2(21):320-3.
31.   Rabkin SW, Chen Y, Leiter L, *et al*. Risk factors correlates of body mass index. *Canadian Medical Association Journal* 1997; 157(Suppl 1):S26-31.
32.   Luepker R. Heart disease. In Wallace R, editor. *Maxey-Rosenau-Last public health and preventive medicine*. 14th ed. Stamford, CT: Appleton & Lange; 1998.
33.   World Cancer Research Fund, American Institute for Cancer Research. *Food, nutrition, and the prevention of cancer: A global perspective*. Washington DC: American Institute for Cancer Research, 1997.
34.   Health and Welfare Canada. *Nutrition Recommendations: The report of the Scientific Review Committee*. Ottawa: Ministry of Supplies and Services, 1990.
35.   Health Canada. 2002. *Canada's food guide to healthy eating*.<www.hc-sc.gc.ca/hpfb-dgpsa/onpp-bppn/food_guide_rainbow_e.html> (November 2002).
36.   Katzmarzyk P, Gledhill N, Shephard R. The economic burden of physical inactivity in Canada. *Canadian Medical Association Journal* 2000; 163(11):1435-40.
37.   Marrett L, Theis B, Ashbury F. Physical activity and cancer prevention. *Chronic Diseases in Canada* 2000; 21(4):143-9.
38.   Statistics Canada. How healthy are Canadians? A summary: 2001 annual report. *Health Reports* 2001; 12(3):1-58. <www.statcan.ca/english/freepub/82-003-XIE/free.htm> (January 2003).
39.   Lee C, Jackson A, Blair S. U.S. weight guidelines: Is it also important to consider cardiorespiratory fitness? *International Journal of Obesity* 1998; 22(Suppl 2):S2-7.
40.   Health Canada. 2000. *Canada's physical activity guide to healthy active living*. <www.hc-sc.gc.ca/hppb/paguide/main.html> (November 2002).
41.   Nestle M, Jacobson F. Halting the obesity epidemic: a public health policy approach. *Public Health Reports* 2000; 115:12-24.
42.   Agriculture and Agri-Food Canada. 1998. *Canada's action plan for food security*. <www.agr.gc.ca/misb/fsb/fsap/fsape.html> (November 2002).
43.   Food Security Bureau. 2001. *Canada's action plan for food security*.<www.agr.ca/misb/fsb/fsap/part2e.html> (November 2002).
44.   United Nations Environment Programme. 2000. *Cartagena protocol on biosafety*. <www.biodiv.org/biosafety/protocol.asp> (November 2002).
45.   Pinker S. Precautionary principle leads to "may contain" clause for genetically modified foods. *Canadian Medical Association Journal* 2000; 162:874.
46.   Health Canada. 1996. *Nutrition for health: An agenda for action*. <www.hc-sc.gc.ca/hppb/nutrition/pube/action/e_overview.html> (November 2002).
47.   Smedley B, Syme S, editors. *Promoting health: Intervention strategies from social behavioural research*. Washington DC: National Academy Press; 2000.
48.   Lee K, Rottensten K. A proposed model for prevention and control of chronic disease: Analogies from communicable diseases. *Public Health and Epidemiology Report* 2001; 21(9):305-11.
49.   Heart and Stroke Foundation of Canada. *Heart disease and stroke in Canada*. Ottawa, 1997.
50.   Health Canada. 2002. *Economic burden of illness in Canada, 1998*. <www.hc-sc.gc.ca/pphb-dgspsp/publicat/ebic-femc98/index.html> (November 2002).
51.   Choinière R, Lafontaine P, Edwards A. Distribution of cardiovascular disease risk factors by socioeconomic status among Canadian adults. *Canadian Medical Association Journal* 2000; 162(Suppl 9):S13-24.
52.   Working Group on Hypercholesterolemia and Other Dyslipidemias. Recommendations for the management and treatment of dyslipidemia. *Canadian Medical Association Journal* 2000; 162(10):1441-7.
53.   Puska P, Tuomilehto J, *et al. The North Karelia Project: Evaluation of a comprehensive community programme for control of cardiovascular disease*. Copenhagen, Denmark: World Health Organization/EURO Monograph Series, 1981.

54. Shea S, Basch CA. Review of five major community-based cardiovascular disease prevention programs. Part 1: Rationale, design, and theoretical framework. *American Journal of Health Promotion* 1990; 4(3):203-13.
55. Shea S, Basch CA. Review of five major community-based cardiovascular disease prevention programs. Part 2: Intervention strategies, evaluation methods, and results. *American Journal of Health Promotion* 1990; 4(4):279-87.
56. Canada Heart Health Surveys Research Group. The Federal-Provincial Canadian Heart Health Initiative. *Canadian Medical Association Journal* 1992; 146(11):1915-6.
57. Health and Welfare Canada. 1992. *Heart health equality: Mobilizing communities for action.* Cat. H39-245/1992 E. <www.hc-sc.gc.ca/hppb/ahi/hearthealth/pubs/equal/eqa01.htm> (November 2002).
58. Harvard Center for Cancer Prevention. Harvard report on cancer prevention. *Cancer Causes Control* 1996; 7:S1-59.
59. Miller A. Planning cancer control strategies. *Chronic Disease in Canada* 1992; 13(1):1-40.
60. Health Canada. 1998. *Lung cancer in Canada.* <www.hc-sc.gc.ca/pphb-dgspsp/publicat/updates/lung-98_e.html> (November 2002).
61. Moloughney B. *Colorectal cancer screening programs: A review of the literature.* Ottawa: Laboratory Center for Disease Control, 1999 February.
62. Simon J. Should all people over the age of 50 have regular fecal-occult blood tests? *New England Journal of Medicine* 1998; 338:1151-5.
63. Canadian Task Force on Preventive Health Care. Colorectal cancer screening: Recommendation statement from the Canadian Task Force on Preventive Health Care. *Canadian Medical Association Journal* 2001; 165(2):206-8.
64. The National Committee on Colorectal Cancer Screening. *Recommendations for a population-based colorectal cancer screening.* <www.hc-sc.gc.ca/pphb-dgspsp/publicat/ncccs-cndcc/ccsrec.htm> (March 2003).
65. Health Canada. 1999. *Breast cancer in Canada.* <www.hc-sc.gc.ca/pphb-dgspsp/publicat/updates/breast-99_e.html> (November 2002).
66. Levine M, Moutquin J, Walton R, *et al.* Chemoprevention of breast cancer: A joint guideline from the Canadian Task Force on Preventive Health Care and the Canadian Breast Cancer Initiative's Steering Committee on Clinical Practice Guidelines for the care and treatment of breast cancer. *Canadian Medical Association Journal* 2001; 164(12):1681-90.
67. Prospero L, Seminsky M, Honeyford J, *et al.* Psychosocial issues following a positive result of genetic testing for BRAC1 and BRAC2 mutations: Findings from a focus group and a needs assessment survey. *Canadian Medical Association Journal* 2001; 164(7).
68. Canadian Task Force on Periodic Health Examination. *The Canadian guide to clinical preventive health care.* Ottawa: Minister of Public Works and Government Services Canada, 1994.
69. Ringash J, Canadian Task Force on Preventive Health Care. Preventive health care, 2001 update: Screening mammography among women aged 40-49 years at average risk of breast cancer. *Canadian Medical Association Journal* 2001; 164(4):469-76.
70. Baxter N. Preventive health care, 2001 update: Should women be routinely taught breast self-examination to screen for breast cancer? *Canadian Medical Association Journal* 2001; 164(13):1837-46.
71. Feightner J. *Screening for prostate cancer.* Canadian Task Force on Preventive Health Care, 1994.<www.ctfphc.org/> (March 2003).
72. Blumenfeld A, Fleshner N, Casselman B, *et al.* Nutritional aspects of prostate cancer: A review. *Canadian Journal of Urology* 2000; 7(1):927-35.
73. McBride M, Gallagher R, Theriault G, *et al.* Power-frequency electric and magnetic fields and risk of childhood leukemia in Canada. *American Journal of Epidemiology* 1999; 149(831-42).
74. Franco E, Duarte-Franco E, Ferenczy A. Cervical cancer: Epidemiology, prevention, and the role of human papillomavirus infection. *Canadian Medical Association Journal* 2001; 164(7):1017-25.

75. Koutsky L, Ault K, Wheeler C, *et al.* A controlled trial of a human papillomavirus type 16 vaccine. *New England Journal of Medicine* 2002; 347(21):1645-51.
76. Clapp R. Environment and health: 4. Cancer. *Canadian Medical Association Journal* 2000; 163(8):1009-12. <www.cmaj.ca/cgi/reprint/163/8/1009> (February 2003).
77. Statistics Canada. *Mortality: Summary list of causes, 1996*, 1996. Cat. 84F0209-XPB.
78. D'Cunha C. 2000. *Taking action on asthma: Report of the Chief Medical Officer of Health.* <gov.on.ca/health/english/pub/pubhealth/asthma/cmoh_asthma.html> (November 2002).
79. Manfreda J, Becklake M, Sears M, *et al.* Prevalence of asthma symptoms among adults aged 20-44 years. *Canadian Medical Association Journal* 2001; 164(7):995-1001.
80. Millar W, Hill G. Childhood asthma. *Health Reports* 1998; 10(3):9-21.
81. Anis A, Lynd L, Wang X, *et al.* Double trouble: Impact of inappropriate use of asthma medications on the use of health care resources. *Canadian Medical Association Journal* 2001; 164(5):625-31.
82. Health Canada. *Health and environment: Partners for life.* Ottawa: Minister of Public Works and Government Services Canada, 1997.
83. Ontario Medical Association. *Ontario Medical Association position paper on health effects of ground-level ozone, acid aerosols, and particulate matter.* Toronto, 1998.
84. D'Cunha C. *Diabetes: Strategies for prevention.* Toronto: Ontario Ministry of Health and Long-Term Care, 1999.
85. Health Canada. 1999. *Diabetes in Canada.* Cat. H49-121/1999. <www.hc-sc.gc.ca/pphb-dgspsp/publicat/dic-dac99/index.html> (November 2002).
86. Health Canada. 2002. *Diabetes in Canada.* 2nd edition. <www.hc-sc.gc.ca/pphb-dgspsp/publicat/dic-dac2/pdf/dic-dac2_en.pdf> (February 2003).
87. Conference Board of Canada. *Physical activity and the cost of treating illness.* Ottawa, 1996.
88. March of Dimes. 2003. *Birth defects.* <www.hc-sc.gc.ca/pphb-dgspsp/publicat/cac-acc02/index.html> (February 2003).
89. Health Canada. 2002. *Congenital anomalies in Canada.* <www.hc-sc.gc.ca/pphb-dgspsp/publicat/cac-acc02/index.html> (February 2003).
90. Ontario Medical Association Committee on Population Health. OMA Position Paper on Second-Hand Smoke. *Ontario Medical Review* 1996; 63(11):29-35.
91. Canadian Paediatric Society, *et al.* 1996. *Prevention of Fetal Alcohol Syndrome and Fetal alcohol effects in Canada.* <www.cps.ca/english/statements/FN/cps96-01.htm> (November 2002).
92. Health Canada. 2002. *Folic acid: Preconception health and folic acid.* <www.hc-sc.gc.ca/english/folicacid/report/prevention.html> (January 2003).
93. Dick PT. Periodic health examination, 1996—Update: 1. Prenatal screening for and diagnosis of Down syndrome. *Canadian Medical Association Journal* 1996; 154(4):465-80.
94. Royal Commission on New Reproductive Technologies. *Proceed with care: Final report of the Royal Commission on New Reproductive Technologies.* Ottawa: Minister of Government Services, 1993.
95. Baird P. Genetic technologies and achieving health for populations. *International Journal of Health Services* 2001; 30(2):407-24.
96. Statistics Canada. 2001. *Arthritis and rheumatism.* <secure.cihi.ca/indicators/en/defin1.shtml#hc> (November 2002).
97. Kelsey J. Musculoskeletal disorders. In Wallace R, editor. *Maxey-Rosenau-Last public health and preventive medicine.* 14th ed. Stamford, CT: Appleton & Lange; 1998.
98. Badley E, Wang P. The contribution of arthritis and arthritis disability to nonparticipation in the labour force: A Canadian example. *Journal of Rheumatology* 2001; 28(5):1077-82.
99. Badley E, Wang, P. Baby boomers and arthritis rates. *Canadian Medical Association Journal* 1999; 160:16.
100. World Health Organization Study Group. *Assessment of fracture risk and its application to screening for postmenopausal osteoporosis.* Geneva: World Health Organization, 1994.

101. Scientific Advisory Board, Osteoporosis Society of Canada. Clinical practice guidelines for the diagnosis and management of osteoporosis. *Canadian Medical Association Journal* 1996; 155(8):1113-33.

102. National Cancer Institute. 2002. *Questions and answers: Use of hormones after menopause.* <newscenter.cancer.gov/pressreleases/estrogenplus.html> (November 2002).

103. Mood Disorder Society of Canada, Association of Chairs of Psychiatry in Canada, Canadian Institute for Health Information, *et al.* 2002. *A report on mental illness in Canada.* <www.hc-sc.gc.ca/pphb-dgspsp/publicat/miic-mmac> (November 2002).

104. World Health Organization. 2001. *Strengthening mental health promotion.* <www.who.int/inf-fs/en/fact220.html> (November 2002).

105. Stephens T, Joubert N. The economic burden of mental health problems in Canada. *Chronic Diseases in Canada* 2001; 22(1):18-23.

106. Centre for Health Promotion. Mental health promotion: What is it? Workshop on Mental Health Promotion, Toronto, June 20-21, 1996.

107. Willinsky C, Pape B. *Mental health promotion.* Toronto: Canadian Mental Health Association, 1997 November.

108. Canadian Alliance on Mental Illness and Mental Health. 2001. *Questions and answers about CAMIMH.* <www.cpa-apc.org/Public/Questions.asp> (November 2002).

109. Canadian Public Health Association. Draft position paper no. 1. Injury prevention and control in Canada: The need for a public health approach and coordinated national leadership. Ottawa. *CPHA Digest* 2002; 26(1):3-8.

110. Potter L, O'Carroll P. Suicide. In Wallace R, editor. *Maxey-Rosenau-Last public health and preventive medicine.* 14th ed. Stamford, CT: Appleton & Lange; 1998.

111. Bosma H, Peter R, Siegrist J, *et al.* Two alternative job stress models and the risk of coronary heart disease. *American Journal of Public Health* 1998; 88:68-74.

112. Hemingway H, Marmot M. Psychosocial factors in the aetiology and prognosis of coronary heart disease: Systemic review of prospective cohort studies. *British Medical Journal* 1999; 318:1460-7.

113. Siegrist J. Adverse health effects of high-effort/low-reward conditions. *Journal of Occupational Health Psychology* 1996; 1:27-41.

114. National Institute of Occupational Safety and Health Working Group. *Stress at work.* Cincinnati: National Institute of Occupational Safety and Health, 1999.

115. Martin J, Wade T. The relationship between physical exercise and distress in a national sample of Canadians. *Canadian Journal of Public Health* 2000; 91(4):302-6.

116. Statistics Canada. Health status of children. *Health Reports* 1999; 11(3):25-34.

117. Health Canada. 2001. *Community programs: 1999-2000 annual review, August 2000.* <www.hc-sc.gc.ca/fnihb/cp/annualreview/injury.htm> (November 2002).

118. D'Cunha C. 2002. *2002 Chief Medical Officer of Health Report — Injury: Predictable and preventable.* <www.gov.on.ca/health/english/pub/ministry/injury_rep02/injury_mn.html> (November 2002).

119. Health Canada. 2001. *Injury section: Interactive Canadian injury statistics.* <www.hc-sc.gc.ca/pphb-dgspsp/injury-bles/index.html> (November 2002).

120. Sibbald B. 2001. *Canada's child death rate from injury among the highest in the OECD.* Canadian Medical Association Journal. <www.cma.ca/cmaj/cmaj_today/2001/02_13.htm> (November 2002).

121. Haddon Jr. W. The changing approach to the epidemiology, prevention, and amelioration of trauma: The transition to approaches etiologically rather than descriptively based. *American Journal of Public Health* 1968; 58:1431-38.

122. Kraus J, Peek-Asa C, Vimalachandra D. Injury control: The public health approach. In Wallace R, editor. *Maxey-Rosenau-Last public health and preventive medicine.* 14th ed. Stamford, CT: Appleton & Lange; 1998.

123. Chapdelaine A, Samson E, Kimberly MD, *et al.* Firearm-related injuries in Canada: Issues for prevention. *Canadian Medical Association Journal* 1991; 145(10):1217-23.

124. Lavoie M, Cardinal L, Chapdelaine A, *et al.* The storage of household long guns: The situation in Quebec. *Chronic Diseases in Canada* 2001; 22(1):24-9.
125. Gabor T, Roberts J, Stein K, *et al.* Unintentional firearm deaths: can they be reduced by lowering gun ownership levels. *Canadian Journal of Public Health* 2001; 92(5):396-8.
126. Government of Canada. 2001. *Highlights of the Firearm Act.* <www.cfc-ccaf.gc.ca/en/general_public/highlights/default.asp> (February 2003).
127. Canadian Centre for Justice Statistics. 2002. *Family violence in Canada: A statistical profile.* Cat. no. 85-224-XIE. <collection.nlc-bnc.ca/100/201/301/statcan/family_violence/> (November 2002).
128. MacMillan H, Wathen C. *Prevention and treatment of violence against women: Systematic review and recommendations.* London: Canadian Task Force on Preventive Health Care, 2001. <www.ctfphc.org/Full_Text/CTF_DV_TR_final.pdf> (February 2003).
129. Health Canada. 2003. *The Canadian incidence study of reported child abuse and neglect.* <www.hc-sc.gc.ca/pphb-dgspsp/cm-vee> (February 2003).
130. Statistics Canada. Family violence: Focus on child abuse and children at risk. *The Daily* 2001, June 28. <www.statcan.ca/Daily/English/010628/d010628b.htm> (January 2003).
131. Podnicks E. National survey of abuse of the elderly in Canada. *Journal of Elder Abuse Neglect* 1992; 4:5-58.
132. Allan B. *Wife abuse: The impact on children.* Ottawa: National Clearinghouse on Family Violence, 1991.

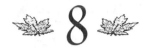

8

COMMUNICABLE DISEASES

Communicable disease is defined as an illness caused by a specific infectious agent or its toxic products that arises through transmission of that agent or its products from an infected person, animal, or reservoir to a susceptible host, either directly or indirectly through an intermediate plant or animal host, vector, or the inanimate environment (1). The beginning of the 20th century was characterized by a progressive decline in morbidity and mortality from communicable diseases in the developed world. The last two decades of the 20th century witnessed a number of emerging and re-emerging infectious diseases — AIDS, outbreaks of viral hemorrhagic fevers (Ebola), hantavirus, and tuberculosis represent examples of the new challenges to public health. Outbreaks of plague in India underscore the failure of healthcare systems to manage previously controlled diseases. Outbreaks of strains of tuberculosis that resist multiple drugs and vancomycin-resistant enterococci (VRE) have raised the spectre of bacteria not susceptible to antibiotics. This prospect was inconceivable 20 years ago, when the U.S. Surgeon General decreed that the war against infectious agents had been won. A recent outbreak of *Escherichia coli* in a contaminated water supply in Walkerton, Ontario, the importation of West Nile virus, severe acute respiratory syndrome (SARS), and anthrax (as a weapon of bioterrorism) in the United States further highlight the importance of infectious diseases.

High-ranking members of the medical and public health communities have expressed their concerns about the dangers posed by communicable diseases. The reasons for the recrudescence of communicable diseases are as broad as the determinants of health. Behavioural intransigence, poverty, war, immigration, environmental desecration, iatrogenesis, and increased international travel figure prominently in the causal underpinnings.

Despite the fears engendered by the extensive publicity given to new communicable diseases, the traditional principles of communicable disease control remain effective. In Canada, immunization programs have significantly decreased the incidence of measles and invasive *Haemophilus influenzae* type b. Infection control, good hygiene, timely surveillance, and outbreak management remain essential components of the

Figure 8.1.   Spectrum of Infectious Disease

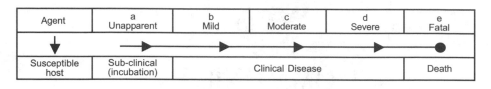

Agent	a Unapparent	b Mild	c Moderate	d Severe	e Fatal
Susceptible host	Sub-clinical (incubation)	Clinical Disease			Death

public health response to communicable diseases.

Notifiable or reportable disease is defined as disease deemed of sufficient importance to public health to require that its occurrence be reported to public health officials (1). All provinces and territories mandate reporting of certain communicable diseases (see list of notifiable diseases in Canada, Chapter 3). Reporting to the federal level is voluntary; however, agreement is reached by consensus of the Advisory Committee on Epidemiology (ACE), which comprises representatives from all provinces and territories.

In Canada, all notifiable disease data are collected systematically by provincial and federal authorities. Interested readers are directed to electronic databases maintained by the Centre for Infectious Disease Prevention and Control in Ottawa, the U.S. Centers for Disease Control (CDC) in Atlanta, and the World Health Organization in Geneva for the most up-to-date data.

1.   BASIC CONCEPTS AND TERMINOLOGY OF COMMUNICABLE DISEASE CONTROL

The investigation and control of communicable diseases (contagious or infectious diseases) requires some knowledge of the spectrum of infectious diseases and the relevant terminology. The spectrum of communicable disease is illustrated by Figure 8.1.

Investigators can characterize the threat of an offending organism by calculating several rates. The **attack rate** is the total number of people who developed clinical disease divided by the population at risk (a+b+c+d+e), usually expressed as a percentage. In Figure 8.1, therefore, the attack rate can be derived by (b+c+d+e)/ (population at risk). The **secondary attack rate** is the number of cases among contacts occurring within the incubation period following exposure to a primary case, in relation to the total exposed contacts; the denominator is thus restricted to the number of susceptible contacts that can be ascertained. This is often used to gauge contagiousness and evaluate disease control measures. The **pathogenicity rate** describes the power of an organism to produce clinical disease in those who are infected; this is expressed as (b+c+d+e)/(a+b+c+d+e). **Virulence** describes the severity of disease produced by the organism in a given host and is expressed as a ratio of the number of cases of severe and fatal infection to the total number clinically infected, or (d+e)/(b+c+d+e). The **case fatality rate** is the proportion of persons contracting the disease who die of it, namely e/(b+c+d+e).

A **reservoir** of infection is a person, animal, or inanimate object in which infectious agents can live and multiply for extended periods of time. **Transmission** of such agents occurs by various means or from one host (human or animal) to another. **Direct** transmission involves the transfer of infectious agents directly from one host to another. **Indirect** transmission can occur through a vehicle, vector, or the air. In **vehicle-borne** transmission, organisms are spread via inanimate materials, objects, or media (e.g., toys, clothes, milk, food). **Vector-borne** transmission may be mechanical (e.g., simple carriage of agents by animals) or biological (e.g., organisms multiplying inside insects). Malaria is an example of biological transmission of parasites from mosquito vectors to human hosts. **Airborne** transmission may occur via droplet nuclei or dust particles.

A **carrier** is defined as an individual who harbours a specific infectious agent usually without overt clinical disease. A carrier state may be of long or short duration, and it may serve as a potential source of infection.

The **communicable period** is the time during which an infectious agent may be transferred from an infected person or vector to another host. **Generation time** is the interval between the entry of infection into the host and its maximal infectivity. **Incubation period** is the interval between infection by an agent and the appearance of the first symptom of the disease. Often generation time is equivalent to the incubation period. **Infectiousness** reflects the ease of disease transmission, and is usually measured by the secondary attack rate.

1.1. OUTBREAKS OF INFECTIOUS DISEASES

An **outbreak** of disease is the occurrence of new cases clearly in excess of the baseline, or normally expected, frequency of the disease in a defined community or institutional population over a given period. An **epidemic** has a synonymous definition, although in common parlance an outbreak usually means an epidemic that is localized, of acute onset, or relatively short in duration. Notable examples of outbreaks include the gastrointestinal illnesses due to *E. coli* in the community of Walkerton during 2000 and the increase in meningococcal disease in a number of provinces during 2000 and 2001. Less publicized are the outbreaks of diseases of moderate morbidity for the general population but of more severe morbidity for those already compromised in health, such as influenza among nursing home residents or viral gastroenteritis among infants and children in day care.

Two other terms are worth noting: endemic and pandemic. **Endemic** refers to the constant presence of a disease or infectious agent within a given geographic area or population subgroup. **Pandemic** refers to an epidemic occurring over a wide area, crossing international boundaries, and affecting a large number of people. The investigation of an infectious disease outbreak requires particular epidemiological methods that establish the cause, risk factors, and modes of transmission of the disease (2).

The control of the outbreak can then be achieved by removing or neutralizing the agent, strengthening the resistance of the host, and interrupting the means of transmission in the environment. Thus, the **agent-host-environment** triad (mentioned in Chapter 1) applies. In addition, the outbreak control response must incorporate appropriate communication and sensitivity to public perceptions of risk, which may differ from expert opinions (see Chapter 9 for risk communication).

1.2.   VERIFICATION OF EXISTENCE OF AN OUTBREAK

As mentioned above, defining whether an outbreak exists requires knowledge of the endemic baseline "normally expected" or the "usual frequency" of cases of the disease in the specified population. Depending on the type of disease and population, the expected frequency may be a certain number per week or month, or none at all. In the early stages of an outbreak, the specific diagnosis of the disease or causative agent is usually not yet known, so the most prominent clinical symptoms are used to identify a possible or suspected case. For example, a nursing home might initially define an outbreak as "three or more residents having three episodes of diarrhea within a 24-hour period," since one or two loose bowel movements may be considered within the expected frequency.

Once an outbreak is suspected, investigators (usually from local public health departments) must first ascertain the history of symptoms and signs of the affected persons, so that an initial **case definition** can be formulated from the most common symptoms or signs. Three elements are generally included in case definition: person, place, and time, i.e. the likely date of onset of illness of the first case (e.g., "any person having onset on or since a specified date, of vomiting, fever higher than 38.5°C and bloody stools"). Laboratory confirmation of the clinical diagnosis is sought as soon as possible — e.g., by culture or serology — and results, when available, can define a case more precisely.

After the case definition has been developed, the extent of the outbreak is determined by active surveillance — that is, active efforts to identify all those who may have been exposed to the infectious agent (population at risk) and who may have illness fitting the case definition. In a community outbreak, this may involve contacting hospital emergency rooms, physicians' offices, and local schools. Typical epidemiological information recorded includes demographics (age, gender, etc.), location (residence, school, or workplace), details about the illness (date and time of onset, symptoms), laboratory tests and treatment (if any), outcome (hospitalized, died, recovered), immunization status (if relevant), and close contacts with other persons. A **line listing** is typically made of all suspected and confirmed cases.

The data from the line listing is used to generate an epidemic curve. The epidemic curve is constructed as a histogram with the number of cases plotted on the vertical axis and their dates or times of onset along the horizontal axis. The **epidemic curve** can visually indicate whether the outbreak has a common (or point) source or whether it is propagated. The location of cases (geographic or institutional) may be depicted as a spot map. Attack rates are often also calculated.

In a **common source outbreak**, individuals become ill because of exposure to a single (common) source of infection; the exposure may be of long or short duration. A **point source** outbreak is of short duration, with the number of cases rising and falling acutely due to short-term exposure to the infectious source, such as food poisoning in a group of persons eating the same item at a church picnic. Hence the epidemic curve would show a single, sharp peak. A **propagated outbreak** may begin with only a few exposed persons but is maintained by person-to-person transmission. The epidemic curve will generally show a series of peaks. A nosocomial (institutional) outbreak of Norwalk-like virus provides a good example of a propagated outbreak. Once the preliminary analysis has the infectious disease risk factor(s) of interest, further investigation (e.g., case control studies) can help define the likely cause and disease transmission pattern, as described in Chapter 2.

1.3. IMPLEMENTATION OF INITIAL CONTROL MEASURES

Depending on the symptoms, the suspected agent, the population at risk, and the location, initial control measures will be adopted. These may include isolation of residents in a facility, augmented hand washing and cleaning, cohort nursing (using the same nursing staff in an institution for cases for the duration of the outbreak), exclusion of symptomatic staff, immunization (e.g., for influenza or measles), prophylactic medication for those exposed or at risk (e.g., rifampin for meningococcal disease), withdrawal of contaminated food from distribution, or issuance of a boil water advisory.

Outbreaks of **nosocomial infections** (i.e., those acquired during stay in a healthcare facility) require an *outbreak management team* to coordinate the efforts of many departments — such as housekeeping, maintenance, dietary, nursing, and medical staff — in implementing investigation and control measures.

Depending on the cause of the outbreak and the mode of transmission, specific control measures (such as immunization or specific improvements in the processes of food preparation) may be implemented. Standard textbooks of epidemiology and infection control contain details regarding the investigation and control of outbreaks (2, 3).

2. IMMUNIZATION

Immunization remains the most important factor in the prevention of infectious disease. Its success in the reduction of morbidity and mortality from infectious diseases is unrivalled by any other medical intervention both in terms of health benefits and cost effectiveness (4). However, there are certain professional and parent groups who perceive a causal association of immunization with certain diseases. Useful material is available for healthcare providers involved in primary care, who are obliged to talk to parents about the benefits and risks of vaccines (5, 6).

This effectiveness depends not only on the efficacy of individual vaccines, but also on the degree of coverage achieved. These factors rely on administrative aspects of the vaccination program as well as on consumer and provider compliance, and the maintenance of potency of the vaccine during transportation and storage. Strategies to improve the effectiveness and efficiency of vaccine delivery programs have been comprehensively reviewed (7, 8). Detailed guidelines are provided by the Canadian National Guidelines for Vaccine Storage and Transportation for the appropriate storage and handling of vaccines (9). According to the Canadian Immunization Guide (10), "it is recommended that all biologicals for immunization be maintained at 2° to 8° Celsius at all times, unless otherwise specified in the product leaflet."

Recommendations are established by Health Canada's National Advisory Committee on Immunization (NACI). Publicly funded vaccines vary by province and territory and hence each publishes its own immunization schedule. Details on adverse reactions from vaccines are regularly reviewed and published by the Centre for Infectious Disease Prevention and Control (11). The recommended schedule for the immunization of infants and children is provided in Table 8.1.

3.   SELECTED VACCINE-PREVENTABLE DISEASES

In the early part of the 20th century, vaccine-preventable diseases were a major cause of morbidity and mortality in Canada, particularly in children. While many of these diseases are now under control in Canada, some remain a major problem throughout the world and thus, the risk of importation into Canada still remains a risk. As a result, these diseases still have the ability to produce significant numbers of cases of preventable illness and death.

While diseases such as tetanus, diphtheria, and polio have been almost eradicated in Canada, sporadic cases and outbreaks of certain diseases that could be prevented by vaccines are still reported. A brief overview of the recent incidence of the major vaccine-preventable diseases in Canada, as well as issues relevant to control, are discussed here. Health Canada's *Canadian National Report on Immunization, 1998,* provides a very good overview of the vaccine preventable diseases in Canada (12).

Pertussis

Pertussis (whooping cough) is an infection of the respiratory tract caused by the bacterium *Bordetella pertussis*. The incidence of pertussis has decreased by more than 90% since the whole-cell pertussis vaccine was introduced in 1943, although periodic outbreaks of pertussis continue to occur in Canada (4). Coverage rates for pertussis immunization have been far lower than other routine immunization (e.g., mumps, measles, and rubella) because of fear of side effects. In 1998, 7,519 cases of pertussis were reported, indicating sub-optimal disease control (12). The severity of the disease has decreased due to widespread vaccination, which affords partial protection. However, the disease has a poorer prognosis in infants under 1 year of age, in whom the case-fatality rate is 1 in 200. In 1994, the Centre for Infectious Disease Prevention and Control revised the optimal management of contacts of sporadic cases and outbreaks of pertussis (13).

Table 8.1.   Recommended Schedule for the Immunization of Infants and Children

Age at vaccination	DTaP[1]	IPV	Hib[2]	MMR	Td[3] or dTap[10]	Hep B[4] (3 doses)	V	PC	MC
Birth									
2 months	X	X	X					X[8]	X[9]
4 months	X	X	X			Infancy or preadolescence (9-13 yrs)		X	X
6 months	X	(X)[5]	X					X	X
12 months				X			X[7]	X	
18 months	X	X	X	(X)[6] OR					
4-6 years	X	X		(X)[6]					
14-16 years					X[10]				

DTaP Diphtheria, tetanus, pertussis (acellular) vaccine
IPV Inactivated poliovirus vaccine
Hib Haemophilus influenzae type b conjugate vaccine
MMR Measles, mumps and rubella vaccine
Td Tetanus and diphtheria toxoid, acellular pertussis, adolescent/adult type with reduced diphtheria and pertussis components
Hep B Hepatitis B vaccine
V Varicella
PC Pneumococcal conjugate vaccine
MC Meningococcal conjugate vaccine

Source: *Canadian Immunization Guide, Sixth edition, page 56*, Health Canada, 2002. © Reproduced with the permission of the Minister of Public Works and Government Services Canada, 2003.

Notes:
1. DTaP (diphtheria, tetanus, acellular or component pertussis) vaccine is the preferred vaccine for all doses in the vaccination series, including completion of the series in children who have received ≥1 dose of DPT (whole cell) vaccine.
2. Hib schedule shown is for PRP-T or HbOC vaccine. If PRP-OMP is used, give at 2, 4 and 12 months of age.
3. Td (tetanus and diphtheria toxoid), a combined adsorbed "adult type" preparation for use in people ≥7 years of age, contains less diphtheria toxoid than preparations given to younger children and is less likely to cause reactions in older people.
4. Hepatitis B vaccine can be routinely given to infants or preadolescents, depending on the provincial/territorial policy; three doses at 0, 1 and 6 month intervals are preferred. The second dose should be administered at least 1 month after the first dose, and the third at least 2 months after the second dose. A two-dose schedule for adolescents is also possible (see chapter on Hepatitis B Vaccine).
5. This dose is not needed routinely, but can be included for convenience.
6. A second dose of MMR is recommended, at least 1 month after the first dose for the purpose of better measles protection. For convenience, options include giving it with the next scheduled vaccination at 18 months of age or with school entry (4-6 years) vaccinations (depending on the provincial/territorial policy), or at any intervening age that is practicable. The need for a second dose of mumps and rubella vaccine is not established but may benefit (given for convenience as MMR). The second dose of MMR should be given at the same visit as DTaP IPV (± Hib) to ensure high uptake rates.
7. Children aged 12 months to 12 years should receive one dose of varicella vaccine. Individuals ≥13 years of age should receive two doses at least 28 days apart.
8. Recommended schedule, number of doses and subsequent use of 23 valent polysaccharide pneumococcal vaccine depend on the age of the child when vaccination is begun (see *Canadian Immunization Guide* page 177 for specific recommendations).
9. Recommended schedule and number of doses of meningococcal vaccine depends on the age of the child (see *Canadian Immunization Guide* page 151 for specific recommendations).
10. dTap adult formulation with reduced diphtheria toxoid and pertussis component.

The new acellular vaccine was licensed in Canada in 1996 and adopted by all provincial and territorial immunization programs by 1998. This vaccine, demonstrated in randomized controlled trials to be safer and more effective than whole-cell preparations, should increase the acceptability and alleviate concerns about safety (14, 15). Increased rates of vaccination against pertussis should result in further reduction in morbidity and mortality. Rates are constantly being monitored to determine the effectiveness of the vaccine.

Measles

Measles is one of the most contagious vaccine-preventable diseases. Complications include otitis media, pneumonia, and diarrhea, and are more frequent in young children. Encephalitis occurs in 1 out of 1,000 cases and can result in permanent brain damage. Death is estimated to occur in 1 of every 3,000 cases in Canada. In 1995, despite high coverage rates, more than 2,300 cases of measles were reported in Canada (16). As a result, the NACI reaffirmed its commitment to eliminating measles and recommended a strategy for measles control in Canada that included a two-dose vaccination program, which was undertaken by all provinces and territories by 1996 (17). This strategy has successfully reduced the incidence of measles in Canada with reports of 12, 29, and 199 cases of measles reported in 1998, 1999, and 2000 respectively (16). Most of the cases reported in Canada since 1998 were imported.

Rubella

The incidence of both rubella and congenital rubella syndrome (CRS) in Canada has significantly decreased with the MMR vaccination of young children. However, outbreaks of rubella continue to occur, and cases of CRS are reported each year. In the past decade, the epidemiology of rubella has also changed with an increasing proportion of cases reported in adolescents and young adults. Approximately 60% of rubella cases occur in persons aged 10 to 39 years. In Manitoba, large outbreaks of rubella occurred in 1992–93 as well as in 1996–97 and involved a total of more than 5,000 cases. Most cases were in young adult males; however, 565 cases were women of child-bearing age.

Only one to two cases of CRS per year were reported between 1996 and 1999 (0.3 to 0.5 cases per 100,000 births) (18). However, serious under-reporting of rubella and lack of identification of CRS are likely responsible for the apparent recent decline in rubella. Female patients should be warned of the dangers associated with rubella infection in pregnancy, if they are not immune. Efforts should be made to improve the rate of prenatal rubella screening and post-natal vaccination to prevent cases of CRS from occurring.

Influenza

Influenza viruses are a major cause of morbidity, mortality, and lost productivity due to work and school absence in the Canadian population. Influenza A strains (H1N1 and H3N2 variants) and influenza B circulate around the globe annually, usually during the winter months. The overall estimated mortality from influenza and pneumonia (a complication of influenza) exceeds that of all vaccine-preventable childhood diseases. In Canada, there are an estimated 6,700 deaths and as many as 75,000 hospitalizations each year from influenza (19). The heaviest toll occurs among those over 65 years of age, although substantial morbidity can occur in younger patients who are immunocompromised or have chronic diseases such as asthma, chronic obstructive pulmonary disease, ischemic heart disease, or diabetes. Medicare and hospitalization costs for influenza in Canada are approximately $500 million per year.

Periodic pandemics of influenza have occurred in the last 100 years. Landmark influenza pandemics occurred in 1918 ("Spanish flu," H1N1), 1957 ("Asian flu," H2N2), 1968 ("Hong Kong flu," H3N2), and 1977 ("Russian flu," H1N1). Since the influenza virus undergoes genetic shifts and drifts, further pandemics are possible. Antigenic shift is a major change in one or both surface antigens (H and/or N) that occurs at varying intervals. Antigenic drift is a minor change in surface antigens that occurs between major shifts.

As immunization of the entire population is the best means of controlling the impact of a pandemic, it is important to promote a high level of influenza immunization between pandemics. Ontario became the first jurisdiction in the world to introduce a universal influenza immunization program in 2000, offering the influenza vaccine free of charge to anyone aged 6 months and older. Such a program contributes greatly to the ability to react in the event of a pandemic as it helps to raise public awareness of the seriousness of influenza and helps to build a community-based infrastructure for vaccination delivery. It has been shown that vaccine uptake is improved if healthcare providers recommend vaccination. Increased efforts in organizing influenza programs, particularly in improving provider compliance with national guidelines for immunization, may improve vaccine coverage.

Pneumococcal Disease

Pneumococcal infection, caused by the bacterium *Streptococcus pneumoniae* (pneumococcus), is a leading cause of death and a major cause of bacterial pneumonia and meningitis among children and the elderly. In Canada, it is estimated to cause 80,000 episodes of pneumonia, 4,000 of bacteremia, and 500 of meningitis each year. Pneumococcal infections account for about 30–50% of hospital admissions for community-acquired pneumonia in adults (20). Although the overall annual incidence rate for infection is 15 cases per 100,000 population, rates are significantly higher in specific age groups at 46 per 100,000 for people aged 65 years and older, 23 per 100,000 for children 2 to 4 years of age, and 108 per 100,000 for children under 2 years of age (4). The overall case fatality rate for invasive pneumococcal disease has been estimated at 11%.

Invasive pneumococcal disease became nationally reportable in January 2000 in order to monitor the burden of illness in the population and to evaluate the effectiveness of the immunization program. A pneumococcal conjugate vaccine for children was licensed in Canada in June 2001, which is recommended by the

NACI for all Canadian children under 2 years of age, and children aged 2 to 5 years who are at high risk for invasive pneumococcal disease (21).

Haemophilus influenzae type b

Haemophilus influenzae type b (Hib) was, until the introduction of an effective vaccine, the leading cause of bacterial meningitis in children. Most cases of Hib meningitis occurred in children under 5 years of age with a rate of infection of 1 in 200. Those with meningitis had a fatality rate of 3–5%, and those who survived had high rates of neurological complications. Since 1986, when national reporting for invasive Hib was introduced, the number of cases ranged from 100 to 650 cases per year. After 1993, with the introduction of the infant conjugate vaccine into all provincial and territorial routine immunization schedules, the number decreased to less than 60 cases per year (12). This illustrates the success of an effective immunization program.

Hepatitis B

The incidence of hepatitis B has declined since the mid 1990s. The incidence of reported cases in Canada in 1994 was 10.6 per 100,000 and has since decreased to 700 cases per year (2.3 per 100,000). The incidence rate is twice as high in males as in females. The highest incidence rate occurs in those aged 30–39 years (6.1 per 100,000), followed by those aged 15–29 years (2.7 per 100,000) and 40–59 years (1.8 per 100,000) (22). The major risk factors in Canada are sexual transmission and intravenous drug use. Vertical transmission (from mother to newborn) and medical and dental occupational transmission (patient to practitioner and vice versa) account for a small proportion of cases.

Hepatitis B is the only sexually transmitted disease for which an effective and safe vaccine is available. Due to the high infectiousness of this virus, the expert consensus in Canada supports universal vaccination against hepatitis B (23). Immunization in late childhood or early adolescence provides maximum protection against sexual transmission of hepatitis B (24). As of 1998, all provinces have universal pre-adolescent hepatitis B vaccination programs.

Varicella

Varicella disease (chickenpox) is a highly contagious viral disease that affects 95% of Canadians, generally before the age of 15 years. The annual incidence of chickenpox approximates the birth cohort and is approximately 344,000 cases per year (95% of cohort). While in healthy children the disease is relatively benign in some children, chickenpox can cause more serious complications including secondary bacterial skin infections, otitis media, mild hepatitis, and thrombocytopenia. The occurrence of invasive group A streptococcal disease (necrotizing fasciitis or "flesh-eating disease") is increased after varicella infection and can lead to a high number of hospitalizations and deaths among children. In adolescents and adults, complications associated with varicella infection are more frequent and include higher rates of pneumonia, encephalitis, and death. Case fatality rates are 10 to 30 times higher in adults than in children. Although adults account for only 5% of all Canadian cases, 70% of varicella-related deaths from 1987 to 1996 were among individuals over 15 years of age. A vaccine against chickenpox was approved for use in Canada in 1999. Among recommended groups for immunization, the NACI recommends the vaccine for all healthy children 12 months of age or older who are susceptible to varicella infection. Prince Edward Island and Alberta currently have routine varicella immunization programs (25).

4. TRENDS IN OTHER SIGNIFICANT INFECTIOUS DISEASES

Tuberculosis

Tuberculosis (TB) is an important bacterial infection, especially in at-risk populations such as those with HIV infection, homeless persons, alcoholics, Aboriginal peoples, and foreign-born individuals from areas where TB is endemic. Since 1987, the previously declining TB rates in Canada have levelled off, with approximately 2,000 new cases and more than 100 deaths reported annually (26). This is due to increased immigration from countries with high TB rates, HIV, and the emergence of drug-resistant TB. Coinfection (concurrent) with HIV and TB has also been a major factor in the resurgence of TB worldwide. Although the rate of TB in Canada is one of the lowest in the world at 7 per 100,000 population per year, the rates in sub-populations still vary. The incidence of TB among Canadian-born non-Aboriginal people is 1 per 100,000 compared to 70 per 100,000 in Aboriginal people (27). In 1996, 76% of reported cases were in Ontario, Quebec, and British Columbia. The rate of TB was highest in the Northwest Territories (53.9 cases per 100,000), which is attributed to the high rates among Aboriginal population (26).

Apart from the difficulties of control in traditional risk groups and HIV-infected people, many immigrants, refugees, and visitors arrive in Canada each year from countries with high rates of TB. The risk of reactivation of disease in those who have previously had it is increased in the foreign-born. Medical practitioners need to be sensitized to the diagnosis and management of TB, particularly as it relates to public health hazards and the emergence of multiple-resistant strains in those non-compliant with chemotherapy. Drug resistance rates have likely increased due to the high number of people arriving in Canada from countries with a high prevalence of drug resistance, but also due to inappropriate or interrupted treatment here in Canada. Multiple drug-resistant (MDR) TB is associated with high mortality rates as well as high costs due to prolonged hospitalization and the cost of second-line drugs.

A major obstacle to tuberculosis control is compliance with medication. A course of therapy requires at least three medications for 6 to 9 months. As the acute symptoms rapidly disappear after 4 to 6 weeks, it is often difficult to persuade people to remain compliant. Strategies such as Directly Observed Therapy (DOT) are effective measures to improve compliance with TB drug therapy, particularly rates of MDR-TB. DOT involves a healthcare worker giving medications to a patient and making sure the patient takes the medication.

Meningococcal Disease

Bacterial meningitis, a serious inflammation of the coverings of the brain and spinal cord, is usually caused by *Neisseria meningitidis*. Death and permanent neurological impairment are the most severe consequences. Meningococcal disease can also manifest as overwhelming septicemia or arthritis. Meningococcal disease is endemic in Canada with disease occurring in cycles of high and low incidence every 10 to 15 years. The incidence of invasive meningococcal disease varies in Canada and is approximately 1 per 100,000 population per year, with the greatest burden of illness in children less than 5 years of age. Between 1985 and 2000, an average of 303 cases were reported each year (28).

Serogroups B and C have been responsible for most cases of endemic meningococcal disease in Canada; however, type C has been primarily responsible for the reported disease clusters and outbreaks. Vaccine is available for type C but not type B. There have been sporadic localized outbreaks and increased activity between 1989 and 1993 and from 2000 to the present (28). Localized outbreaks involving predominantly adolescents and young adults have been reported by five provinces and include patients who have been previously vaccinated. Targeted vaccination programs for specific age groups (mostly for people between the ages of 10 and 29 years) have been announced in the localities with clusters or outbreaks.

Despite improved therapeutic management, about 20 people die — mostly infants — from complications every year. The overall case-fatality rate in recent years has been less than 11%, as compared with more than 30% in the 1950s and 1960s.

Hepatitis C

Most hepatitis C infections are clinically inapparent, but up to 90% of infections become chronic. It is estimated that 300,000 Canadians have been infected with this virus. Although there has been an exponential increase in the number of reported cases since 1995, this is likely a result of increased laboratory detection and reporting of disease rather than an increase in new infections.

Hepatitis C is transmitted through blood or body fluids contaminated with the virus. Since the blood bank screening of hepatitis C in 1990, the major mode of transmission of hepatitis C is currently the sharing of drug injection equipment. Other risk factors associated with transmission are needle sharing, tattooing, body piercing, and needle stick injuries, if the items used in such activities are contaminated with infected blood or body fluids. There is a low but measurable rate of vertical and sexual transmission. Currently no vaccine exists. Prevention efforts are focused on prevention of high-risk behaviours, screening of blood donors, and encouraging the use of clean needles (29).

Invasive Group A Streptococcus

Invasive Group A Streptococcus became prominent when Quebec politician Lucien Bouchard underwent a leg amputation due to necrotizing fasciitis. The condition appears to be caused by a heightened immune reaction to the presence of a specific protein in certain strains of Group A Streptococcus. The incidence of the disease is low in the population. However, there is compelling evidence that it can be spread from person to person. The disease is reportable to public health authorities in some provinces.

Respiratory Syncytial Virus

Respiratory syncytial virus (RSV) is a common virus that circulates annually and often precedes the influenza virus. It is an important cause of morbidity and mortality for very young children and the elderly, and is associated with increased hospitalization for both groups. RSV has increasingly been implicated in nursing home outbreaks of respiratory illness and may be a factor in the increase in winter mortality of the elderly at a magnitude that rivals influenza (30). Although no vaccine exists, institutional infection control measures can limit the spread of RSV infections and reduce morbidity and mortality.

5. ANTIBIOTIC RESISTANCE

The emergence of antimicrobial resistance in the past two decades has become a major healthcare issue both in the community and hospital setting in Canada. The late 1980s and 1990s witnessed the development of antibiotic resistance of several common bacteria including penicillin-resistant *Streptococcus pneumoniae* (PRSP), methicillin-resistant *Staphylococcus aureus* (MRSA), vancomycin-resistant enterococci (VRE) and the extended-spectrum beta lactamase-producing bacteria (ESBL) e.g., *Klebsiella pneumoniae, Klebsiella oxytoca,* and *Escherichia coli*. Although there has been some improvement in decreasing some levels of antibiotic resistance, the prevalence of other resistant bacteria have risen dramatically. According to the Canadian Bacterial Surveillance Network, resistance rates of *Streptococcus pneumoniae* — the most common cause of otitis media in children and community-acquired pneumonia in adults — have decreased from the peak of more than 14% resistance to penicillin in 1998 to 10% in 2001 (31). This contrasts with other countries where resistance rates of *Streptococcus pneumoniae* are still rising. However, the incidence of MRSA has increased 3 to 4 times since 1995 (31).

The determinants of antibiotic resistance are complex. Iatrogenic factors such as the prescription of antibiotics to treat viral infections and host factors such as non-compliance with full course of treatment with antibiotics play a role in fostering resistance. The extensive use of antibiotics in feedstock has also been implicated. Agent factors such as the dissemination of resistance among different bacteria have been documented conclusively (32).

The consequences of antibiotic resistance are sobering: persons with antibiotic-resistant infections suffer higher morbidity and mortality rates and have longer and more expensive hospitalizations. Antibiotic development is expensive and requires considerable time for appropriate testing. Currently, there are few promising new antibiotic medications on the development horizon. The control of antibiotic resistance requires enhanced epidemiological and laboratory surveillance, rational prescription practices by physicians, increased compliance by individuals requiring therapy, and adherence to infection control practices in hospitals, nursing homes, and childcare facilities.

6.   VECTOR-BORNE DISEASES AND RABIES

Vectors such as mosquitoes and ticks are responsible for a small but important proportion of communicable diseases. Lyme disease is not as prevalent in Canada as in the United States. There is a small endemic focus of ticks infected with *Borrelia burgdoferii* in southern Ontario. Mosquito-borne illnesses such as Western Equine Encephalitis occur in sporadic outbreaks depending on environmental conditions. Vector-borne illnesses such as malaria, dengue fever, and yellow fever are major global causes of morbidity and mortality. There is some evidence linking changes in global climate to the expansion of the range of vector-borne diseases (33).

West Nile virus (WNV), historically found in Africa, Asia, Europe, and the Middle East, was identified for the first time in the United States in 1999. Carried and spread by mosquitoes, it can cause fatal inflammation of the spinal cord and brain (encephalitis) in certain birds, horses and humans. Between September 2002 and February 2003, WNV infection was confirmed in dead birds and horses in Nova Scotia, Quebec, Ontario, and Manitoba, and 91 confirmed cases of human infection, 150 probable cases, and eight deaths have been reported in Ontario and Quebec (34).

Rabies is a fatal viral illness. Due to a combination of an effective vaccine available for post-exposure prophylaxis, as well as excellent control of rabies in domesticated animals, human rabies cases have been a rare event over the last two decades. Southern Ontario had the highest rates of wildlife rabies in the world, until oral vaccine was given to wild foxes. A raccoon strain of rabies was predicted to cross the United States into Canada in 1995, which prompted an aggressive and successful campaign of vaccinating wild raccoons through bait drops and trap-vaccinate-and-release programs.

7.   FOOD-BORNE AND WATER-BORNE ILLNESS

Food and water remain important and often unrecognized sources of communicable disease (see Chaper 9). In 2000, an outbreak of gastroenteritis in

Walkerton marked the first documented outbreak of *Escherichia coli* 0157:H7 infection associated with a treated municipal water supply in Canada. More than 2,000 cases were associated with this outbreak (35). In 2001, water-borne outbreaks of *Cryptosporidium* infection affected between 5,800 and 7,100 in North Battleford, Saskatchewan (36), and Kamloops, British Columbia. These outbreaks underscore the necessity for vigilance to ensure that municipal water supplies are maintained at the highest level of quality.

Food-borne illness is a common cause of morbidity in the population. Common organisms associated with food-borne gastroenteritis are *Escherichia coli*, *Salmonella, Staphylococcus aureus,* and *Bacillus cereus*. Reports of food-borne illness to public health authorities are underestimated. This is because the vast majority of food-borne illness does not come to medical attention, or no stool cultures are taken.

With the increased global nature of the food industry, serious illness and multi-provincial outbreaks have been associated with contaminated food. Hamburger disease, caused by *E. coli* 0157:H7, has resulted in severe gastroenteritis and hemolytic uremic syndrome. A large outbreak in the U.S. was traced to a contaminated shipment of ground beef. A large, geographically dispersed *Salmonella* outbreak in the United States was traced to contaminated ice cream from Minnesota. In 2001, an outbreak of *Salmonella* in Canada was traced to contaminated almonds. Over the past few years, *Cyclospora* has been responsible for outbreaks in Canada and the United States.

The Centre for Infectious Disease Prevention and Control and the Health Protection Branch convened the 1996 National Consensus Conference on Food-borne, Water-borne, and Enteric Disease Surveillance to develop a plan to better control human illness from these sources (37).

8.   SEXUALLY TRANSMITTED DISEASES

8.1.   INCIDENCE

In general, socioeconomic conditions and changes in lifestyle in North America are likely to have contributed to the observed increase in sexually transmitted diseases (STDs) in Canada. The 1960s brought new affluence, and with it more leisure time, social mobility, and changes in sexual behaviour. In addition, improved availability of birth control methods decreased the probability of unwanted pregnancy. These changing social norms and the emergence of viral sexually transmitted diseases — e.g., genital herpes infection in 1980s, HIV/AIDS in the 1990s, and human papilloma virus as a cause of cervical cancer — resulted in a major cause of morbidity and mortality in adults.

Chlamydia trachomatis
Genital chlamydia, gonorrhea, and AIDS account for more than half of the reported cases of all notifiable diseases combined. Infection with genital *Chlamydia*

trachomatis, a bacterial infection, has emerged as the most frequent STD in recent years in Canada, now occurring over seven times more frequently than gonorrheal infections and responsible for more than 46,000 reported cases of STD during 2000 (38). The rise in the number of reported cases is partly related to an increase in screening for infection, awareness of the disease, an increase in partner notification as well as better diagnostic techniques, resulting in increased reporting. Chlamydia infection became nationally notifiable only in 1990. The disease is most prevalent among sexually active adolescents, particularly females aged 15 to 24 years. In 2000, rates of infection for women in that age group were highest in females 15 to 19 years (1236/100,000) followed by females aged 20 to 24 years (1179/100,000). These rates are compared to 212/100,000, the national rate for all females (38). Serious long-term consequences for females are pelvic inflammatory disease, ectopic pregnancy, and infertility.

Gonorrhea and Syphilis

The incidence of gonorrhea and syphilis has increased slightly over the past few years. Gonorrhea reports rose from 4,522 in 1997 to 6,222 in 2000. In 2000, almost half of all reported cases of gonorrhea in Canada were among 15-24 year olds (38). This trend has remained the same for years. Most women (70%–80%) with gonorrhea have no clinical symptoms. Cases often go undetected.

A few years ago, the elimination of syphilis in Canada seemed a possibility; however, regional increases of disease threaten this effort. The syphilis rate in Canada was 0.4 to 0.6 cases per 100,000 from 1994 to 2000, but increased to a projected 0.9 cases per 100,000 in 2001. Incidence rates are increasing among both males and females. This increase is partially attributed to recent outbreaks in population subgroups including sex trade workers in British Columbia, heterosexuals in the Yukon, and men who have sex with men (MSM) in Calgary, Ottawa, and Montreal. This recent increase emphasizes the need for enhanced case finding and management, as well as rapid outbreak response (39). The incidence of congenital syphilis is related to young maternal age, ethnicity (Aboriginal), lack of prenatal care, and failure of healthcare professionals to repeat non-treponemal tests in the third trimester of pregnancy.

Interactions among all bacterial STDs (chlamydia, gonorrhea, and syphilis) and HIV have been estimated to increase the transmission of HIV. Since early treatment and detection can have a major impact on the transmission of HIV, it is increasingly important to control the incidence and spread of bacterial STDs.

HIV/AIDS

AIDS is caused by the human immunodeficiency virus (HIV), which is transmitted by four routes: by sexual contact with an infected partner, via infected blood and blood products, from an infected mother to her unborn child perinatally, and via contaminated needles and syringes shared among intravenous drug abusers. Sexual contact is the most frequent route for both men having sex with men (MSM) and heterosexuals. Unprotected anal and vaginal intercourse poses a great risk. Not all individuals exposed to HIV are at risk of infection; the factors influencing this are poorly understood. With rare exceptions, most patients have seroconverted (that is, antibodies have developed in the blood as a result of infection) by 6 months after exposure, the majority seroconverting within two to six weeks. Evidence from virus isolation studies indicates that the majority of individuals who are HIV-antibody positive have the virus in their lymphocytes. All people with reactive HIV serology must be considered infectious. However, because some infected individuals may not develop the HIV antibody or may be in the incubation period, any person who has been exposed or belongs to a high-risk group should be considered potentially infectious regardless of serologic status.

AIDS was first identified in Canada in 1979, and became a reportable disease in Canada in 1982. Cumulatively from January 1985 up to December 2001, there were 50,277 positive HIV tests, 18,034 AIDS cases, and 12,619 deaths in Canada. After a rapid rise through the 1980s, the number of new AIDS cases in Canada peaked at 1,859 in 1993 and then declined steadily to 297 in 2001. However, although the decline in the annual number of AIDS cases that started in 1995 is continuing, the rate of decline has slowed and the curve in now levelling off (40).

As the incidence of AIDS cases has decreased, the number of deaths due to HIV/ AIDS also decreased from 1,614 in 1995 to 297 in 2001. The number of deaths has decreased more quickly than the incidence rate, indicating that people with HIV are progressing at a slower rate and that people with an AIDS diagnosis are living longer. One of the factors that may be contributing to this is the advent of highly active antiretroviral therapy (HAART) (41).

Changes in risk behaviour have also been observed. While prior to 1995, HIV/ AIDS affected primarily MSM, now injection drug users (IDU) and heterosexuals are increasingly becoming affected. In 2000, 10.1% of those diagnosed with AIDS were adult women and 1.2% were children. Slightly more than half (50.8%) of the cases diagnosed among adults in 2000 were attributable to MSM, 21.7% were associated with injection drug use, and 1.2% were attributed to tainted blood and blood products (40). The proportion of Aboriginal people with AIDS has increased from 3.5% in 1995 to 7.3% in 1997 and to 12.3% in 1999 (42). Globally, the HIV pandemic continues unabated. In sub-Saharan Africa, 2.4 million deaths due to AIDS were estimated in 2000. Rates of HIV infection in users of intravenous drugs, in new immigrants from AIDS-endemic countries, and in the sexual partners of these groups have established the disease in the socio-economically disadvantaged and their next generation.

HIV/AIDS affects a growing number of women. HIV/AIDS among women is of concern because of the potential for transmission to their infants. Of all cumulative reported AIDS cases in women, 33.9% are attributed to heterosexual contact, 23.2% to injecting drug use, and 9.6% to recipients of blood and blood products. Studies of HIV seroprevalence in child-bearing women in Canada show rates of 3.2 per 100,000. There were 207 cases of AIDS diagnosed in children under age 15 by June 2001, with 83% being the result of perinatal transmission. Prenatal HIV testing of pregnant women is encouraged in several provinces (43). AIDS is also associated with increases in tuberculosis morbidity. Between 2% and 5% of all AIDS cases have tuberculosis as well.

8.2.   TRADITIONAL STD PREVENTION

STD services attempt to control STDs by secondary prevention involving diagnosis and treatment, and primary or secondary prevention for contacts. Patients with gonorrhea, syphilis, or chlamydia may be asymptomatic, making diagnosis difficult. The other problems associated with control are difficulties in the follow-up of contacts, poor compliance with treatment regimens by patients, and the lack of physician reporting of cases. Contact tracing provided by public health staff is often more effective than that provided by medical practitioners. Current treatment schedules for STDs are established by Health Canada (44). Each province and territory circulates specific guidelines for the treatment of STDs.

Effective prevention for one sexually transmitted disease is likely to have an effect on others. Condom use is successful for not only preventing HIV, but also reducing rates of syphilis, gonorrhea, chlamydia, and unplanned pregnancies. STD prevention is rapidly evolving and new developments include female condoms (vaginal pouches).

8.3.   HEALTH PROMOTION IN SEXUAL HEALTH

The concept of **healthy sexuality** is one mode of primary prevention. Healthy sexuality is comfort with one's own sexuality, body characteristics, and self-efficacy in making decisions related to sexuality, such as contraception, pregnancy, and prevention of sexually transmitted disease. Developing positive sexual health involves a multifaceted approach of health education, self-esteem, and decision-making skills for behavioural change, as well as communication of specific knowledge, such as methods of birth control (oral contraception and barrier methods) and STD prevention (safer sex techniques).

Education and communication in this area must be innovative and sustain the interest of youth. Although young people appear to have adequate knowledge about STDs, they are unlikely to interpret risks personally and will take the view that "it cannot happen to me" (45). Public health units have developed a variety of resources on safer sex in an attempt to reach youth. Efforts to provide better communication about sexual health and services with high-risk groups have been developed. These include more accessible clinics (such as locating clinics in high schools (46) and providing other user-friendly types of facilities in shopping malls), reaching homeless youth in the community through outreach workers, and community development. For example, a healthy public policy approach would encourage schools to provide condom machines in washrooms. Community development, as exemplified by gay communities, can result in widespread behaviour change. The continued incidence of HIV infection in the 1990s and continuing through 2002 — especially in groups previously largely unaffected — remains a major concern, as is the chlamydia epidemic.

8.4.   SEXUAL HEALTH AND AIDS

Strategies to control AIDS have focused on preventing the spread of HIV infection and providing multi-drug therapy early. Strategies to control sexual transmission of the virus include the promotion of behavioural change to encourage the use of condoms for safer sex. Partner notification must also be undertaken in all cases of AIDS and HIV infection. Local public health authorities are involved with referrals for clinical evaluation, testing, treatment and health education. To prevent transmission by infected blood and blood products, the Canadian Blood Services screens all donors and tests each unit of blood or blood product collected for a variety of transmissible diseases including HIV and hepatitis C. Sperm and organ donors are screened for the presence of HIV antibody. The Krever Commission of Inquiry on the Blood System in Canada comprehensively reviewed the issues of the transmission of HIV through blood and blood products (47).

Strategies for preventing the spread of HIV among drug users involve the use of **harm reduction** techniques (see Chapter 1) such as the establishment of needle exchanges (where clean equipment can be obtained) and the training of intravenous drug users in disinfecting their equipment using bleach kits (48). Furthermore, recommendations have been made for healthcare personnel to adopt **universal precautions** for handling body fluids (see Chapter 10). The administration of the antiviral agent AZT is successful in reducing the rate of maternal transmission of HIV infection to newborns (49). Protease inhibitors have given rise to the hope that HIV can become a manageable chronic disease. A vaccine for HIV remains a distant hope. Primary prevention should still be regarded as the best possible way to prevent the spread of HIV.

Testing those at risk for HIV has assumed importance largely as a means of reinforcing the need for adopting safer sex behaviour as well as allowing early HIV treatment. Guidelines for HIV testing that involve pre- and post-test counselling have been established and disseminated because it is important that people being tested understand the disease and the implications of the test.

The components of health promotion (as established in the Ottawa Charter for Health Promotion) have been applied to AIDS in terms of comprehensive and integrated action in the 1990s (50). The implementation of healthy public policy, aimed at minimizing structural discrimination against those who are HIV infected, reduces the alienation of those needing health and social services. A social environment supportive of safer sex practices, such as the use of condoms (and safer intravenous drug use), can use the principles of social marketing. Personal skills in safer sexual behaviour can be developed by applying the communication-education theory, particularly in communications to at-risk groups, such as outreach programs and small group sessions. Promotion of the strengthening of communities has enhanced behaviour change and behavioural norms in at-risk groups. Other strategies for the last component of the Ottawa Charter approach — the reorientation of the health system emphasizing a community approach — have already been discussed.

Global experience in AIDS prevention indicates that population-based strategies need to be supplemented with messages adapted to the specific culture and practices of those at risk. Peer-led education models and the use of influential celebrities can broadcast messages tailored to the particular concerns of those who perceive themselves to exist outside the mainstream. A recent review of AIDS prevention has emphasized the effectiveness of community-based strategies in the prevention of AIDS (51).

9.   EMERGENCY PREPAREDNESS AND BIOTERRORISM

Anthrax cases reported in the United States in 2001 have heightened public awareness of bioterrorism. **Bioterrorism** can be described as the use of a microorganism with the deliberate intent of causing infection in order to achieve certain goals. With increased availability of biological agents and the technical capacity to produce them, bioterrorism may become the weapon of choice in the future (52). However, the concept of biological warfare is not new, and preparations for a possible bioterrorist attack had been undertaken even before the 2001 attacks. In 1999, the U.S. Centers for Disease Control and Prevention (CDC) suggested that six microorganisms posed the greatest threat to public health: *Variola major* (smallpox), *Bacillus anthracis* (anthrax), *Yersinia pestis* (plague), *botulinum toxin* (botulism), *Francisella tularensis* (tularemia), and *filovirus/arenavirus* (hemorrhagic fevers) (53). The last naturally acquired case of smallpox in the world occurred in October 1977. The World Health Organization certified global eradication of the disease in 1980. Prior to 1980, smallpox was a reportable disease in Canada. Although smallpox no longer occurs naturally, there is a concern that stockpiles may exist elsewhere in the world (besides designated laboratories) and that terrorists may access these sources.

While the probability that such attacks will occur in Canada is low, if there is an attack the consequences could be severe. Projections based on a CDC model using Canadian data predicts that, under certain conditions, an anthrax attack on 100,000 Canadians could result in 50,000 anthrax cases, 32,875 deaths, 332,500 hospitalization days, and a cost of $6.5 billion (52).

Emergency preparedness plans are necessary for emergency services and the public health system to respond effectively and in a coordinated manner. The outbreak of severe acute respiratory syndrome (SARS) in several Canadian cities in 2003, highlighted the importance of coordinated efforts on the part of local, provincial and federal governments, as well as international health agencies. In Canada, plans are developed by provincial and territorial ministries of health, regional and local health departments, and Health Canada's Centre for Emergency Preparedness and Response and collectively they have set out detailed strategic plans, which are available in case of emergency (54). Components of an effective response include the development of protocols for investigation of suspicious packages (e.g., box, letter) that might contain bioterrorist material; the development and implementation of a disease-tracking system to detect unusual health events or patterns of illness that may be associated with bioterrorism; the need for training for healthcare providers and laboratory staff in the identification, and diagnosis of diseases that may be caused by bioterrorism agents; and the development of a resource-distribution strategy to determine availability, storage, and distribution of supplies including vaccine or antibiotics (52). Strategies for dealing with an outbreak of infectious disease not due to bioterrorism (e.g., pandemic influenza, SARS) also lend themselves to preparation for a bioterrorist event.

10. SUMMARY

Despite the widespread availability of most vaccines, outbreaks of communicable diseases such as measles, meningitis, and tuberculosis continue to occur in Canada and are associated with significant mortality and morbidity.

Although vaccine preventable diseases have declined, sporadic cases and outbreaks of a number of infectious diseases are being reported. These include:

- *Pertussis:* Periodic whooping cough outbreaks continue to occur. The virulence of this bacteria has decreased due to widespread vaccination which affords partial protection.
- *Measles:* Since the introduction of a two-dose immunization strategy in all provinces by 1996, the incidence of measles in Canada has decreased. Most cases reported in Canada since 1998 have been imported.
- *Rubella:* Incidence of rubella and congenital rubella syndrome has decreased, although outbreaks continue to occur. An increased proportion of cases have been reported in adolescents and young adults.
- *Influenza and pneumococcal disease:* These are especially significant in winter. The mortality from influenza (particularly in the elderly) and pneumococcal infections (a possible complication of influenza infection) exceeds that of all vaccine-preventable childhood disease.
- *Meningococcal disease:* Bacterial meningitis is an inflammation of the covering of the brain and spinal cord that primarily affects children, especially infants; however, outbreaks involve mostly adolescents and young adults. There have been sporadic localized outbreaks and increased activity during 1989–93 and from 2000 to present.
- *Haemophilus influenzae type b:* After the introduction of the new conjugate vaccine for infants, the number of cases decreased to fewer than 60 cases per year.
- *Hepatitis B:* The incidence of this sexually transmitted disease has declined from 10.6 per 100,000 in 1994 to 2.3 per 100,000, likely due, in part, to the universal immunization of school-aged children.
- *Tuberculosis:* This is a significant chronic infection in a number of at-risk populations (e.g., alcoholics, persons with HIV, immigrants, and Aboriginal peoples).

Vector-borne diseases, although rare in Canada, are an important cause of morbidity and mortality worldwide. Food-borne disease contributes significantly to the burden of morbidity from communicable disease in Canada. Food-borne and water-borne diseases can be caused by bacteria, viruses, and rare parasites.

The effectiveness of vaccination in protecting individuals depends both on the efficacy, or performance of the vaccine under ideal conditions, and on the degree of coverage achieved. Primary immunization for infants and children against diphtheria, whooping cough, tetanus, poliomyelitis, and *Haemophilus influenzae* type b starts at the age of 2 months and is given at 4 and 6 months, with booster doses at 18 months and at 4 to 6 years of age. Measles, mumps, and rubella vaccine is given after the first birthday and before school starts.

Genital chlamydia, gonorrhea, and AIDS now account for more than half of the reported cases of all notifiable diseases combined. Infection with genital chlamydia has emerged as an epidemic STD in recent years in Canada. The disease is most prevalent among sexually active young women aged 15 to 24. Despite effective antibiotic therapy, there has been a rise in the incidence of gonorrhea in the past two decades and a persistence of syphilis.

AIDS incidence appears to have levelled off, but continues to rise among intravenous drug users. Carriers of HIV will develop AIDS within 11 years after infection. AIDS is caused by HIV, which is transmitted by four routes: by sexual contact with an infected partner, via infected blood and blood products, from an infected mother to her unborn child and perinatally, and through the use of contaminated needles by intravenous drug abusers. Strategies to control the sexual transmission of the virus include promoting behavioural change to limit the number of sexual partners and the use of condoms for safer sex.

Bioterrorism is the use of a microorganism with the deliberate intent of causing infection in order to achieve certain goals. With increased availability of biological agents and the technical information required to produce them, bioterrorism may become the weapon of choice in the future. Health Canada's Centre for Emergency Preparedness and Response has detailed strategic plans which are available in case of emergency.

11. REFERENCES

1.   Last J. *A dictionary of epidemiology*, fourth ed. Toronto: Oxford University Press, 2001.
2.   Chin J. *Control of communicable diseases in man*, 17th ed. Washington DC: American Public Health Association, 2000.
3.   Giesecke J. *Modern infectious disease epidemiology*, 2nd ed. New York: Oxford University Press, 2002.
4.   National Advisory Committee on Immunization. *Canadian immunization guide*. Ottawa: Minister of Supply and Services Canada, 5th edition, 1998. <www.hc-sc.gc.ca/pphb-dgspsp/publicat/immguide/index.html> (October 2002).
5.   Immunization Action Coalition. 2003. <www.immunize.org> (February 2003).
6.   Canadian Public Health Association. 2003. *Canadian Immunization Awareness Program*. <www.immunize.cpha.ca/english/index.htm> (February 2003).
7.   Gyorkos T, Tannenbaum T, Abrahamowicz M. Evaluation of the effectiveness of immunization delivery methods. *Canadian Journal of Public Health* 1994; 85(S1):S14-S29.

8. Tannenbaum T, Gyorkos T, Abrahamowicz M. Immunization delivery methods: Practice recommendations. *Canadian Journal of Public Health* 1994; 85(S1):S37-S47.

9. National Advisory Committee on Immunization. National guidelines for vaccine storage and transportation. *Canada Communicable Disease Report* 1995; 21(11):93-7.

10. National Advisory Committee on Immunization. *Canadian immunization guide*. Ottawa: Minister of Supply and Services Canada, 2002. 6th edition. <www.hc-sc.gc.ca/pphb-dgspsp/publicat/cig-gci> (January 2003).

11. Pless R, Duclos P. Reinforcing surveillance for vaccine-associated adverse events: The Advisory Committee on Causality Assessment. *Canadian Journal of Infectious Disease* 1996; 7:98-9.

12. Health Canada. Canadian National Report on Immunization, 1998. *Paediatric and Child Health* 1999; 4 (suppl. C).

13. National Advisory Committee on Immunization. Statement on management of persons exposed to pertussis and pertussis outbreak control. *Canada Communicable Disease Report* 1994; 20(22):193-9.

14. Greco D, Salmuso S, Mastrantonio P, *et al*. A controlled trial of two acellular vaccines and one whole cell vaccine against pertussis. *New England Journal of Medicine* 1996; 334:341-8.

15. Gustafson L, Hallander H, Olin P, *et al*. A controlled trial of two component acellular and a whole cell pertussis vaccine. *New England Journal of Medicine* 1996; 334:349-55.

16. Shapiro H, Weir E. Measles in your office. *Canadian Medical Association Journal* 2001; 164:1614.

17. National Advisory Committee on Immunization. Supplementary statement on measles elimination in Canada. *Canada Communicable Disease Report* 1996; 22(2):9-15. <www.hc-sc.gc.ca/hpb/lcdc/publicat/ccdr/96vol22/dr2202ea.html> (October 2002).

18. Canadian Paediatric Society. *Canadian Paediatric Surveillance Program: 1999 results*. Ottawa: Canadian Paediatric Society, 2000. <www.cps.ca/english/CPSP> (October 2002).

19. Canadian Consensus Committee on Influenza. Canadian Consensus Conference on Influenza. *Communicable Disease Report* 1993; 19(17):136-46.

20. Canadian Consensus Committee on Pneumonia. Preventing pneumococcal disease. *Canadian Journal of Infectious Diseases* 1999; 10 (suppl. 1).

21. National Advisory Committee on Immunization. Statement on recommended use of pneumococcal conjugate vaccine. *Canada Communicable Disease Report* 2002; 28(ACS-2):1-32. <www.hc-sc.gc.ca/pphb-dgspsp/publicat/ccdr-rmtc/02vol28/28sup/acs2.html> (October 2002).

22. Zhang J, Zou S, Giulivi A. Hepatitis B in Canada. Report on Viral Hepatitis and Emerging Bloodborne Pathogens in Canada. *Canada Communicable Disease Report* 2001; 27S3. <www.hc-sc.gc.ca/pphb-dgspsp/publicat/ccdr-rmtc/01vol27/27s3/27s3e_e.html> (October 2002).

23. Infectious Diseases and Immunization Committee, Canadian Paediatric Society. Hepatitis B in Canada: The case for universal vaccination. *Canadian Medical Association Journal* 1992; 146(1):25-7.

24. Gold R. Hepatitis B vaccine: Revisited. *Pediatric Child Health* 1996; 1:95-6.

25. National Advisory Committee on Immunization. NACI update to statement on varicella vaccine. *Canada Communicable Disease Report* 2002; 28(ACS-3):1-7. <www.hc-sc.gc.ca/pphb-dgspsp/publicat/ccdr-rmtc/02vol28/28sup/acs3.html> (October 2002).

26. Long R, Njoo H, Hershfield E. Tuberculosis: 3. Epidemiology of the disease in Canada. *Canadian Medical Association Journal* 1999; 160:1185-90.

27. Fanning A. Tuberculosis: 1. Introduction. *Canadian Medical Association Journal* 1999; 160:837-9.

28. National Advisory Committee on Immunization. Statement on recommended use of meningococcal vaccines. *Canada Communicable Disease Report* 2001; 27(ACS-6):2-36. <www.hc-sc.gc.ca/pphb-dgspsp/publicat/ccdr-rmtc/01vol27/27sup/acs6.html> (October 2002).

29.   Zou S, Tepper M, Giulivi A. Hepatitis C in Canada. Report on Viral Hepatitis and Emerging Bloodborne Pathogens in Canada. *Canada Communicable Disease Report* 2001; 27S3:1-64. <www.hc-sc.gc.ca/pphb-dgspsp/publicat/ccdr-rmtc/01vol27/27s3/27s3f_e.html> (October 2002).

30.   Nicholson K. Impact of influenza and RSV on mortality in England from January 1975 to December 1990. *Epidemiology and Infection* 1996; 116:51-63.

31.   Conly J, Paton S, Forward K, *et al.* 2002. *Reduction in oral antimicrobial consumption in Canada.* <www.ccar-ccra.org/PDF/Reduction.pdf> (October 2002).

32.   Travis J. Reviving the antibiotic miracle. *Science* 1994; 264:360-2.

33.   Epstein P, Rogers D, Sloof R. Satellite imaging and vector-borne disease. *Lancet* 1993; 341:1404-6.

34.   Health Canada, Population and Public Health Branch. 2002. *West Nile Virus Surveillance Information.* <www.hc-sc.gc.ca/pphb-dgspsp/wnv-vwn> (February 2004).

35.   Waterborne outbreak of gastroenteritis associated with a contaminated municipal water supply, Walkerton, Ontario, May–June 2000. *Canada Communicable Disease Report* 2000; 26(20):170-3. <www.hc-sc.gc.ca/hpb/lcdc/publicat/ccdr/00vol26/dr2620eb.html> (October 2002).

36.   Stirling R, Aramini J, Ellis A, *et al.* Waterborne Cryptosporidiosis outbreak, North Battleford, Saskatchewan, Spring 2001. *Canada Communicable Disease Report* 2001; 27(22):185-92. <www.hc-sc.gc.ca/pphb-dgspsp/publicat/ccdr-rmtc/01vol27/dr2722ea.html> (October 2002).

37.   Summary of the National Consensus Conference on Foodborne, Waterborne, and Enteric Disease Surveillance. *Canada Communicable Disease Report* 1996; 22(11):81-4. <www.hc-sc.gc.ca/hpb/lcdc/publicat/ccdr/96vol22/dr2211ea.html> (October 2002).

38.   Health Canada. 2002. *STD Data Tables.* <www.hc-sc.gc.ca/pphb-dgspsp/std-mts/stddata1201/index.html> (October 2002).

39.   Health Canada. 2002. *STD EPI Update.* <www.hc-sc.gc.ca/pphb-dgspsp/publicat/epiu-aepi/std-mts/infsyph_e.html> (October 2002).

40.   Health Canada. 2002. *HIV and AIDS in Canada, Surveillance report to June 30,* 2002. <www.hc-sc.gc.ca/pphb-dgspc/publicat/aids-sida/haic-vsac0602/pdf/haic-vsca0602.pdf> (March 2003).

41.   Grossman D, Glazier R. *HIV Services Planning Report.* Toronto: St. Michael's Hospital, Department of Family and Community Medicine, 2000.

42.   Health Canada. *HIV and AIDS in Canada: Surveillance report to December 31, 1999.* Ottawa: Laboratory Centre for Disease Control, 2000.

43.   Health Canada. *HIV and AIDS in Canada: Surveillance Report to June 30, 2001.* Ottawa, Population and Public Health Branch, 2001.

44.   Health Canada. *Canadian STD guidelines.* Ottawa: Minister of Public Works & Government Services Canada, 1998.

45.   Bowie W, Warren W, Fisher W, *et al.* Implications of the Canada Youth and AIDS Study for health care providers. *Canadian Medical Association Journal* 1990; 143(8):713-6.

46.   Rafuse J. MDs, nurses play major role in success of "Sexuality Clinics" at Ottawa high schools. *Canadian Medical Association Journal* 1992; 146(4):593-6.

47.   Krever H. *Commission of Inquiry on the Blood System in Canada (Krever Commission Report).* Ottawa: Health Canada, 1997. <www.hc-sc.gc.ca/english/protection/krever> (October 2002).

48.   Des Jarlais D. Harm reduction: A framework for incorporating science into drug policy. *American Journal of Public Health* 1995; 85(1):10-1.

49.   Connor E, Sperling R, Gelber R, *et al.* Reduction of maternal-infant transmission of human immunodeficiency virus type 1 with zidovudine. *New England Journal of Medicine* 1994; 331(18):1173-80.

50. Nutbeam D, Blakey V. The concept of health promotion and AIDS prevention: A comprehensive and integrated basis for action in the 1990s. *Health Promotion International* 1990; 5(3):233-42.
51. Coates T, Aggleton P, Gutzwiller F. HIV prevention in developed countries. *Lancet* 1996; 348:1143-8.
52. Bioterrorism and public health. *Canada Communicable Disease Report* 2001; 27(4):29-31. <www.hc-sc.gc.ca/pphb-dgspsp/publicat/ccdr-rmtc/01vol27/dr2704ea.html> (October 2002).
53. Centers for Disease Control and Prevention. Biological and chemical terrorism: Strategic plan for preparedness and response recommendations of the CDC strategic planning working group. *Morbidity and Mortality Weekly Report* 2000; 49(RR-4):1-14.
54. Health Canada. 2002. *Bioterrorism and Emergency Preparedness.* <www.hc-sc.gc.ca/english/protection/biotech/bioterrorism.htm> (October 2002).

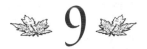

9

ENVIRONMENTAL HEALTH

1. GENERAL FRAMEWORK

In recent years, there has been increasing recognition of the interdependence of human health and the health of the global ecosystem, with its many life forms. Much of this awareness has been generated by community-based environmental advocacy groups such as Greenpeace and Pollution Probe, as well as by Aboriginal peoples, who have all highlighted the importance of the environment. Historically, the field of environmental health has usually dealt with food and water safety, and with the inspection and investigation of environmental hazards that may arise from inadequate sanitation. In most of Canada (apart from areas such as Aboriginal reserves where physical facilities may be grossly inadequate), provision of sanitation, potable water supply, and food free from gross contamination have been largely achieved despite tragedies like Walkerton, Ontario (1), where poor management of the municipal water supply and a lack of provincial safeguards resulted in several unfortunate deaths and many illnesses. There is, however, growing concern over the status of the environment and the consequences of environmental pollution, particularly of chemical and biological contamination. This concern is not only limited to the effects on human health but also to the viability of ecosystems in general and many species in particular.

Public attention has been captured by recent reports detailing the effects of acid rain on forest and aquatic ecosystems, climatic changes resulting from the greenhouse effect, the depletion of the ozone layer, the effects of marine pollution on aquatic life, and the long-term effects of consuming genetically modified foods. Public interest has also been heightened as a result of numerous reports linking environmental exposure to adverse human health outcomes. Environmental factors may contribute to the development of breast cancer, and the reported decrease in the sperm count in some developed nations has led to increased research of the role of chemical contamination on human reproductive capacity (2).

There is a growing awareness of possible links between illness and many features of industrialized society (3). Indoor air quality has been investigated in many modern buildings, following reports of symptoms in employees or residents and resulting in a newly identified illness pattern: the sick building syndrome. The evacuation of Saint-

Basile-le-Grand near Montreal in August 1988, following the fire-related release of polychlorinated biphenyls (PCBs) and the 1997 fire of a warehouse containing plastic in Hamilton, Ontario, are examples of events that focused public attention on emergency response measures and the control aspects of environmental health.

Environmental health may be defined as the study of conditions in the natural and built (physical) environment that influence human health and well-being. Because the impact of the environment on human populations is widespread, a variety of disciplines and practitioners contribute to the field of environmental health, including clinical medicine (4). While other disciplines assess the impact of environmental agents or hazards on the individual patient, the focus of study in environmental health is the impact of these agents on the health of the population.

The environment as it affects health can be divided into working and non-working categories. The workplace environment is often associated with high-level exposure of a population predominantly of adult age and in good health. In contrast, non-workplace environmental exposures are generally low level and may be chronic. The population at risk consists of persons at the extremes of age, developing fetuses, and the ill or immunocompromised. Thus, although many of the pathogenic agents are similar, there is an arbitrary distinction between working and non-working environmental health. The specific concerns relating to the working environment (occupational health) are addressed in Chapter 10. An overview of environmental health in Canada is given in the publications by Health Canada entitled *A Vital Link: An Overview of Health and the Environment in Canada* (5), *Health and Environment: Partner for Life* (3), and *Environment and Health: A Handbook for Health Professionals* (6). A series of articles in the *Canadian Medical Association Journal* on environment and health provide important information for clinicians (7-14). Another series of articles in the *Canadian Medical Association Journal* on environmental health is also very informative (15-21).

Despite the uncertainty associated with many environmental health problems, healthcare providers are considered to be the most credible source of information regarding the health effects of environmental exposures. Consequently, it is important for every healthcare provider to be familiar with the concepts employed and the issues involved in environmental health.

This chapter will explore the concepts of risk assessment (using toxicological data with exposure estimates) as well as the concepts of risk management and communication. Several topical issues will be explored including physical agents, climate change, air and water quality, and chemical toxicity. An approach to creating a healthy environment, which focuses on healthy public policy and managing environmental accidents, will conclude the chapter.

2.   METHODS AND TOOLS

The study of environmental health issues relies heavily on the disciplines of toxicology, microbiology, and epidemiology. **Toxicology**, the science of poisons (toxins), attempts to identify adverse effects of substances on health and to predict harmful dosages. One of the fundamental tenets of toxicology is that any substance can be a poison if given in a large enough dose. By contrast, a carcinogen may have no threshold dose below which it no longer causes cancer. **Microbiology** deals with the scientific study of microorganisms e.g., bacteria, viruses, and fungi. The other discipline, **epidemiology**, as previously defined in Chapter 2, is the study of the distribution and determinants of health and disease in human population. Although these disciplines provide a vast amount of information on specific environmental health hazards, the interpretation of these data for regulatory decisions is often difficult (22). This section addresses some of these difficulties.

There are a variety of problems in the measurement of a specific toxic agent. The levels are often difficult to determine, both in the human body and in the ambient (surrounding) environment. As technology progresses, the detection of minute quantities of chemicals is enhanced, but the interpretation of their significance to human health may remain difficult. When a level is measurable, often it does not reflect the concentration in the target organ of interest; rather, it represents a crude attempt to assess dose by measuring tissue fluid levels (usually blood). Often the agent itself is not toxic but is metabolized to toxic end products within the body. When ambient levels can be defined, the dose-response relationship at low levels is often difficult to predict because i) most toxicological data are obtained from high-dose animal experimentation or ii) most epidemiological data from occupational exposure. Extrapolation to low doses is uncertain, and there are several models to choose from. Often an arbitrary safety factor is applied to the threshold dose to derive an acceptable intake (exposure) level for humans. This safety factor attempts to account for both inter- and intra-species variation.

The study of some adverse health outcomes, particularly mutagenic and carcinogenic effects, is complicated by the long latency period following exposure. During the latency period for most cancers, exposures to causal agents may be terminated or periodic. Adverse outcomes may manifest only in a small fraction of the exposed population. This again makes epidemiological analysis difficult (23). Furthermore, the confounding effects of multiple exposures often mask the effects of a specific agent. The relationship between agents grows even more complex when one accounts for synergistic, promoting, or attenuating interrelationships of chemical mixtures (24). The study of environmental health is also complicated by the fact that many adverse outcomes are non-specific and subjective. The upper respiratory and conjunctival symptoms of the sick building syndrome, for example, are difficult to quantify objectively. Analysis becomes more difficult when one considers that such non-specific and ill-defined psychosomatic symptoms have also been induced by fear of ill effects from the environment (25). One study reviewed the strengths and weaknesses of a number of epidemiological studies related to environmental concerns and found the weaknesses were a lack of certainty of exposure to putative agents, large potentially exposed populations, and relatively common adverse health effects(26).

Recent research has extended the domain of concern about persistent chemicals in the environment to include reproductive and neurobehavioural outcomes. There is an emerging body of literature that examines the effects of chemicals on the hormone systems of humans and animals (27, 28). For example, in Sydney, Nova Scotia, there is continuing controversy regarding the local tar ponds, which are made up of the waste byproducts of coke production and qualify as the largest toxic waste site in North America (711,200 metric tonnes of toxic sludge). This waste site is situated in a tidal estuary that empties into the Atlantic Ocean. Laboratory testing has revealed high levels of toxic chemicals such as arsenic, molybdenum, benzopyrene, antimony, naphthalene, lead, toluene, tar, benzene, kerosene, copper, and polyaromatic hydrocarbons (PAHs). Cape Breton (where Sydney is located) has the highest rates of lung, breast, and stomach cancer in Nova Scotia, and Nova Scotia has the highest rate of cancer in Canada (29). Local area residents also experience chronic symptoms such as ocular irritation, headaches, dry throats, and diarrhea, which they feel are attributable to exposure to the tar ponds. The federal, provincial, and municipal governments are funding initiatives to clean up the area.

2.1.   ESTABLISHING TOXICITY

Every day, each of us is exposed to a variety of environmental and behavioural risks. The leading authorities responsible for identifying and assessing the risks to human health posed by the environment include Health Canada, Environment Canada, provincial and territorial ministries of health and environment, local and regional public health units, and various professional groups. These bodies evaluate the political, economic, societal, and technological implications of the risk and identify the options for managing risks according to the best available evidence. They then develop the policies, regulations, and other measures for protection of the public.

Risk assessment is the first approach to assessing health risks posed by contaminants. Two closely associated concepts, risk management and risk communication, deal with actions taken to reduce risk and to communicate with the public about perceived environmental hazards. Another method, outlined in Chapter 2, deals with the investigation of clusters of non-communicable diseases, such as congenital defects or cancer in the community due to putative environmental agents.

There are four major steps in the risk assessment of any environmental contaminant: hazard identification, exposure assessment and monitoring, dose-response assessment, and risk determination.

2.2.   RISK ASSESSMENT

Hazard Identification
In identifying hazards, it is important to consider any potentially adverse effects of the exposure, particularly the organ system affected and the severity of potential harm. Information is obtained from laboratory, genetic, animal, and human epidemiological studies. The U.S. Environmental Protection Agency's IRIS database (Integrated Risk Information System) is an excellent information resource that contains information about human health effects that may result from exposure to various substances found in the environment (30, 31).

Exposure Assessment and Monitoring

Exposure can be defined as any contact between a substance and an individual. An exposure pathway has five components:

- the source of contamination;
- the environmental media;
- the point of exposure;
- the receptor populations; and
- the route of exposure.

With this general framework in mind, it is possible to develop a model of the variety of possible exposures and their potential impact on humans. The principal environmental media for the exposure to contaminants are water, food, soil, and air. The major routes of exposure for humans are inhalation, ingestion, and dermal contact. Once these factors are characterized, it is possible to calculate an estimated daily intake (EDI), which is the sum of the estimated dose from all possible exposure routes. Because data are often not available for all routes of exposure or the toxicology of all contaminants, it is often necessary to make assumptions about the estimated dose that a person may have achieved. The averaging process that occurs may not take into account variability with respect to differences in body weight or duration of exposure, and may not precisely estimate consumption rates for food and water.

Toxicological studies are used to determine the dose response relationship between a substance and its potential health effects. An essential component of a health risk assessment is the concept of a threshold. Animal data from toxicological studies and data derived from epidemiological data on humans are used to determine the level of exposure at which no observable adverse effects occur (NOAEL) or the lowest dose at which a measurable adverse effect occurs (LOAEL). Once the LOAEL or NOAEL has been estimated, it is possible to estimate a tolerable exposure level to a contaminant, called the **tolerable daily intake** (TDI). A non-threshold model indicates that any exposure is likely to result in some adverse effect. The concept of dose response is particularly important for carcinogenic chemicals for which it may be necessary to specify exposures with an acceptable degree of risk: less than one chance in a million for an individual to develop cancer over a lifetime (if exposure cannot be eliminated entirely).

These estimates are always uncertain, however, so the TDI usually includes a safety factor. Depending on the extent of the laboratory and epidemiological studies available and the adverse effects that the substance can cause, the safety factor may range from 100 to several thousand or more. The estimated daily intake from the various exposure routes can be compared to the tolerable daily intake in order to determine whether an individual or population is exposed to greater than acceptable exposures. If this occurs, then risk management strategies, as outlined below, can be implemented.

There are a large number of potentially harmful exposures from environmental sources, and monitoring the levels of selected potential exposures is necessary. However, it is not feasible to monitor all potential exposures, so selected indicators are usually chosen for surveillance purposes. Identification of potential contamination of nutritional sources includes the monitoring of breast milk for contaminants such as dioxins and

PCBs and the levels of these contaminants in fish and animals in local environments where subsistence fishing and hunting is practised by Aboriginal peoples.

Health Canada has published Guidelines for Canadian Drinking Water Quality since 1968. The sixth edition was published in 2002 (32). These are designed to ensure that the water is free from pathogenic organisms, harmful chemicals, and radioactive matter and that it is palatable. **Maximum acceptable concentrations** (MACs) for a wide range of chemicals, aesthetic objectives, and microbiologic characteristics for water have been defined. The microbiological assessment of drinking water generally involves assessment for coliform organisms as a marker of fecal contamination. In recreational water, the presence of *Escherichia coli* at specified levels is regarded as an indicator of fecal contamination (33). Although viruses have been implicated in water-borne disease outbreaks, no specific virological standards have been developed. The turbidity of water is assessed for aesthetic purposes and as a way of monitoring for sudden changes in source water due to contamination or for upsets in the treatment process. Turbidity can also interfere with the detection methods for bacteriological quality and with the disinfection process.

MACs are also applicable in assessing individual air contaminants. The Air Quality Index described in Chapter 3 only addresses six important pollutants that are related particularly to acute health effects. Evidence of long-range transport and deposition of air-borne contaminants such as mercury and organochlorine pesticides indicates the need for the measurement and surveillance of other air-borne pollutants (34).

Risk Determination

In risk determination, it is important to consider the following:
- the potential toxicity of the substance, and the likely effects on human health;
- the actual or estimated exposure and the dose-response relationship; and
- the measure of uncertainty inherent in this calculation.

2.3.   RISK MANAGEMENT

Risk management is the series of steps that follows risk assessment and is integral to creating healthy public policy (see Section 4). It involves decision making and implementation of options for management of the identified risk. For example, in the consideration of food contaminants, if a potential daily intake exceeds the tolerable daily intake, then certain risk management options are considered. The options include:
- establishing guidelines or promulgating specific regulations controlling the toxic substance or substances;
- restricting the sale or distribution of food produced in an area that may have been identified as the source of the contamination; and
- recommending changes in dietary habits.

Before initiating any specific action in Canada, however, the federal Health Products and Food Branch must assess its advantages and disadvantages. For example, the removal of certain foods from the market or recommendations to change dietary habits could deny those people at risk of an essential source of nutrition, which might cause a more serious health problem than that associated with the chemical contaminant e.g., consumption of wild foods by First Nations' peoples.

2.4. RISK COMMUNICATION

The communication of risk in relation to environmental hazards, and to public health hazards in general, depends on an important concept: the perception of risk by the lay public often differs from that of scientific experts. Experts tend to express risk in terms of the actual numbers affected and numerical probabilities. The lay public tends to perceive risk according to the degree of unfamiliarity of the threat and whether there is a threat of a catastrophe involving serious adverse events (particularly death) for many people at one time. The model for this concept of risk perception is the **factorial model**, the two factors being fear of the unknown and dread. These factors can be quantified on two-dimensional axes. For example, in Canada nuclear installations score very highly on both of these factors (both x and y axes), and public reaction to any possibility of an environmental threat is likely to be high. Another principle of risk communication is that the potential risk of an environmental health hazard should be expressed in readily understandable terms. For example, expressing the risk of cancer from a contaminant in drinking water as less than one chance in a million over the lifetime of an individual is more useful than using scientific language.

In general, however, the public has difficulty with the expression of risk as a probability; people generally prefer to know whether the agent does or does not pose a risk to health (the **risk dichotomy** concept). Since it is usually impossible to dichotomize risk so absolutely, effective risk communication may involve informing the public that the measured level of the agent is either above or below a certain guideline or regulated level. It is nevertheless essential to have an accurate understanding of the perception of risk in the community and an accurate understanding of the range of risk acceptable to the community. Otherwise, reassurance may be perceived as false and not truly addressing the degree of concern and stress in the community. The relevant aspects of risk perception and communication have been well summarized (35).

3. ENVIRONMENTAL HEALTH ISSUES

In the following section, some environmental agents that have been associated with ill health are described. The sources of the agents, routes of human exposure, adverse effects, and approaches to control are included here.

3.1. OUTDOOR AND INDOOR ENVIRONMENTS

3.1.1. Ionizing Radiation

There are two types of radiation: ionizing and non-ionizing. Ionizing radiation is emitted from radioactive substances and is capable of producing ions in matter, including cellular matter, causing altered cell physiology. More than 80% of the radiation to which humans are exposed is produced from natural sources, whether from the radioactive elements in the earth's crust, cosmic radiation, or from ingested or inhaled isotopes. With the exception of radon, non-background radiation exposure is primarily an occupational hazard for certain categories of workers and is discussed in greater detail in Chapter 10.

Radon

Radon is a naturally occurring radioactive gas that forms as a decay product of uranium 238. Uranium is a trace element found in all soil. As part of the radioactive decay process, radon produces four progeny that emit alpha radiation. Human skin acts as a barrier, but inhaled radon progeny deposit alpha particles internally in the localized area of the bronchial epithelium, which eventually may lead to lung cancer. Due to its accumulation indoors, radon is more of a concern as a form of indoor air pollution, although it is present in the ambient environment as well. Radon gas passes from porous soil into buildings through cracks in basement floors and walls. Given that most of an individual's time is spent indoors, there is a potential health risk from natural sources of radon. Health Canada has recommended that the Canadian guideline for existing homes for radon should be 20 picocuries per litre, and 4 picocuries per litre for newly constructed homes. When the level of radon is in doubt, houses must be individually tested for radon levels; extrapolation from neighbouring homes is not adequate though regional variation provides some clues.

Estimates of the lung cancer risk following household radon exposure have been extrapolated from studies of lung cancer incidence in uranium miners. The relative risk for exposed households has been estimated to range between 1.1 and 1.5. It has also been estimated that up to 15% of lung cancer deaths may be attributable to domestic radon exposure (36). Occupational standards have been set for exposure to radon for uranium miners and for dwellings in uranium mining communities. In dwellings with high levels, simple measures such as increasing basement ventilation and sealing cracks and holes decrease radon concentrations effectively. Tobacco smoking increases an individual's chance of getting lung cancer with radon exposure. Combined radon exposure and tobacco smoking increases an individual's chance of getting lung cancer.

Living Near Nuclear Facilities

Nuclear accidents at Chernobyl, Ukraine, and Three Mile Island, Pennsylvania, have raised public anxiety and affected perceptions of the safety of living in close proximity to nuclear facilities. The major issue is better communication among the public, healthcare providers, and authorities, based on an expanded knowledge base about radiation effects and the realistic potential for exposure on an ongoing basis (which is minimal) (37). Many factors can influence the health effects of radiation, including the type of radiation, the rate at which energy is deposited in tissues, the dose of radiation administered and received by tissues, and the radiation sensitivity of the affected tissue. The total dose is also important. The effects of high-dose radiation are well documented and are described in Chapter 10. Less is known about low-dose exposure. A study of the rates of childhood leukemia in the vicinity of nuclear facilities in Ontario (Chalk River, Port Hope, Elliot Lake, Pickering, and Bruce) demonstrated only a slightly increased number of observed leukemia deaths. In the United Kingdom, the higher incidence of childhood leukemia has raised the issue of paternal exposure to possible workplace hazards but, so far, there is little evidence to support this hypothesis for paternal radiation exposure (38, 39).

3.1.2. Non-ionizing Radiation

Electromagnetic Fields
The use of electricity creates two kinds of invisible fields: electric and magnetic. Electric fields are produced by voltage, magnetic fields by current. Together they are referred to as electromagnetic fields, a form of non-ionizing radiation. In Canada, the strongest electric field normally encountered by the public is about 10 kilovolts per metre and is found under high-voltage transmission lines. Other sources of exposure to electric fields are electric blankets, computers, fluorescent lighting, household appliances, and wiring. From most of these sources the electric field strength seldom exceeds 1 kilovolt per metre. The strongest domestic magnetic fields are those produced by hair dryers.

Considerable research has been carried out on the health effects of exposure to electromagnetic fields. A recent Canadian study demonstrated excess of cancers only for a small subset of workers employed in very high exposure settings. In general, the research failed to indicate an excess of cancer for those exposed at lower levels (40, 41). Considerable media attention has focused on the potential adverse health effects of cellular phones. Cellular phones emit low-level radio frequency radiation in the microwave range, which is unlikely to cause cancer when absorbed by human tissues. There has been no consistent link found between cellular phone use and brain cancer (42). Because this technology is so new, however, the long-term effects of exposure are still not known. The U.S. Food and Drug Administration thus advises those who still have concerns to minimize their exposure by choosing digital rather than analogue phones and maximizing the distance between themselves and the phone antenna (43).

Cellular phones have been shown to interfere with bone-anchored hearing aids (44). They also have the potential to interfere with cardiac pacemakers, although this is not considered to be a contraindication to the use of cellular phones in those with pacemakers because the effect is seen only when the phone is held very close to the pacemaker (45). Pacemaker wearers are advised not to keep their phone in a breast pocket directly over their pacemaker.

Legislation banning the use of cellular phones while driving has been passed in many countries including Australia, Denmark, and Japan. New York was the first state in the United States to impose a ban, which took effect in November 2001. Newfoundland and Labrador announced a ban that went into effect early in 2003, and such a ban is under consideration by Ontario legislature (see Chapter 4). A 1997 study of Toronto drivers demonstrated a quadrupled risk of collision while drivers were on the telephone. Opponents of legislation point to the fact that since the study was conducted, cellular telephone use in Toronto has skyrocketed with no corresponding increase in collisions (46).

3.1.3.   Light Pollution

There is growing concern about illumination from electric lighting in the urban environment. Some people believe that, apart from wasting energy and obscuring the dark night sky, which is a part of the natural environment, this excess light disrupts human circadian rhythms. This in turn is thought to interfere with the natural endocrine system and thus possibly contribute to the increased number of cases of breast cancer seen in industrialized nations (47).

3.1.4.   Noise Pollution

Noise has been shown to act as a general stressor leading to changes such as increases in blood pressure, heart rate, and vasoconstriction. Noise also induces irritability. It is not believed to be a direct cause of mental illness but might accelerate and intensify the development of latent mental disorders. The evidence relating noise to mental illness is scanty and much of it is based only on clinical impression. Despite its weaknesses, the evidence points to possible negative effects of community noise on mental health, manifested in the presence of medical drug use, psychiatric symptoms, and mental hospital admission rates (48).

3.2.   CLIMATE CHANGE, GREENHOUSE GASES, AND GLOBAL WARMING

Air pollution and subsequent global warming are growing concerns for Canada, as well as the rest of the world, due to their potential to cause widespread adverse health effects and devastating climate changes. The Intergovernmental Panel on Climate Change, which is supported by 200 governments aroung the world, was formed to deal with this issue.

Energy from the sun drives the earth's weather and climate, and heats the earth's surface; in turn, the earth radiates energy back into space. Atmospheric greenhouse gases (water vapor, carbon dioxide, and other gases) trap some of the outgoing energy, retaining heat like the glass panels of a greenhouse. Without this natural "greenhouse effect," temperatures would be much lower than they are now, and life as known today would not be possible. Instead, due to greenhouse gases, the earth's average temperature is a more hospitable 15°C. However, problems may arise when the atmospheric concentration of greenhouse gases increases.

Some greenhouse gases occur naturally in the atmosphere, while others result from human activities. Naturally occurring greenhouse gases include water vapor, carbon dioxide, methane, nitrous oxide, and ozone. Certain human activities, however, add to the levels of most of these naturally occurring gases: 1) carbon dioxide is released to the atmosphere when solid waste, fossil fuels (oil, natural gas, and coal), and wood and wood products are burned; 2) methane is emitted during the production and transport of coal, natural gas, and oil, from the decomposition of organic wastes in municipal solid waste landfills, and from the raising of livestock; and 3) nitrous oxide is emitted during agricultural and industrial activities, as well as during combustion of solid waste and fossil fuels. Very powerful greenhouse gases that are not naturally occurring include hydrofluorocarbons (HFCs), perfluorocarbons (PFCs), and sulphur hexafluoride (SF6), which are generated in a variety of industrial processes. Each greenhouse gas differs in its ability to absorb heat in the atmosphere. HFCs and PFCs are the most heat-absorbent. Methane traps over 21 times more heat per molecule than carbon dioxide, and nitrous oxide absorbs 270 times more heat per molecule than carbon dioxide.

Carbon dioxide emissions from the combustion of fossil fuels are one of the major concerns causing global warming through the greenhouse effect. Since the beginning of the industrial revolution, atmospheric concentrations of carbon dioxide have increased nearly 30%, methane concentrations have more than doubled, and nitrous oxide concentrations have risen by about 15%. These increases have enhanced the heat-trapping capability of the earth's atmosphere. Sulphate aerosols, a common air pollutant, cool the atmosphere by reflecting light back into space; however, sulphates are short-lived in the atmosphere and vary regionally. Scientists generally believe that the combustion of fossil fuels and other human activities are the primary reason for the increased concentration of carbon dioxide.

A steady increase in global temperatures affects the environment by changing weather patterns, which in turn affects the habitat and food systems that plants, animals, and people rely on for survival. Global warming could adversely affect human health by increasing morbidity and mortality from heat stroke as well as by creating more favourable conditions for infectious disease to spread (9). Increased temperatures will also create more favourable conditions for photochemical smog and subsequently more adverse health effects.

As a consequence of these issues, efforts to decrease the use of fossil fuels have assumed a higher priority on the environmental health agenda at all levels of government. Under the Kyoto Protocol on Climate Change, industrialized countries must reduce their collective emissions of greenhouse gases by 2012. Canada has committed itself to reduce greenhouse gas emissions by 6% from 1990 levels by 2012. Canada signed the Kyoto Protocol at the United Nations in New York in 1998, and ratified it in 2002.

3.2.1. Air Pollution

Air pollution exists when certain substances are present in the atmosphere in sufficient concentrations to cause adverse affects. Natural sources include volcanoes and forest fires. In Canada, air pollution results primarily from the combustion of fossil fuels, particularly by cars and some industrial processes, with release into the atmosphere of various oxides of sulphur, nitrogen, and carbon. In addition, a variety of toxic trace elements (lead, cadmium, beryllium, asbestos) have also been detected. There are three major categories under the rubric of air pollution causing similar health effects.

Smog

The word "smog" was coined several decades ago, derived from the combination of the words "smoke" and "fog," to describe the brownish yellow haze that sometimes hangs over urban areas. It is primarily a combination of ground level ozone and inhalable particulates. Combustion contributes a large part of the oxides of nitrogen. Smog may also contain acidic air pollutants, nitrogen oxides, sulphur oxides, and carbon monoxide. It usually occurs in urban areas but suburbs and rural communities are also affected. Ground-level ozone tends to form under conditions of bright sunlight, high temperature, and a stationary air mass when volatile organic compounds and oxides of nitrogen combine. Therefore, the afternoons and early evenings of hot summer days are peak smog periods; by late in the day, the sun's rays have "baked" the exhaust from motor vehicles and industries into smog. Inhalable particulate matter concentrations depend less on temperature and can occur throughout the day as well as result in winter smog episodes, when ozone levels are much lower.

Ozone Pollution

Ozone is not directly released into the atmosphere in significant amounts, but forms when nitrogen oxides and volatile organic compounds (VOCs) react in the presence of sunlight or — to a much lesser degree — electrical discharges such as lightning storms. Nitrogen oxides are produced when fossil fuels are burned in motor vehicles, power plants, furnaces, and turbines. In Ontario, for example, vehicle emissions account for about 60% of total nitrogen oxide emissions. VOC emissions result from incomplete combustion of gasoline and from evaporation of petroleum fuels, industrial solvents, paints, and dry-cleaning fluids.

Acid Rain

Acid rain refers to hydration of oxides of sulphur and nitrogen, which transforms nitrogen oxides into nitric acid and sulphur oxides into sulphuric acid. These compounds can remain suspended in the atmosphere (pre-depositional) or can fall to earth as precipitation (depositional). The chief sources of sulphur dioxide ($SO2$) are industrial emissions, although exhaust from vehicles using high sulphur fuels also plays an important role. The negative impact on plant and aquatic ecosystems has been widely studied (49).

Impact of Air Pollutants on Health

Smog adversely affects lung function even in healthy adults and also damages vegetation (17). Ground-level ozone is the principal ingredient of smog. The health effects of smog resemble those of ozone. However, because smog is a mixture of pollutants, its effects can vary, and the impact of one pollutant may be intensified when the pollutant is combined with another. The Great London Fog of 1952 demonstrated an association between cardiorespiratory mortality and sulphur dioxide concentrations. Particulate matter smaller than 10 microns (PM-10s) are easily deposited in the lungs and are also implicated in contributing to respiratory morbidity.

Ozone in the troposphere has been associated with a decreased functional capacity of the lungs and tied to increased hospital admissions for respiratory ailments (17). Adverse health effects may be exacerbated in those suffering from respiratory diseases and those engaging in heavy exercise when the air quality is poor. Children and the elderly may also be particularly vulnerable to the effects of ozone. It has been reported that 16,000 early deaths and many hospital visits in Canada each year are related to air pollution. Canada's healthcare system could save an estimated $8 billion over the next 20 years by taking action to improve air quality (50). The Ontario Medical Association estimates that health and economic costs (due to lost production due to employee illness) of air pollution costs in Ontario alone top $1 billion annually (51). In a recent report on the state of air pollution in Ontario, the Ontario Medical Association expressed concern that despite knowledge of the adverse health effects of air pollution, ozone levels are continuing to increase, and levels of particulates, VOCs, and oxides of nitrogen are relatively unchanged. The increase in ozone levels may be due, in part, to the trend of the increasing annual national temperature in Canada since this promotes the reaction of VOCs and oxides of nitrogen (NOx) to produce ozone. Ontario has some of the highest maximum ozone levels in Canada (52). More research is required to identify and understand the health effects of various chemical combinations and of long-term exposure to low levels of smog (53).

Strategies Dealing with Outdoor Air

A number of strategies have been developed to minimize air pollution. The Air Quality Index (AQI) is a useful indicator of overall air quality, based on pollutant measurements of some or all of the six common air pollutants (see above). It is based on individual readings of the common air pollutants and is reported as a single score. There are five categories of AQI readings: 0–15 very good, 16–31 good, 32–49 moderate, 50–99 poor, and 100 and over very poor. Values in category of poor and very poor are associated with adverse effects on the human and animal populations, whereas a score in the moderate range may cause some adverse effects on very sensitive people such as those who have serious respiratory or cardiac problems (54). The Air Pollution Index (API) is a special component of the AQI and provides 24-hour running averages of sulphur dioxide and particulate matter. The government can order major emitters of these pollutants to reduce or suspend operations in the event that the API reaches unacceptable levels. The AQI is available on line and is a useful resource for people with cardiac or respiratory problems to help them avoid being outdoors when the air quality is particularly poor.

The establishment of emission standards for all sources has contributed to control of air pollution, including those for cars (for which catalytic converters and other technologies have been introduced), and many industrial sources including ferrous foundries, and asphalt-paving producers, power plants, and smelters. A number of pollution abatement technologies have been developed to address specific pollutants, and progress has been made on some emissions. Optimal use of road and transit systems are objectives to be achieved and are being addressed in initiatives such as the Healthy Cities approach as a part of healthy public policy in Toronto (see Chapter 1). Healthy public policy in the environmental context has great potential for involving major stakeholders vital to the development and implementation of workable solutions to pollution. Many proposed solutions have enormous cost implications. Round-table conferences on environmental issues involving industry, and government have been held in a number of provinces, which illustrate a collaborative approach. The enforcement of legislation has led to penalties for non-observance of regulations regarding some environmental pollution, although these are not considered severe enough by some interest groups. The implementation of the Kyoto Protocol will have a measurable impact on reducing air pollution nationally and globally.

3.3.   OZONE DEPLETION

Ozone (O3) is a gas in the stratosphere that forms a layer that protects the earth from harmful ultraviolet radiation. There is growing concern about ozone depletion in the stratosphere causing an increased incidence of skin cancer of all types, including melanoma. Ultraviolet radiation is thought to have other health effects, such as causing cataracts and other ophthalmic conditions, and depressing the immune function, which may increase susceptibility to cancers. The ozone layer is destroyed when synthetic chemicals such as chlorofluorocarbons (CFCs) and halons are released into the atmosphere during the production, use, and disposal of products such as air conditioners, plastic foams, and solvents. In the presence of sunlight in the atmosphere, these molecules split and the resulting chlorine reacts with the ozone, breaking it down.

A number of strategies have been introduced to address ozone depletion. The Montreal Protocol on Substances that Deplete the Ozone Layer, which was adopted in 1987 by developed and developing nations to stop producing CFCs, has had considerable success. It is estimated that without the Montreal Protocol, by 2050 ozone depletion would be about 10 times worse than current levels (55, 56). The import, manufacture, and export of ozone-depleting substances are under the control of the *Ozone-Depleting Substances Regulations, 1998 (57)*. Other initiatives are the conservation, recovery, and recycling of ozone-depleting chemicals. Environment Canada publishes a weekly ozone index with appropriate recommendations, such as limiting the amount of time spent in direct sunlight to avoid sunburn in persons with fair skin. The UV index measures the sun's ultraviolet (UV) rays, using a scale that runs from 0 (lowest intensity) to 12 (highest). When the index exceeds 7, some people can get sunburned in 15 minutes. In addition, skin-protection precautions are also promoted, such as wearing hats and protective clothing and using sunscreen.

3.4.   INDOOR AIR POLLUTION

Indoor air quality has been scrutinized, following complaints of adverse health effects and discomfort in occupants of sealed buildings. A variety of non-specific health effects have been identified, including eye and upper respiratory tract irritation, as well as headache, fatigue, and nausea. Other building-associated illnesses include Pontiac fever (an influenza-like illness) and Legionnaires' disease. A variety of indoor pollutants can be measured, originating from building materials, furnishings, heating, and human activities. Indoor pollutants also originate from the external environment. The most frequent pollutants include tobacco smoke, volatile organic compounds, formaldehyde, and other gases. The degree of ventilation and entry rate of fresh air, as well as the reaction rate between chemicals, determines the concentration of indoor pollutants. Other factors such as temperature and humidity are important for comfort. Psychological factors also play a role.

There is a correlation between levels of carbon dioxide in indoor air, a measurable surrogate marker, and the prevalence of complaints about indoor air quality. At levels of CO_2 less than 500 parts per million (ppm) there are usually no complaints; from 500 to 1,000 ppm, occasional complaints, and more than 1,000 ppm, many complaints. While a CO_2 level of 1,000 ppm is not in itself dangerous, it does indicate poor air quality with inadequate ventilation. Identification and control of sources and increasing the fresh air circulation (versus recirculated air) should be the first response to complaints of poor indoor air quality. There is a tendency to avoid precise measurement of actual contaminants, as these have not proved helpful in reducing adverse health effects to data. The National Building Code, which was updated in 1995, sets standards for residential mechanical ventilation systems and for adequate ventilation. Exposure guidelines have been published for indoor air (58).

Associated with indoor air quality is the recent identification of the health hazards of passive smoke exposure, which are discussed in Chapters 7 and 10.

The role of indoor moulds in causing non-specific illness has received a great deal of media attention recently. The concern started due to reports that *Stachybotrys* was linked with cases of pulmonary hemosiderosis in infants. Further studies have shown this link to be inconclusive, although the public's fear of mould in their homes and classrooms has continued to grow. Mould's ability to infect human tissues and to elicit an allergic response has been described well in the literature but does not explain the myriad of symptoms, such as memory loss and dizziness, that people feel are due to mould. Keeping spaces clean, dry, and well ventilated hinders mould growth. Cleaning damp surfaces with vinegar and baking soda or bleach also prevents mould growth (59).

4.   WATER QUALITY

Ensuring a safe potable water supply has long been a prerequisite for public health. The issue was brought to the forefront in 2000, when the municipal drinking water supply in Walkerton, Ontario, became contaminated with *Escherichia coli* 0157:H7. Seven people died and more than 2,300 became ill. The contamination resulted from a combination of the spreading of manure near a well and improper disinfection of the water supply through inadequate chlorination. The problem was compounded by a lack of monitoring of water quality (1). One year later, a *Cryptosporidium* outbreak due to a sub-standard water treatment plant in North Battleford, Saskatchewan, again highlighted the problem of indifference to public health safety aspects of drinking water (60). One of the other concerns raised has been the overflow of waste products containing biological contaminants into water systems from mega farms (e.g., pig farms). As indicate earlier, guidelines for Canadian drinking water quality are established by Health Canada in conjunction with provinces. The quality and safety of bottled water is regulated under Canadian *Food and Drug Act*.

Recently, people have become concerned about chemical contamination of water. There are more than 70,000 industrial chemicals, and hundreds of new chemicals are developed each year. Many of these chemicals, including household detergents, fail to biodegrade, resulting in their accumulation in soil and water. It is estimated that drinking water accounts for less than 1% of our total exposure to persistent pollutants, with most of our intake coming from food (3).

In response to the public's increasing use of bottled water and devices to treat municipal water, the City of Toronto Department of Public Health undertook a risk assessment of drinking water in 1990 (61). Bacterial contamination was not found in tap water, but was found in both device-treated and bottled water. Trace chemical contaminants were found in all three types of water; however, tap water was considered superior overall due to the variability of the chemical contaminants in the other water sources and the lack of guidelines for acceptable levels. Four groups of chemicals caused some concern in tap water. Lead usually enters drinking water when it is standing in lead water pipes (but not in plastic pipes) and can be avoided if recommendations are followed (see below). Aluminum levels are largely present as a result of added alum, for which alternative technologies can be adopted. Potentially carcinogenic and mutagenic trihalomethanes (THMs) are produced when chlorine is added to the water for disinfection and reacts with organic matter. A number of other organic compounds, such as haloacetic acids, have also been detected in trace levels, for which further investigation is required. Alternatives are available such as the use of pre-ozonation for disinfection to reduce the need for chlorine, although such alternatives also produce various toxic byproducts. Chlorination is the principal method for disinfecting drinking water in Canada and the risks posed by generation of THMs are greatly outweighed by the reduction of pathogen risks through disinfection.

In many parts of Canada, fluoride is added to drinking water to prevent tooth decay. The recommended level of flouride in drinking water is 0.8 mg to 1.0 mg per litre (32). Levels as low as 0.7 mg/L can cause discolouration of children's teeth (dental fluorosis) (62). Chronic exposure to very high levels of fluoride can be associated with skeletal fluorosis, a progressive disorder in which bones increase in density while becoming more brittle. In severe cases, this may lead to rigidity of the spine, skeletal deformities, and increased risk of bone fractures. Health Canada estimates that the average fluoride levels to which Canadians are exposed are at least 20% lower than the levels at which adverse effects on the skeleton are anticipated. There is no evidence that fluoride exposure leads to heart disease, cancer, thyroid problems, birth defects, miscarriages, or hearing or vision problems (3).

Interest in water quality and its possible human health effects has also focused on the Great Lakes, due to the known persistence of toxic chemicals arising from industrial and commercial production and use. In 1985, the Great Lakes Water Quality Board identified 11 pollutants as critical on the basis of their persistence, their ability to bioaccumulate in living organisms and cause adverse human and environmental health effects, and because they were already subject to extensive regulation. These critical pollutants are PCBs, dichlorodiphenyltrichloroethane (DDT) and its breakdown products, aldrin and dieldrin, toxaphene, dioxins (2,3,7,8-TCDD), furans (2,3,7,8-TCDF), mirex, mercury, benzopyrene, hexachlorobenzene, and alkylated lead. Current knowledge of the level of contamination in open waters and in aquatic biota has come from the findings of studies by Environment Canada, Health Canada, and the Department of Fisheries and Oceans. Although the Great Lakes are a polluted ecosystem, the levels of toxic chemicals in open waters were found to be well below Canadian and international drinking water standards. Sediment studies demonstrated that pollution by synthetic organic chemicals and heavy metals peaked in the 1960s and early 1970s, declining in the 1980s. Levels of PCBs, DDT, dieldrin, hexachlorobenzene, toxaphene, and benzopyrene in herring gull eggs and fish have not declined significantly since 1985 for any of the Great Lakes (63).

5.   FOOD QUALITY

Although Canada's food supplies are considered to be among the safest in the world, environmental contamination of food continues to be a concern. Food contamination accounts for up to 95% of our daily intake of persistent toxic chemicals whereas air contributes approximately 15% and drinking water contributes very little. *The Health and Environment Handbook for Health Professionals* is an excellent source for information on food quality(6). Common concerns about the quality of food are the use of pesticides and chemicals during food production and handling, the use of drugs such as antibiotics and hormones to treat livestock, use of food additives and preservatives, quality of sport-caught fish, genetically modified foods, and food irradiation (see Chapter 4). Major sources of food contamination in Canada are microbial contamination, environmental contamination, naturally occurring contaminants, pesticide residues and chemicals in meat and milk products, and food additives and preservatives. The common microbial contamination in raw foods are *Salmonella*, *Campylobacter*, and *Escherichia coli* (see Chapter 8). The only certain way to eliminate bacterial contamination of raw foods is to irradiate them, a practice not currently followed in Canada. Safe handling and cooking practices can significantly reduce or even eliminate bacteria in foods. Persistent chemicals such as PCBs, dioxins, and some pesticides (e.g. DDT, dieldrin, mirex) as well as methyl mercury, cadmium, and lead are of concern because of their tendency to accumulate in the fat or organs of fish and wildlife. Fish and small insects absorb these chemicals directly from contaminated water and concentrate them in target tissues, such as fat. Larger predators consume these small organisms and the concentration of the contaminants increases up the food chain, which is known as **biomagnification**. For example, in Ontario, the Ministry of Environment monitors levels of contaminants in fish by species and water body and uses this data to offer recommended consumption levels in the "Guide to Eating Ontario Sport Fish" (64).

The presence of persistent organochlorine residues in foods is another area of concern. The Canadian Food Inspection Agency is responsible for testing foods to ensure that the residues are below the maximum residue limits. There are many naturally occurring contaminants in food, including polycyclic aromatic hydrocarbons (from broiling and smoking), aromatic amines (from broiling and frying), nitrosamines, mycotoxins (from moulds), antioxidants in prepared foods, and alkaloids in plants and herbs. Food additives include both natural and artificial compounds that are added to a particular food for a specific reason. According to the Canadian *Food and Drugs Act* and Regulations, any chemical substance added to food during processing or storage, which could, either by itself or through its byproducts, affect the characteristics of a food or become part of it, is considered a food additive. Some common food additives are preservatives, leavening agents, flavour enhancers, colour additives, sulphites, and emulsifiers, stabilizers, and thickeners. The use of antibiotics and growth hormone for domestic animals is controversial. These substances are thought to be bioactive in food when it reaches the consumer. There is also a concern that this practice may contribute to the growing problem of antibiotic resistance. Issues related to genetically modified foods are described in Chapter 4.

6.   TOXIC CHEMICALS

Only a small number of chemicals in use today have had adequate toxicological testing prior to their introduction. Less than 1% has an established threshold limit value to regulate occupational exposure. Furthermore, older toxicity testing data available may be limited to tests for mutagenicity and acute toxicity, although reproductive, immunological, neurotoxic, and other chronic tests are required of new consumer chemicals. A review of the adverse health outcomes of the differing classes of chemicals is beyond the scope of this chapter. Instead, this section will examine a small number of the most prominent chemical classes in relation to environmental health.

6.1.   METALS

Many metals are essential human micronutrients. At higher doses, however, these elements can have serious toxic effects (see Chapter 10). Environmental exposures to metals have been documented as a cause of disease in humans.

Lead
Source and Exposure. Lead is a naturally occurring metal that has been used since prehistoric times. Lead exposure occurs chiefly through ingestion, although inhalation is the exposure pathway in those who are occupationally exposed. Drinking water and food are sources of environmental exposures to lead. Automobile emissions were a significant source of exposure until 1975, when unleaded gasoline was introduced in Canada. Industrial emissions now exceed automobile emissions. Lead paint is an important source of exposure for children. The older the home, the more likely it is to have lead-based paint, which is an important potential source of lead exposure in people who renovate homes. Domestic drinking water may be contaminated through the leaching of lead from water pipes and lead solder. Hobbies that put people at increased risk of lead exposure include pottery, artistic painting, stained-glass making, glass or metal soldering, target shooting, electronic soldering, and construction of bullets, slugs, or fishing sinkers.

Health Effects and Control. Lead is absorbed into the bloodstream and deposited in bone and other tissues. The toxicity of lead is multisystemic. Acute exposure to large amounts of lead may cause abdominal pain, hemolytic anemia, nephropathy, and encephalopathy. Chronic exposure may result in constitutional complaints as well as abdominal cramps, central nervous system effects ranging from impaired concentration to encephalopathy, peripheral motor neuropathy, microcytic anemia with basophilic stippling, nephrotoxicity, and adverse reproductive outcomes including miscarriage, low birth weight, and impaired neurological development. In the general population, two groups — the unborn child and children up to 6 years of age — are at a greater risk of the adverse health effects of lead. During pregnancy, lead can cross the placenta and reach the unborn child. Neurological development may be compromised because there is no blood-brain barrier. Young children are a high-risk group for several reasons: they take in more lead per unit of body weight than adults, develop at a rapid rate, and are more susceptible to the adverse effects of lead. Children also absorb a higher proportion of ingested lead (50%, compared to 10% in adults). Over the past decade, some researchers have found that exposure to even low levels of lead prior to birth or during infancy and early childhood can cause impaired intellectual development, behavioural disturbances, decreased physical growth, and hearing impairment. High levels of lead exposure have been linked to increased spontaneous abortion and stillbirth rates in female workers (18). Elevated lead levels can be detected by a simple blood test. There are guidelines recommended by the joint Federal/Provincial Advisory Committee on Environmental and Occupational Health that dictate the tolerable level of lead for individuals and the community. When these levels are exceeded, intervention is appropriate: identification of the source of exposure, control of the source, or removal of individuals from further exposure. Municipal water treatment removes lead effectively and the alkalization of water can reduce leaching from corroded pipes. To avoid post-treatment exposure, if water is left standing for more than a few hours, taps should be flushed until the water is as cold as it will get; if lead levels at point-of-use exceed recommended levels, then replacement of lead pipes and lead solder by municipalities and homeowners may be necessary.

Mercury

Source and Exposure. Mercury is a naturally occurring metal that is found in cinnabar ore. It is used in the manufacture of chlorine and caustic soda, in electrical equipment, and in thermometers and other instruments. It is released into the environment through natural degassing of the earth's crust as well as through industrial releases. Organic mercury (predominantly methyl mercury) is the form that is most toxic to humans, and it may be formed by the action of microorganisms on elemental mercury landing in areas of flooding, direct water emissions, or considerable air deposition. A well-known example is the incidence of neurological and teratogenic consequences following contamination of Minamata Bay in Japan with organic mercury.

Most exposure to mercury today occurs through the eating of fish. Fish bioconcentrate mercury in their muscle tissue by a factor of 10 to 100,000. Canadians who rely on subsistence fishing and do not heed consumption guidelines are at particular risk of exposure to mercury. Surveys of mercury levels (in hair and blood) undertaken in 350 Aboriginal communities revealed a disturbing prevalence of elevated mercury levels in 2.5% of communities (5). Pregnant women who consume large quantities of mercury-contaminated fish are at risk of exposing their unborn children to mercury. Health Canada advises Canadians to limit consumption of shark, swordfish, and fresh and frozen tuna to one serving per week. Pregnant women, women of childbearing age, and young children should eat no more than one serving per month (20). These fish are near the top of the food chain and often have higher levels of mercury than those found in most other commercial fish.

Health Effects and Control. Unlike elemental and inorganic mercury, organic mercury is rapidly absorbed from the gut. Acute intoxication can cause paresthesia, ataxia, impaired vision and hearing, psychosis, and kidney damage. Chronic low-dose poisoning results in an asymptomatic period (of some months), during which time the mercury penetrates cell membranes and binds with proteins and sulphhydryl groups. Liver and kidney damage can occur, as can central nervous system impairment of sensory, coordinating, and visual functions. The brain of the developing fetus is particularly at risk if exposed to high levels of circulating maternal organic mercury. Possible effects include retarded physical growth and coordination, cerebral palsy, and more subtle effects on coordination, behaviour, and intelligence quotient (65).

Cadmium

Source and Exposure. Cadmium is a relatively rare element in the earth's crust; however, as a result of industrial and municipal wastes, it is accumulating in the soil at a rate of 1% increase per year. Cadmium is used in the process of electroplating metals, as a stabilizer for plastics, in batteries, and in high-technology industries (e.g., the manufacture of television tubes and nuclear reactor shields). It is also released in the burning of fossil fuels, incinerator discharges, and cigarettes. It is one of the five most common leachates in water near hazardous waste sites.

Plants taking up cadmium from contaminated soil and the use of sewage sludge as fertilizers for feed crops result in bioconcentration of cadmium in vegetables, poultry, and beef. Incinerator deposits settle on crops, which augment the levels found in plants. Fish also bioconcentrate cadmium. Most exposure to cadmium therefore occurs by food intake. However, cigarette smokers who smoke a pack a day can double their usual intake of cadmium (4).

Health Effects and Control. Cadmium is known to cause lung cancer in humans. Acute exposure may cause respiratory distress (after inhalation) or gastroenteritis (after ingestion). Chronic exposure leads to kidney damage and multiple system effects including emphysema, liver and tesitculare damage, immune system, and central nervous system damage as well as painful itai-itai disease from the accumulation of cadmium in bones (66).

Aluminum

Source and Exposure. Aluminum is one of the most common elements in the earth's crust. Food ingestion is responsible for 96% of the usual human aluminum intake, drinking water for 3.5%, and antacids and other consumer products for the remainder.

Health Effects and Control. The potential health effects of aluminum in drinking water are the cause of ongoing controversy, particularly in relation to its putative role in Alzheimer's disease, the most common cause of dementia. At this point, however, no role for aluminum in causing the disease has been established (67), according to the causal association criteria described in Chapter 2.

6.2. POLYCHLORINATED BIPHENYLS AND DIOXINS

Polychlorinated Biphenyls (PCBs)

Source and Exposure. PCBs are a class of highly stable, non-corroding, and relatively non-flammable chemicals first manufactured on a commercial scale in 1929. For several decades, they were used extensively in a wide range of industrial applications, especially the manufacture of electrical and heat exchange equipment. In the past, PCBs have also been used in such products as inks, oil, sealants, caulking compounds, and carbonless copy paper. In the 1970s, concerns over health and the environmental impact of PCBs led to their substitution by other compounds and eventually to a North American ban in 1977 on the manufacture, importation, and most non-electrical uses of PCBs. Electrical uses of PCBs are now being phased out, with stringent requirements for their handling and disposal.

Studies have found trace levels of PCBs everywhere in the environment even though they are no longer being manufactured. This is because PCBs do not readily break down. This persistence, coupled with their tendency to accumulate in the fat of living organisms, means that they are often present and biomagnified in the food chain. Humans are regularly exposed to minute amounts of PCBs in food, air, and water (20). Ingestion is the most common route of entry. As a result, all humans have a low level of PCBs in their body fat and blood. Uncontrolled fires involving PCBs can pose a significant threat to human health. When PCBs are heated, they are transformed into an array of dangerous chemicals, including furans and occasionally dioxins.

Health Effects and Control. Sustained, high-level exposure to PCBs has been associated with adverse health effects. These include a severe form of acne (chloracne), eye discharge, swelling of the upper eyelids, hyperpigmentation of the nails and skin, numbness of limbs, weakness, muscle spasms, chronic bronchitis, and decreased birth weight and head circumference in newborns. These health effects were identified following an incident in Japan in 1968 involving the accidental mixing of PCBs with cooking oil. Scientists generally agree that short-term, low-level exposure to PCBs is unlikely to have a significant health impact on adults. However, there is potential cause for concern over long-term exposure to low concentrations (65).

Long-term, high-level PCB exposure has been linked to an increased incidence of cancer, particularly liver cancer. This is based on studies of humans exposed to high concentrations of furan-contaminated PCBs. Laboratory rats exposed for a lifetime to high levels of a PCB mixture also developed liver cancer.

The association between prenatal exposure to PCBs and neurocognitive effects in children is controversial. Transplacental transfer has been documented and was predictive of low birth weight, smaller dimensions of the infant, neonatal hypotonia and hyporeflexia, and cognitive, motor, and behavioural development deficits. There is no evidence of any harmful effects from the small amounts of PCBs found in breast milk. Healthcare professionals advise that the known benefits of breastfeeding outweigh any potential risks that may be associated with PCBs in human milk.

PCBs bioconcentrate in fish, and those who eat fish regularly are thus at risk of PCB exposure. Aboriginal people who survive on subsistence fishing are at risk if they do not heed guidelines. As mentioned previously, PCBs are being phased out following legislation banning their production. However, transport and storage of existing wastes containing PCBs pending destruction are also regulated under the *Transportation of Dangerous Goods Act* and Canada's *Environmental Protection Act*, respectively, as well as under provincial legislations.

Dioxins and Furans

Source and Exposure. Dioxins are a family of toxic substances called polychlorinated dibenzo-para-dioxins. A second family of closely related toxic substances known as polychlorinated dibenzofurans is very often present with dioxins. Dioxins and furans, which have never been purposely manufactured, are byproducts of the production of certain chemicals (such as some pesticides and wood preservatives) of the chlorine-bleaching process used in some pulp and paper mills, and of the incomplete combustion of materials that contain both chlorine atoms and organic matter. Although they are most often human-made, some natural occurrences, such as forest fires, are believed to contribute to the presence of dioxins and furans in the environment.

People living in industrialized nations are constantly exposed to minute amounts of dioxins and furans in food, air, water, soil, and some consumer products. Scientists have shown that food is the major source of dioxins and furans for humans.

Health Effects and Control. Because dioxins and furans are soluble in fat, they can accumulate in the bodies of all animals, including humans. The remarkable loss of reproductive capability in fish-catching birds and wildlife in the Great Lakes area in the 1970s may have been associated with dioxins and furans. Recent scientific studies indicate that high levels of dioxins and furans can significantly damage the health of laboratory animals, including weight loss, skin disorders, effects on their immune system, impaired liver function, induction of liver enzymes, impaired reproduction (including birth defects), and increased numbers of tumours. Effects on humans are equivocal. No conclusive link has been established between human exposure to dioxins and furans and effects such as cancer or abnormal reproduction. Establishing levels of exposure to dioxins and furans that might be considered acceptable for the general population is controversial.

Despite the lack of direct evidence that current exposures to dioxins and furans in Canada contribute to health problems in humans, the government of Canada recognizes that these compounds are undesirable environmental contaminants and that, where possible, their unintentional production should be limited. The Healthy Environments and Consumer Safety Branch of Health Canada monitors dioxin levels in a variety of foods, human breast milk, water, and some paper products. The federal government no longer permits the sale and use of pesticides containing 2,3,7,8-TCDD (a form of dioxin) and has regulated the content of other dioxins in pesticides remaining on the market. The government of Canada, in conjunction with the provinces, has also established codes of practice to reduce contamination by the wood preservation industries. These efforts to control sources of dioxins and furans have had a positive impact. One indicator of this is that levels of dioxins and furans in human breast milk have been declining (68).

6.3 PESTICIDES

Pesticides are unique as a class of environmental agents because they are deliberately added to the environment for the express purpose of killing some form of life. They have been categorized as economic poisons because they have some important beneficial effects on food supply and on health. For example, the use of insecticides has eliminated or controlled vector-borne disease in many parts of the world.

Both acute and chronic human health effects related to pesticide exposure have been identified (19). The acute effects are primarily occupational in origin. Among the variety of delayed health effects associated with pesticides, the carcinogenic and reproductive effects of Agent Orange have been more noticeable. This compound, which contains the herbicide 2,4,5-T and combined with the potent carcinogen 2,3,7,8-TCDD (a dioxin), was sprayed over many of the Vietnamese field camps, jungles, and roadways during the Vietnam war. Studies of exposed U.S. Vietnam veterans have revealed an excess of soft-tissue sarcomas and lymphomas. Studies of the teratogenic consequences of Agent Orange exposure have produced inconclusive results. The International Agency for Research on Cancer (IARC) considers the pesticides chlordane-heptachlor, DDT, dieldrin, and HCH-lindane as possible human carcinogens. There is some suggestion that pesticides may be capable of inducing Parkinson's-like disease in humans (19).

Pesticide residues contaminate food products and can concentrate in the ecological food chain. Almost every human body is born with measurable organochlorine pesticide levels, related to widespread use of pesticides. The delayed effects of pesticide exposure are difficult to investigate as exposures are universal and not easily measured; a latency period applies to all carcinogenic outcomes, and there are no unexposed control groups. Given these difficulties, epidemiological researchers have increasingly turned to reproductive effects. Several municipalities in Canada have used their powers to limit many cosmetic uses of pesticides in their jurisdictions. The federal government has also created the Pest Management Regulatory Agency to monitor the impact of pesticides on food supply and their effects on human health (see Chapter 13). The *New Pest Control Product Act* has more stringent requirements for manufacturers to provide safety data on their product and post-registration surveillance (69).

7. MULTIPLE CHEMICAL SENSITIVITY

Multiple chemical sensitivity (MCS) is an ill-defined constellation of non-specific symptoms (e.g., nausea, headache, eye irritation) and is thought by many to be caused by exposure to various chemicals at very low levels of exposure (i.e., below the levels at which they are usually considered to be toxic). Significant controversy surrounds the diagnosis of MCS. One descriptive study in a rural North Carolina community described a prevalence of 33% of MCS in their study population (70). Without doubt, people with MCS are very often distressed and functionally disabled. There is a paucity of good epidemiological evidence, however, to support the theory that the various symptoms and distress seen in MCS can be attributed to chemical exposures alone. More likely, the condition is multifactorial in origin with psychosocial as well as physical risk factors, a theory supported by evidence of improvement in MCS patients after undergoing cognitive behavioural therapy (71-73).

8.   CREATING A HEALTHY ENVIRONMENT

With increasing recognition of the importance of the ecosystem has come respect for the maintenance of the integrity of the environment for its intrinsic value, as well as for its purpose in meeting human needs. A number of strategies have been developed and are discussed below. They include the broad framework of healthy public policy in relation to the environment, sustainable development, the management of waste, and response to environmental emergencies. Strategies to protect human health in relation to the environment include both direct and indirect approaches. An example of a direct strategy is to establish guidelines for human exposure to toxic substances. An indirect strategy is to reduce the production of chlorofluorocarbon, which will help sustain the atmosphere's integrity and thus benefit human health.

8.1.   HEALTHY PUBLIC POLICY

Healthy public policy aims at mobilizing many segments of the community to reduce the adverse health effects on humans that may result from deleterious environmental exposures. The measures include intersectoral and interdepartmental action, legislation, regulations and guidelines, community organization, education, and advocacy (see Chapter 1). A unifying approach to public policy in environmental protection has developed in the form of the concept of sustainable development. Specific strategies are discussed below. First, however, it is instructive to review the population-based theoretical position that provides the rationale for healthy public policy approaches in relation to the environment. In a continuous distribution of exposures, large numbers exposed to small risk from environmental exposure generate the bulk of the resulting disease(74). In comparison, there are far fewer cases among those at high risk due to extreme exposure than there are, for example, among those in an occupational setting. The solution to reducing exposures to substances that have the most potential to generate the most illness includes mass measures, as well as paying attention to those at high risk.

8.1.1. Regulations and Guidelines

Global

Many of the current initiatives to deal with environmental issues are undertaken at an international level for sustainable development and waste management. The United Nations, non-governmental organizations such as Greenpeace, and various international governmental organizations are instrumental in raising awareness and developing accords in this area. Examples include international agreements on banning whale hunting and the Montreal and Kyoto protocols.

Federal

Jurisdictional responsibility for environmental issues is shared between the federal and provincial/territorial governments, and areas of overlap are usually resolved through close cooperation. The *Canadian Environmental Protection Act* is the cornerstone of federal environmental legislation. It provides the framework for protection from hazardous substances, enforcement tools, and powers to reduce pollution and to eliminate and regulate emissions of toxic substances. It ensures that substances not specifically covered under other legislation meet Canadian standards in the areas of human health and safety and environmental protection. Environment Canada enforces the Act, and Health Canada contributes to the development of regulations and guidelines.

Other pieces of federal legislation relevant to environment and health are the *Food and Drugs Act* and Regulations (Health Canada), the *Pest Control Products Act* (Agriculture and Agri-Food Canada), and the *Hazardous Products Act* and Regulations (Canada Customs and Revenue Agency and Health Canada). There is, however, fragmentation at this level of government. The federal government is also entirely responsible for setting national policy with regard to environmental pollutants, such as atmospheric sulphur or nitrogen dioxides (which cause smog and acid rain) that can travel across provincial or international boundaries.

The environmental assessment and review process is formalized in the *Canada Environmental Assessment Act*. This process is used to identify and review the implications to multiple sectors, including health, of all projects, with both public and professional input being obtained. For example, the location of dams and of nuclear facilities are both major issues in Canada, and environmental assessments are a means of identifying implications for the whole ecosystem as well as for human health. Provinces have also developed environmental assessment processes and regulations.

Federal government departments also make health-based guidelines for air, drinking, and recreational water. These are not enforceable but are used by many jurisdictions as guidelines for developing their own regulations. Guidelines have the advantage of a capacity for greater responsiveness compared to legislation but have the disadvantage of unenforceability. The new Canada-wide standard being used to address some pollutants may change this.

Provincial and Territorial

The provinces and territories have primary responsibility for the quality of local air and water, the quantity and types of emissions allowed by industries, the disposal of toxic waste products, and the identification and management of environmental health hazards. For example, Ontario's *Environmental Protection Act* and its amendments require control of pollutants below any level known to produce a hazard or discomfort to humans or livestock, to damage vegetation, or to cause corrosion of soil or buildings. Provinces and territories are also responsible for setting soil contamination guidelines. Provincial and territorial ministries of the environment play a primary role in this field, but share responsibilities with the ministries of labour, natural resources, and health, among others. As with the federal level, the provincial and terrritorial levels of responsibility in relation to environment and health are fragmented.

Municipal

Local municipalities and special purpose local/regional agencies are usually responsible for safe food in restaurants, monitoring of drinking and recreational water quality, private septic system placement and maintenance, sewage and solid waste collection and disposal, noise control, animal control, land use planning, traffic control, and building inspection. They use both provincial legislation and local bylaws to enforce various parts of their programs. Many have taken initiatives such as recycling programs and are at the forefront of cleaning up the environment to improve health. Local government can request the province to pass enabling legislation to allow local regulations regarding environmental hazards to be developed and implemented.

Role of Public Health

Public health departments usually have municipal and provincial mandates for the enforcement of regulations regarding safe food and water, sanitation, and other environmental hazards such as restriction of smoking in public places. In addition, the role of public health in environmental issues is frequently that of an honest broker — getting the stakeholders to the table, providing information on health effects, legitimizing concerns and issues by encouraging expression of these by stakeholders, and then negotiating solutions that address the concerns of all parties to the extent possible. A stakeholder is a party affected in some way, frequently economic, by a decision or issue, or who has a mandate or responsibility for involvement; the public or non-government organizations or advocacy groups are major stakeholders. The role of public health departments is described in more detail in Chapter 15.

Intersectoral Initiatives

In Canada, there have recently been a number of initiatives undertaken in relation to the environment that have included many departments of government and other sectors. For example, the Great Lakes Action Plan involves four federal departments: Environment Canada, Department of Fisheries and Oceans, Agriculture and Agri-Food Canada, and Health Canada. The purpose of the plan is to renew and strengthen planning, cooperation, and coordination between Canada and Ontario in implementing actions to restore and protect the ecosystem, to prevent and control pollution into the ecosystem, and to conserve species, populations and habitats in the Great Lakes Basin ecosystem.

Another example of healthy public policy related to environmental health is Canada's Green Plan, which incorporates community involvement and education, legislation, and participation by stakeholders in partnerships to improve the environment. The environment is likely to be placed on the agenda of many sectors, both private and government. The federal government and the provinces and territories are committed to this plan to clean the air, water, and land; to eliminate the dumping of toxic substances into the environment; to sustain forestry, agriculture, and fisheries development; to protect 12% of Canada as park space; to preserve the integrity of the Arctic and the global environment, including reducing greenhouse gases; to develop partnerships in environmental literacy; and to prepare for environmental emergencies.

8.1.2. Sustainable Development

Sustainable development is defined as development that meets the needs of the present without compromising the ability of future generations to meet their own needs. It refers to use of resources, direction of investments, the orientation of technological development, and institutional development in ways which ensure that the current development and use of resources do not compromise the health and well-being of future generations (75). Certain widely held human values and practices, such as support for population growth, increased production of goods and services, increasing material expectations, and the belief in technology have caused specific ecological phenomena that threaten human health. The major issues are global warming and climatic change with possible consequent food shortages and change in distribution of vector-borne diseases, ozone pollution, ecosystem contamination, and resource depletion. Sustainable development is a conceptual model that incorporates a number of generic approaches to reverse the deterioration of the earth, to prevent pollution beyond the point where natural systems cannot cope, to conserve natural resources by sparing or reducing use or by recycling and reuse (with municipal recycling programs a positive indication of action in this area), and to sustain yield, whereby renewable resources are used at a rate that does not exceed their continued replenishment. Earlier sections in this chapter describe relevant control strategies.

Waste Management

Waste management involves the disposal, destruction, or storage of solid waste and sewage (and industrial discharges and nuclear waste). More recently, it has begun to include other waste management practices to reduce the volumes of waste produced, such as recovery from the waste stream and the adoption of a sustainable environment framework. Canadians produce more 30 million tons of solid waste per year, of which 8 million tons are considered hazardous waste. There are three main approaches to solid waste disposal in Canada: burial, ideally in modern sanitary landfills that satisfy criteria relating to aesthetics, health, and the monitoring and prevention of leaching (which is the diffusion of substances into groundwater from the landfill site); incineration (in which controlled combustion is used to stabilize and eliminate hazardous material, convert organic into inorganic matter, and kill pathogens); and transformation, for example, anaerobic digestion by microorganism or pyrolysis (chemical decomposition caused by combustion in an oxygen-starved environment), which can reduce waste volume by 91%. Sewage is treated in Canada in municipal sewage treatment plants (except from areas where septic tanks are used). After a process of screening and settling, the resulting sludge is processed to form biosolids, which are spread on agricultural land, stored in a landfill or processed to form sludge cakes that are then incinerated. Effluent liquids are chlorinated and discharged into bodies of water, causing concerns as to the possible effects of chlorinated organic compounds (such as trihalomethanes and chloramines) on aquatic life.

The best way to manage waste is for society — including government, industry, and individuals — to produce less of it, by following the **"4 Rs"**: reduce, reuse, recycle, and recover (3). Reducing the consumption of goods is the most effective waste management strategy, because it results in less waste and consumes less energy. Reusing products is the next best option. Examples of this strategy include returnable beverage bottles, garage sales, and used furniture and clothing outlets. Recycling involves using material from old products to make new products; commonly recycled materials include newspapers, aluminum cans, glass containers, plastics, cardboard, and auto parts. Recovery involves harvesting energy or economically worthwhile components from waste materials. Industrial-scale examples include heat energy generated from the incineration of solid wastes and methane gas recovered from composting organic wastes. It is estimated that after recycling plastic, glass and metal containers, and paper products, backyard composting could reduce the volume of remaining residential waste in Canada by up to 60%.

Special provision is made for disposal of hazardous waste with support for household hazardous waste drop-off programs and location of new hazardous waste destruction facilities (e.g., for PCBs) and supporting technology.

8.2.   MANAGING ENVIRONMENTAL ACCIDENTS

The management of life-threatening incidents involving exposure to toxic chemicals (such as in Bhopal, India) or radiation exposure (such as in Chernobyl, Ukraine) is difficult. It requires collaboration from several levels of government and at times from international experts in ways similar to the handling acts of bioterrorism (see Chapter 8). Most of these incidents are not so dramatic but are nonetheless serious. To evaluate unknown health effects, the first step is to evaluate the problem, documenting evidence and obtaining accurate information on the nature and magnitude of the hazard. The second step is to contain the problem, coordinating efforts with responsible public and private agencies. The third step is to assess health effects, focusing on specific outcomes, when the exposure is known, and on the primary organ systems of concern (dermal, respiratory, hepatic, neurological, and renal) and carcinogenic and fetotoxic effects when the exposure is not known (76).

9. SUMMARY

Environmental health may be defined as the study of conditions in the natural and human-made environment that can influence health and well-being. The focus of study in environmental health is the impact of environmental or hazardous agents on the health of the population, and it can be divided into workplace and non-workplace categories. The workplace environment (occupational health) is often associated with high-level exposure, with the exposed population being predominantly of adult age and in good health. In contrast, non-workplace environmental exposures are generally low level and often chronic. The population at risk contains the extremes of age, developing fetuses, and ill or immunocompromised persons.

The study of environmental health relies on epidemiology, toxicology, and microbiology. Epidemiology is the study of the distribution and determinants of health and disease in human population. Toxicology, the science of poisons, identifies adverse effects and predicts harmful dosages. One of the fundamental tenets of toxicology is that any substance can be a poison if given in a large enough dose. Microbiology deals with the scientific study of microorganisms, e.g., bacteria, viruses, and fungi.

Canadians are exposed to toxic substances through a variety of sources, including food, water, air, soil, and consumer products. Risk assessment, management, and communication are strategies for dealing with health risks posed by the environmental contaminants. There are four major steps in the risk assessment of any environmental contaminant. These are hazard identification, exposure determination and monitoring, dose-response determination, and risk determination. Risk management follows risk assessment and involves making decisions and implementing options for managing the identified risk. The communication of risk in relation to environmental hazards depends on the perception of risk by the public versus the perception of risk by experts.

Environmental health issues focus on the outdoor and indoor environment, water quality, food quality, and toxic chemicals. Factors in the outdoor and indoor environments that affect health consist of ionizing radiation, electromagnetic fields, noise pollution, light pollution, air pollution, ozone pollution and ozone depletion. Ionizing radiation, emitted from radioactive substances and the natural background, alters cell physiology. Due to conflicting research results, it is not yet clear whether or not electromagnetic fields are a health hazard. The main sources of exposure to these fields are high-voltage transmission lines, computers, electric blankets, fluorescent lighting, and household appliances. The adverse health effects of noise and light pollution are just starting to be considered and more research in these areas is needed. Air pollution results primarily from the incomplete combustion of fossil fuels, particularly by truck and motor vehicles. Recently, the depletion of ozone in the stratosphere has caused an increased incidence of skin cancer of all types including melanoma, cataracts, and depressed immune function. Acid rain refers to the oxidation of the sulphur and nitrogen precursors to acidic compounds. Carbon dioxide emissions from the combustion of fossil fuels are causing global warming through the greenhouse effect. Global warming has the potential to cause very significant climatic changes, which could, in turn, adversely affect humans through a variety of mechanisms. Smog is a combination of ground level ozone and inhalable particles and is a potent respiratory irritant that causes many hospital visits and early deaths each year. Increases in mortality and morbidity have been temporarily associated with periods of high atmospheric concentrations of pollutants. Thousands of hospital admissions and emergency room visits each year are due to the effects of air pollution.

With respect to water quality, the major chemical contaminants in water are PCBs, dioxins, furans, mercury, lead, and pesticides. Biological contamination of municipal drinking water supplies is of growing concern, in light of the recent tragic events in Walkerton, Ontario, and North Battleford, Saskatchewan.

With respect to food quality, the major concerns are contamination of food by microbial organisms, environmental contaminants, pesticide residues, chemicals, and food additives and preservatives.

Toxic chemicals include metals (such as lead, mercury, aluminum), PCBs, and dioxins. The toxicity of lead is multisystemic. PCBs and dioxins do not readily break down and hence persist in the environment. Because of this persistence, coupled with their tendency to accumulate in the fat of living organisms, they bioaccumulate in higher concentrations in those organisms near the top of the food chain. The same phenomenon of bioconcentration is also true of mercury.

A number of strategies have been proposed in order to create a safer environment, including those undertaken at the global level. These strategies consist of healthy public policy, waste management, and managing environmental accidents. Healthy public policy mobilizes many segments of the community to reduce the adverse health effects on humans that may result from deleterious environmental exposures. Measures include regulations and guidelines, education and advocacy, legislation, and community organization. Policies that support sustainable development also contribute to healthy public policy by trying to reverse the deterioration of the earth, prevent pollution, promote conservation, and sustain yield. It is the concept of productive economic activity that leaves resources in the natural environment intact. Waste management involves the disposal, destruction, or storage of solid waste, and sewage. The three main approaches to solid waste disposal in Canada are burial, incineration, and transformation. The best way to manage waste is for society to produce less and to reduce, reuse, recycle, and recover. The management of life-threatening exposures to toxic chemicals requires collaboration among several levels of government, and involves evaluating the problem, containing the problem, and assessing the health effects.

10.   REFERENCES

1.   Walkerton Inquiry. *Report of the Walkerton Inquiry: Parts I and II*. Toronto: Publication Ontario, Government of Ontario, 2002.
2.   de Krester D. Declining sperm counts. *British Medical Journal* 1996; 312(7029):457-8.
3.   Health Canada. *Health and environment: Partners for life*. Ottawa: Minister of Public Works and Government Services Canada, 1997.

4. Cole D, Kearney J. Blood cadmium, game consumption, and tobacco smoking in southern Ontario anglers and hunters. *Canadian Journal of Public Health* 1997; 88(1):44-6.

5. Health Canada. *A vital link: Health and the environment in Canada*. Ottawa: Health and Welfare Canada, 1992.

6. Health Canada. 1998. *The health and environment handbook for health professionals*. <www.hc-sc.gc.ca/ehp/ehd/catalogue/bch_pubs/98ehd211/98ehd211.htm> (January 2003).

7. McCally M. Environment and health: An overview. *Canadian Medical Association Journal* 2000; 163(5):533-5.

8. Speidel J. Environment and health: 1. Population, consumption and human health. *Canadian Medical Association Journal* 2000; 163(5):551-6.

9. Haines A, Michael A, Epstein P. Environment and health: 2. Global climate change and health. *Canadian Medical Association Journal* 2000; 163(6):729-34.

10. De Gruijl F, van der Leun J. Environment and health: 3. Ozone depletion and ultraviolet radiation. *Canadian Medical Association Journal* 2000; 163(7):851-5.

11. Clapp R. Environment and health: 4. Cancer. *Canadian Medical Association Journal* 2000; 163(8):1009-12.

12. Leaning J. Environment and health: 5. Impact of war. *Canadian Medical Association Journal* 2000; 163(9):1157-61.

13. Solomon G, Schettler T. Environment and health: 6. Endocrine disruption and potential human health implications. *Canadian Medical Association Journal* 2000; 163(11):1471-6.

14. Chivian E. Environment and health: 7. Species loss and ecosystem disruption – the implication for human health. *Canadian Medical Association Journal* 2001; 164(1):66-9.

15. Weir E. Identifying and managing adverse environmental effects: a new series. *Canadian Medical Association Journal* 2002; 166:1042-43.

16. Marshall L, Weir E, Abelsohn A. Identifying and managing adverse environmental effects: 1. Taking an exposure history. *Canadian Medical Association Journal* 2002; 166:1049-55.

17. Abelsohn A, Stieb D, Sanborn MD. *et al*. Identifying and managing adverse environmental effects: 2. Outdoor air pollution. *Canadian Medical Association Journal* 2002; 166:1161-67.

18. Sanborn MD, Abelsohn A, Campbell M, *et al*. Identifying and managing adverse environmental effects: 3. Lead exposure. *Canadian Medical Association Journal* 2002; 166:1287-92.

19. Sanborn MD, Cole D, Abelsohn A, *et al*. Identifying and managing adverse environmental effects: 4. Pesticides. *Canadian Medical Association Journal* 2002; 166:1431-36.

20. Abelsohn A, Gibson B, Sanborn MD, *et al*. Identifying and managing adverse environmental effects: 5. Persistent organic pollutants. *Canadian Medical Association Journal* 2002; 166:1549-54.

21. Abelsohn A, Sanborn MD, Jessiman B, *et al*. Identifying and managing adverse environmental effects: 6. Carbon monoxide poisoning. *Canadian Medical Association Journal* 2002; 166:1685-90.

22. Cole D, Upshur R, Gibson B. Detective work: Scoping the environmental burden of human illness. *Alternatives* 1999; 25(3):26-32.

23. Morgenstern H, Thomas D. Principles of study design in environmental epidemiology. *Environmental Health Perspectives Supplements* 1993; 101(s4):23-37.

24. Carpenter D, Arcaro K, Spink D. Understanding the human health effects of chemical mixtures. *Environmental Health Perspectives Supplements* 2002; 110 Supplements(1):25-42.

25. Eyles J, Taylor S, Baxter J, *et al*. The social construction of risk in a rural community. *Risk Analysis* 1993; 13:282-90.

26. Frank JW, Gibson B, McPherson M. Information needs in epidemiology: Detecting the health effects of environmental chemical exposure environment. In Fowler CD, Grim AP, Munn RE, editors. *Information needs for risk management*. Toronto: University of Toronto Press; 1988.

27. Cocco P. On the rumours about silent spring: Review of the scientific evidence linking occupational and environmental pesticide exposure to endocrine disruption health effects. *Cadernos de Saude Publica* 2002; 18(2):379-402.

28.   Colburn T, vom Saal F, Soto A. Developmental effects of endocrine disrupting chemicals in wildlife and humans. *Environmental Health Perspectives* 1993; 101:378-84.

29.   Sierra Club of Canada. 2003. *Hell on Earth — and in Canada*. <atlantic.sierraclub.ca/CB.htm> (January 2003).

30.   National Center for Environmental Health. 2003. *National Report on Human Exposure to Environmental Chemicals*. <www.cdc.gov/nceh/dls/report/factsheets/default.htm> (January 2003).

31.   U.S. Environmental Protection Agency. 2003. *Integrated risk information system.* <www.epa.gov/iris> (January 2003).

32.   Federal-Provincial Subcommittee on Drinking Water of the Federal-Provincial Committee on Environmental and Occupational Health. 2002. *Guidelines for Canadian drinking water quality.* 6th ed. <www.hc-sc.gc.ca/ehp/ehd/catalogue/bch_pubs/dwgsup_doc/dwgsup_doc.htm> (January 2003).

33.   Federal-Provincial Working Group on Recreational Water Quality of the Federal-Provincial Advisory Committee on Environmental and Occupational Health. *Guidelines for Canadian recreational water quality.* Ottawa: Minister of Supplies and Services, 1992.

34.   Macdonal R, Barrie L, Bidleman T, *et al.* Contaminants in the Canadian Arctic: Five years of progress in understanding sources, occurrence, and pathways. *The Science of the Total Environment* 2000; 254(2-3):93-234.

35.   Covelho V. Risk perception and communication. *Canadian Journal of Public Health* 1995; 86(2):78-9.

36.   Lubin J, Tomasek L, Edling C, *et al.* Estimating lung cancer mortality from residential radon using data for low exposures of miners. *Radiation Research* 1997; 147:126-37.

37.   Klich B. Medical symposium explores radiation risks and public concern. *Ontario Medical Review* 1992; 59(10):23-30.

38.   Draper G, Little M, Sorhan T, *et al.* Cancer in the offspring of radiation workers: A record linkage study. *British Medical Journal* 1997; 315(7117):1181-8.

39.   McLaughlin J, King W, Anderson T, *et al.* Paternal radiation exposure and leukaemia in offspring: The Ontario case-control study. *British Medical Journal* 1993; 307(6910):959-66.

40.   Miller A. Planning Cancer Control Strategies. *Chronic Disease in Canada* 1992; 13(1):1-40.

41.   Ahlbom I, Cardis E, Green A, *et al.* Review of the epidemiologic literature on EMF and health. *Environmental Health Perspectives* 2001; 109(Suppl 6):911-33.

42.   Frumkin H. Cellular phones and risk of brain tumors. *Cancer Journal for Clinicians* 2001; 51(2):137-41.

43.   Food and Drug Administration, U.S. *Cell phones facts.* <www.fda.gov/cellphones/wireless.html#2> (March 2003)

44.   Kompis M. Electromagnetic interference of bone anchored hearing aids by cellular phones. *Acta Oto-laryngologica* 2000; 120(7):855-9.

45.   Hayes D. Interference with cardiac pacemakers by cellular telephones. *New England Journal of Medicine* 1997; 336(21):1473-9.

46.   Canadian Safety Council. 2002. *Cell phone use skyrockets while road fatalities drop? Where's the evidence to ban car phone?* <www.safety-council.org/news/media/releases/feb6-cell.html> (September 2002).

47.   Stevens R. Lights in the built environment: Potential role of circadian disruption and endocrine disruption and breast cancer. *Cancer Causes and Control* 2001; 12(3):279-87.

48.   Berglund B, Lindvall T, Schwela D. *Guidelines for Community Noise*: World Health Organization, 1999. <www.who.int/peh/noise/guidelines2.html> (February 2003).

49.   Naus M. Health effects of acid rain exposure. *Ontario Disease Surveillance Report* 1988; 9(17):296-8.

50.   Last J, Troton K, Pengelly D. *One breath away: The health effects of air pollution and climate change*: David Suzuki Foundation, 1998.

51.   Ontario Medical Association. *The illness cost of air pollution: A summary of findings.* Toronto, 2000.

52. Ontario Medical Association. 2002. *Ontario's air: Years of stagnation.* <www.oma.org/phealth/smogmain.htm> (September 2002).
53. Ontario Medical Association. *Health effects of ground level ozone.* Toronto, 1998.
54. Government of Ontario. 2002. *What is the Air Quality Index.* <www.airqualityontario.com/science/aqi_description.cfm> (January 2003).
55. Gindi M. Ultraviolet radiation: A public health perspective. *Public Health and Epidemiology Reports Ontario* 1992; 3(9):136-40.
56. United Nations Environment Programme. 2001. *Backgrounder: Basic facts and data on the science and politics of ozone protection.* <www.unep.org/ozone/reprts.shtml> (September 2002).
57. Environment Canada. 1996. *Canada's ozone layer protection program: A summary.* Ottawa. <www.ec.gc.ca/ozone/odsr/english/index.html> (September 2002).
58. Federal-Provincial Advisory Committee on Environmental and Occupational Health. *Exposure guidelines for residential indoor air quality.* Ottawa: Ministry of Supply and Services, Government of Canada, 1995.
59. U.S. National Center for Environmental Health. 2002. *Questions and answers on Stachbotrys cartarum and other molds.* <www.cdc.gov/nceh/airpollution/mold/stachy.htm> (September 2002).
60. North Battleford Water Inquiry CLR. 2002. *Report of the Commission of Inquiry into matters relating to the safety of the public drinking water in the city of North Battleford, Saskatchewan.* Battleford. <www.northbattleforwateinquiry.ca/inquiry/inquiry.htm> (September 2002).
61. Department of Public Health, City of Toronto. *The quality of drinking water in Toronto: A review of tap water, bottled water, and water treated by a point-of-use device.* Toronto: City of Toronto, 1990.
62. Locker D. 1999. *Benefits and risks of water fluoridation: An update of the 1996 Federal-Provincial Sub-committee report.* <www.gov.on.ca/MOH/english/pub/ministry/fluoridation/fluor.pdf> (January 2003).
63. Environment Canada. 1996. *The state of Canada's environment, 1996.* <www2.ec.gc.ca/soer-ree/English/SOER/1996report/Doc/1-9-1.cfm> (September 2002).
64. Government of Ontario, Ministry of the Environment. 2003. *The 2001-2002 guide to eating Ontario sport fish.* <www.cne.gov.on.ca/envision/guide> (February 2003).
65. Rice D. Neurotoxicity of lead, methylmercury, and PCBs in relation to the Great Lakes. *Environmental Health Perspectives* 1995; 103 (Suppl 9):71-87.
66. Olson K, editor. *Poisoning and drug overdose.* 3rd ed. Stamford, CT: Appleton & Lange; 1999.
67. Flaten T. Aluminum as a risk factor in Alzheimer's disease, with emphasis on drinking water. *Brain Research Bulletin* 2001; 15(55(2)):187-96.
68. Hoover S. Exposure to persistent organochlorines in Canadian breast milk: A probabilistic assessment. *Risk Analysis* 1999; 19(4):527-45.
69. Health Canada. 2002. *New Pest Control Product Act.* <www.hc-sc.gc.ca/pmra-arla/english/legis/pcpa-e.html> (January 2003).
70. Meggs W, Dunn K, Bloch R, *et al.* Prevalence and nature of allergy and chemical sensitivity in a general population. *Archives of Environmental Health* 1996; 5(4):275-82.
71. Graveling R, Pilkington A, George J, *et al.* A review of multiple chemical sensitivity. *Occupational and Environmental Medicine* 1999; 56(2):73-85.
72. Sparks P, Daniell W, Black D, *et al.* Multiple chemical sensitivity syndrome: A clinical perspective. 1. Case definition, theories of pathogenesis, and research needs. *Journal of Occupational Medicine* 1994; 36(7):718-30.
73. Staudenmayer H. Psychological treatment of psychogenic idiopathic environmental intolerance. *Occupational Medicine* 2000; 15(3):627-46.
74. Rose G. Environmental factors and disease: The man-made environment. *British Medical Journal* 1987; 294(6577):963-5.

75.   Nutbeam D. *Health promotion glossary*. Geneva: World Health Organization, 1998.

76.   Guidotti T. Managing incidents involving hazardous substances. *American Journal of Preventative Medicine* 1986; 2(3):148-54.

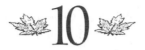

10

OCCUPATIONAL HEALTH AND DISEASE

Most adults spend a considerable amount of time at their workplace and are exposed to a variety of work-related situations. Some of these situations are pleasant, but others expose the workers to stressful situations, and also to physical, chemical, mechanical, ergonomic, and biological hazards. The effects of these hazards are not always immediate and some have a long latency period. This chapter deals with the impact of the workplace environment as it relates to Canadian workers.

1.   OCCUPATIONAL HEALTH

Occupational health is defined as the maintenance and promotion of health in the work environment. The delivery of occupational health services involves physicians, nurses, hygienists, engineers and safety officers, ergonomists, chiropractors, physicists, and technicians. The jurisdiction for enforcement of occupational health legislation lies with the provinces. Exceptions to this are 16 federally regulated industries covered under the Canada Labour Code, such as the grain industry and the transportation industry. Because of this provincial jurisdiction, there are variations in legislation and regulations governing occupational health across Canada. However, the principles of the worker's right to know, the worker's right to refuse dangerous work, and the need for workers and management to participate on joint safety and health committees exist across most of the country. The joint safety and health committee is an important bipartite forum where employees and employers can manage issues of concern.

The work environment contains a wide range of potential environmental exposure grouped as chemical (e.g., solvents, poisons), physical (e.g., radiation, noise), biological (e.g., blood products, viruses), mechanical and ergonomic (e.g., repetitive strains, awkward posture), and psychosocial (e.g., stress, isolation). Protecting the worker from exposure to these factors requires a commitment on the part of management to ensure that activities are carried out in the areas of health promotion (worker education and work design), health protection and disease prevention (protecting workers from hazards and monitoring the health of the worker), and rehabilitation (returning the worker to safe, meaningful, productive work).

1.1.   CANADIAN WORKFORCE

Although most of Canada's wealth has traditionally come from natural resources, today it is a modern country with most of its workers employed in the service sector. In 2001, there were approximately 16.2 million people in the workforce, 11.7 million of whom were employed in service industries. Although men outnumber women in the total workforce — 8.8 million to 7.5 million — there is a slightly higher representation of women in service industries (6.3 million women to 5.4 million men). This is due to the fact that men are to a greater extent over-represented in the goods-producing industry: 3.2 million men to 1.0 million women. Statistics Canada defines the goods-producing industry as including manufacturing, construction, utilities, agriculture, and the other primary industries (fishing, trapping, logging, mining, quarrying). All other sectors of industry, including government, are considered services. The gender distribution of workers in the following employment sectors is as follows: manufacturing, 2.4 million total, of whom 71.5% are male; construction, of whom 0.9 million (89.8%) are male; and agriculture, of whom 0.2 million (70.8%) are male. The sex distribution suggests that gender is a determinant with respect to type of workplace injury encountered (1).

1.2.   HEALTH INDICATORS AMONG CANADIAN WORKERS

The Association of Workers' Compensation Boards of Canada (AWCBC) collects information from the provincial and territorial workers' compensation boards (WCBs). Common classifiable occupational injuries and diseases that cause time-loss injuries are musculoskeletal injuries, injuries to nerves, spinal cord and bones, superficial wounds, nervous system and sense organ disease, digestive system disease and disorders, and mental disorders and syndromes.

In 2000, there were 392,502 lost-time injuries and 882 fatalities related to activity in the workplace. This amounts to an incidence rate of 2.5 lost-time workplace injuries per 100 workers and a workplace fatality rate of 5.5 per 100,000 workers. On average, this works out to 2.4 fatalities every day.

Of the total 392,502 lost-time injuries in 2000, 29% occurred in manufacturing, 11% in the retail trade, 10% in the health and social service industries, 8% in the construction industry, and the remainder 42% in other sectors. Of the 882 fatalities, 209 (24%) occurred in manufacturing, 148 (17%) in construction, 122 (14%) in transportation and storage, and 98 (11%) in mining, quarrying, and oil wells. The highest annual incidence of occupational fatality rates per 10,000 workers employed in Canada for 2000 were as follows: mining, 5.7; fishing and trapping, 4.4; logging and forestry, 3.2; construction, 1.7; transportation, 1.5; and manufacturing, 0.9 (1, 2).

The economic impact of occupational injuries is measurable in both direct and indirect costs (see Chapter 5). Compensation payments to workers by WCBs for 2000 totalled approximately $5 billion, of which $2.1 billion was paid out by Ontario's WCB (the highest of all the provinces and territories); as indirect costs generally equal compensation claims, the estimated cost to the Canadian economy for 2000 is at least $10 billion (3).

Injuries account for 90% of all compensated cases by WCBs; the remainder are occupational diseases (2, 3).

1.3. ISSUES RELATED TO OCCUPATIONAL HEALTH DATA

Injury and illness prevention are among the most important issues in occupational health. The lack of coordinated data collection in Canada has long been recognized as a major hindrance to the prevention of occupational injury and illness (4-6). One of the problems is deciding who should be responsible for collecting this information — a difficult problem as occupational health falls under federal, provincial, and territorial jurisdictions, and potential occupational exposure data are collected from hospitals, primary care physicians, emergency room visits, medical examiner reports, health surveys, death certificates, occupational medicine specialists, industry, cancer registries, health insurance firms, and WCBs. In fact, WCBs provide the bulk of the information, with cancer registries and health insurance firms providing most of the rest of the information. Unfortunately, these sources of information remain largely unrealized. WCB data tend to be imperfect; the data focus mostly on the illness of the worker with little information on any substances to which all workers were exposed in the same work situation, i.e., pooled exposure data. Information is collected from the WCBs through the AWCBC.

Epidemiological studies require unique patient-identifying data, accurate medical diagnosis, acceptable causes of disease, and defined industry and occupation coding — none of which is accepted as the standard today.

An additional problem exists with the interpretation of epidemiological data, even if data collection is satisfactory, as there is the confounding effect of non-occupational disease. For example, when researchers try to determine the causation between coal mining and lung cancer, smoking becomes an extremely powerful confounding factor. This makes for challenging study design as well as problematic WCB compensation claims in miners who smoke.

In addition to lifestyle, there is also the issue of genetic, or inherent, disease. For instance, not all asthma in workers is due to exposure to sensitizers, such as diisocyanates. A segment of these asthma cases would have developed even without sensitizing exposures in the workplace. The realization of the confounding effect of non-occupational disease presents a special problem in occupational epidemiology. As the stakes are high from the worker's perspective with respect to compensation for illness, it is very important for both worker and employer that the employer performs the proper preplacement and periodic health screening examinations.

2. OCCUPATIONAL HEALTH RESOURCES

Occupational health resources are based in government, industry, educational institutions, union-based centres, and hospitals. The federal government's jurisdictional responsibility in occupational health is mainly for federal employees and a few special sectors, such as banks, nuclear power, and transportation. The federal government relies on two ministries to set standards and provide appropriate health services: Labour Canada and Health Canada. The provinces have the most responsibility for occupational health. At the provincial level, regulatory responsibility lies with one or more departments or ministries (the Ministry of Labour is usually the lead agency; others with responsibility are the Ministry of Mining and the Ministry of Health). Services are provided to the civil service by the Ministry of Government Services. Major industries have corporate medical departments where company-hired healthcare professionals are responsible for the surveillance and monitoring of workers as prescribed by law and corporate policy. The range of healthcare professionals hired depends on the size and complexity of the industry or corporation and may include a physician, nurse, industrial hygienist, psychologist, chiropractors, and physiotherapists. Educational institutions, hospitals, union-based centres, and consultants provide some, if not all, occupational health services on a fee-for-service basis or through other payment mechanisms. The occupational health services provide health promotion and health protection (primary prevention), management of injury and illness (secondary prevention), and rehabilitation services (tertiary prevention).

There are no legislated requirements for specific health and safety expertise in the workforce. Consequently, there is a wide variation in the skill set available for ensuring a safe and healthy work environment. In smaller companies there may be no one assigned the role of a health and safety professional. In larger companies there may be a large healthcare staff, often led by a physician, which could include industrial hygienists, nurses, and technicians. Generally, at any particular site an occupational health nurse or a safety professional serves in the day-to-day health and safety function. A physician may be called upon to provide diagnostic information or act as a consultant with respect to return-to-work programs or health surveillance. The industrial hygienist is usually concerned with monitoring the environment for workplace hazards and protecting the worker from these hazards. Engineers play a role in designing any process with safety in mind, substituting dangerous materials, and implementing changes to the work environment to protect the worker with engineering controls where necessary. Clearly, however, these are generalizations and, except where mandated by professional requirements (e.g., diagnosing disease by physicians and designing equipment by professional engineers), there is a great deal of variability in what various degrees of training can bring to the workforce.

The specifics of corporate responsibility to workers' safety are determined to a large part by the provincial legislation; however, there are three aspects that are universal across the country. The first is the concept of **due diligence**. That is, the employer must demonstrate that reasonable steps were taken to become familiar with the inherent dangers in the workplace and that action was taken to ensure that the workplace was safe. Ignorance is no excuse for an unsafe workplace if it can be demonstrated that no effort was made to understand the hazards of the workplace.

Second, the federally legislated **Workplace Hazardous Materials Information System (WHMIS)** applies across Canada (see Chapter 13). The WHMIS is intended to ensure that workers are protected from hazards in the workplace by labelling all chemical substances in the workplace, educating all workers at the work site with respect to the WHMIS program, and by keeping a centralized record of all hazards in the workplace on Material Safety Data Sheets (MSDSs), which detail important information on handling hazardous substances and cleaning up spills properly(7).

Third, provincial occupational health and safety acts mandate the existence of *joint health and safety committees*. These committees are composed of representatives drawn from both management and workers. Their purpose is to identify workplace health and safety hazards and to communicate their concerns to management in writing. Workers must be granted time, with pay, to prepare for and attend committee meetings and to participate in inspections of the workplace.

2.1. HEALTH PROMOTION AND HEALTH PROTECTION

As already explained, the prevention of injury and illness is very important for maintaining the physical, mental, and social well-being of employees in the workplace. The goal of **primary prevention** is to take action in the workplace so that the worker is protected from injury and illness. These interventions can take place at the source, along the path, or at the worker level. Ideally, of course, this is the preferred level of prevention and includes such activities as identifying hazards in the workplace (**hazard identification**), assessing the actual level of risk associated with the identified hazards (**risk assessment**), and reducing exposure to environmental stressors in the workplace (through risk control and risk communication), similar to those described in Chapter 9. **Risk control** is achieved through the reduction of exposure, which can be achieved in a variety of ways, such as engineering practices; an example is substitution — the replacement of a hazardous substance with one that is less hazardous, such as replacing silica powder with a silica-free inert powder in the moulding trade. Other engineering practices include enclosure — the physical containment of hazards — and exhausting (or ventilation). Enclosure and exhausting are sometimes collectively referred to as segregation methods to reduce worker exposure.

Industrial engineers use several methods for setting standards for the exposure limits to hazardous substances in the work environment. When legislation recognizes these limits, they constitute legal standards. Where levels are not defined, the acceptable code of practice is usually based on a 40-hour work week (i.e., 8 hours a day). Industrial engineers rely on **threshold limit values** (TLVs). TLVs place a limit on exposure as measured by **time-weighted averages** (TWAs). The TWA concentration is calculated for a conventional 8-hour workday and a 40-hour workweek, which is what most workers are exposed to repeatedly, day after day, without adverse effect. The American Conference of Governmental Industrial Hygienists sets guidelines for these values, based on the assumption that a small percentage of workers will suffer adverse effects as a result of exposure at the set TLV and TWA, and publishes them (8). The values are revised if the scientific literature provides justification. In Ontario, there is a list of designated substances that are considered to be particularly hazardous (see Table 10.1). Legislated regulations specify the procedures for control of each substance. Employers must assess the likelihood of worker exposure and, in conjunction with

Table 10.1   Designated Substances in Ontario

Acrylonitrile	Coke Oven Emissions	Mercury
Arsenic	Ethylene Oxide	Silica
Asbestos	Isocyanates	Vinyl Chloride
Benzene	Lead	

Ontario's Joint Health and Safety Committee, institute a control program that includes engineering controls, work practices, hygiene practices, record keeping, and medical surveillance, if applicable. Administrative strategies for controlling exposure include job rotation, whereby employees rotate through jobs that have exposure to hazardous materials and minimize exposure to certain repetitive tasks. Work practice strategies include clean working procedures and wetting down surfaces contaminated with dust. Personal protection equipment for the worker is the control strategy of last resort, because it is expensive to purchase and maintain, training is generally required, and equipment must be individually fitted. Nonetheless, personal protection equipment can be very effective provided the worker wears the equipment. Non-compliance is commonly a problem in the workplace, as personal protection equipment is often uncomfortable to wear and the long-term benefits of improved health are often not perceived as desirable as the relief afforded in removing the equipment.

2.1.1.   Healthy Lifestyle Promotion

Health promotion in the workplace has emerged as an effective approach, enabling access to the substantial number of people in the workplace not only for prevention of work-associated health problems, but also for wellness programs that incorporate attention to lifestyle and other health determinants (9-11). These determinants include the broad, systemic, and social conditions or environments that influence employee health. Specific work practices, job design, work process, and lifestyle may need change. A comprehensive approach beyond lifestyle, based on community development and healthy public policy strategies, as discussed in Chapter 1, is relevant. For example, provision of a daycare centre on-site and flexible work hours facilitate the health of female employees of child-rearing age. Small group development and community organizing can enhance worker empowerment. Joint collaboration among employers and workers, beyond the collective bargaining process, helps fulfill employee needs as well as achieve organizational goals.

Health promotion programs in the workplace have many potential benefits to offer the employer as well as the employees. These benefits include reduction of employee healthcare costs, disability, and turnover; enhancement of the company image; and improving employee productivity (12).

The federal government has developed the Corporate Model of a Workplace Health System for interested employers (13). Employers can request a survey of workers' health and health concerns to determine their health needs. The survey is then analyzed and recommendations made, in conjunction with management, through a workplace health committee that then develops prevention programs for prevalent problems or risk factors. Recently, the emphasis has moved away from providing expensive gymnasiums and equipment, which were part of the initial response to health promotion in the workplace by larger companies. They now often include dietary advice, including attention to the type of items offered by the cafeteria (if one is provided), stress management, and smoking cessation counselling, as well as opportunities for enhancing fitness and broader changes to the work environment as discussed above (11).

Smoking cessation programs have been extensively studied and are one of the few lifestyle programs that are justifiable to employers based on cost effectiveness alone, as the investment in the program is less than the savings achieved through a reduction in absenteeism from smoking-related illnesses. Other healthy lifestyle programs include blood pressure reduction, weight loss, alcohol and caffeine moderation, and cholesterol reduction.

Employee assistance programs (EAPs) help employees deal with stress. They provide for a third party to be available for counselling services to help employees deal with workplace and home problems (which may include stress of relationships, financial issues, or drug or alcohol abuse).

2.2. DISEASE PREVENTION

The goal of disease prevention (primary and secondary prevention) is to monitor workers' health in order to prevent the development of disease. Secondary prevention in occupational health involves the use of preplacement and periodic examinations. The preplacement examination findings help in establishing an individual's baseline characteristics. Periodic examinations facilitate early, and often presymptomatic, diagnosis and may also serve as an early indicator of the effectiveness of plant hygiene controls.

It must be emphasized that the periodic exams are not the regular check-ups performed by the family physician but are highly selective examinations that focus on the organ systems at risk due to specific hazards in the work environment. This includes directed histories (with emphasis on specific symptoms), directed physicals, and appropriate physiological, biochemical, and imaging studies. For example, a worker exposed to lead will have a physical examination that focuses on mental function and signs of renal failure, in addition to routine biochemical analysis of hemoglobin and kidney function, and to check the blood lead level. Another aspect of secondary prevention in the workplace is the issue of employee screening for substance abuse. Mandatory pre-employment and random testing have been introduced in many industries in the United States. The Canadian Medical Association (CMA) is opposed to routine pre-employment drug testing and recommends that random drug testing among employees be restricted to safety-sensitive positions and undertaken only when measures of performance and effective peer or supervisory observation are unavailable (14). Although a great many drugs can be detected in urine, the tests do not indicate when the substance was used, as levels may persist for weeks. There is also individual variation between levels detected and extent of impairment of work performance, which is the most germane issue. The most commonly abused substance, alcohol, is generally not tested for as the emphasis has been on detecting illicit drugs. The issue generates much concern with regard to civil liberties.

If substance abuse is detected, whether by organized screening or by observation of impaired performance, such as may occur with alcoholism, an organizational response is warranted. This includes provision of counselling and cessation programs, and many employers offer employee assistance programs for those with alcohol problems.

2.3.   REHABILITATION

Tertiary prevention in occupational health refers to the treatment of injury or illness with the safe return to the workforce in the most timely and appropriate manner. A rapid return to the workplace reflects the employer's desire to reduce costs associated with a worker's absence while convalescing and the employee's desire to be a functioning and productive member of society. The cornerstones of a successful rapid return-to-work philosophy include the prompt initiation of treatment and rehabilitation and the return to the workplace as soon as possible, using a modified program where appropriate. A modified program is work that has been selected to accommodate any limitations that the worker may have while recovering. The CMA has published guidelines for the physician's role in helping the worker to a safe return to meaningful work following injury or illness. These focus on the physician's role in diagnosing and treating injury or illness, advising the worker, communicating, and working with the worker and the employer to facilitate the return to productive employment (15, 16).

Following a work-related injury or illness, the individual may be temporarily or permanently disabled. If these individuals are covered under their provincial workers' compensation act, financial compensation is available for rehabilitation services.

2.3.1.   Workers' Compensation Board

The injury and disease related to work are compensable in all provinces and territories. The agency that deals with compensation in most provinces is called the Workers' Compensation Board (WCB); in Ontario it is called the Workplace Safety and Insurance Board. Workers' compensation falls within the jurisdiction of provincial statutes, although the general principles are uniform across Canada. The main features are as follows: the WCB is autonomous, employers pay for costs, and the WCB decides benefits. First aid, medical treatment, lost time, and rehabilitation are covered for most workers; negligence is not considered a factor — it is a no-fault insurance system, and workers abdicate their right to sue the employer. The employer must notify the WCB within a specified time (ascribed in legislation) of an employee's becoming injured and is responsible for first aid to the worker and transport to hospital. The treating physician should submit a report to the WCB (in Quebec reporting is mandatory). In addition to treatment, the WCB offers rehabilitation consisting of physiotherapy, occupational therapy, counselling, social work, and chiropractic services for accepted claims.

3. COMMON OCCUPATIONAL EXPOSURES

The balance of this chapter provides a brief overview of the clinical aspects of common occupational exposures and diseases. More detailed clinical reviews are available in textbooks on occupational medicine, some of which are included in the bibliography (17-19).

The occupational health history must be a routine component of any health history (17, 20). When occupational disease is suspected, the history should be suitably detailed. Generally speaking, there are two main parts: a work history, which includes exposure and controls, and a health history, which reviews the symptoms in order to determine any relationship to work. While this history is being elicited, other significant environmental exposures (such as hobbies or travel history) should also be ascertained. Although occupational diseases have their origin in the working environment, it should be noted that similar diseases can also be caused by non-occupational exposures, the distinction being the location of the exposure.

The agents that cause occupational disease may be divided into five broad groups: chemical, physical, biological, mechanical and ergonomic, and psychosocial. At the time of diagnosis, certain conditions must be fulfilled before attributing causality to the workplace as described in Chapter 2. These conditions, where applicable, include adequate concentration and duration of exposure, absorption by the body, appropriate temporal sequence, and consistency of ill-health effects with the putative exposure. The list of occupational diseases may be endless. However, this chapter focuses on those deemed significant because of their frequency of occurrence in Canada or the severity of the disability produced. Known or highly suspected carcinogens in the workplace are listed in Table 10.2.

3.1. CHEMICAL AGENTS

3.1.1. Organic Dusts

Organic dusts contain carbon and are largely derived from substances of animal or plant origin. Common examples are dusts and fibres arising from the handling or manufacture of wood, bone, shell, fur, skins, hides, leather, brooms, straw, flour, grain, tobacco, jute, flax (linen), hemp, cotton, wool, felt, carpets, rag, paper, or sweepings.

Most organic dusts do not cause lung disease of a specific disabling nature. Many are irritants to the upper respiratory passages and to the conjunctivae and skin, causing bronchitis, conjunctivitis, and dermatitis. However, many organic dusts may cause sensitization and induce occupational asthma in exposed workers. Workers may exhibit no outward symptoms until they are exposed to a dust to which they have been sensitized, and develop an allergic reaction characterized by a decrease in the vital capacity of the lung from a normal level of about 5 litres to 2.5 or 3 litres as well as a

Table 10.2.   Examples of Known Carcinogens in the Workplace

Carcinogen	Target organ in humans
Aflatoxins	Liver
Aluminum production	Lung, bladder, and others
4-aminobiphenyl	Bladder
Arsenic and arsenic compounds	Lung, skin
Asbestos	Lung, pleura, peritoneum
Benzene	Hematopoietic system
Benzidine	Bladder
Beryllium	Lung
Bis(chloromethyl) ether	Lung
Cadmium	Lung
Chromium VI	Lung
Coal-tar pitches	Skin, lung, bladder
Coke production	Skin, bladder, respiratory tract, kidneys, large intestine, pancreas
Erionite	Pleura
Ethylene oxide	Lymphatic, hematopoietic
Mineral oils	Skin
Mustard gas	Pharynx, lung
2-Naphthylamine	Bladder
Neutrons	Leukemia, ovarian, mammary, lung, liver
Nickel and nickel compounds	Nasal cavity, lung
Plutonium 239 and decay products	Various
Radon	Lung
Shale oils	Skin
Silica, crystalline	Lung
Solar radiation	Skin
Soots	Skin, lung, esophagus, liver, hematopoietic system
Talc containing asbestiform fibres	Lung
2,3,7,8-Tetrachloro-dibenzo-p-dioxin	Lung, soft tissue
Tobacco smoke	Lung, bladder, oral cavity, pharynx, larynx, esophagus
Vinyl chloride	Liver, lung, blood vessels
X and gamma radiation	Hematopoietic system, mamary, lung, thyroid

Source: Adapted from R. Clapp. Environment and health: 4. Cancer. *Canadian Medical Association Journal* 2000; 163(8):1009-12. <www.cmaj.ca/cgi/reprint/163/8/1009> (February 2003).

decrease in the timed forced expiratory ventilation fractions (FEV1) indicating bronchiolar spasm. They may complain of wheezing, and dyspnea (shortness of breath). Such adverse effects are usually relieved by cessation of the exposure, and tend to recur when the person returns to the job. A typical history includes symptoms of cough, wheezing, or shortness of breath, worsening during the workweek with improvement on weekends and holidays.

Other substances such as isocyanates may also cause occupational asthma. In fact, isocyanates are the most common cause of occupational asthma in many industrial jurisdictions.

3.1.2. Mineral Dusts

No dust can be regarded as entirely harmless; however, for practical purposes mineral dusts can be divided into two classes: active and inert. The majority of dusts encountered, industrially or otherwise, are relatively inert. Some of the inert dusts may cause radiological pulmonary shadowing from the deposition of radio-opaque material in the lungs, without initiating fibrosis or loss of pulmonary function. Their main importance lies in the problem they present in differential diagnosis. Siderosis, which is due to the deposition of iron dust in the lung, is probably the most frequently encountered non-disabling pneumoconiosis.

Among the active dusts, silica and asbestos are the chief offenders in producing disabling pulmonary disease in this country. It has been conclusively established that the vast majority (more than 90%) of the particles that reach the alveoli are less than 3 microns (3/1000 mm) in diameter. Most particles larger than 3 microns either settle out of the air before it is breathed or are trapped in the secretions of the nose and throat and are eliminated or swallowed. As a rule, dusts vary greatly in size, depending to some extent upon the mechanical processes involved in their production, for example, wet versus dry drilling of hard rock.

Silica

With regard to the numbers of people exposed and cases of disability produced, free silica (silicon dioxide, SiO_2) is the chief cause of pulmonary dust disease; in contrast, combined silica (silicate, SiO_3) is probably inert. Silica is the main constituent of sand, sandstone, and granite, and is present in iron ore and coal. Exposure to crystalline silica occurs in several occupations (such as hard rock mining, sandblasting, and granite cutting). The three most common crystalline forms of silica encountered in the workplace environment are quartz, tridymite, and cristobalite (21). The approximate average duration of exposure required for the development of silicosis varies widely for different occupations, from five years in unprotected sandblasting to 30 years in moulders and granite cutters. The prolonged inhalation of dusts containing free silica may result in a disabling pulmonary fibrosis known as silicosis. Silicosis, usually a nodular pulmonary fibrosis, is the disease most associated with exposure to respirable crystalline silica (particle size less than 10 microns (22). It is characterized by generalized fibrotic changes and the development of miliary nodules in both lungs and by shortness of breath, decreased chest expansion, lessened capacity for work, absence of fever, increased susceptibility, or reactivation of tuberculosis (some or all of these symptoms may be present), and x-ray findings that show rounded opacities, localized initially to upper lung fields, and "egg shell" calcification of hilar lymph nodes in a minority of cases.

In diagnosing silicosis, one must ascertain whether the worker was exposed to silica and, if so, whether sufficient exposure to cause the disease occurred. The x-ray on its own is of little value in determining disability and in fact may be misleading.

In 1996, the International Agency for Research on Cancer added silica to the list of group I substances described as carcinogenic to humans. It is, however, still unclear whether silica exposure in the absence of silicosis carries increased risk for lung cancer (23).

Asbestos

Canada is one of the principal asbestos-producing countries in the world. There are many types of asbestos, including chrysotile, amosite, and crocidolite. Canada produces mainly chrysotile, which is chiefly hydrated magnesium silicate that occurs as a white fibrous ore. The fibres, when separated, may be spun into yarn and woven in much the same manner as ordinary textiles, or they may be ground and mixed with other materials to form insulating boards or sheets. Exposure to the dust occurs in the crushing, carding, spinning, and weaving of the material, and in the manufacture of brake linings and insulating products.

The essential lesion in asbestosis is a diffuse fibrosis, which probably begins as a "collar" around the terminal bronchioles. Usually, at least 4 to 7 years of exposure are required before a serious degree of fibrosis occurs. There have, however, been cases reported in workers exposed to extremely high levels of asbestos for less than 1 month. Asbestosis does not cause predisposition to tuberculosis as seen in silicosis. Lung cancer is a known complication of asbestos exposure. Asbestosis does not need to be present in order for a diagnosis of lung cancer due to asbestos exposure to be made. The sentinel malignancy for asbestosis is mesothelioma, which has a long latency period (24).

Coal

Graphite is a crystalline form of carbon; ash-free anthracite coal is an amorphous form of the same element. In their pure state, these dusts cause no fibrosis of the lung. As they occur in nature, however, graphite and anthracite frequently contain considerable amounts of free silica, and exposed workers may develop a modified form of silicosis or coal worker's pneumoconiosis characterized by small, diffusely scattered, stellate patches of fibrosis, each surrounded by an area of focal emphysema. Like true silicosis, coal worker's pneumoconiosis may be disabling. The incidence of the disease is proportional to the concentration of silica dust in the air and to the length of exposure.

3.1.3. Heavy Metals

Lead

The use of lead is widespread in industry. The occupations that expose workers to the highest levels of lead are the manufacture of storage batteries and the reclamation of scrap metal. Exposure also occurs in soldering operations and lead burning, in the manufacture of paints containing lead, and in the sanding of surfaces coated with lead paints. Other exposures occur in the printing trade, the breaking up of ships coated with lead paints, the glazing of pottery, the manufacture and use of certain insecticides, and the blending of tetraethyl lead gasoline additive. The environmental aspects of lead contamination are described in Chapter 9.

The toxicity of lead compounds depends upon several factors: the solubility in body fluids, the size of the particles (solubility is inversely proportional to particle size), and conditions under which the compound is used. Where a lead compound is used as a powder, atmospheric contamination is reduced if the powder is kept damp. Of the various lead compounds, the carbonate, the monoxide, and the sulphate are considered to be more toxic than metallic lead or other lead compounds.

Acute lead poisoning is rarely encountered in industry today. Chronic lead poisoning occurs from the inhalation or ingestion of small amounts of lead dust, fumes, or vapours over a relatively long period of time. The early diagnosis of lead poisoning is often difficult since the presenting symptoms are non-specific (see also Chapter 9). To make a diagnosis of occupational lead poisoning, the following criteria must be met: there must be a history of significant exposure to lead at work, there must be clinical signs and symptoms compatible with lead poisoning, and there must be supportive laboratory evidence (i.e., increased blood lead levels). It also requires the medical professional to be cognizant of the possibility of the occupational hazard of lead in order to consider the diagnosis.

Ideally, prevention of lead poisoning consists of avoiding exposure to lead. Minimum requirements for surveillance of workers exposed to lead consist of a periodic medical examination and periodic inquiry into general health, together with blood lead level measurements.

Mercury

Mercury and mercury compounds are used widely in many industries. For example, they are used in the manufacture of scientific instruments and industrial chemicals, in the photographic industry, in the pharmaceutical industry, in dentistry, in power generators, and in the manufacture of amalgams with copper, tin, silver, and gold. The effects of mercury toxicity are described in Chapter 9.

Cadmium

Today the largest use of cadmium is in the electroplating industry. Almost all industrial exposures are due to the inhalation of fumes emitted in smelting impure zinc, in distilling cadmium sponge, or in welding or burning cadmium-plated metal. The effects of acute and chronic cadmium toxicity are described in Chapter 9.

Nickel

Nickel is used in the manufacture of alloys of iron, chromium, and tungsten. Its salts are also used widely. In industry, exposure occurs through the inhalation of the dusts and fumes that are byproducts of the production of the metal. Nickel and its salts are not considered to cause systemic poisoning. Cases of lung and sinus cancer have been found in greater than normal numbers among men employed in calcining and sintering operations. However, the most common effect resulting from exposure to nickel compounds is the development of a contact allergic dermatitis ("nickel itch") seen most commonly in people doing nickel plating.

3.1.4. Volatile Solvents and Organic Materials

Use of solvents is ubiquitous in many industries. Most solvent exposure occurs through inhalation and skin absorption. The effects of solvent exposure are similar to those that occur with alcohol intoxication. Benzene is one of the most toxic solvents used commercially. It is a natural component of petroleum and is added to gasoline as an octane enhancer and as an anti-knock agent. In acute poisoning, the worker rapidly develops a disturbance of the central nervous system that may manifest itself as headache, nausea, dizziness, convulsions, or coma. In non-fatal cases, recovery is usually complete. With chronic exposure, aplastic anemia or leukemia may develop. Toluene and xylene are closely related chemically to benzene but are less toxic and do not produce the same effects; however, these have been contaminated with benzene in the past.

Chlorinated hydrocarbons are used widely in oils, greases, and waxes. They are generally nonflammable, and their toxicity to the liver and kidney ranges from very high to very low. Carbon tetrachloride is the most toxic of this group. Following exposures to high concentrations, the worker may become unconscious and, if exposure is not terminated, death can follow from respiratory failure. Exposure to lower concentrations, insufficient to produce unconsciousness, usually results in severe gastrointestinal upset and may progress to serious kidney and hepatic damage. The use of solvents such as n-hexane, methyl butyl ketone, and 1,1,1-trichloroethane has been associated with peripheral sensory neuropathy (25).

Methyl Alcohol

Methyl alcohol is used as a solvent in the manufacture of lacquers, varnishes, shellac, and cleaning and polishing materials. In industry, exposure occurs mainly through inhalation of the vapour, but also via absorption through the skin. Severe exposure leads to dizziness, unconsciousness, cardiac depression, and, eventually, death. In mild to moderate exposure, blurring of vision, photophobia, and conjunctivitis, followed by blindness, may occur secondary to the metabolism of methyl alcohol to toxic formic acid.

3.1.5. Gases

Industrial gases may be divided into three groups: those irritating to the upper respiratory tract (e.g., ammonia, sulphur dioxide), those that are toxic (e.g., carbon monoxide, arsine), and those that are asphyxiants and displace oxygen (e.g., methane, nitrogen).

Sulphur Dioxide

Sulphur dioxide (SO_2) occurs widely in industry. High concentrations produce immediate irritation of the eyes and coughing and cannot be tolerated for very long. Continued exposure may result in edema of the larynx and lungs, and bronchopneumonia. Repeated exposure to the gas results in nasopharyngitis, bronchitis, shortness of breath on exertion, increased fatigue, and alteration of the sense of taste and smell.

Carbon Monoxide

Carbon monoxide (CO) is produced by the incomplete combustion of carbon-containing materials. Poisoning is most commonly from automobile exhaust, and from poorly designed or poorly ventilated gas burners in stoves or heaters.

Carbon monoxide combines with hemoglobin in blood to form carboxyhemoglobin, which limits the ability of hemoglobin to carry oxygen to the body's tissues. With concentrations up to 10% of carboxyhemoglobin in the blood, there are rarely any symptoms. Concentrations of 20% to 30% cause shortness of breath on moderate exertion, flu-like symptoms, and slight headache, and could be missed if clinician is not alert to diagnosis. Concentrations from 30% to 50% cause severe headache, mental confusion and dizziness, impairment of vision and hearing, and collapse and fainting on exertion. Unconsciousness results with concentrations of 50% to 60%, and death may follow with continued exposure. Concentrations of 80% result in almost immediate death. There is usually no cyanosis (blue skin), as one might expect from the presence of deoxygenated hemoglobin); because carboxyhemoglobin is a bright red compound, the lips may take on a healthy red appearance.

Hydrogen Sulphide (Sour Gas)

Hydrogen sulphide (H_2S) is a colourless gas that has an offensive odour that smells like rotten eggs. However, the gas rapidly paralyzes the olfactory nerve endings, so that heavy exposure may occur without the patient being aware of it (which is perhaps the biggest danger of hydrogen sulphide in the workplace). It presents as a byproduct in industry (such as the petroleum industry where sulphur-rich crude is processed). Additionally, it is a hazard in sewers, mines, wells, and tunnels. Hydrogen sulphide causes cellular asphyxia by inhibiting the cytochrome oxidase system, in the same way that cyanide does (26). High concentrations may cause upper-airway irritation and pulmonary edema. Exposure to very high concentrations causes immediate death.

Silo Filler's Disease

Silo filler's disease is due to poisoning by oxides of nitrogen. A silo is an airtight structure in which green crops such as corn and clover are pressed and kept for fodder. The decomposition of organic material produces oxides of nitrogen, which can cause pulmonary edema. These may clear or slowly accumulate in the lungs where hydration to nitric acid results in delayed onset of a chemical pneumonitis (26). Pathology may demonstrate bronchiolitis obliterans. X-rays show a diffuse fine nodular infiltrate in the lungs, concentrated in the suprahilar area.

Environmental Tobacco Smoke

Tobacco smoke contains more than 4,000 different chemicals, 103 of which have been shown to be poisonous to human health (see Chapter 7). The International Agency for Research on Cancer (IARC) has determined that 43 of these are also carcinogenic in animals. Exposure to environmental tobacco smoke has been shown to cause heart disease, lung disease, nasal sinus cancer, lung cancer, asthma exacerbation, and lower respiratory tract infections. There is preliminary evidence that suggests that it may also play a role in causing stroke, breast cancer, cervical cancer, and miscarriages. Exposure to environmental tobacco smoke is responsible for as many as 7,800 deaths per year in Canada, with at least one third occurring in Ontario. Environmental tobacco smoke is a major source of benzene exposure to those working in restaurants and bars (27). The federal government and most provincial jurisdictions have a formal law or regulation that restricts smoking in the workplace to a varying extent. Only Prince Edward Island and Nova Scotia have no such legislation. The *Non-Smokers' Health Act* (1988) provides partial protection to federal workers from second-hand smoke in the workplace (28).

3.2. PHYSICAL AGENTS

3.2.1. Excessive Noise

The effects produced by excessive noise may include impaired hearing (usually referred to as noise induced hearing loss), fatigue, increased blood pressure, decreased efficiency, and emotional disturbances. Noise can be measured by a sound level meter, which determines the intensity of a sound in the immediate environment in terms of decibels. Ordinary conversation varies from 35 to 65 decibels. The normal threshold of audibility is 0 decibels. Intensity above 80 decibels is annoying and noise levels of 100 to 130 decibels have been found to cause temporary and permanent deafness, even after short-term exposure. Levels above 130 decibels are painful to the ear.

Although industrial noise is usually a combination of sounds at different frequencies, it is still possible to establish the main source of a noise and take appropriate steps to eliminate or reduce it. Initial loss of acuity occurs for sounds at high frequencies, particularly those around 4,000 cycles per second (Hz). A reading of 4000 Hz on an audiogram is characteristic of noise-induced hearing loss. Brief exposures to high noise levels result in temporary hearing loss, with recovery over several days to weeks. However, exposure to sustained noise levels of 85 decibels or higher for several months may result in permanent partial impairment of hearing. In general, the greater the loss of acuity in the speech frequencies, the more seriously the person is handicapped. Often the first time that someone may notice a hearing problem is during a telephone conversation.

In assessing the importance of noise in producing hearing loss, a careful search must be made to rule out other conditions. There is considerable individual susceptibility to the effects of noise. Preplacement and periodic audiograms are essential for employees working in high noise levels. It is necessary also to distinguish between occupational impairment and the normal deterioration in hearing that occurs with advancing age (presbycusis). Noise may be prevented or eliminated by one or more of the following methods: elimination of noise at its source, isolation of noisy operations, reduction of noise by sound insulation, and use of personal protective devices against noise.

Preliminary studies in animals reveal physiological reactions such as elevations in heart rate, blood pressure, and peripheral resistance. These are the same non-specific effects seen with any type of stress. There is a possibility that chronic exposure to noise may lower susceptibility to other diseases that are regarded to be consequences of chronic stress. There is, however, no conclusive evidence to date that exposure to noise levels below the threshold to cause hearing impairment causes any impairment of health, and more research in this area is being done.

3.2.2. Temperature and Humidity

Excessively high temperature and humidity occur in many industries, principally as a result of the heat and moisture produced by industrial processes. A high external temperature may accentuate this during the summer months. Very high temperatures may bring about heat cramps, heat exhaustion, or heat stroke.

Heat Cramps

Heat cramps, which are due to sodium chloride depletion, may occur in people who sweat profusely as a result of heavy physical work performed in hot environments. The characteristic symptoms consist of spasmodic contractions of the muscles of the extremities and abdominal wall. The body temperature is usually normal or slightly elevated, the pulse rate slightly increased, the blood pressure normal, and the skin moist. Nausea and vomiting may occur. The cramps disappear completely and rapidly following intravenous injection of physiological saline and can be prevented by oral administration of salt and water.

Heat Exhaustion

This usually occurs in hot weather, with the initial symptoms being fatigue, headache, and dizziness. These may progress to a state of unconsciousness or collapse. The body temperature may be low or elevated (although not exceeding 39°C), the skin may be moist, the pulse is rapid and weak, and the blood pressure is usually low. The clinical picture is the same as shock.

Heat Stroke

Heat stroke is often called sunstroke when the cause is the radiant heat from the sun. In industrial workers, it occurs most frequently during prolonged heat waves. The condition is due to failure of the temperature-controlling centre of the hypothalamus. The onset may be sudden, with the outstanding symptom being a high body temperature over 40.5°C. The pulse is rapid (except in the late stages) and the blood pressure is elevated. Other characteristics include laboured respiration, hot and dry skin (as compared to the damp skin of heat exhaustion), flushed face, depressed nervous system, incontinence, vomiting, and coma. The state of coma may last for hours or days.

Cold

Exposure of extremities to the cold can cause chilblains or precipitate attacks of Raynaud's disease in susceptible individuals. Raynaud's phenomenon is an idiopathic, paroxysmal, bilateral, asymmetrical cyanosis of digits, due to arterial or arteriolar contractions, brought on by cold or emotions. Re-warming the affected part reverses the temporary damage. Frostbite is a more severe and largely irreversible form of local cell injury. Upon thawing, hyperemia and increased capillary permeability cause edema, swelling, and thrombosis, which can be followed by ischemia and gangrene in the digits.

3.2.3. Abnormalities of Air Pressure

Exposure to abnormally high atmospheric pressures occurs in diving operations and in occupations where compressed air shafts and caissons are used, as in construction of tunnels, bridge piers, and building foundations. Workers are exposed to air pressures exceeding the hydrostatic pressure of water at the depths in which they work. Rapid gain in altitude can also cause adverse health effects as a result of the body's difficulty in adjusting to reduced oxygen availability at high altitudes. Acute Mountain Sickness (AMS) may present as headache, fatigue, loss of appetite, nausea, vomiting, difficulty sleeping, or confusion at altitudes above 2500 metres. In severe cases, it may progress to pulmonary or cerebral edema and death (29).

Decompression Sickness

Most frequently encountered by industrial workers, symptoms usually appear within the first few hours following rapid decompression, which leads to the formation of bubbles of nitrogen gas that block off the blood supply to various parts of the body, including the spinal cord. The most common symptom is severe pain in the muscles and joints of the arms and legs ("the bends"). Other symptoms include epigastric pain, skin mottling or itching, retrosternal burning with paroxysmal cough, dyspnea, paralysis of skeletal muscle, and shock. Death may occur rapidly or may follow secondary complications. Prevention consists of limiting the lengths of time a worker may stay in compressed air at specified pressures, and requiring adequate periods for decompression after each work period.

Barotrauma

This occurs as the result of rapid changes in atmospheric pressure. A sudden increase in pressure with a blocked Eustachian tube may result in otic barotrauma (rupture of the tympanic membrane), whereas a sudden decrease, with blocked nasal sinuses, may cause sinus barotrauma. A similar effect can occur in other gas-containing cavities (e.g., intestines), if the external air pressure is suddenly decreased.

3.2.4. Radiation

Radiation exposure occurs from x-rays (medical and dental) primarily but also from radon progeny, radioactive minerals in building materials, phosphate fertilizers, smoke detectors, and nuclear power plants. There are two types of radiation: ionizing and non-ionizing.

Ionizing Radiation

Ionizing radiation consists of x-rays, gamma rays, alpha particles, beta particles, and neutrons. **X-rays** are streams of photons that have great penetrability and move at high speed. **Gamma rays** are higher energy photons that have greater penetrability. **Beta particles** are electrons that can penetrate several centimetres of body tissue. **Alpha particles** are positively charged helium nuclei and have poor penetration. They can be easily impeded but deposit a lot of energy in a short track. **Neutrons** are uncharged particles that exist independently only for a fraction of a second.

Exposure to x-ray and gamma radiation is measured in grays (1 Gy = 100 rads, or radiation absorbed dose) while the unit sievert (1 Sv = 100 rem, or roentgen equivalent in man) expresses a dose equivalent. The exposure of radiation workers is limited to 20 mSv (2 rem) per year averaged over a five-year period (the background radiation exposure varies by geographical location but is about 0.03 rem per year in North America). This exposure limit is set by the Atomic Energy Control Board of Canada, which is responsible for most regulations in the radiation field. As a result of these regulations, all atomic radiation workers must wear dosimeter film badges to measure exposure.

The type and severity of the injury caused by ionizing radiation depend on the extent of the tissue exposed and on the particular tissue that absorbs the radiation. The lymphoid tissue appears to be the most sensitive to radiation. The effects of ionizing radiation may be subdivided into somatic and genetic. The acute somatic effects are known as radiation sickness; this varies in severity from mild skin erythema (redness) to severe illness with death occurring within a week of exposure. The latter follows exposures of greater than 50 Sv. Nausea and vomiting develop within an hour of such exposures; these may subside for a few days, only to be followed by the return of nausea, vomiting, diarrhea, fever, bleeding, and ulceration of the mucous membranes. The blood lymphocyte count declines and secondary infection may occur. Death is usually the result of intestinal or hematopoietic injury. Treatment of acute radiation sickness is so far only palliative.

The delayed somatic effects of ionizing radiation include leucopenia, anemia, sterility, fetal injury, bone necrosis, and sarcomata (as occurred among dial painters who ingested radium paint during World War I), lung cancer (reported among uranium miners in Czechoslovakia and Colorado), chronic atrophic dermatitis, hyperkeratoses, epitheliomata, leukemia, breast and thyroid cancer (reported among survivors of Hiroshima and Nagasaki), and production of cataracts by neutron exposure. Except for leukemia, a long latency period of 15 to 25 years is characteristic of malignancies secondary to radiation exposure.

With respect to the genetic effects of ionizing radiation, there are few human data. The majority of both natural and radiation mutations are of recessive inheritance, and the probability of their becoming manifest in future generations is small. In follow-up studies on the survivors of the Japanese bombings, so far there has been little evidence of a deleterious effect on succeeding generations.

Non-Ionizing Radiation

Non-ionizing radiation refers to emission from those parts of the electromagnetic spectrum where emitted photons generally have insufficient energy to produce ionization of atoms. These forms of radiation include microwave, television and radio waves, visible light, and infrared and ultraviolet radiation, among others. Important workplace forms of non-ionizing radiation are ultraviolet and infrared radiation.

Ultraviolet (UV) Radiation. Occupational exposure to ultraviolet rays occurs chiefly from sunlight in workers such as farmers and construction workers. The risks are acute (sunburn) or delayed (skin cancer or cataract). Exposure to sunlight is associated with an increased risk of non-melanocytic skin cancer. These tumours occur predominantly on the skin of the face and neck, which is most commonly exposed to sunlight, although the distribution of basal cell carcinomas is not as closely related to the distribution of exposure to the sun as is that of squamous cell carcinomas. People who work primarily outdoors have higher mortality from these cancers, and there is some evidence that outdoor workers have a higher incidence. In contrast, the associations between melanoma and total exposure to the sun over a lifetime or in recent years are inconsistent (30).

Welding is a source of ultraviolet radiation exposure. The intensity of the ultraviolet radiation increases with the temperature of the welding process. Exposure may also occur in the use of ultraviolet rays for inspecting razor blades, blue prints, and golf balls. Ultraviolet rays are also used in the diagnosis and treatment of skin diseases such as psoriasis.

UV radiation primarily affects the eyes, skin, and superficial blood vessels. Symptoms appear 4 to 12 hours after exposure, with skin developing erythema, followed by freckling and pigmentation. The eyes may react by developing ophthalmia with acute conjunctivitis, lacrimation, photophobia, and burning. In severe cases, corneal ulceration, iritis, and cataracts may develop.

Infrared Radiation. Infrared radiation (heat radiation) is given off by everything with a temperature of greater than absolute zero but is of a concern in high temperature processes such as welding, glass blowing, foundry work, and other occupations where metal and glass are heated to a molten state. In these processes, there may be a concomitant exposure to ultraviolet rays and to excessive light radiation. Infrared rays are used in industry in the heating and drying of many materials, e.g., painted and lacquered objects and automobiles.

Infrared radiation causes a vasodilatation of the skin and stimulation of cellular activity. In excessive doses, it produces an erythema followed by pigmentation and freckling. The most serious effect of prolonged exposure to infrared radiation is the development of cataracts.

Video Display Terminals (VDTs). Problems experienced by operators of video display terminals (VDTs) are often complex. They are associated with the equipment in use, the environment, and the work habits of the operator (31). VDT users have more visual, musculoskeletal, and stress-related complaints than other workers. Proper ergonomic standards (e.g., appropriately designed work spaces, approved office furniture and machines, adequate lighting and glare reduction, regular rest breaks, and suitable environmental conditions) should be encouraged in the workplace to maximize the comfort of the VDT operator (32).

The National Institute for Occupational Safety and Health (NIOSH), the U.S. Army Environmental Hygiene Agency, and others have measured radiation emitted by VDTs. The tests show that levels for all types of radiation are below those allowed in current standards. In fact, some measurements show radiation levels so low that they cannot be distinguished from general environmental radiation (background radiation). Currently, NIOSHA has no reliable information that any birth defects have ever resulted from a pregnant woman working at a VDT. Health Canada and the World Health Organization (WHO) have come to same conclusion (31, 33).

3.2.5. Electricity

The effects of electrical currents upon the body depend on external and individual conditions. The severity of the damage is proportional to the strength and duration of the current. In general, the higher the voltage, the greater the current that will pass through the body. The strength of the current will be increased if the skin is damp or wet. The current mostly affects the organs through which it passes. When the current passes through the brain, the patient may be rendered unconscious. Death is caused by ventricular fibrillation, failure of the respiratory centre, or prolonged tetanus of the respiratory muscles resulting in suffocation. Exposure to as little as 35 volts has been known to cause death. If the current does not pass through any of the vital organs, other parts of the body may be affected. This may result in functional or structural damage, which may be either temporary or permanent. Permanent disability is usually the result of electrical burns in tissues directly affected by the current. A discussion of electromagnetic fields that are generated by electric current and are indirect effects of electricity to which workers may be exposed is given in Chapter 9.

3.3. BIOLOGICAL AGENTS

These include bacteria, rickettsia, viruses, fungi, and protozoa. Diseases caused by such agents may be regarded as occupational in origin when the nature of the work involves exposure to the organism. Thus tuberculosis may be accepted as an occupational disease when it occurs in healthcare professionals whose daily work has caused them to be exposed to mycobacterium tuberculosis. Most occupational diseases of infectious origin occur in groups of employees exposed to animals or birds, such as abattoir workers, veterinarian, and pet shop workers. An example of this type of biological disease (undulant fever) is given below. Of more recent concern, however, are blood-borne infections such as AIDS and hepatitis B in the workplace, particularly (but not exclusively) in the healthcare setting. Blood is increasingly being recognized as a potentially toxic substance.

Blood-borne Occupational Diseases

The occurrence of occupationally acquired blood-borne infection depends on the frequency and types of hazardous exposures, the risk associated with each type of discrete exposure, and the prevalence of infection in the patient population. The prevalence of potentially infectious individuals within the Canadian general population varies depending on the virus involved: hepatitis B (HBV) (< 0.5%), hepatitis C (HCV) (1%), and HIV (0.15%). Their prevalence in population subgroups, such as intravenous drug users, can be substantially higher (34, 35). The other factors are discussed below.

Hepatitis B surface antigen can be found in virtually all body secretions and excretions; however, only blood (and serum-derived fluids), saliva, and semen and vaginal fluids have been shown to be infectious. The risk of a healthcare worker contracting HBV from occupational exposure is significant; the categories of healthcare workers (e.g. surgeons, nurses, pathologists, blood bank staff) who have the greatest exposure to blood-borne pathogens are at most risk. In Canada, there were three cases of compensated occupational hepatitis in healthcare workers in 1998. Nurses and nursing supervisors were the healthcare professional group most affected (36).

Regarding HIV infection, although the proportion of healthcare workers infected is similar to the general population, there is a statistically greater proportion of infected healthcare workers with no known risk factors or an undetermined transmission category. The risk of transmission of HIV to healthcare workers from HIV-infected patients by needlestick exposure is approximately 3%. The rate of seroconversion following a mucous membrane exposure is 0.09%. There has been one occupational HIV percutaneous transmission documented in Canada (36).

Universal precautions, also known as body substance precautions, are intended to prevent parenteral, mucous membrane, and non-intact skin exposures of healthcare workers to blood-borne pathogens. These precautions have been recommended and widely introduced (37), although there is some concern about their effectiveness in preventing the occupational spread of HIV. A surveillance study by Canada's Federal Centre for AIDS indicated that healthcare workers were exposed to blood despite protection, but seroconversions did not occur (38). The basic tenet of universal precautions is that all specimens should be regarded as hazardous and treated with equal care. The National Committee for Clinical Laboratory Standards has published effective recommendations that include the prevention of sharp instrument injuries, the use of protective barriers, and immediate washing of hands and surfaces contaminated by blood and other fluids to which universal precautions apply. These measures are intended to supplement existing practices of hand washing and use of gloves to prevent infection. Universal precautions apply to blood and other body fluids containing visible blood and tissues, but do not apply to feces, nasal secretions, sputum, sweat, tears, urine, and vomit unless they contain visible blood.

A further current issue in relation to occupational spread of HIV is the reciprocity of the rights of patients and healthcare workers with regard to HIV testing (39). There is a slight potential risk for patients contracting HIV from infected practitioners, given that there is reasonable evidence that three patients were infected by a dentist (40). This type of transmission is, however, regarded as a rare occurrence. Guidelines for the continuing practice of HIV-positive physicians have been produced in a number of jurisdictions. The Centre for Infectious Disease Prevention and Control has advised that mandatory testing of healthcare workers and patients for HIV is not currently warranted due to the extremely small risk of HIV transmission in this setting and the impracticality of this measure (40-42).

As an adjunctive measure to prevent blood-borne infection, pre-exposure hepatitis B vaccinations are recommended for healthcare workers who are potentially exposed to blood. Compliance among healthcare workers for hepatitis B vaccination has been high. Protocol for appropriate post-exposure hepatitis B includes testing, passive immunization, and active vaccination (43). Many provinces have developed protocols to reduce the incidence of blood-borne infections in hospitals and other healthcare settings. The introduction of the HBV vaccine and universal precautions contributed to a 95% decrease in the occupational transmission of HBV to American healthcare workers from 1983 to 1995 (44).

Undulant Fever (Brucellosis, Malta Fever)

Undulant fever is an acute infectious disease characterized by a prolonged febrile course with irregular remissions and exacerbation. A member of the brucella group of microorganisms causes it. The causative agent is ingested from contaminated food and drink, particularly milk, butter, and cheese from infected goats and cows. Those who handle infected meat and meat products also contract it. The majority of cases occur in farmers, milkers, and abattoir workers. The average incubation period is two weeks, with the onset being gradual. Fever, anorexia, constipation, loss of weight, and generalized muscle and joint pains are common characteristics.

Anthrax

Anthrax is an infectious disease caused by *Bacillus anthracis*, a large gram-positive, spore-forming bacillus transmitted to humans by contact with infected animals or contaminated animal products. Rare cases of inhalation anthrax have developed in workers during the processing of contaminated materials such as woolens, hides, or bone meal (45). Several cases of occupational inhalational anthrax have recently occurred in the U.S. with exposure that was assumed to have occurred through contaminated mail in acts of biological terrorism (see Chapter 8) (46).

3.4.   MECHANICAL AND ERGONOMIC AGENTS

Tenosynovitis and Bursitis

The inflammation of tissues near joints occurs as a result of chronic repetitive movements, exertions, impacts, pressure, or the resumption of aggressive work after an extended break (e.g., winter layoff for bricklayers). The resulting inflammation often manifests clinically as tenosynovitis, bursitis, and myositis, causing pain and swelling in the tendons, joints, or muscles subjected to the strains. In the treatment of occupational tenosynovitis and bursitis, transfer to other work or removal from the job is important so that the affected part can be put at rest.

Hand-Arm Vibration Syndrome

The clinical effects resulting from prolonged use of piston-operated vibrating tools have been recognized for some years. Portable vibrating tools are of two main types:

the piston-operated pneumatic tools, such as road and rock drills, chipping hammers, or riveting hammers, and the newer rotating tools that consist of a handle through the centre, which is a rotating spindle, and are driven by an electric motor or compressed air. Both types of tools may be carried in the hands. In either case, the vibrations of the tool are transmitted to the hands and arms of the operator.

The most common effect is a disturbance of the blood vessels of the fingers (Raynaud's phenomenon). The condition may develop within only months of exposure to the vibrations but usually requires longer exposure. The condition may not become apparent until after exposure to vibration has ceased. Exposure to cold is the precipitating factor inducing the vasospastic attacks. Another associated feature of traumatic vasospastic disease is the effect on the neurological system, which includes pain and tingling in the extremities, and loss of grip strength. Both the vascular and neurological symptoms may be lessened by the use of calcium channel-blocking medication. It is imperative that the worker be removed from the offending environment to prevent further progression of the disease.

Carpal Tunnel Syndrome

Carpal tunnel syndrome is the most frequent compression or entrapment neuropathy. It is characterized by pain in the hand and lower arm associated with disturbances in sensation and grip strength. It is caused by compression of the median nerve as it passes through the wrist (carpal) tunnel formed by bones of the wrist and transcarpal ligament. The worker often complains that the pain in the lateral three digits is worse at night or when driving, and is relieved by shaking the hands vigorously. In the workplace, it is associated with jobs involving repetitive wrist flexion and extension with forceful gripping and vibration. Typical jobs are meat packers, seamstresses, automobile and aircraft assembly line workers, and clerical workers. A change in the way that a worker performs the work is essential to avoid recurrence. Many other common conditions may be responsible for carpal tunnel syndrome including pregnancy, diabetes, rheumatoid arthritis, and hypothyroidism.

Occupational Low Back Pain

Occupational low back pain is a very common disorder and a leading cause of disability. Low back pain disorders are associated with work-related lifting, forceful movements, and whole-body vibration as well as working in awkward positions. Psychosocial factors, such as job satisfaction, personality traits, perception of intensified workload, and job control are also associated with low back pain. Strategies for preventing low back pain include ergonomic interventions as well as education and exercise (see Chapter 16) (47).

3.5.   PSYCHOSOCIAL AGENTS

Stress-induced illness in the workplace is increasingly recognized as a serious problem (48), with at least one WCB compensating for workplace stress-induced illness. The recent downsizing that has occurred in North America has lead to rapidly changing patterns of work organization and employment, which, in turn, provide the right conditions for stress to build. According to the World Health Organization, up to half of all workers in industrialized countries judge their work to be "mentally heavy." Psychological stress caused by time pressure and hectic work has become more prevalent during the past decade. Various tools have been used to measure work stress, including the Karasek job content questionnaire (49), based on a job strain model that proposes high work stress is a combination of high responsibility and little control on the job. Stress may be attributable to increase in work load, lack of control, heavy responsibility, monotonous work or work that requires constant concentration, shift work, job insecurity, and work under the threat of violence as, for example, police or prison work. Additionally, there are the stressors specific to particular jobs such as working in geographical isolation (such as at a remote outpost) or shift work. Workplace-induced stress is increasingly being seen to have high indirect costs in terms of decreased productivity due to job dissatisfaction, mental illness, and increased absenteeism. The WHO estimates that mental illness is on a par with heart disease and cancer as a key cause of disability (50). There also appears to be overlap between stress and physical factors in determining the course of various work-related musculoskeletal problems. Psychological stress and overload have been associated with sleep disturbances, burnout syndromes, and depression. There is also epidemiological evidence of an elevated risk of cardiovascular disorders, particularly coronary heart disease and hypertension (see Chapter 1) (51). Psychosocial factors are thought to contribute to various chronic pain syndromes (52). Severe psychological conditions such as post-traumatic stress disorder may be seen among the workers involved in serious catastrophes or major accidents where human lives are threatened or lost (53).

Discrimination against several designated groups (women, Aboriginal peoples, visible minorities, and the disabled) is prevalent in the Canadian workforce. This works on several levels: by excluding these individuals from entering the workforce, and by hindering their promotion; by lack of suitable work for level of training (underemployment), which is particularly common among recent immigrants from developing countries with professional qualifications; and by both overt and systemic racism in the workplace. Discrimination increases the general level of stress in the workplace, and causes considerable demoralization and financial strain. Federal and provincial legislations attempt to address the issues of employment equity.

4. SKIN DISEASES

As indicated earlier, occupational diseases represent a small proportion (10%) of all lost time compensations due to work related illnesses compared with injuries, which make up 90%. Skin diseases constitute a major portion of compensated occupational disease and are relatively common in certain workplaces. They may be the result of chemical, physical, or biological classes of environmental exposures. The skin forms a major component of the interface between the work environment and the worker unless the worker is completely protected by barrier clothing. Occupational skin disease may be categorized into contact dermatitis, occupational acne, pigmentation disorders, neoplastic disorders, and miscellaneous disorders.

Contact dermatitis may be irritant or allergic. Irritant contact dermatitis comprises the majority of contact dermatitis and is a result of direct injury to the skin as with many industrial materials including but not limited to acids, alkalis, metal compounds, detergents, petroleum products, oxidizing agents, solvents, and frequent hand washing with water with or without soap. Immunology does not play a role in the development of irritant contact dermatitis. On the other hand, allergic contact dermatitis, which comprises the minority of contact dermatitis, is the result of an immune reaction to a chemical agent. The presence of allergic contact dermatitis cases may be confirmed by patch testing, which shows the delayed hypersensitivity (i.e., the reaction to the agent occurs after 48 to 96 hours).

Occupational acne is the result of exposure to various agents that cause a chronic inflammatory process in the pilosebaceous follicles. Agents implicated in the development of occupational acne include oil, fats, and tars. Chloracne is the pathognomonic marker of exposure to halogenated aromatic hydrocarbons, including polychlorinated biphenyls (PCBs), dioxins, and organochlorine pesticides. Pigmentation disorders may result in staining, hyperpigmentation, or hypopigmentation. Examples of exposures that result in staining include aniline dyes, picric acid, nitric acid, coal tar, and silver. Exposure to phytotoxins, ionizing radiation, or ultraviolet light may result in hyperpigmentation. Phenols and hydroquinones, on the other hand, may result in hypopigmentation. Radiation, ultraviolet light, arsenic, and polyaromatic hydrocarbons are some of the agents associated with the development of skin cancer.

Exposure to different extremes of temperature may result in miscellaneous skin disorders, for example, chilblains, immersion foot, and frostbite as a result of exposure to cold, and sunburn and toasted skin syndrome as a result of exposure to heat.

5.   SUMMARY

Occupational health may be defined as the maintenance and promotion of health in the working environment. In 2001, there were approximately 16.2 million people in the workforce, 11.7 million of whom were employed in service industries. The annual incidence of occupational injuries in the Canadian workforce is about 2.5%. Injuries account for 90% of all compensated cases by workers' compensation boards; the remaining 10% comprises occupational diseases. In 2000 alone, $5.0 billion was paid out by WCBs in Canada.

The specifics of corporate responsibility to workers' safety are determined to a large part by provincial legislations. There are three aspects of legislation that are universal across the country: due deligence, application of WHMIS, and existence of joint health and safety committees in workplace.

Primary prevention in occupational health first involves substitution of the hazardous material with something safer, and, if this is not possible, then segregation is attempted, including ventilation. Personal hygiene and protective equipment are used if the measures outlined above are not feasible. Industrial engineers use several methods for setting standards for the exposure limits to hazardous substances in the work environment. When legislation recognizes these limits, they constitute legal standards. Where levels are not defined, the acceptable code of practice is usually set on a 40-hour work week (i.e., eight hours a day). Industrial engineers rely on *threshold limit values* (TLVs). TLVs place a limit on exposure as measured by *time-weighted averages* (TWAs). Secondary prevention in occupational health involves the use of preplacement and periodic examinations that are usually directed to a specific exposure or workplace substance (e.g., blood lead for lead exposure). Another aspect of secondary prevention in the workplace is the issue of employee screening for substance abuse. Tertiary prevention involves treatment, rehabilitation, and retraining under the auspices of workers' compensation. The injury and disease related to work are compensable in all provinces and territories by WCBs; workers' compensation falls within the jurisdiction of provincial statutes, although the general principles are uniform across Canada. The main features are as follows: the WCB is autonomous; employers pay for costs; the WCB decides benefits; negligence is not considered a factor; first aid, medical treatment, lost time, and rehabilitation are covered for most workers; it is a no-fault insurance system; and workers who receive compensation abdicate their right to sue the employer.

The agents causing occupational disease may be divided into five broad groups: chemical, physical, biological, mechanical or ergonomic, and psychosocial. In order to establish causality between the workplace and the health problem there must be adequate concentration and duration of exposure, absorption into the body, appropriate temporal sequence, and consistency (among multiple reports) of ill-health effects with the exposure.

Chemical agents include organic dusts, heavy metals, solvents, industrial gases, and environmental tobacco smoke. Mineral dusts include silica, asbestos, and coal. Prolonged inhalation of free silica leads to silicosis, which predisposes to tuberculosis infection. In asbestosis, the essential lesion is a diffuse fibrosis. Heavy metals include lead, mercury, cadmium, and nickel. Lead is perhaps the most important metal both because it is ubiquitous and because poisoning may result in serious disability. There are two types of poisoning: acute and chronic. Acute lead poisoning results from exposure to a large dose, over a short period of time, usually occurring as a result of accidental ingestion of lead salts. Chronic lead poisoning occurs from the inhalation or ingestion of small amounts of lead dust, fumes, or vapours over a relatively long period of time. Volatile solvents and organic materials also affect the health of the worker. Benzene is one of the most toxic solvents used commercially. The toxicity of chlorinated hydrocarbons varies from very high to very low, attacking the liver and kidney. Carbon tetrachloride is the most toxic of the group. Methyl alcohol may cause dizziness, unconsciousness, blindness, cardiac depression, and eventually death.

Physical agents have the potential of harming the worker. The effects produced by excessive noise may include fatigue, impaired hearing, increased blood pressure, decreased efficiency, and emotional disturbances. Industrial noise is a combination of sounds of different frequencies. Very high temperatures may bring about heat cramps, heat exhaustion, or heat stroke. Exposure of hands, feet, ears, and nose to the cold can cause chilblains or precipitate attacks of Raynaud's phenomenon. The most common effect resulting from repeated vibration exposure is vasospastic disturbance of the blood vessels of the fingers, leading to blanching of the digits on exposure to cold. Muscular stiffness, soreness, blisters, and cramps are clinical signs of the adverse effects of repeated motion on certain body parts. Decompression sickness and barotrauma are examples of the body's reaction to abnormalities of air pressure.

Another physical agent is radiation. The ultimate effect of ionizing radiation is damage to, or death of, the cells. The type and severity of the injury depends on the extent of the tissue exposed and on the particular tissue that absorbs the radiation. Non-ionizing radiation comprises ultraviolet rays (UV), infrared, microwave, and radio and television waves. Problems experienced by operators of video display terminals are visual, musculoskeletal, and stress-related complaints. VDTs do not cause radiation risk or cause birth defects in pregnanant woman using them. Electrical currents travelling through the body damage tissues through which they pass.

Biological agents include bacteria, viruses, fungi, protozoa, and rickettsia. Disease caused by these organisms may be regarded as occupational in origin when the nature of the work involves exposure to the organism. Since quite a few diseases are spread via blood (e.g., AIDS, hepatitis B, hepatitis C), it is also recognized as a potentially toxic substance. The occurrence of occupationally acquired blood-borne infection depends on the frequency and types of hazardous exposures, the risk associated with each type of discrete exposure, and the prevalence of infection in the patient population. Anthrax is a rare disease in humans that is occasionally seen in those working with contaminated animal products such as hides or bone meal.

Mechanical and ergonomic agents cause soft-tissue injuries such as tenosynovitis and bursitis. They can also cause hand-arm vibration syndrome and carpal tunnel syndrome. Many of these conditions are the result of repetitive movements, excessive force, awkward postures, or poorly designed physical working environments. They can be prevented or alleviated by change of job or change in the way tasks are performed, or by medication.

Psychosocial agents contribute to health-related problems in the workplace. Stress may be attributed to workload, responsibility, or fear of job loss, geographical isolation, or shift work. Stress clearly incurs high indirect costs in the form of absenteeism, poor productivity, and mental illness. Post-traumatic stress disorder is also a recognized condition that can be related to occupation.

Skin diseases comprise a major portion of compensated occupational disease. Occupational skin disease may be categorized into contact dermatitis, occupational acne, pigmentation disorders, and neoplastic disorders.

6.   REFERENCES

1.   Statistics Canada. *Historical labour force statistics*, 2001. Cat. No. 71-201-XPB.
2.   Association of Workers' Compensation Boards of Canada. *Work injuries and diseases, 1998-2000*. Mississauga: Association of Workers' Compensation Boards of Canada, 2001.

3.   Association of Workers' Compensation Boards of Canada. 2002. *Key statistical measures, 2000.* Mississauga. <www.awcbc.org/english/board_pdfs/key_2000.pdf> (September 2002).

4.   Markham JW, Kirkbride J, Pelmear P. Health surveillance data. *Occupational Health in Ontario* 1986; 7(4):192-204.

5.   Ross JB. Prevention of occupational disease: Problems of data collection for adequate surveillance. *Canadian Medical Association Journal* 1992; 147(10):1443-5.

6.   Spiegel S, Yassi A. Occupational disease surveillance in Canada: A framework for considering options and opportunities. *Canadian Journal of Public Health* 1991; 82:294-9.

7.   Health Canada. 2002. *Workplace hazardous materials information system.* <www.hc-sc.gc.ca/hecs-sesc/whmis/index.htm> (November 2002).

8.   American Conference of Governmental Industrial Hygienists. *Threshold limit values and biological exposure indices for 1996-1997.* Cincinnati: American Conference of Governmental Industrial Hygienists, 1997.

9.   Pegus C. Effect of the Heart At Work Program on awareness of risk factors, self-efficacy, and health behaviors. *Occupational and Environment Medicine* 2002; 44(3):228.

10.   Derouche F. Promoting health in the workplace. *Ontario Prevention Clearinghouse News* 1992; 3(4):1-2.

11.   Erfurt J, Foote A, Mex A, et al. Improving participation in worksite wellness programs: Comparing health education classes, a menu approach, and follow-up counselling. *American Journal of Health Promotion* 1990; 4(4):270-8.

12.   Aldana S. Health promotion programs, modifiable health risks, and employee absenteeism. *Occupational and Environmental Medicine* 2001; 43(1):36-46.

13.   Health Canada. 2002. *Corporate health model: A guide to developing and implementing the workplace health system in medium and large businesses.* <www.hc-sc.gc.ca/hecs-sesc/workplace/publications/corporatehealth_guide/model.htm> (September 2002).

14.   Canadian Medical Association. Drug testing in the workplace. *Canadian Medical Association Journal* 1992; 146(12):223A-B.

15.   Canadian Medical Association. The physician's role in helping patients return to work after an illness or injury. *Canadian Medical Association Journal* 1997; 156(5):680A-C.

16.   Physician Education Project in Workplace Health. 2000. *Injury/Illness and return to Work/ Function.* <www.wsib.on.ca/wsib/wsibsite.nsf/public/HealthPhysiciansGuideRTW> (October 2002).

17.   LaDou J. *Occupational and environmental medicine,* Second ed. Norwalk: Appleton & Lange, 1997.

18.   Rom W, editor. *Environmental medicine.* 2nd ed. Baltimore: Lippincott, Williams, and Wilkins, 1998.

19.   Brooks S. *Environmental medicine.* St. Louis: Mosby, 1995.

20.   Newman L. Occupational illness. *New England Journal of Medicine* 1995; 333(17): 1128-34.

21.   National Institute for Occupational Safety and Health. *Criteria for a recommended standard: Occupational exposure to crystalline silica.* Atlanta, GA: National Institute for Occupational Safety and Health, U.S. Department of Health, Education, and Welfare, Health Service, and Mental Health Administration, 1974.

22.   National Institute of Occupational Safety and Health Working Group. *Health effects of occupational exposure to respirable crystalline silica.* Atlanta, GA: National Institute for Occupational Safety and Health, Centers for Disease Control and Prevention, 2002. DHHS(NIOSH) 2002-129.

23.   American Thoracic Society. 2002. *Adverse effects of crystalline silica exposure.* <www.thoracic.org/adobe/statements/silica1-8.pdf> (September 2002).

24.   Parkes W. *Occupational lung disorders,* 3rd ed. Oxford: Butterworth-Heinemann, 1994.

25.   House R, Wills M, Liss G. Paresthesias and sensory neuropathy due to 1,1,1-trichloroethane. *Archives of Environmental Health* 1994; 49:196-99.

26.   Olson K, editor. *Poisoning and drug overdose*. 3rd ed. Stamford, CT: Appleton & Lange; 1999.

27.   Basrur S. 2002. *Ten key carcinogens in Toronto workplaces and environment: Assessing the potential for exposure, Summary report, 2002*. <www.city.toronto.on.ca/health/cr_index.htm> (September 2002).

28.   Ontario Tobacco Research Unit. 2001. *Protection from second-hand tobacco smoke in Ontario: A review of the evidence regarding best practices*. <www.otru.org/pdf/special_ets_eng.PDF> (November 2002).

29.   Shlim D. 2000. *High altitude medicine guide*. <www.high-altitude-medicine.com/AMS> (January 2003).

30.   International Agency for Research on Cancer. 1992. *Solar and ultraviolet radiation*. <www-cie.iarc.fr/htdocs/monographs/vol55/solar-and-uv-radiation.htm> (January 2003).

31.   National Institute of Occupational Safety and Health. 2001. *Safety and health program for video display terminal (VDT) operators*. <www.niehs.nih.gov/odhsb/notes/note11.htm> (September 2002).

32.   Canadian Medical Association. Video display terminals. *Canadian Medical Association Journal* 1986; 135(6):688A.

33.   Health Canada. 2002. *Safety of exposure to electric and magnetic fields from computer monitors and other video displays terminals*. <www.hc-sc.gc.ca/english/iyh/products/vdt.html> (September 2002).

34.   Health Canada. 2001. *Inventory of HIV incidence and prevalence studies in Canada*. <www.hc-sc.gc.ca/pphb-dgspsp/publicat/hips-ipvc01/pdf/hivinventory_e.pdf> (February 2003).

35.   Preventing the transmission of bloodborne pathogens in health care and public service settings. *Canada Communicable Disease Report* 1997; 23(Suppl 3):i-iv,1-43.

36.   Prevention and control of occupational infections in health care. *Canada Communicable Disease Report* 2002; 28(Suppl 1):1-264.

37.   Laboratory Center for Disease Control. Update: Universal precautions for the prevention of human immunodeficiency virus, hepatitis B virus, and other blood-borne pathogens in health care settings. *Canadian Disease Weekly Report* 1988; 14(27):117-23.

38.   Federal Centre for AIDS. *National surveillance of occupational exposure to the human immunodeficiency virus*. Ottawa: Federal Centre for AIDS, 1992.

39.   McQueen M. Conflicting rights of patients and health care workers exposed to blood-borne infection. *Canadian Medical Association Journal* 1992; 147(3):299-302.

40.   Canadian Medical Association. Update: Transmission of HIV infection during invasive dental procedures. *Canadian Medical Association Journal* 1992; 146(4):519-21.

41.   Tyndall M, Schecter M. HIV testing of patients: Let's waive the waiver. *Canadian Medical Association Journal* 2000; 162(2):210-1.

42.   Hoey J. CMA rescinds controversial policy. *Canadian Medical Association Journal* 2000; 163(5):594.

43.   National Advisory Committee on Immunization. *Canadian immunization guide* 6th edition. Ottawa: Minister of Supply and Services Canada, 2002. <www.hc-sc.gc.ca/pphb-dgspsp/publicat/cig-gci> (October 2002).

44.   Mahoney F, Stewart K, Hu H, *et al.* Progress toward the elimination of hepatitis B virus transmission among health care workers in the United States. *Archives of Internal Medicine* 1997; 157:2601-3.

45.   Goldman J, Bennett J, editors. *Cecil textbook of medicine*. 21st ed. Philadelphia: W.B. Saunders; 2001.

46.   Bush L, Abrams B, Beall A, *et al.* Index case of fatal inhalation anthrax due to bioterrorism in the United States. *New England Journal of Medicine* 2001; 345(22):1607-10.

47.   Bowler R, Cone J, Cone J, *et al. Occupational medicine secrets*. San Francisco: Hanley & Belfus.1999.

48. Cole D, Ibrahim S, Shannon H, *et al.* Work and life stressors and psychological distress in the Canadian working population: A structural equation and modelling approach to analysis of the 1994 National Population Health Survey. *Chronic Diseases in Canada* 2002; 23(4):91-9.

49. Karasek R, Brisson C, Kawakami N, *et al.* The job content questionnaire (JCQ): An instrument for internationally comparative assessment of psychosocial job characteristics. *Journal of Occupational Health Psychology* 1998; 3(4):322-55.

50. Murray CJ, Lopez AD, editors. *The global burden of disease: A comprehensive assessment of mortality and disability from diseases, injuries, and risk factors in 1990 and projected to 2020.* Cambridge, MA: Harvard University Press; 1996.

51. Shields M. Shift work and health. Ottawa. *Health Reports* 2002; 13(4).

52. Torp S, Riise T, Moen B. The impact of psychosocial work factors on musculoskeletal pain: A prospective study. *Journal of Occupational and Environmental Medicine* 2001; 43(2): 120-6.

53. World Health Organization. 1994. *Global strategy on occupational health for all: The way to health at work.* <www.who.int/environmental_information/Occuphealth/strategy2.htm#Situation2> (September 2002).

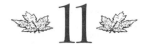

PERIODIC HEALTH
EXAMINATIONS

Since the release of Marc Lalonde's "A New Perspective on Health of Canadians" (1), there has been increased emphasis on disease prevention and health promotion through various strategies such as health education, taxation, regulations, and modification of lifestyles. Physicians have also increasingly focused on early detection of diseases and early interventions. In this chapter, major clinical activities, specifically the periodic health examination, are discussed.

The **periodic health examination** has been defined as a group of activities that encompass both primary and secondary prevention in order to determine a person's risk of developing disease and to identify early, asymptomatic disease. Primary prevention has been defined by the Canadian Task Force on Preventive Health Care as measures, such as immunization, reduction of exposure to risk factors, and modification of behaviours, that aim to prevent the occurrence of disease. Secondary prevention aims at identifying asymptomatic individuals with early-stage disease when early identification and treatment promises better outcomes than identification through presentation with symptoms (2). The presumed reasons for periodic health examinations, including annual examinations, include prevention of specific diseases and conditions by risk factor identification and intervention, early identification and treatment of disease, establishment of a baseline examination, and development of the patient-doctor relationship.

In the past, the practice of annual examination has been criticized on many grounds, such as its ritualistic nature, content and frequency, low yield, irrelevance to the needs of different age groups, and the inclusion of tests and procedures with scanty evidence of effectiveness or efficacy. It was in this context that the Canadian Task Force on the Periodic Health Examination was established by the Conference of Deputy Ministers of Health in 1976. It has since been renamed the Canadian Task Force on Preventive Health Care.

1.   CANADIAN TASK FORCE ON PREVENTIVE HEALTH CARE

1.1.   TERMS OF REFERENCE

The terms of reference for the Task Force are relatively straightforward (3). Its purpose was

- to identify the main killing or disabling conditions, unhealthy states, and unhealthy behaviours that affect Canadians and to determine which could possibly be prevented according to present knowledge.
- to consider evidence for the benefit of early detection or prevention of killing or disabling conditions and unhealthy states and unhealthy behaviours in the non-complaining individual. (If early detection or prevention was judged to be beneficial, the particular condition was termed preventable.)
- to define groups at high risk for specific preventable conditions, states, and behaviours.
- to design health protection "packages" shown to be effective — or, in special circumstances, desirable on other grounds — that should become part of periodic health examinations at defined ages and for defined population groups.
- to make recommendations on the procedures, content, frequency, and appropriate providers of periodic health examinations and preventive interventions at defined ages and for defined population groups.
- to propose specific measures for evaluating the effectiveness and efficiency of the recommended plan for periodic health examinations that would permit recurring reassessment and improvement.

The Task Force concluded that it would be better to identify preventable conditions of importance to each age group, and to assess the detection manoeuvres and preventive interventions related to each condition. Its main recommendation is therefore that the routine annual check-up be abandoned in favour of a selective approach that is determined by a person's age and sex. The Task Force recommends a specific strategy comprising a lifetime healthcare plan based on a set of age- and sex-related **health protection packages**. Recommendations are based on the available scientific evidence. Evidence takes precedence over consensus. With the emphasis on evidence, recommendations need to be updated and can be altered as new scientific information emerges. This innovative approach has since been adopted in other countries including the United States (4, 5).

The Task Force received many submissions and held several discussions with different groups. Based on these, the Task Force has made recommendations over the past 25 years and published a compendium of all the topics and recommendations in 1994 in *The Canadian Guide to Clinical Preventive Health Care* (6). As new information becomes available, the updates are published in the *Canadian Medical Association Journal* and on the Task Force's Web site (7).

2.   RECOMMENDATIONS

A major objective of the Task Force is to help physicians choose tests, immunizations, counselling strategies, and other preventive interventions of proven utility and to avoid those that lack scientific evidence of value. In recent years there have been a growing and diverse set of methods for ranking evidence (8). However, the methodology used by the Task Force has had two key features: recommendations made on graded strength based on the quality of the published medical evidence, and placing the greatest weight on the features of study design and analysis that eliminate or minimize biased results (2).

2.1.   QUALITY OF PUBLISHED EVIDENCE

The effectiveness of intervention is graded according to the quality of evidence obtained, as follows:

I-1: Evidence obtained from at least one properly randomized controlled trial.

II-1: Evidence obtained from well-designed controlled trials without randomization.

II-2: Evidence obtained from well-designed cohort or case-control analytical studies, preferably from more than one centre or research group.

II-3: Evidence obtained from comparisons between times or places with or without the interventions. Dramatic results from uncontrolled experiments (such as the results of the introduction of penicillin in the 1940s) could also be regarded as this type of evidence.

III: Opinions of respected authorities, based on clinical experience, descriptive studies, or reports of expert committees.

However, there is a growing and diverse set of methods for ranking evidence. While the Task Force uses one properly randomized control trial for grade I evidence, other advocates of evidence-based medicine now place positive evidence gathered from meta-analysis and systematic reviews at the top (9).

2.2.   GRADES OF RECOMMENDATIONS

On the basis of the quality of published evidence, the Task Force makes clear graded recommendations for preventive healthcare maneuvres for different conditions to be included in the periodic health examination for each age group and differentiated where applicable by sex. Recommendations are classified as follows:

A: There is good evidence to support the recommendation that the condition be specifically considered in a periodic health examination.

B: There is fair evidence to support the recommendation that the condition be specifically considered in a periodic health examination.

C: There is poor evidence regarding the inclusion or exclusion of the condition in a periodic health examination, but recommendations may be made on other grounds.

D: There is fair evidence to support the recommendation that the condition be excluded from consideration in a periodic health examination.

E: There is good evidence to support the recommendation that the condition be excluded from consideration in a periodic health examination.

Because the effectiveness of treatment or of the preventive measure for a condition was so important, the final recommendation for each condition relied heavily on an assessment of the evidence. Thus a class A recommendation was rarely made in the absence of grade I evidence regarding effectiveness of treatment or prevention. However, there is one exception to this rule: when a clinical intervention was shown, in grade II terms, to save the lives of victims of a previously universally fatal condition. For example, if malignant hypertension is left untreated, all affected patients will die, but if treated, most will survive; thus grade II evidence is sufficient for a class A recommendation. Such examples are rare, however, and grade I evidence was required for the highest recommendation for most conditions.

One of the challenges that has arisen with the recommendations is the large number of class C recommendations that, due to inconclusive scientific evidence, leave clinicians to make decisions regarding such preventive manoeuvres on other grounds. Recently, the Task Force has provided some guidelines for decision-making on class C recommendations (2). These include:

- increasing patient involvement in decision-making;
- minimizing harm;
- advocating major change only on strong proof of need;
- avoiding unnecessary labelling;
- avoiding expensive manoeuvres of unclear benefit;
- focusing on conditions with a high burden of illness; and
- being attentive to special needs of high-risk groups.

3.   HEALTH PROTECTION PACKAGES

Appendix A contains health protection packages, which are up to date as of June 2001, for various age groups and both sexes. Updates are published in the *Canadian Medical Association Journal* and on the Canadian Task Force on Preventive Health Services Web site (7). In some instances, the recommendation is intended only for a designated high-risk group. A number of recommendations also relate to counselling patients about specific risk behaviour and different types of counselling practices have been described (10). Other preventive health practices are also important for physicians, such as fitness to drive vehicles or airplanes and pre-employment examinations of workers (11, 12) (see also Chapter 10).

4.   COMPLIANCE

Studies on the use of guidelines have shown that the following factors increase compliance with guidelines: evidence-based recommendations rather than consensus-based ones, clear language rather than vague, and non-controversial topics rather than controversial (13). A number of studies of compliance with the Canadian Task Force on Preventive Health Care indicate that many of these recommendations are nonetheless still not being optimally implemented (14-17). Clinical practice guidelines, even when based on sound evidence, may conflict with the perceived needs and expectations of patients and physicians (18). Those who develop the guidelines need a good understanding of the values of patients and physicians to create better, more effective communication strategies. Most (90%) of primary care physicians have been found to comply with the Task Force's recommendations for breast examination, mammography, cervical smears, and initial counselling against smoking, but in the context of an annual general physical examination rather than integrated into routine patient care (19).

5.   SUMMARY

Since 1974, increased emphasis has been placed on disease prevention and health promotion through various strategies. These strategies include determining an individual's risk for disease, health education, modification of lifestyle and risk behaviours, and early detection and intervention by physicians.

This chapter discussed the periodic health examination and the Canadian Task Force on Preventive Health Care. The Task Force, initially named the Canadian Task Force on the Periodic Health Examination, was established in 1976 to assess the effectiveness of the annual check-up. Some of the terms of reference for the Task Force included the design of effective health protection packages, the definition of groups in the population at high risk for specific preventable conditions, and the consideration of the benefits of disease prevention and early detection manoeuvres. The Task Force concluded that it would be more efficient to identify preventable conditions of importance to each age group and sex, and the appropriate intervention for these conditions. Hence, it recommended abandoning routine annual check-ups in favour of a selective approach determined by a person's age and sex. The Task Force emphasized available scientific evidence rather than consensus opinion. It also recognized that since there is constantly new scientific information that may alter its recommendations, new conditions to the health protection packages may have to be added and recommendations may also change over time.

The Task Force, using explicit criteria for evaluating the effectiveness of preventive healthcare interventions, uses a standard methodology. This methodology has two key features: recommendations made on graded strength based on the quality of the published medical evidence, and placing the greatest weight on the features of study design and analysis that eliminate or minimize biased results. The Task Force has developed health promotion packages for various age groups and for both sexes that are continually updated over time(see Appendix A). Studies show that most of primary care physicians comply with the Task Force's recommendations for breast examination, mammography, cervical smears, and initial counselling against smoking, but in the context of an annual general physical examination rather than integrated into routine patient care.

6. REFERENCES

1. Lalonde M. *A New Perspective on the Health of Canadians*. Ottawa: Ministry of Supply and Services, 1975.
2. Canadian Task Force on Preventive Health Care. 1997. *History and Methods*. <www.ctfphc.org> (October 2002).
3. Canadian Task Force on Periodic Health Examination. The Periodic Health Examination. *Canadian Medical Association Journal* 1979; 121(99):1193-254.
4. U.S. Preventive Services Task Force. 2002. *Guide to Clinical Preventive Services*. 3rd edition, 2000–2002. <www.ahrq.gov/clinic/cps3dix.htm> (October 2002).
5. U.S. Preventive Services Task Force. *Guide to Clinical Preventive Services*, 2nd ed. Washington, DC: U.S. Department of Health and Human Services, 1996.
6. Canadian Task Force on the Periodic Health Examination. *The Canadian Guide to Clinical Preventive Health Care*. Ottawa: Minister of Supply and Services Canada, 1994. <www.hc-sc.gc.ca/hppb/healthcare/pubs/clinical_preventive/> (October 2002).
7. Canadian Task Force on Preventive Health Care. 2002. *Quick Tables of Current Recommendations*. <www.ctfphc.org> (October 2002).
8. Phillips B, Ball C, Sackett D, *et al*. 2001. *Levels of evidence and grades of recommendations*. <www.minervation.com/cebm2/docs/levels.html> (January 2003).
9. Centre for Evidence-Based Medicine. 2003. *Learning EBM*. <minerva.minervation.com/cebm/> (January 2003).
10. Elford R, MacMillan H, Wathen C. *Counseling for risky health habits: A conceptual framework for primary care practitioners*. London, ON: Canadian Task Force on Preventive Health Care, 2001. CTFPHC Technical Report No. 01-7. <www.ctfphc.org/Sections/Counseling.htm> (October 2002).
11. Canadian Medical Association. *Determining medical fitness to drive: A guide for physicians*, 6th ed. Ottawa: Canadian Medical Association, 2000. <www.cma.ca/staticContent/HTML/N0/l2/publications/catalog/driversguide/> (October 2002).
12. Canadian Medical Association. *Fit for Flying? A Guide for Mandatory Medical Reporting*. Ottawa: Canadian Medical Association, 1986.
13. Fitzgerald M. Implementing guidelines to improve TB control. World Conference on Lung Health, International Union against Tuberculosis and Lung Diseases, Paris, France, 2001.
14. Grimshaw J, Russel I. Effect of clinical guidelines on medical practice: A systematic review of rigorous evaluation. *Lancet* 1993; 1993(342):1317-22.
15. Battista RN. Adult Cancer Prevention in Primary Care. *Canadian Medical Association Journal* 1983; 73:1036-9.
16. Battista RN. Practice guidelines for preventive care: The Canadian experience. Canadian Task Force on the Periodic Health Examination. *Canadian Medical Association Journal* 1993; 149(12):1795-800.
17. Battista RN, Palmer CS, Marchand BM, *et al*. Patterns of preventive practice in New Brunswick. *Canadian Medical Association Journal* 1985; 132:1013-5.
18. Beaulieu M, Hudon E, Roberge D, *et al*. Practice guidelines for clinical prevention: Do patients, physicians, and experts share common ground? *Canadian Medical Association Journal* 1999; 161(5):519-23.
19. Smith HE, Herbert CP. Preventive practice among primary care physicians in British Columbia: Relation to recommendations of the Canadian Task Force on the Periodic Health Examination. *Canadian Medical Association Journal* 1994; 150(6):871-9.

"Health is a political construct, not a biological or technical process."

Author Unknown

PART
THREE

THE HEALTHCARE SYSTEM

The traditional Canadian values of social justice and equity that are reflected in our political system have shaped the healthcare system. This part provides an overview of the healthcare system and the constant turmoil it faces due to jurisdiction dispute between federal and provincial governments. It begins with the evolution and history of health care in Canada, and describes the federal, provincial, and local delivery structures for funding, resource allocation and accountability, and includes a special description on Quebec. It also covers healthcare professionals and their role in the system. For several years, Canada has been voted as among the top countries to live in, thanks in no small manner to our healthcare system.

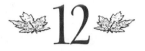

EVOLUTION OF NATIONAL HEALTH INSURANCE

The choice each country makes with respect to health policy reflects the extent to which it is a just and caring society (1). For example, in countries where individual choices are valued above the societal goods and government involvement is considered an infringement on personal rights, as in the United States, the healthcare system is to a large extent private. However, in countries where liberal socialism exists and where health care is viewed as an individual right and social good, the healthcare system is mainly financed and delivered by the public sector, such as in the United Kingdom. In Canada, where a large majority of people hold dear the values of social justice and equity but still believe to some degree in individualism, certain important or expensive components of the healthcare system are in the public sector and others are in the private domain (2).

Political leaders and health ministries of every country are faced with a series of decisions about how best to meet the healthcare needs of their populations. Conceptually, the organization of a healthcare system can be divided into how health services are delivered to those in need and how payments for the provision of these services are financed. The terms "public" and "private" are not precise but are often used to describe healthcare systems. "Virtually every country employs some combination of financing and delivery models, relying on various public-private combinations in various sectors of the health care system or for various groups of the nation's population" (3).

In general terms, "public" refers to government involvement while "private" is generally thought of as what lies beyond the boundaries of government. In Canada, the public sector can be divided into four levels of government:

- national (federal government);
- provincial/state (province or territorial);
- regional (e.g., regional health authority); and
- local (e.g., municipality).

Private is generally thought of as what lies beyond the boundaries of government to include both the family and the market. The private sector can be thought of as including both not-for-profit organizations and for-profit organizations. The private sector can also be divided into four different levels:

Table 12.1.   Public Sector and Private Sector Involvement in Healthcare Systems

Financing	Delivery Sector	
	Public	Private
Public	Financing and delivery of services are handled by a public agency (e.g., Sweden).	The public pays for services through taxes or social security and the services are delivered by private not-for-profit and for-profit agencies (e.g., Canada and Australia).
Private	The cost is charged directly to users through private insurance or directly to the individual and services are provided in public facilities.	Private insurance or the patient pays for services, which are provided in private not-for-profit and for-profit facilities (e.g., United States).

Source: Adapted from C Blanchette, E Tolley. *Public- and private-sector involvement in health-care systems: A comparison of OECD countries*. Ottawa: Depository Services Program, Government of Canada 1997, revised 2001 <dsp-psd.communication.gc.ca/Collection-R/LoPBdP/BP/bp438-e.htm> (September 2002).

- corporate for-profit, which must return profits to shareholders;
- small business/entrepreneurial;
- charitable/not-for-profit, which can use varying combinations of paid staff and volunteers; and
- family/personal.

The first two levels would be termed private for-profit and would range in size from individual businesses (e.g. physician offices) to large investor-owned corporations (e.g., pharmaceutical companies.). The third level involves private not-for-profit organizations that can range from small groups relying on volunteers (e.g., Meals on Wheels) to large organizations with multimillion dollar budgets and thousands of employees (e.g., teaching hospitals). However, the boundaries between not-for-profit and for-profit can be blurred, particularly if a private sector organization is performing a public function or relying on public funds (4). Examples include Canadian hospitals as well as the regulatory bodies that police health professionals with private money in the public interest (such as the College of Medical Laboratory Technologists of Ontario, which collects members' dues).

In this context, there are three other items that must be understood: financing (how services are paid), delivery (how services are provided to recipients of care), and allocation (how resources flow from those who finance care to those who deliver it and are described in detail in Chapter 14). Indeed, it is the combination of varying delivery and financing models that makes each individual health system unique. Table 12.1 illustrates the different combinations of public and private sector involvement in healthcare systems.

This chapter provides an overview of the organization of the delivery and financing of the Canadian medicare system, offers a review of its historical evolution, and, finally, describes the organization of the delivery and financing of healthcare systems of other industrialized nations.

The contemporary Canadian healthcare system combines a system of private service delivery (in which health providers are self-employed rather than employees of the state) with publicly financed care (through a single-source provincial government payer). Additionally, due to the division of federal-provincial responsibilities at the time of Confederation, Canada does not have a single health system, but rather ten provincial and three territorial health systems with uniform federal guidelines. The current legal foundation of Canada's health system is based on three statutes: the *Constitution Act,* 1867, which deals primarily with the jurisdictional power between federal and provincial governments, the *Canada Health Act* (CHA) of 1984, and the *Canada Health and Social Transfer Act* (CHST) of 1996. The CHA outlines the national terms and conditions, whereas the CHST sets the conditions for fiscal transfers from the federal government to the provinces and territories. To understand these particular Canadian features, and how they evolved from a free enterprise system of medicine, one first must examine the historical development of health care in Canada and how collective Canadian values have shaped and continue to shape the healthcare system (2, 5-7).

1. HEALTH CARE PRIOR TO 1950

1.1. HEALTH AND THE BRITISH NORTH AMERICA ACT

In 1867, Canada's Confederation was proclaimed in the *British North America Act* (BNA Act, now known as the *Constitution Act*, 1867), our most fundamental constitutional document. At that time, the government's role in the healthcare system was minimal. Most Canadians had to rely on their own resources for medical care, and hospital services were provided only by charitable trusts and religious organizations. Naturally, those who drafted the BNA Act and even the Fathers of Confederation could not predict the volume of industrial and technological growth, or the healthcare needs for the coming years. The only references to health matters in the BNA Act are found in section 91, which enumerates the power of the federal government, and section 92, which enumerates provincial powers.

Section 91 defines the primacy of the federal economic role including the regulation of trade, taxation, external affairs, defence, quarantine, immigration, criminal law, and the powers of reservation and disallowance. **Section 92** defines the provincial social role including social welfare, education, civil law, and agriculture. This list of powers neither is exhaustive nor does it include any expansion of state role into areas such as health anticipated at the time Section 91 and 92 were written. The *Constitutional Act* and subsequent interpretations of it gave the provinces jurisdiction over most health services. The federal government was given jurisdiction only for those specific populations mentioned in the *Constitutional Act*. These include aboriginal peoples with whom the federal government has signed treaties, the armed forces, the RCMP, immigrants or refugees at certain stages in the immigration process, those living in the territories, and a few other small groups. From 1867 to 1919, the Department of Agriculture covered any federally related health concerns (8). Table 12.2 outlines the historical evolution of the role of federal government involvement in personal health care in Canada.

Since the establishment of the first federal health department, the role of the federal government has expanded. This increased role will be discussed in the next chapter.

1.2.   1867 TO 1948

The origin of publicly financed medical care and hospital care can be traced to Saskatchewan. In 1914, the rural municipality of Sarnia, Saskatchewan, experimented with a form of medical care insurance by offering physicians a retainer to practise in the area. This plan guaranteed the physician certain remuneration and allowed for a practice on a fee-for-service basis. The experiment was so successful that two years later the provincial government passed the *Rural Municipality Act*, which permitted any rural municipality in Saskatchewan to levy property taxes to retain doctors who provided primary medical care and public health services in that area. This legislation encouraged doctors to settle in the province. By 1946, there were about 100 of this sort of publicly supported plan in Saskatchewan, and they continued to operate for some years. Similar but less extensive plans were adopted by Manitoba in 1921 and by Alberta in 1926.

In 1916, Saskatchewan took one of the first steps to break down the tradition of municipal responsibility for hospital care by passing the *Union Hospital Act*, which permitted municipalities to merge into hospital districts for building and maintaining hospitals. In the following year, legislation gave municipalities the right to collect taxes to finance hospital care for their residents. By 1946, many local plans were operating in the province.

Newfoundland in the 1930s is another example of government involvement in health. The province faced many of the same health service challenges as Saskatchewan — namely a sparse population, small population centres, and remote distances. However, the situation was complicated by the fact that most access to remote communities was over sea, not over land. All these factors led to the introduction of the Cottage Hospital and Medical Care Plan in 1934, which provided out-port care by having doctors and nurses regularly visit the communities by sea.

The first attempt to develop a national health insurance program was in 1935, when the conservative federal government of Prime Minister R.B. Bennett proposed the *Employment and Social Insurance Act* to collect taxes in order to provide certain social security benefits, including health benefits. However, the provinces challenged the Act because it encroached on their jurisdiction. The provincial governments were so concerned with Bennett's proposals that they took the matter to the British Privy Council for a constitutional determination. The program was ruled *ultra vires* in 1937, meaning it was outside of the federal government's area of responsibility. This was the

Table 12.2.   Historical Evolution of Federal Government Involvement in Personal Health Care

1867 Confederation	*British North American Act* (now *Constitution Act*, 1867); no involvement.
1935-1945	Proposed national health care and security legislation; the idea of legislation rejected by provinces.
1944	Veterans Affairs Health Care Programs which provides veterans and dependents with health and social programs.
1947	Saskatchewan introduced a public insurance plan for hospital services
1948	National Health Grants; beginnings of infrastructure for national health insurance.
1957	Equalization Program which addresses horizonnal imbalances between provinces and territories
1957	*Hospital Insurance and Diagnostic Services Act*; universal hospitalization for acute care.
1961	Saskatchewan extended public health insurance to cover physicians services outside hospitals
1966	*Canada Assistance Plan (CAP)* introduced by the federal government, a cost-sharing plan for comprehensive welfare programs. The plan also covered certain health services
1966	*Medical Care Act*; unIversal coverage for physicians' services.
1977	*Established Programs Financing Act* and Extended Health Care Services; revised financial arrangements and coverage for additional services.
1979	Medical Services Branch
1984	*Canada Health Act*; consolidation of previous two acts with some revisions.
1985-86	Territorial Formula Financing (TFF) was introduced to replace a system of annual grants negotiated by federal and territorial governments.
1996	*Canada Health and Social Transfer Act;* consolidation of finances under previous arrangement of *Established Programs Financing Act*, Canada Assistance Plan, and postsecondary education.
1997	Report of National Forum on Health
1997	*Health Transition Fund*
1999	*Social Union Framework Agreement* signed by the Prime Minister and all premiers and territorial leaders except Quebec
1999	Announcement in the Federal Budget of a new five-year funding arrangement for CHST
1999	1999 Federal Budget announced key steps to strengthen health care in Canada, improve the health of Canadians and enhance health research
2000	*Primary Health Care Transition Fund*
2002	Reports by Kirby Commission and Romanow Commission
2003	Health Care Renewal Accord, federal government commits new funding for health care renewal and reform

first formal determination that health was a provincial responsibility. The Supreme Court of Canada later upheld this position.

After World War II, countries all over the world were caught up in reconstruction, which brought about certain promising changes that bettered the lives of people in some countries, particularly in the western world. This process influenced the provision of social services — especially in the areas of health, education, and welfare.

At the same time, it was extremely difficult for provincial governments and major Canadian hospitals to find adequate financial resources to provide health services. Health care costs were rising. There were technological advances and the union movement was influencing the hospital workforce. The federal government's attempts to deal with the problem failed because the issue became entangled with jurisdictional dispute between the federal and provincial governments. Between 1942 and 1944, the Select Committee on Social Security of the House of Commons received reports on social security, the Report of the Advisory Committee on Health Insurance, and a draft bill for comprehensive national health insurance. After considering these reports, the Select Committee produced a specific proposal for a broad program of social security, including health insurance based on shared costs and a phased introduction. This proposal was presented to the provincial governments in 1945 at the Dominion-Provincial Conference on Post-War Reconstruction, but was rejected because the provinces and federal governments could not agree on the financial arrangements.

Meanwhile, Saskatchewan decided to proceed on its own. In 1947, it became the first province to introduce a hospitalization plan for all residents, financed by a combination of premiums and general taxes. Other provinces followed. British Columbia introduced its universal hospital insurance program in 1949, and Alberta initiated a limited plan in 1950. Newfoundland and Labrador joined Confederation in 1949 and one of the conditions of joining was the maintenance of its Cottage Hospital Plan.

2.   THE HEALTHCARE SYSTEM BETWEEN 1948 AND 1977

2.1.   NATIONAL HEALTH GRANTS

Recognizing constitutionally that the federal government could not unilaterally move forward with a national health system, the politicians and the bureaucrats decided they could advance their agenda by means of cash incentives to the provinces. Since provinces had jurisdiction over health, the role of the federal government was restricted to assistance in paying the bills. However, the federal government could steer the healthcare system by imposing conditions whenever it shared the cost of programs.

The first step was the enactment of the *National Health Grants Act* of 1948. This act marked the entry of the federal government into the health field. Under it, grants-in-

Table 12.3. Equalization Transfers for 2001–2002

Province	B.C.	Sask.	Man.	Que.	N.B.	N.S.	P.E.I.	Nfld.
$ Millions	488	325	1,158	4,678	1,174	1,260	248	1,019

Source: Department of Finance Canada, Keeping Equalization "Up to Date" <www.fin.gc.ca/transfers/transfers_keeping_up_e.html> (September 2002).

aid were provided to the provinces for a variety of public health services: hospital construction, laboratory services, and professional training for public health. The federal government viewed these grants as the fundamental prerequisites of a nationwide system of health insurance. Later, other grants were added but, except for professional training grants and public health research grants, they were all gradually abolished after the introduction of Canadian medicare and the contemporary provincial health insurance programs.

2.2. THE EQUALIZATION PROGRAM

Initiated in 1957, the Equalization Program is renewed every five years by legislation. Its purpose is to address the horizontal imbalances among provinces and territories. This program enables provincial and territorial governments to provide their residents with reasonably comparable levels of public services at reasonably comparable levels of taxation. The equalization payments are calculated according to a formula set out in federal legislation. The basis of the equalization entitlements has changed over time (9). Equalization payments are unconditional in that the receiving provinces are free to spend them on public services according to their own priorities. Unlike the other federal transfers, the Equalization Program is entrenched in the Canadian Constitution and is one of the few federal programs exempted from restraint measures over the past few years (10).

Equalization transfers for 2001 and 2002 can be found in Table 12.3. Not every province and territory is eligible for this federal transfer. Alberta and Ontario did not qualify for equalization in fiscal year 2001– 02 as they are above the threshold for equalization.

2.3. THE HOSPITAL INSURANCE AND DIAGNOSTIC SERVICES ACT OF 1957

There have been several federal acts related to health and hospitals passed since 1950; one of the first was the *Hospital Insurance and Diagnostic Services Act* (HIDS), passed by Parliament in 1957 and enacted in 1958. HIDS provided for federal cost sharing of all services delivered in hospital except for those provided by physicians in those provinces with a universal hospital insurance plan. Five provinces immediately agreed to the terms of the Act. By 1961, it was operating in all provinces and territories and covered 99% of the population of Canada. Its main purposes were to establish and maintain services and facilities that would lead to better health and health care for the population as a whole by providing, as its name implies, hospital care and diagnostic services. Although all residents of Canada were eligible for hospital insurance coverage, the federal law excluded services for those already eligible for similar benefits under other federal or provincial legislation, such as workers covered by workers' compensation legislation or veterans covered by the *Pensions Act*.

One basic principle influenced the development of hospital insurance legislation: the belief that existing traditions should be maintained as far as possible. Therefore, the pattern of hospital care and ownership that existed before 1957 was retained, and provincial autonomy in health care was not affected. The policy of provincial autonomy allowed each province to decide on its own administrative methods, while ensuring a basic uniformity of coverage throughout the country.

2.3.1. Terms and Conditions

HIDS stipulated that the following must be insured services provided to inpatients:
* Accommodation and meals at the standard or public ward level;
* Necessary nursing service;
* Laboratory, radiology, and other diagnostic procedures;
* Drugs, biological products, and related preparations;
* Use of operating room, case room, and anesthetic facilities, including necessary equipment and supplies;
* Routine surgical supplies;
* Use of radiotherapy facilities, where available;
* Use of physiotherapy facilities, where available; and
* Such other services as specified in the agreement.

At the option of each province, any of the above could also be provided as insured outpatient services. Provinces may include additional benefits in their plans without affecting the federal-provincial agreements. The Act also made hospital insurance portable for residents who temporarily left their home province, although coverage was subject to provincially regulated limits. In many cases, elective hospitalization outside the province required prior approval, which could be withheld in some provinces if equivalent services were available.

2.3.2. Methods of Financing

The federal contribution paid to the provinces for insured services amounted to approximately 50% of the costs of those services. The cost sharing in this legislation involved a federal contribution of:
* 25% of per capita cost of inpatient services in Canada, plus
* 25% of per capita cost of inpatient services in province.

Shared costs under the agreements with the provinces excluded most hospital construction costs but could include the cost of movable equipment and most fixed equipment specifically required by hospitals. Each province determined how its share of the costs would be financed; most financed their share out of general revenue, but some provinces also imposed premiums or certain authorized charges.

HIDS was replaced by the *Canada Health Act* in 1984, which has similar provisions.

2.4. THE MEDICAL CARE ACT OF 1966

2.4.1. Events Leading to the Medical Care Act of 1966

Hospital insurance paved the way for medical care insurance. Saskatchewan once again was the first province to experiment with a compulsory, government-sponsored medical care insurance program. The program's principles were prepayment, universal coverage, and acceptability both to providers and receivers of services. The legislation received royal assent in November 1961, and, despite a strike by physicians, the program was implemented on July 1, 1962. British Columbia, Alberta, and Ontario adopted their own medical insurance programs between 1963 and 1966.

In 1965, the federal government's Royal Commission on Health Services (appointed in 1960, chaired by the Honourable Emmett M. Hall, Justice of the Supreme Court of Canada) completed the most comprehensive assessment of health services undertaken to that date. It found that nearly 60% of Canadians had some form of insurance against the costs of medical care, but for approximately 30% of those insured, this coverage was inadequate. The commission recommended strong federal government leadership and financial support for medical care. However, it also recommended that the operating controls of the program be decentralized under the provincial governments. General standards and guidelines were suggested as part of the federal government's conditions, but the commission recommended that each province should be permitted wide latitude in its program. It also made closely related recommendations for greatly expanded support for teaching, research, and other facilities for training healthcare personnel. In the summer of 1965, a new federal proposal based on the recommendations of the Hall Commission was introduced at a federal-provincial conference (11).

2.4.2. Enactment of the Medical Care Act of 1966

After a series of discussions between the federal and provincial governments, the *Medical Care Act* of 1966 was enacted and implemented in 1968. By 1971, all provinces had set up programs that complied with the Act. Under the *Medical Care Act*, each province received a federal government contribution equal to half of the average per capita medical care costs incurred by all provinces, multiplied by the number of insured people in that province. As the average cost in poorer provinces was lower than in richer provinces, these cost-sharing arrangements gave larger proportion of payments to the poorer provinces. Hence, the federal contribution as a proportion of the total cost for medical care varied among provinces. In 1975–76, the proportion ranged from 40.8% in British Columbia and 49.2% in Ontario, to 67.7% in Prince Edward Island and 75.6% in Newfoundland. All physicians' services and some additional services provided by dentists and chiropractors were covered. To be eligible for federal contributions, the provincial medical services plan was required to meet criteria very similar to those in HIDS, which were called the "Four Points": medical insurance must be comprehensive, universal, portable, and publicly administered.

2.4.3.   Terms and Conditions

Comprehensive Coverage

At a minimum, the plan was to provide coverage for all services rendered by medical practitioners, without dollar limit or exclusions, provided there was medical need, unless coverage was available under other legislation. The plan was to be administered so that no financial limitation prevented an insured person from receiving necessary medical care. Certain surgical-dental procedures by dental surgeons (when rendered in hospital) were included from the beginning, and other professional services were added as the provincial government considered fit. Each province could provide additional insured benefits but without federal cost sharing.

Universality

The plan was to be uniformly available to all eligible residents (no fewer than 95% of the population must be covered). Each province determined whether its residents should be insured on a voluntary or compulsory basis. Provinces were allowed to charge premiums to the enrollees in the program. No discrimination according to previous health, race, age, or non-membership in a group was permitted, but partial or complete premium subsidization for low-income groups or the elderly was allowed, if all qualifying residents were treated equally. Similarly, utilization charges at the time of service were not precluded by the federal legislation if they did not impede, either by their amount or by the way they were applied, reasonable access to necessary medical care, particularly for low-income groups.

Portability

Under the *Medical Care Act*, benefits were portable when the insured person was temporarily absent from the province, whether travelling anywhere in the world or changing jobs, retiring, or moving from one province to another, provided the individual remained enrolled in the program and paid premiums in those provinces that charged premiums. When an insured resident moved to another province, the province of origin would provide medical care benefits during any waiting period imposed by the medical insurance plan of the destinations. No province could impose a waiting period longer than three months before a new resident was entitled to obtain coverage. Some provinces required that people obtain approval before having elective (i.e., non-emergency) care outside their province. In general, provinces limited the amount payable for medical services received out of province to the amount payable for similar services in the person's province.

Public Administration

The plan was non-profit and administered by a public agency accountable to the provincial government for its financial transactions.

The above criteria gave each province substantial flexibility in determining the administrative arrangements for the operation of its medical care insurance plan and in choosing its financing plan (through premiums, sales tax, or other provincial revenues, or a combination thereof). Federal contributions to the provinces under this program totalled $1.7 billion by the fiscal year 1975–76.

Like HIDS, this act was replaced by the *Canada Health Act* in 1984, which has similar provisions.

3.   1977–1984: NEW FINANCING OF HEALTHCARE PROGRAMS AND THE CANADA HEALTH ACT

By the middle of the 1970s, the shared-cost health programs had become a critical problem for both the federal and provincial governments. The chief point of contention between the two levels of government was increasing healthcare costs as the cost was transferred from the private sector to the public sector. In 1976, total health expenditures in Canada exceeded $13 billion. Because these programs were open-ended (i.e., the federal government paid the provinces about half of the cost for insured hospital and medical care costs), they impeded federal governmental program planning in other fields. The provincial governments were also dissatisfied because, while the most expensive costs of health care were shared, other important and innovative aspects (such as the development of community-based services instead of general hospital care) were not shared. To alleviate this, a new agreement on financing arrangements was reached at the Conference of First Ministers in December 1976. The legislation was enacted on March 31, 1977, as the *Federal-Provincial Fiscal Arrangements and Established Programs Financing Act* (EPF), 1977, and included extended healthcare services.

3.1.   ESTABLISHED PROGRAMS FINANCING ACT, 1977

3.1.1.   Description of Financing Arrangements

As of April 1, 1977, federal contributions to the provinces and territories for the established programs of hospital insurance, medical care, and post-secondary education were no longer directly related to provincial costs. About 70% of all the EPF transfers were designated for the health component, while the remaining 30% went to education. This breakdown was arbitrary, because EPF was a "block" funding mechanism. In other words, unlike the shared-cost programs, EPF transfers were not determined based on the province's expenditures on health care and education. In addition, each province was free to allocate the EPF transfers according to its own priorities.

EPF total transfers, or entitlements, had two components: a tax transfer and a cash transfer. Cash transfers to the provinces corresponded to monetary or financial contributions paid periodically by cheque, while the federal government also accorded a certain tax room to the provinces through the transfer of tax points. To do this, the federal government reduced its tax rates while the provinces increased their rates by an equivalent amount. This procedure resulted in a reallocation of revenue between the two levels of government: federal revenue was reduced by an amount equivalent to the increase in the provincial governments' revenues. The fiscal burden on taxpayers remained the same because, although they paid more provincial tax, they paid less federal tax.

These financing arrangements initially provided each province with more money than it might have received with the previous cost-sharing formula but the increase was tied to the GNP and population growth. There was greater equality among the provinces in what they received from the federal government per capita and they had greater flexibility in the use of their own funds and federal contributions. The arrangements were more stable for both levels of government. Program administration was simplified because federal auditing of provincial records was no longer required. The terms of the financing arrangements were to be indefinite, but a provision in the legislation permitted the federal government to terminate the arrangements with three years' notice.

Originally, the basic payment under the EPF was calculated on an initial per capita amount determined in 1975–76, which was then adjusted each year according to an escalator that considered the rate of growth per capita in the gross national product (GNP). To determine the total value of a province's EPF entitlement, the initial amount was multiplied by the escalator and then by the population of that province. The EPF contained a clause to the effect that for five years the federal government would not modify the formula in any way that would have adverse effects on the provinces and territories without their consent.

The escalator was modified on several occasions from the mid 1980s to the mid 1990s. In 1983–84 and 1984–85, the education escalator was capped at 6% and 5% respectively. If the formula based on the per capita growth in the gross domestic product, or GDP, had been used, the amount would have increased by 9% in 1983–84 and by 8% in 1984–85. For all other years, the escalator for post-secondary education was the same as for healthcare insurance. From 1986–87 to 1989–90, the escalator used to calculate total EPF payments was reduced by 2%. After this period, and until 1994–95, per capita transfers were frozen at their 1989–90 levels, so that the total amount of transfer payments increased only in accordance with population growth in each province (about 1%). For 1995–96, the escalator was decreased by 3% and the result was a negative escalator (almost –1.0%, according to the Federal-Provincial Relations Division of the Department of Finance); this meant a decrease in per capita transfers, given the fact that GDP growth was less than 3% (12).

The federal government had attached broad conditions to its cash payments in order to guarantee adequate standards of health care across the country. The conditions were the same as those used for hospital and medical care insurance since the beginning: comprehensiveness, universal coverage, portability of benefits, and non-profit administration by a public agency.

The CHST in 1996, which has similar provisions, replaced the EPF.

3.1.2. Extended Healthcare Services

Under the EPF, the federal government made a financial contribution for extended healthcare services. Payments began on April 1, 1977. The Extended Health Care Services Program allowed the federal government to make block-funded contributions (one payment to cover all services) to the provinces in order to assist them in providing nursing homes (intermediate care), adult residential care, converted mental hospitals, health-related aspects of home care, and ambulatory health care.

This program had three purposes:

- to provide the provinces with financial assistance for providing less costly forms of health care in conjunction with the insured services of the *Hospital Insurance and Diagnostic Services Act* and the *Medical Care Act*;
- to encompass most of health and institutional health services within a similar block-funding financial arrangement; and
- to provide the provinces with greater flexibility.

Funding for 1988–89 was approximately $48 per capita ($1.27 billion), with the same terms as those of the EPF (i.e., based on the growth of GNP and the population). Since this program was viewed as complementary to basic hospital and medical care insurance, the only condition of payment was that the provinces furnish the federal minister of health with information required by the federal government for its international obligations, national planning and standards, and information exchanges with the provinces.

In 1995–96, the last year of the EPF, provinces and territories received a total of $22 billion in EPF entitlements (cash and tax), 71.2% of which was intended for health care and the rest for post-secondary education. This arrangement was replaced by the CHST in 1996, which has similar provisions.

Territorial Formula Financing (TFF)

Territorial Formula Financing (TFF) was introduced in 1985–86 to replace a system of annual grants negotiated by federal and territorial governments. The TFF enables the territories to provide a range of public services comparable to those offered by provincial governments. TFF is an unconditional cash transfer based on the difference between the expenditures needs and revenue means of the territorial governments, a formula designed to fill gaps.

In 2001–02, the federal government transferred almost $1.5 billion to the three territorial governments: $510 million to the Northwest Territories, $611 million to Nunavut, and $346 million to the Yukon (13).

3.2. THE CANADA HEALTH ACT

The EPF no longer tied federal payments to particular forms of health services, which reduced the effect of imposed federal steering. During the late 1970s, healthcare costs increased faster than the GNP, leading the provinces to bear greater costs due to increase in demand for health care and relatively lower contributions by the federal government. As a result, the provinces introduced measures of cost containment such as restraints on raising physicians' fees. An increasing number of physicians responded to this by extra-billing their patients (14), that is, billing patients above the fee schedules, which were negotiated with their provincial health insurance plans. These factors led to charges from the public and interest groups that medicare was being eroded. The federal government established another commission to review the Canadian healthcare system, led again by the Honourable E.M. Hall, who had reviewed the healthcare system in early 1960s.

In 1980, Mr. Justice Hall published the results of this health services review, which emphasized the issue of accessibility of services (15). He concluded that extra-billing threatened to violate the principle of uniform terms and conditions and would prevent access to services for some people. He therefore recommended that this practice be banned and that fair compensation for physicians' services to be determined through negotiation between physicians and governments, with binding arbitration if negotiations failed. Those physicians unwilling to accept the plan as payment in full would be required to practise entirely outside the plan, as was already the case in Quebec. They would bill their patients directly, and patients would be responsible for the full cost of the service.

In 1981, the Parliamentary Task Force on Federal-Provincial Fiscal Arrangements, an all-party task force of members of Parliament, published a review of the EPF, entitled *Fiscal Federalism in Canada* (16). This report included a review of the problems in delivering health care and fulfilling various program conditions outlined in the original hospital and medical care insurance acts. As well, it addressed the question of whether health care in Canada was underfunded and recommended, as had Mr. Justice Hall, that a national health council be formed that would be independent of government and of healthcare providers. This council would act as a coordinating body for defining, planning, and implementing health policy for Canada. Such a council could monitor whether the conditions of the various healthcare programs were being met.

3.2.1.   Enactment of the Canada Health Act, 1984

Following these two major reports, the federal government introduced proposals for a new *Canada Health Act* in May 1982, which was enacted on April 1, 1984, with support from all political parties.

3.2.2   Criteria, Provisions, and Conditions of the Canada Health Act

The *Canada Health Act* (CHA) combined and updated the 1957 *Hospital Insurance and Diagnostic Services Act* and the 1966 *Medical Care Act*. It reaffirmed national principles but added specific restrictions to discourage any form of direct patient charges and to provide citizens of all provinces and territories access to health care regardless of their ability to pay.

The CHA sets out nine requirements that provincial and territorial governments must meet through their public healthcare insurance plan in order to qualify for federal funding under the 1977 EPF. These nine requirements consist of five criteria, two provisions, and two conditions. The five criteria are as follows:

- Public administration: the program must be administered on a non-profit basis by a public authority accountable to the provincial government.
- Comprehensiveness: the program must cover all medically necessary hospital and medical services, and surgical-dental services rendered in hospitals.
- Universality: 100% of the eligible residents must have access to public healthcare insurance and insured services on uniform terms and conditions.
- Portability: provinces and territories must cover insured health services for their citizens while they are temporarily absent from their province of residence or Canada; the home province must pay for out-of-province services at the host province rates and must pay for out-of-country services at the home province rates.
- Accessibility: reasonable access to insured health services must be neither obstructed, either directly or indirectly, by financial charges nor discriminated against on the basis of such factors as income, age, and health status.

The two provisions of the Act specifically discouraged financial contributions by patients, either through user charges or extra-billing for services covered under the provincial healthcare insurance plans.

However, the Act makes a distinction between insured health services (i.e., those that have been deemed medically necessary) and extended healthcare services. Medically necessary services are defined only in the broad sense of the term in the Act. Section 2 states that *insured health services*, which must be fully insured by provincial healthcare insurance plans, comprise:

- hospital services that are medically necessary for the purpose of maintaining health, preventing disease, or diagnosing or treating an injury, illness or disability, and include accommodation and meals, physician and nursing services, drugs, and all medical and surgical equipment and supplies;
- any medically required services rendered by medical practitioners; and
- any medically or required surgical-dental procedures that can only be properly carried out in a hospital.

Section 2 of the Act also stipulates that *extended healthcare services* include intermediate care in nursing homes, adult residential care service, homecare service, and ambulatory healthcare services. Because these services are not subject to the two provisions relating to user charges and extra-billing, they can be charged at either partial or full private rates. In addition, provincial healthcare insurance plans may cover other health services, such as optometric services, dental care, assistive devices, and prescription drugs, which are not subject to the Act, and for which provinces may demand payment from patients. The range of such additional health benefits that are provided under provincial government plans, the rate of coverage, and the categories of beneficiaries vary greatly from one province to another

Penalties for defaults under the CHA are linked to federal transfers to the provinces. The financial penalties stipulated in the Act vary depending on whether a default is directly related to extra-billing and user charges or involves failure to satisfy any of the five criteria (17). The federal Department of Finance has been responsible for making payments to the provinces and territories since the enactment of the CHST on April 1, 1996. The CHST replaced the 1977 EPF and the Canada Assistance Plan (CAP) in 1996. However, the Minister of Health is responsible for determining the amounts of any deductions or withholdings pursuant under the CHA (17).

As indicated above, one of the conditions of the CHA was a partial withholding of funds from provinces that allowed extra-billing and user charges. Ontario, Alberta, Manitoba, Saskatchewan, and New Brunswick allowed extra-billing. With the introduction of the CHA, these provincial governments had to enact legislation to ban extra-billing or they would loose revenue from the federal government. This stipulation strained relations between the two levels of governments and also between provincial governments and their respective medical associations. For example, in 1986, when Ontario introduced legislation banning extra-billing, some physicians in that province went on strike. However by 1987, all provinces had banned extra-billing. The Canadian healthcare system was moving toward an increased federal role especially in the areas of formulation, monitoring, and enforcement of program conditions.

4.   OTHER HEALTH PROGRAMS FINANCED BY THE GOVERNMENT

Canada Assistance Plan (1966)

Under the Canada Assistance Plan (CAP), the federal government paid 50% of the cost of cash assistance and health and welfare services to people in need. CAP involved cash transfers only, except for Quebec, which received a special five-point tax abatement on personal income (17). The program was administered by provincial governments, which were free to offer a wide range of healthcare benefits. The range of benefits varied from province to province, but could include such services as eyeglasses, prosthetic appliances, dental services, prescribed drugs, homecare services, and nursing home care. The only eligibility requirement specified was that of need, determined by an assessment of budgetary requirements, client income, and resources. Provinces are required to provide assistance irrespective of province of origin. The eligibility requirements and rates of assistance were set by the provinces and adjusted to the local conditions and needs of special groups. The provinces had to establish appeal procedures for decisions relating to the provision of assistance.

From the beginning of the plan's operation and until 1990, CAP transfers were open ended; the federal government kept pace with whatever the provinces decided to spend and transfers were accordingly not subject to any limits. In 1990–91, the federal government placed a ceiling on financing, usually called the "cap on CAP." More specifically, a 5% limit for 1990–91 and 1991–92 was placed on annual increases in the contributions made to the three provinces that received no equalization payments (Alberta, British Columbia and Ontario); the other provinces were not subject to any limit. In February 1991, the federal government extended the ceiling until 1994–95.

Then, in its February 1994 budget, for 1995–96 it froze the amounts paid under CAP to all provinces at the 1994–95 level (12).

The CHST replaced CAP in 1996.

Vocational Rehabilitation of Disabled Persons (1952)

The Vocational Rehabilitation of Disabled Persons program has been administered by Health Canada since April 1, 1973. Under it, the federal government contributes 50% of the costs to all provinces, except Quebec, of providing a comprehensive range of services for the vocational rehabilitation of physically and mentally disabled people. Services include social and vocational assessment; counselling; training; maintenance allowances; the provision of tools, books, and other equipment; remedial and restorative treatments; and the provision of prosthetic and orthotic appliances, wheelchairs, and other mobility aids.

5. FROM THE CANADA HEALTH ACT TO THE SOCIAL UNION

5.1. THE CANADA HEALTH AND SOCIAL TRANSFER ACT (1996)

In 1996, the CHST replaced federal transfers for social assistance under the CAP, and for health and post-secondary education under the EPF (described above) (4). The CHST is a block fund designed to give provinces enhanced flexibility in designing and administering efficient healthcare and social programs while upholding basic principles of medicare and safeguarding social programs. The *Budget Implementation Act, 1995* (Bill C-76) specified the amount of this new transfer and broke it down by province for 1996–97. Since then, the *Federal-Provincial Fiscal Arrangements Act*, which now governs the CHST, has been modified on five different occasions by the following pieces of legislation: Bill C-31 (1996); Bill C-28 (1998); Bill C-71 (1999); Bill C-32 (2000); and Bill C-45 (2000) (12). The CHST is similar to the EPF in structure, including a direct cash transfer from the federal government and federal tax concessions that allow provincial governments to raise additional revenues from taxes without increasing the overall tax burden on taxpayers. Unlike the EPF, the CHST legislation specifically guaranteed a floor for each transfer for a number of fiscal years, in order to protect against unexpected economic fluctuations that might reduce the total entitlement or significantly increase the value of the tax transfer, which would decrease the cash transfers to the provinces. Initially, this floor was set to be no less than $11 billion. Bill C-28 (1998) raised the floor to $12.5 billion for 1997–98 and beyond. The CHST's cash floor provision was abolished in 1999 as the amended legislation (Bill C-71) provided a level of cash transfer over and above the $12.5 billion limit. Many commentators argue that, unlike the EPF, which aroused fears that the cash transfers might reach zero, the CHST ensures that a monetary contribution will be made to the provinces and thereby preserves the federal government's power to mandate.

Table 12.4.   Contribution of Federal Government toward Canada Health and Social Transfer, 1994-2003

$ Million	1994–1995	1995–1996	1996–1997	1997–1998	1998–1999	1999–2000	2000–2001	2001–2002	2002–2003
	EPF/CAP			CANADA HEALTH AND SOCIAL TRANSFER					
Cash	18,700	18,500	14,700	12,500	12,500	14,500	15,500	18,300	19,100
Tax	10,700	11,400	12,200	13,300	14,300	15,600	16,400	16,100	16,600
Total	29,400	29,900	26,900	25,800	26,800	30,100	31,900	34,400	35,700

Source: Health Canada: Canada Health and Social Transfer "<www.hc-sc.gc.ca/english/media/releases/2002/health_act/chst.htm>January 2003

As Table 12.4 shows, federal cuts to CHST from 1995 to 1997 led to a significant reduction in the total CHST entitlement for the purposes of health care, post-secondary education, and social assistance. The effects are more proportionately observed in the cash component because the tax transfer continued to grow.

From 1995–96 to 1996–97, the total CHST entitlement (expressed in current dollars) decreased by nearly $3 billion, a reduction of almost 10% (see Table 12.4). In the following fiscal year, the total CHST entitlement was reduced again by $1.1 billion (or 5%). The cash component of the CHST declined even more steeply by $3.8 billion (or 20%) from 1995–96 to 1996–97 and by $2.2 billion (or 15%) from 1996–97 to 1997–98. The changes legislated in Bill C-28 reversed these downward trends, while Bill C-71, Bill C-32, and Bill C-45 together led to substantial growth in both the total CHST entitlement and the CHST cash transfer. In 1999–2000, the total CHST entitlement reached its peak level of 1995–96, but the CHST cash component did not match its 1993–94-peak level until 2002–03.

However, when converted into constant 1993–94 dollars, the total CHST entitlement did not surpass the 1995–96 level until 2001–02, and did not achieve its peak level of 1993–94. In other words, although Bill C-28, Bill C-71, and Bill C-45 resulted in real growth in cash transfers, this growth does not allow for the full restoration of the federal cash funding provided prior to the creation of the CHST.

5.2.   SOCIAL UNION: NEW PRESCRIPTION FOR CANADIAN HEALTH CARE

The social union framework forms the basis of a new partnership between the federal government and the provinces and territories. On February 4, 1999, the Prime Minister and all premiers and territorial leaders, except Quebec, signed the agreement on the Social Union Framework (18). As stated in this document, under this umbrella, the federal and provincial/territorial governments will concentrate their efforts to modernize Canadian social policy.

At the First Ministers' Meeting in September 2000, the Government of Canada and all provinces and territories agreed to a new prescription for Canadian health care (19). The first ministers declared that Canadians will have publicly funded health services that provide quality health care and that promote the health and well-being of Canadians in a cost-effective and fair manner. To achieve this, they made the following commitments. Their governments will:

- support the principles of universality, accessibility, comprehensiveness, portability, and public administration for insured hospital and medical services;
- continue to renew healthcare services by working with other governments, communities, service providers, and Canadians;
- promote those public services, programs, and policies that extend beyond care and treatment and that make a critical contribution to the health and wellness of Canadians;
- further address key priorities for healthcare renewal and support innovations to meet the current and emerging needs of Canadians;
- expand the sharing of information on best practices and thereby contribute to continuing improvements in the quality and efficiency of healthcare services;
- report regularly to Canadians on health status, health outcomes, and the performance of publicly funded health services, and the actions taken to improve these services; and,
- work in collaboration with Aboriginal people, their organizations, and their governments, to improve their health and well-being.

New federal funding was also made available to accompany the agreements on health renewal and early childhood development, including $23.4 billion of new federal investments over five years to support agreements by First Ministers on Health Renewal and Early Childhood Development (ECD) (19). To ensure stable, predictable, and growing funding in the CHST, the federal government would legislate over $21 billion of additional cash over the next five years. This included a new $2.2 billion investment for ECD.

In order to accelerate and broaden health renewal, the government of Canada would also invest in three targeted areas reflecting agreed priorities:

- It would invest a total of $1 billion in 2000–01 and 2001–02, through transfers to the provinces and territories, for new medical equipment. Of this amount, $500 million would be immediately available to enable the acquisition of necessary diagnostic and treatment equipment.
- It would invest a further $800 million over four years, beginning in 2001–02, in a renewed Health Transition Fund to support innovation and reform in primary care.
- It would invest $500 million immediately in an independent corporation mandated to accelerate the development and adoption of modern systems of information technology, such as electronic patient records, so as to provide better health care.

The progress in the healthcare system in Canada has been incremental due to jurisdictional disputes and divided federal-provincial responsibility. For the past half-century, Canadians have witnessed acrimonious stands taken by both levels of government on how to reform the healthcare system and the changes have been slow. In the beginning of this century, the federal government and a number of provinces had appointed commissions and committees to review their healthcare systems and recommend blueprints for reform in health care; these are described in Chapter 18.

In late 2002, the Commission on the Future of Health Care (the Romanow Commission) and the Senate Committee Report on the Health of Canadians (the Kirby Commission) recommended the need for specific reforms in the Canadian healthcare system and an infusion of new funds (2, 20). When the First Ministers met in February 2003, they agreed on an action plan to improve access to quality care for all Canadians (21). The Government of Canada agreed to provide $34.8 billion over five years: to relieve immediate pressure on the healthcare system; for a new Health Reform Fund for primary care, home care, and catastrophic drug coverage; for the purchase of diagnostic and medical equipment, and investment in information technology; and to increase funding to address the health of Aboriginal people to reduce health inequity. The First Ministers also agreed to prepare an annual public report on primary care, home care, and catastrophic drug coverage commencing in 2004, and they agreed to create a health council that will report regularly to Canadians on the quality of their health care.

6.   DESCRIPTION OF THE FINANCING AND DELIVERY OF HEALTH CARE IN SELECTED COUNTRIES

The first sections of this chapter traced the evolution of Canada's medicare system from Confederation in 1867 to the present. What started as a minimal state role in a privately financed and mostly privately delivered system has evolved into a largely publicly funded system referred to by many as Canada's public policy success story (1). The evolution of the Canadian healthcare system as it faces its many current challenges, however, is not yet over. Some of the main issues currently facing the system are described in subsequent chapters in this book.

The 1990s were a decade of restructuring of healthcare systems, both in North America and abroad. Triggered largely by fiscal considerations and concerns about increases in costs, virtually every government in the industrialized world sought to reform its healthcare system (22). In its review of recent health system reforms, the Organisation for Economic Co-operation and Development (OECD) lists the following key goals of healthcare reform (22):
- adequacy and equity in access to health services;
- income protection;
- macroeconomic efficiency;
- microeconomic efficiency;
- appropriate provider autonomy; and
- freedom of choice for consumers.

Reform measures were introduced to contain costs and enable healthcare resources to be used more efficiently. In general, these changes have meant reduced public coverage, decreased publicly funded services, and increased out-of-pocket payments. The private sector is now more involved in health care. Increasingly, the public and private sectors are working conjointly to fund and deliver health care. This section will describe the national

Table 12.5.   A Comparison of Healthcare Spending, Resources, and Health Status for Selected Countries

Country	Total expenditure on health as % of GDP	Public sector expenditure on health as % of GDP	Percentage of population covered	Inpatient care as % of total expenditure on health	Total inpatient care beds per 1,000 population	Practicing physicians (density per 1,000 population)	Infant mortality, deaths per 1,000 live births	% of the population over 60 years of age[a] Male/Female		Life expectancy (in years) Male/Female	
								M	F	M	F
Australia	8.6	6.0	100	43.3	8.5	2.5	5.0	15	18	75.9	81.5
Canada	9.3	6.5	100	43.1	4.1	2.1	5.3	15	19	76.1	81.5
France	9.3	7.1	99.5[b]	44.8	8.5	3.0	4.6	18	23	74.6	82.2
Germany	10.3	7.8	92.2[b]	34.0	9.3	3.5	4.6	20	27	74.5	80.5
Japan	7.5	5.8	100	37.6	16.5	1.9	3.6	21	26	77.2	84.0
New Zealand	8.1	6.3	100	N/A	6.2	2.2	6.8[b]	14	17	75.2	80.4
Sweden	7.9	6.6	100	N/A	3.8	3.1	3.5	20	25	76.9	81.9
UK	6.8	5.7	100	N/A	4.2	1.7	5.7	18	23	74.8	79.7
US	12.9	5.8	45[b]	41.3	3.7	2.7	7.2	14	18	73.8	79.5

Source: Adapted from OECD, 2002. Health Data 2001 <www.oecd.org> (April 2002). Estmates based on 1998 data unless otherwise indicated.
[a] Information on the percentage of individuals over age 60 taken from United Nations, Statistics Division and Population Division, 2003. Indicators on youth and elderly populations, 2001.
[b] Based on 1997 OECD data.

values of different coutnries as reflected in how their health systems are financed and delivered, and the roles played by the public and private sectors.

Table 12.5 provides a comparison of healthcare spending, resources, and health status indicators statistics for selected countries.

6.1.   THE UNITED KINGDOM (A PUBLIC/PUBLIC MODEL)

The United Kingdom has the same parliamentary system as Canada. However, unlike Canada, the United Kingdom is a unitary state comprising England, Scotland, Wales, and Northern Ireland. Each nation is responsible for managing its own healthcare system. The principles upon which the healthcare systems function are basically the same.

The British National Health Service (NHS) has existed since 1948 as a publicly financed and centralized system providing free universal access to health care. It was the first publicly funded and publicly owned health system to appear in Western Europe. With 6.8% of GDP spent on health in 1998 (see Table 12.5), the U.K. consistently spends less on health care than most of its European or North American neighbours.

6.1.1.   Finance

The NHS is a universal system of national health insurance financed mainly through central government general taxation. The NHS funds 84% of healthcare spending, which is a higher proportion than in Canada where the public sector funds 70% (20). The NHS is financed mainly through central government general taxation, together with an element of national insurance contributions made by employers and employees. It provides comprehensive coverage not only for professional services, but also for hospitalization and other benefits such as drugs, dental care, eyeglasses, and hearing aids. Eligibility for medical benefits is universal based only on citizenship, and care is provided free of charge at time of delivery. There are no user charges for physician services, specialist services, and hospital services. User charges do apply to prescription drugs and to dental and optical services. User charges account for only 3% of the total NHS financing. Unlike Canada, the United Kingdom allows individuals to purchase private health insurance that covers the same benefits as the NHS if providers working outside of the NHS provide these services. Approximately 11.5% of the population has private insurance (20).

6.1.2.   Delivery

Delivery from 1948 to 1997
Prior to the 1989 reforms, the NHS was publicly financed and delivered. Regional budgets for hospitals and community care services were set up on a per capita basis adjusted for demographic and other factors, and passed on to hospitals and other facilities via district health authorities (HAs). The HAs were the organizers and providers

of care. Hospitals were run by the HAs and received global lump sum budgets, ultimately set by the central government. General practitioners (GPs) were self-employed and paid according to a central contract involving a mix of capitation, fee for service, and other payments. GPs provided ambulatory services and acted as gatekeepers for non-emergency hospital care and referrals to specialists. Hospital staff physicians (specialists) were salaried, but were allowed part-time private practice. They billed the private health insurance plans for the services of their private practice.

Delivery after the Reforms of 1989 and 1991

Until 1989, the UK's healthcare system was almost entirely public delivery, with the NHS owning and operating most health facilities. Although largely successful in keeping down macro-level costs, the system was criticized for being overtly bureaucratic and unresponsive to patient needs — complaints frequently heard about public delivery systems.

Reforms were proposed in the 1989 white paper titled *Putting People First*. These reforms were subsequently enacted in 1990 legislation and implemented beginning in 1991. The goal was to maintain the public financing role but to have providers of specialist services compete in a quasi or internal market for secondary health care by separating them from purchasers. This type of reform was known as the purchaser-provider split. There were two types of purchasers — district health authorities (HAs) and general practitioner (GP) fund-holders. HAs and GP fund-holders contracted with the hospital trusts for the quantity and type of services to be provided and for the fees that the hospitals were to be paid.

The separation of the purchaser and provider functions affected the relationship between the regional health authorities and the hospitals. The HAs ceased to manage hospitals and become responsible, as purchasing organizations, for contracting with the NHS hospitals and private providers to deliver the services required by their resident population.

The NHS allocates money for health services to regional health boards, which, in turn, disburse funds among the district HAs in their region. There are 100 HAs in the NHS (23). Each is allocated a budget to purchase health services for its population, by entering into service contracts with local self-governing hospital trusts. Service contracts were awarded on a competitive basis based on service cost and quality. Hospitals were transformed into NHS trusts, or not-for-profit organizations within the NHS but outside of the control of the regional health authorities.

The establishment of the GP fund-holding system modified the organization and shape of the general family practices. Under this system, large groups of GPs (serving 7,000 or more people) were given a "fund" of two spending categories: the cost of drugs prescribed to their patients and the cost of certain kinds of specialist and hospital treatment. GP fund-holders were responsible for managing a budget, which was used to secure hospital and primary care services and pharmaceuticals for their enlisted patients. Prior to more recent reform, 3,500 GP fund-holders existed in the NHS covering over half of the population (23).

In 1997, the government announced the termination of the internal market system and introduced a new approach that relies on cooperation and partnership rather than emphasizes competition and financial performance (23). The structure of the new NHS was outlined in a 1997 white paper and enshrined in the 1999 *Health Act*. The NHS plan is to be implemented over a 10-year period and commits to a 6.3% increase in funding over five years to 2004 (24). The Modernisation Board was set up to advise the Secretary of State for Health and the ministerial team on implementing the plan. The board is made up of representatives from healthcare institutions, such as the royal colleges, clinical staff, and managers from within the NHS and patient representatives.

Specific changes to the NHS to date include the following (24):

- An increase in the number of critical, general, and acute beds, an increase in the number of nurses working in the NHS (approximately 10,000 in England), and the replacement and the installation of 52 new computer tomography (CT) cancer scanners.
- As of April 2002, England's 95 HAs were replaced by 28 larger health authorities. The new HAs will manage the NHS locally, providing a link between the Department of Health and the NHS. They will also ensure that national priorities (such as programs for improving cancer service) are integrated in the local health services.
- The GP fund-holding system was abolished in favour of Primary Care Trusts (PCTs), which are group practices of merged GP fund-holders. PCTs are larger than GP fund-holders, covering between 50,000 to 250,000 people in designated geographic areas (20). The creation of the PCT does not affect the ways GPs are reimbursed.
- Quality management is given greater emphasis under the heading of clinical governance, which includes policies for managing risk and tackling poor performance, greater accountability, and a commitment to life-long learning.
- National standards were introduced. National Service Frameworks (NSF) are being established to improve quality and to reduce unacceptable variations in service. The National Institute for Clinical Excellence was created in 1999 to produce and disseminate clinical guidelines.
- The Commission for Health Improvement was established to monitor the implementation of standards set by the NSF.
- NHS Direct, a 24-hour telephone helpline operated by nurses was created to offer advice on self-care or to refer callers to the appropriate services.
- Walk-in centres staffed by nurses were introduced to offer advice and treatment for minor ailments seven days a week.

More recent changes have occurred in the NHS and have shifted the focus from market-oriented competition to concerns about quality management and accountability.

Private Healthcare Delivery

There are approximately 230 independent medical/surgical facilities and hospitals in the United Kingdom. In the private settings, physicians are paid fee-for-service either directly by the patient, who then may be reimbursed by a private insurance company (if the patient is a policyholder) or by the private hospital or clinic at which the services were provided. Private sector care is specialized and is mainly used for elective surgical procedures such as hernias and hip replacements. Recently, there has been some growth in this sector in rather more complex procedures such as coronary bypass grafts and other heart procedures.

There is little privately financed primary care in the UK. It is estimated that only 3% of GPs work in the private sector. The reason for this is that they are not allowed to see patients on their NHS list privately or to issue NHS prescriptions (20).

6.2.   THE UNITED STATES (PRIVATE/PRIVATE MODEL)

At the other end of the public/private continuum from the UK's largely public sector healthcare system lies the healthcare system of the United States. The U.S. has a federalist system of government consisting of a national government and 50 state governments. Each level of government plays some role in the financing or delivery of healthcare services. As in Canada, the national government provides health services to specific groups of the population, including military personnel, veterans with service-related disabilities, Native Americans (American Indians and Alaskan Natives), and inmates of federal prisons. The U.S. government has the authority to raise taxes and appropriate funds for the purpose of the general welfare of the population, including health care. The Health Care Financing Administration in the Department of Health and Human Services is responsible for administering the healthcare insurance programs Medicare and Medicaid and the recently enacted State Children's Health Insurance Program (SCHIP). The U.S. government is also responsible for regulating the healthcare insurance provided by employers and managed care organizations participating in federally subsidized health care.

The responsibilities of state governments with respect to health care include the licensing of hospitals and healthcare personnel, the provision of public health services (sanitation, water quality, etc.), and the provision of mental health services. States can raise their own revenue by various types of taxes and there is no federal limit on their taxing powers. State governments must conform to federal regulations in order to receive funds from the national government under Medicaid and SCHIP. They are also responsible for regulating private healthcare insurance, including managed care organizations, as well as Blue Cross/Blue Shield.

Although the federal and state governments provide public coverage for health care, the U.S. healthcare system remains unique around the world as it strongly relies on the private sector to provide healthcare coverage as well as deliver health services.

The U.S. healthcare system is a very fragmented, pluralistic system with health services provided by a loosely structured system organized at the local level. Recently, private insurance companies have set up vertically integrated networks of care for their subscribers. Although several publicly funded and delivered healthcare programs exist in the U.S., 55% of health care is financed and delivered privately.

The U.S. spends more on health care than any other industrialized country in the world. In 1998, the U.S. spent 13.6% of its GDP, or $4,178 per capita, on health — more than twice the per capita average of the countries surveyed by the Organisation for Economic and Co-operation and Development (see Table 12.5) (20).

6.2.1. Finance

There are multiple methods of financing health services in the U.S. including both private funds and public funds. The majority of healthcare funding comes from private sources including private health insurance and out-of-pocket payment. The private health insurance industry covers three quarters of the population (e.g., Blue Cross/Blue Shield, private insurance companies, corporate self-insurance, managed care plans). Insurance coverage is largely employment-based and entirely voluntary. Small employers generally cannot afford to offer their employees insurance coverage, and even large companies do not cover most part-time and contractual workers.

Both the national and state governments provide public funds for health care. The three publicly funded government plans are Medicare, Medicaid, and SCHIP. Medicare is a federally subsidized program for those over age 65, some people with disabilities, and people with chronic renal diseases. Benefits that are not generally transferable outside Medicare fall into two parts: Part A, a hospital insurance program for the populations mentioned above, and generally requiring contributions by participants for a minimal period of their working lives; and Part B, an optional social security arrangement for medical care insurance that covers some of the costs of services provided by medical practitioners and certain other benefits.

Medicare is delivered through two different mechanisms. First, under the original Medicare plan the federal government contracts with private insurance companies (there are about 55) to process and pay claims. Many offer their clients Medigap, a supplemental insurance policy that helps to fill the gaps in the plan (co-insurance, deductibles, and other out-of-pocket costs). Some Medigap policies also cover services not covered by Medicare, such as prescription drugs. Some 80% of Medicare beneficiaries are enrolled in the original plan.

Second, since 1997, Medicare can be provided through "Medicare+Choice." This option offers access to managed care plans — such as health maintenance organizations (HMOs) and preferred provider organizations (PPOs) — as well as to medical savings accounts or other private healthcare insurance options (HMOs and PPOs are discussed later). Medicare managed care plans have the following characteristics.

- They must provide all of the services that are offered under the original Medicare plan.
- They can offer a variety of additional benefits, such as preventive care, prescription drugs, dental care, hearing aids, eyeglasses, and other items not covered by the original Medicare plan. Costs for these extra benefits vary greatly among plans.
- They usually impose restrictions on the choice of providers. For example, clients enrolled in an HMO will only be able to seek care from doctors and hospitals employed or owned by the HMO.

Given these restrictions on the freedom to choose, these plans permit savings in comparison to the average cost of the original Medicare coverage. Those who enrol in the HMO option are charged a lower premium to belong to Medicare Part B.

Medicaid is a series of state programs with federal cost sharing. Eligibility for Medicaid benefits is based on income- and means-tested criteria, and is determined by county welfare boards. Basic benefits cover inpatient and outpatient hospital services, laboratory and radiology, basic physician medical services, and skilled nursing facility coverage for people over age 21. Each state is responsible for the administration, establishment of eligibility standards, type and scope of services, and the reimbursement for services. As a result, Medicaid programs vary from state to state.

In 1997, the federal government initiated SCHIP to expand healthcare coverage to otherwise uninsured children. This program allows for the coverage of children from working families with incomes too high to qualify for Medicaid and too low to afford private health insurance.

A growing proportion of the population is uninsured. It is currently estimated that 15.5% of the population in the U.S. have no health insurance (20). In addition, a significant proportion of the U.S. population are under insured, meaning that they have some insurance coverage but there is no limit on out-of-pocket costs.

6.2.2. Delivery

In the U.S., the dominant system of health services delivery is private and usually for-profit. Public services are usually limited to providing care to special groups such as veterans, the mentally ill, or the poor. Some jurisdictions (cities or counties) operate public hospitals and community health centres as a social safety net, although many such institutions are now under fiscal pressure and are being downsized or closed.

Ambulatory care physicians in private practice are paid a fee-for-service, usually by their patients, who are subsequently reimbursed by their insurance plans. Physicians working in private practice can, and usually do, extra-bill above levels reimbursed by insurance companies. Physicians under Medicare are reimbursed based on a fee-for-service. This has been changing since 1997 with the introduction of the Medicare+Choice program. With the advent of managed care as an option for Medicare patients, other methods of reimbursement such as capitation are becoming more common. Physicians participating in Medicaid must accept the reimbursement level set by the state and are not allowed to extra-bill. Those physicians working in managed care organizations, such as HMOs or PPOs, are generally paid on a capitation or salary basis, but a wide assortment of plans and payment arrangements are possible. An HMO offers health services provided by selected doctors and hospitals. In exchange for a monthly fee, enrolees receive care as needed. A PPO is a simplified form of HMO that provides incentives to its enrolees to use a limited number of selected providers at a reduced cost.

Most recently, there has been a rapid movement toward integrated delivery structures, and the managed care portion of the market has grown.

There are two main concerns driving recent health reform efforts in the U.S. (25). The first, as in the majority of OECD countries, is a concern with rapidly growing healthcare expenditures. The difference between the U.S. and other OECD countries is not one of substance, but of degree. The second major trend, unique to the U.S., is the growing proportion of the population that is entirely uninsured. For this reason, the *Health Security Act* of 1993 was proposed in the U.S. by President Bill Clinton (26). The Clinton plan would have included mandatory, universal healthcare coverage for all U.S. citizens and legal residents with a public-private mix of funding and responsibility, but Congress defeated it. In 1996, Clinton signed a law prohibiting insurance companies from denying coverage to any applicant based on pre-existing medical conditions. Although still a far cry from the original, more ambitious plan, the Clinton administration felt that this was the first step in an ongoing reform process.

In addition to the national reforms proposed by Clinton and others, individual states have also undertaken significant reform efforts. Most notable among these efforts are the Oregon Plan and health reforms in California.

Briefly, the State of Oregon's reform efforts aimed at extending Medicaid coverage to a wider net of the state's poor, while at the same time limiting the number and type of services that would be covered. Service rationing was decided through a process of broad public consultation, and was based on the social value and perceived effectiveness assigned to each service.

6.3.   AUSTRALIA (MIXED MODEL)

Like Canada, Australia has a federal system of government. Health care in Australia is a shared responsibility between the national (or Commonwealth) government and sub-national governments (six states and two territories). (The information in this section comes from Australia's Department of Health and Aged Care (27) except where otherwise noted.)

The Commonwealth government is responsible for public policy making at the national level in the fields of public health, research, and national health information management. The Commonwealth government operates Medicare, the national, publicly funded healthcare insurance plan in Australia, and regulates the private healthcare insurance industry. It also finances and regulates residential aged care (nursing homes) and, together with the states and territories, funds and administers some community-based and home care.

The state and territory governments have primary responsibility for the management and delivery of publicly insured health services within their jurisdiction. As such, they deliver public acute and psychiatric hospital services and a wide range of community and public health services including school health, dental care, and maternal and child health. The state and territory governments are also responsible for the regulation of healthcare providers as well as for the licensing and approval of private hospitals. Healthcare funding by states and territories is derived mostly from grants from the Commonwealth government, as well as from general taxation and user charges.

Local governments are responsible for health promotion and disease prevention programs (such as immunization) and environmental health services (such as sanitation and hygiene).

6.3.1. Finance

In 1998, national health spending in Australia accounted for 8.6% of the GDP (see Table 12.5). Health care in Australia is financed by a mix of public and private funding arrangements. Public funding accounts for 69.3% of the total health spending (20).

Medicare in Australia is a compulsory regime that provides universal coverage to all citizens. Public funding for health care is derived from general taxation plus a dedicated healthcare levy of 1.5% on taxable income above a certain income threshold. Taxpayers with high incomes who do not have private health insurance pay an additional 1% of taxable income. Public healthcare insurance is broader in Australia than in Canada because it provides universal access to the doctor of choice, for out-of-hospital care, free public hospital care, and subsidized pharmaceuticals. In contrast to Canada, user charges and extra-billing may be required for publicly insured health services.

Within the Medicare arrangement, there is a range of measures such as safety nets and direct billing in order to protect individuals and families from unnecessarily high out-of-pocket costs. Medicare funds health care through annual block grants to the states and territories. The amounts of the grants are negotiated in five-year agreements with the states and territories, which in return do not allow user charges for public hospital services.

Australian Medicare is made up of three main components: public hospital funding, the Medical Benefits Scheme (covering fees for private practitioner services), and the Pharmaceutical Benefits Scheme. The Medical Benefits Scheme (MBS) ensures access to physician services outside of hospitals. The MBS lists a wide range of physician services and stipulates the fee applicable to each item (the "scheduled fee"). The scheme reimburses only 85% of the doctors' scheduled fees. In other words, Australian physicians may extra-bill. A safety net provision applies: once patients have paid A$276 in physician fees in a given year (about C$240), they are exempt from further charges. Private insurance is not allowed to provide coverage for physician services that are publicly insured or for the gap between Medicare and the fee charged by the doctor. Relatively few physicians bill patients more than 85% of the MBS schedule. Social security recipients and veterans are not required to pay any extra-billing.

The extent of public coverage for hospital care depends on whether a patient elects to be a public patient or a private patient. Full coverage for hospital care is provided to public patients in hospitals owned by the state or territory or in private non-profit hospitals. Public patients are also entitled to free hospital care in for-profit hospitals, which have made arrangements with governments to care for such patients. However, when an individual chooses to be a private patient in a public hospital (in which case the patient can choose his or her own doctor) or goes to a private hospital, the federal (Commonwealth) government pays only 75% of the scheduled hospital-based physician fee. All other costs are the responsibility of the patient. The safety net that applies to physician services under the MBS and limits the amount paid by the patient for one year does not apply to Medicare benefits for hospital services. Private healthcare insurance is allowed to cover the difference between 75% of the scheduled fee and the actual fee charged. Private insurers can also provide additional benefits for hospital accommodation and other hospital charges.

The Pharmaceutical Benefits Scheme (PBS), which is based on a national drug formulary, provides free access to drugs prescribed outside of hospital, subject to annual thresholds. About 75% of all prescriptions issued in Australia are subsidized under the PBS.

As in Canada, some services are not covered under Australian Medicare, such as cosmetic surgery and services provided under workers' compensation insurance. Private insurance can cover allied health and paramedical services (such as physiotherapists' and podiatrists' services), as well as some aids and devices. Unlike Canada, private insurers may cover the same benefits as under the public plan. Australians can supplement their Medicare benefits through private healthcare insurance, but they cannot opt out of the publicly funded system since they continue to pay their taxes. The federal government regulates private healthcare insurance and it requires that premiums be community rated. A common premium exists for all enrolees regardless of their health status. This means that high-risk individuals such as the elderly or chronically ill cannot be charged higher premiums. The federal government has also introduced a number of tax-based measures to encourage people to purchase private healthcare insurance so that they can continue to enrol in private insurance plans. It offers holders of private health care insurance a 30% refundable tax credit.

The Lifetime Health Cover was also introduced in July 2000. Under this system, individuals aged 30 years or less who purchase private healthcare insurance pay lower premiums throughout their life than someone who joins later in life. This initiative is expected to reduce premium rates by encouraging more of younger and healthier people to take out private insurance and by discouraging people from joining prior to treatment and leaving following the treatment. Overall, there are about 40 private healthcare insurance funds registered in Australia (20).

Residential care for seniors is financed by the federal government by means of subsidies paid to service providers, based on the level and type of care needed by the individual. The federal and state and territory governments jointly fund community care services for the frail and the disabled.

6.3.2   Delivery

As in Canada, the majority of doctors are self-employed. Most primary care provided by general practitioners in private practice is reimbursed on a fee-for-service basis. A small proportion of physicians are salaried employees of Commonwealth, state and territory, or local governments. General practitioners in primary care act as gatekeepers, with access to specialist medical services being available only on their referral.

A mix of public and private institutions provides hospital care. Public hospitals are the major providers of care in Australia. Public hospitals include hospitals established by state and territory governments and hospitals established by religious or charitable bodies but now directly funded by government. Specialists in public hospitals are either salaried or paid per session. Salaried specialist doctors in public hospitals can treat some patients in these hospitals as private patients, charging fees to those patients and usually contributing some of their fee income to the hospital.

There are a small number of private for-profit hospitals built and managed by private firms that provide public hospital services under arrangements with state and territory governments. However, most acute care beds and emergency outpatient clinics are in public hospitals.

Private hospitals tend to provide less complex non-emergency care, such as simple elective surgery. However, some private hospitals are increasingly providing complex, high technology services. Like public hospitals, some private facilities provide same-day surgery and other non-inpatient operating room procedures.

A significant proportion of other healthcare providers are self-employed. In addition, there are many independent pathology and diagnostic imaging services operated by doctors.

6.4. FRANCE (MIXED MODEL)

In 2000, France's healthcare system was ranked number one among the 191 member countries surveyed by the World Health Organization (WHO). According to WHO, France's system provides "the best overall health care" (28). France spent 9.3% of its GDP on health care in 1998 (see Table 12.5). Its system is complex and pluralistic and charges more in the form of individual user fees than other European countries.

France has a centralized government, where the national government maintains all power. The government decides what kinds of care are to be reimbursed and to what extent, defines the responsibilities of the various actors, and ensures that the entire population has access to care. The government is also responsible for defending patients' rights by drafting and enforcing relevant policy. It is therefore responsible for safety within the healthcare system. Health authorities controlled by the government decide on the number and size of hospitals, as well as the amount and allocation of highly technical equipment (CT scanners). They also organize the supply of specialized wards (e.g., transplants, neurosurgery) and ensure the provision of care at the regional level (29).

6.4.1. Finance

Health system finance in France is the responsibility of several entities and organizations, both public and private. In general, health services in France are paid by open-ended, compulsory health insurance funds called the Caisses nationales, which operate within the national social security scheme. These insurance funds are financed by compulsory, income-related payroll taxes and provide almost universal (99% of the population) coverage. The payroll tax is split between employers, who contribute 12.6% of the employees' income to the caisses, and employees, who contribute 6.8% of their income. The caisses are semi-autonomous, non-governmental bodies responsible for administering the insurance scheme. Membership is based on occupation. There is one large fund called the Régime général de la Sécurité sociale (General Social Security System), covering the majority (80%) of all workers and their dependants, as well as pensioners. Fifteen smaller caisses cover the remaining 20% of workers for self-employed workers, farmers, and special groups such as miners and transport workers.

In addition to the compulsory coverage provided by the caisses, 80% of the population voluntarily purchases supplementary private insurance to top up the coverage provided by the universal system. Supplementary health insurance is provided by private insurance companies or by non-profit, charitable societies called mutuelles. These provide reimbursement for user charges (called ticket moderateur), extra-billing, and a few benefits not covered by the caisses. They are financed through a voluntary payroll deduction of 2.5% of income. Supplementary private insurance is paid for through actuarial based, voluntary premiums.

Mutuelles also finance a system of safety-net care for the very poor or those with unstable employment. They comprises roughly 5% of France's population.

The Ministère de la santé provides funds from general taxes for community health services (e.g., immunizations) and for capital development of public hospitals.

Insurance companies offer payment in the form of reimbursement to patients for most ambulatory care, while paying most physicians directly for hospital care. The health insurance is comprehensive, including services rendered at home, at a doctor's office, or in a hospital. Included are home care, dental and nursing care, drugs and prostheses, and replacement income during illness. No disease is excluded. Cost sharing applies to most services provided by public programs, constituting approximately 17% of all healthcare expenditures in France. Of all the western European countries, only France requires such a high level of cost sharing by individuals for the health services they receive. The extent and the nature of the co-payments depend on the type of care. As part of this cost-sharing scheme, there is a ticket moderateur levied for every service provided. This user fee is set at 30% of the negotiated fee for physician visits; 20% for hospital care; 0, 35% and 65% for medicines depending upon individual's income and employment status; and 40% for laboratories (29). About 10% of insured people who are chronically ill or receiving long-term care do not have to pay the user fees for prescription drugs and those individuals with supplementary private insurance can be reimbursed.

In 2000, a means-tested, public supplementary insurance program called Couverture maladie universelle (CMU) was implemented to ensure the poor have access to health care. For those whose income is below a certain threshold (about 10% of the population is eligible), this insurance covers all public co-payments and offers lump-sum reimbursement for eyeglasses and dental prostheses. Healthcare professionals are not allowed to charge more than the public tariff or the lump sum for CMU beneficiaries, which means that, in theory, access to care is free of charge (29).

6.4.2. Delivery

Healthcare services in France are provided through a mixed public and private delivery system: Sixty-five percent of the hospital beds are part of the public sector and 35% are private — some private, non-profit; others private, for-profit (30). Public hospitals in France are large, well equipped, and designed to offer comprehensive care including emergency and trauma care. Private hospitals, conversely, are usually much smaller and designed to provide specialist care such as obstetric services, elective surgery, or long-term care. Public hospitals are supported by global budgets set according to the workload of the hospital using a formula based on diagnostic-related groups (DRGs). Private hospitals, however, are paid on a per diem rate. A uniform hospital information system has been implemented to monitor the various establishments' activity. Gradually, all public and private establishments are switching to DRG payment systems (30).

Physicians in private hospitals are considered private entrepreneurs, getting paid on a fee-for-service basis by their patients, and comprise about two thirds of all hospital physicians. The remaining one third of physicians work in public hospitals or in private non-profit hospitals, are public employees who receive a salary, and are also allowed a private practice on a part-time basis outside their hospital practice. The majority (80%) of ambulatory physicians work in private practice. The remainder are employed by the health insurance scheme, by charitable societies, or by official authorities responsible for providing services to the poor. Half of the physicians are specialists.

Access to care in France is unlimited: patients can see as many physicians as often as they like. Patients do not need referrals to see specialists, and in general, there is no gate-keeping system of any kind.

6.5. GERMANY (MIXED MODEL)

Germany is a federal republic consisting of a federal government and 16 state governments known as Länder. Responsibility for health care is a shared responsibility between all levels of government including the federal and state governments and local authorities. To ensure a uniform standard of service throughout Germany, the federal government has enacted federal laws covering many areas of the healthcare system. National healthcare policy rests essentially on the principles of statutory social insurance (often referred to in Germany as the Bismarck model). The federal government has the authority to regulate the Krankenkassen (health insurance funds, described below) and private healthcare insurance. It is also responsible for long-term care policy as well as for reference pricing policy with respect to prescription drugs.

The Länder are responsible for implementing laws passed by the federal government, exercising administrative responsibilities such as supervision of councils of health professions as well as planning and financing of investment in the hospital sector (31). They own many hospitals, along with local governments and charitable organizations, and are responsible for maintaining all hospital infrastructures in their jurisdiction, independent of actual ownership. Länder have the authority to finance medical education and supervise healthcare professionals. They are also responsible for public health, health promotion, and disease prevention (20).

Germany has the largest economy in Europe and spends 10.3% of its GDP on health care; this is slightly higher than the OECD average (see Table 12.5). The public share of overall healthcare spending is higher in Germany (75%) than in Canada (70%). Private sector funding in Germany accounts for the remaining 25%.

6.5.1. Finance

The organization of health insurance falls into three different schemes: health insurance funds, private for-profit healthcare insurance, and public coverage by the federal government for military personnel, police officers, and social welfare recipients. Health care is financed primarily through a system of open-ended non-governmental social insurance funds called health insurance funds. There are approximately 453 such funds covering the healthcare costs of roughly 90% of the population (20).

Krankenkassen are private not-for-profit organizations structured on a regional and/or occupational basis. Membership is compulsory for employees with a gross income lower than 39,600 (approximately C$65,500) and is voluntary for those above this income level. The financing of Krankenkassen is based on contributions made by both employees and employers. Money is collected through income-related payroll taxes at a rate of 13.5% of individual income; half is paid by the employer and half by the employee (20). Contributions for individuals who are unemployed, retired, disabled, or below the poverty line are made by local Krankenkassen and local governments. Most individuals are not free to choose which fund to join. This decision is made according to the individual's place of residence and occupation. These funds are called Reichversicherungsordnung funds (state insurance regulation funds) and include local/regional Krankenkassen, industrial funds, crafts funds, rural funds, sailors' funds, miners' funds, and blue-collar or white-collar workers' funds.

Individuals who have stable employment and earn over a certain income per month can choose which fund to join. Their membership is usually in voluntary sickness funds called Ersatzkassen.

Contribution to a sickness fund includes coverage for unemployed spouses and all dependants, whether children or adults. This is called the solidarity principle, by which a member's contribution remains the same whether that person is single or has dependants or non-working family members who are co-insured.

Krankenkasse members may also be required to pay user charges for certain services. User charges are determined by national legislation and currently apply to prescription drugs, dental care, hospital services, rehabilitation services, and ambulance transportation. User charges are subject to an annual threshold: once they have reached this limit, fund members are exempt from further charges. Some individuals are exempted from paying any user charges, such as those with low income, those receiving unemployment benefits or on social welfare, children, and the chronically ill. Individual out-of-pocket expenses comprise 11% of total health expenditures (20). Physicians are allowed to extra-bill only their private patients; the practice of extra-billing remains very limited.

Private healthcare insurance is available to individuals whose annual gross income is greater than 39,600 (approximately C$65,000) and who have voluntarily opted out of their Krankenkasse. At present, 52 private insurance companies offer private coverage. Since re-entry of privately insured people into Krankenkassen is not permitted under ordinary circumstances, private insurers are obliged to offer an insurance policy with the same benefits at a premium no higher than the average maximum contribution to the funds. Premiums in the private healthcare insurance sector are risk-related and reflect the medical history of the insured individual. Unlike Krankenkassen, private healthcare insurers require that separate premiums be paid for spouses and dependants (20).

Private healthcare coverage is also available to self-employed people who are excluded from the Krankenkassen. Private insurers also provide coverage to public servants, who are also excluded from participating in the funds as their healthcare bills are reimbursed at 50% by the federal government (private insurance covers the remainder). Finally, private healthcare insurance can offer supplementary benefits to members of the Krankenkassen (which are not legally allowed to offer these extra benefits).

Overall, Krankenkassen covers 88% of the German population: 74% are mandatory members and their dependants, while 14% are voluntary members and their dependants. Some 9% of the German population are covered under private healthcare insurance, mostly high-income earners; another 2% are insured by governmental insurance (police officers, military members, etc.). Less than 1% of the population has no healthcare insurance at all (20).

Contributions to the Krankenkassen constitute the main source of financing health care in Germany (70%). User charges by patients fund the next largest share (12%), while the balance of funding comes from general taxation (7%), private healthcare insurance (7%), and other sources (4%). General taxation is used to reimburse some of the healthcare expenditures incurred by public employees, persons on welfare, and subsidies for the farmers' funds(20).

Krankenkassen cover a comprehensive array of health services mandated by federal legislation to prevent different levels of coverage. Benefits include physician services, hospital, diagnostic services, prescription drugs, ambulatory medical care, dental care, medical devices, transport, home nursing services, rehabilitation services, psychotherapists, medical services by non-physicians (physiotherapists, speech therapists, occupational therapists, etc.), and income support during sick leave (20).

6.5.2. Delivery

The German healthcare delivery system is a mixed public and private one that is fairly heavily regulated. A national body, called Die Sachverständigenrat für die Konzertierte Aktion im Gesundheitswesen (the Advisory Council for Concerted Action in Health Care) is responsible for setting guidelines with respect to the rate of growth of healthcare spending. These guidelines must be taken into account in the determination of hospital budgets and physician remuneration.

There are three types of hospitals: publicly owned hospitals (39%); private, voluntary, non-profit hospitals usually owned by charities or religious groups (40%); and private, proprietary, for-profit hospitals usually owned by doctors individually or in groups (21%) (20). The state government is responsible for developing all hospital plans, which determine the number of hospitals in a region, which specialties are necessary, and the number of beds.

In the 1990s, the federal government introduced several changes to hospital financing. Remuneration of hospitals now consists of three parts: a general per diem typically covering food and lodging, a ward-specific compensation for additional resources spent in a given hospital department, and a lump-sum remuneration for specialized treatment services (such as cancer treatment and organ transplants).

Doctors employed in public hospitals are paid on a salary basis. Non-profit hospitals and the doctors working in them receive payment in the same fashion as their public hospital counterparts. Arrangements in the private for-profit hospitals are somewhat different. These doctors are paid on a fee-for-service basis according to a schedule that is laid out by the federal government. A part of each fee received by doctors working in private for-profit hospitals is given to the hospital.

Ambulatory physicians — both GPs and specialists — do not generally have admitting privileges to hospitals, and hospital physicians generally cannot provide outpatient care. An exception to this strict division exists in the private sector, where ambulatory care physicians (mostly specialists) can rent hospital beds from private hospitals to allow for inpatient treatment of their patients. Individuals are allowed free choice of GPs and specialists, and a person is admitted to hospitals by referral from an ambulatory care doctor; the hospital is usually the one closest to the person's residence. At the beginning of each year, in each state, the health insurance funds and the regional medical associations negotiate an overall remuneration package. Then, the medical associations distribute this total allotment according to a uniform value scale. This scale lists all medical services that can be provided by physicians and allocates a point value to each service. For example, a telephone consultation is assigned 80 points, a home visit 360 points, and lab or diagnostic work between 360 and 900 points. At the end of each quarter, every office-based physician invoices the association for the services delivered. Physicians, however, do not know exactly how much they will earn because the monetary value of a single service may decline if physicians are performing too many services in any one category. Although the Krankenkassen and private insurers use the same scale for remunerating primary care physicians, each assigns different point values. Private insurers generally provide a higher remuneration for the same services compared to the Krankenkassen. The physician is paid quarterly by the fund based on caseload — that is, on the volume and mix of services provided. The fees are calculated not in absolute terms but according to the number of value-point services provided in comparison with other physicians. Thus, at the time of service provision, the physician also does not know the actual cost.

Physicians treating privately insured patients are not subject to budget caps as occurs with Krankenkassen. Therefore, physicians obtain a higher remuneration when treating privately insured individuals in Germany. Furthermore, it is permissible for physicians to extra-bill privately insured patients.

Primary care physicians are paid on a fee-for-service basis. As in Canada, physicians cannot extra-bill patients insured under Krankenkassen.

7.   SUMMARY

Conceptually, the organization of healthcare systems can be divided into how health services are delivered to those in need and how payments for the provision of these services are financed. The terms public and private are not precise but are often used to describe healthcare systems.

In general terms public sector refers to government involvement while private sector is generally thought of as what lies beyond the boundaries of government. The public sector can be divided into four levels of government: national (in Canada, the federal government), provincial or state (in Canada, province or territory), regional (e.g., regional health authority), and local (e.g., municipality).

Private is generally thought of as what lies beyond the boundaries of government to include both the family and the market. The private sector can be thought of as including both not-for-profit organizations and for-profit organizations. The private sector can also be divided into four different levels: corporate for-profit, which must return profits to shareholders; small business/entrepreneurial; charitable/not-for-profit, which can use varying combinations of paid staff and volunteers, and family/personal.

The *Constitution Act* of 1867 gave the federal government a minimal role in the healthcare system. Section 91 defines the primacy of the federal economic role including the regulation of trade, taxation, external affairs, defence, quarantine, immigration, criminal law, and the powers of reservation and disallowance. Section 92 defines the provincial role in social welfare including health, education, civil law, and agriculture. However, the federal government has become involved in health care by sharing the cost of programs and thus steering the healthcare system. Since 1950, a number of federal acts have been passed, most significantly the *Hospital Insurance and Diagnostic Services Act* (HIDS) of 1957 (which provided universal hospitalization) and the *Medical Care Act* of 1966 (which provided universal coverage of necessary medical services). The federal government shared 50% of the cost of these programs with the participating provinces, provided the provinces and territories met four criteria: universality, portability, comprehensiveness, and public administration. All provinces and territories participated in these programs. In the 1970s, the shared cost of health programs became a critical problem for the federal and provincial governments alike and this led to the legislation of the *Federal-Provincial Fiscal Arrangements and Established Program*

Financing Act (EPF) of 1977. In this act, the federal government agreed to pay the provinces by the transfer of income tax points and cash contribution linked to an increase in the GNP instead of the previous 50% cost sharing. The EPF no longer tied federal payments to a particular form of health services, thus reducing the federal steering effect.

During the early 1980s, critical reviews of national health insurance programs and financing arrangements led to the 1984 enactment of the *Canada Health Act*. This act amalgamated the HIDS and the *Medical Care Act*. It also established five criteria that provincial health programs must meet in order to be eligible for the full cash portion of the federal government contribution, namely public administration, comprehensiveness, universality, portability, and accessibility. The Act also banned extra-billing, and by 1987 all the provinces had complied. It appeared that the Canadian healthcare system was moving toward an increased federal role, especially in the areas of formulation, monitoring, and enforcing of program conditions. However, as a result of budgetary deficits, the federal government was forced to reduce transfer payments for health care and post-secondary education to the provinces. Bills C-96, C-69, and C-20 were enacted to freeze the cash flow to the provinces, resulting in a diminished federal role in enforcing healthcare policy. In an attempt to stabilize the amount of federal health and social transfers to the provinces and maintain a role in health, the federal government passed the *Canada Health and Social Transfer Act* in 1996 — a block grant to the provinces covering health care, higher education, and social programs. Since 1999 the federal government has increased its financial contribution to sustain and reform the health care system.

Although it appears that Canada has a national medicare program, this is incorrect: health care is actually a provincial responsibility. The involvement of the federal government is through financial contributions, which enables the federal government to establish national standards. As a result, Canada has ten provincial and three territorial healthcare systems that are structured on federal guidelines and provide mainly sickness care and, to a lesser extent, preventive practices carried out by physicians. However, the jurisdictional dispute between the provinces and the federal government in the health sector has become a source of increasing tension. The primary objective of the social union initiative is to reform and renew Canada's social services and to reassure Canadians that their pan-Canadian social programs are strong and secure.

The healthcare systems of Australia, the United Kingdom, the United States, France, and Germany are described, and similarities and differences with Canada's healthcare system are highlighted.

8.   REFERENCES

1.   Mhatre S, Deber R. From equal access to health care to equitable access to health: A review of Canadian provincial health commissions and reports. *International Journal of Health Services* 1992; 22(4):645-66.
2.   Romanow R. *Building on values: The future of health care in Canada*. Ottawa: Commission on the Future of Health Care in Canada, 2002.

3. Deber R, Narine L, Baranek P, *et al.* The public-private mix in health care. In National Forum on Health Secretariat, *Striking a balance: Health care systems in Canada and elsewhere*. Ottawa: Canada Communications Group, 1998.
4. Health Canada. Health System and Policy Division. *Canada Health and Social Transfer: Backgrounder*. Ottawa: Health Canada, 1996.
5. Vayda E, Deber R. The Canadian health care system: An overview. *Social Science and Medicine* 1984; 18(3):191-7.
6. Department of National Health and Welfare. *Review of health services in Canada*. Ottawa: Government of Canada, 1976.
7. National Forum on Health. *Vol. 1: The Final Report of the National Forum on Health*. Canada Health Action: Building on the legacy. Ottawa: Minister of Public Works and Government Services, 1997.
8. Chénier N. 1999. *Health policy in Canada*. Library of Parliament, Research Branch, 1994, revised 1999. <dsp-psd.pwgsc.gc.ca/Collection-R/LoPBdP/CIR/934-e.htm> (September 2002).
9. Department of Finance Canada. 2002. *The Equalization Program*. <www.fin.gc.ca/FEDPROV/eqpe.html> (September 2002).
10. Department of Finance Canada. 2002. *Federal transfers to provinces and territories: Questions and answers*. <www.fin.gc.ca/budget99/multimedia-e/fedprov3-e.html> (September 2002).
11. Taylor M. *Health insurance and Canadian public policy: The seven decisions that created the Canadian health insurance system*. Kingston: McGill-Queen's University Press, 1978.
12. Madore O. 2001. *The Canada Health and Social Transfer: Operation and possible repercussions on the health care sector*. Ottawa: Library of Parliament, Research Branch. <dsp-psd.pwgsc.gc.ca/Collection-R/LoPBdP/CIR/952-e.htm> (September 2002).
13. Department of Finance Canada. 2002. *What is territorial formula financing?* <www.fin.gc.ca/FEDPROV/tffe.htm> (September 2002).
14. Heiber S, Deber R. Banning extra-billing in Canada: Just what the doctor didn't order. *Canadian Public Policy* 1987; 13:62-74.
15. Hall EM. *Canada's national-provincial health program for the 1980s: A commitment for renewal*. Ottawa: Health and Welfare Canada, Special Commissioner, 1980.
16. Parliamentary Task Force on Federal-Provincial Fiscal Arrangements. *Fiscal federalism in Canada*. Ottawa: Ministry of Supply and Services, 1981.
17. Madore O. 2001. *The Canada Health Act: Overview and options*. Library of Parliament, Research. <dsp-psd.pwgsc.gc.ca/Collection-R/LoPBdP/CIR/944-e.htm> (September 2002).
18. First Ministers' Meeting. 1999. *A framework to improve the social union for Canadians*. <www.scics.gc.ca/cinfo99/80003701_e.html> (October 2002).
19. First Ministers' Meeting. 2000. *Communiqué on health*. <www.scics.gc.ca/cinfo00/800038004_c.html> (October 2002).
20. Kirby M, LeBreton M. 2002. *The health of Canadians: The federal role. Interim report, volume 3: Health care systems in other countries*. Standing Senate Committee on Social Affairs, Science and Technology. <www.parl.gc.ca/37/1/parlbus/commbus/senate/com-e/SOCI-E/rep-e/repjan01vol3-e.htm> (September 2002).
21. Health Canada. 2003. *First Ministers' Accord on Health Care Renewal*. <www.hc-sc.gc.ca/english/hca2003/accord.html> (February 2003).
22. Abel-Smith B, Mossialos E. Cost-containment and health care reform: A study of the European Union. *Health Policy* 1994; 28:89-132.
23. Koen V. *Public expenditure reform: The health care sector in the United Kingdom*. Economics Department Working Papers No. 256, Organization for Economic Co-operation and Development, 2000.

24.   United Kingdom. National Health Service. 2002. *The NHS explained: Priorities — The NHS plan.* <www.nhs.uk/thenhsexplained/priorities.asp> (September 2002).

25.   Organisation for Economic Co-operation and Development. *U.S. health care at the crossroads.* Health Policy Studies No. 1. Paris: OECD Publications, 1992.

26.   Angell M. The beginning of health care reform: The Clinton plan. *New England Journal of Medicine* 1993; 329(21):1569-70.

27.   Australia. Department of Health and Aged Care. *An overview of health status, health care, and public health in Australia.* Canberra: Publication Production Unit, Commonwealth Department of Health and Aged Care, 1999.

28.   Lenain P. Santé to the French health system. *OECD Observer* 2000, October 19. <www.oecdobserver.org/news/fullstory.php/aid/356/Sant%E9_to_the_French_health_system_.html> (September 2002).

29.   Couffinhal A, Paris V. 2001. *Utilization fees imposed to public health care systems users in France.* Workshop organized for the Commission on the Future of Health Care in Canada, November 2002. <www.credes.fr/En_ligne/WorkingPaper/ecogen/userschar.pdf> (September 2002).

30.   Couffinhal A. The French health care system: A brief overview. Presentation prepared for the meeting of the Permanent Working Group of European Junior Doctors, October, 2001.

31.   Germany. Federal Ministry of Health. 2001. *Health care reform 2000.* <www.bmgesundheit.de/engl/healthcare.htm> (October 2002).

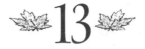

FEDERAL AND PROVINCIAL HEALTH ORGANIZATIONS

Under the *Constitutional Act, 1867*, the federal government had almost no power in personal health care. However, through a number of financial arrangements, the government influenced two major areas: medical care and hospital care. This chapter deals with the major functions of federal and provincial governments in this context. It describes how both levels of government cooperated to work at arm's length so as to avoid intruding on each other's jurisdiction. These joint ventures have particularly benefited the smaller provinces and territories, which do not always have the resources to mount in-depth studies or planning processes.

1.   HEALTH CANADA: FEDERAL HEALTH ORGANIZATION

As seen in Chapter 12, under the terms of Confederation the federal government had relatively little jurisdiction over health care. In 1872, the Department of Agriculture had primary responsibility for federal health activities, which were gradually dispersed among several departments: Agriculture, Inland Revenue, and Marine and Fisheries. In 1919, the Department of Health was established by an act stating that its duties, powers, and functions "extend to and include all matters relating to the promotion or preservation of the health, social security and social welfare of the people of Canada over which the Parliament of Canada has jurisdiction." In 1929, the Department of Soldiers' Civil Re-establishment was discontinued and the Department of National Health became the Department of Pensions and National Health. In 1945, it was split into Health and Welfare Canada and the Department of Veterans' Affairs. At that time, the task of Health and Welfare Canada was two-fold: to promote, preserve, and restore the health of Canadians, and to provide social security and social welfare to Canadians. In June 1993, the department was reorganized and welfare responsibilities were moved to what is now called Human Resources Development. The remaining department is now known as Health Canada.

Health Canada is responsible for helping the people of Canada maintain and improve their health. In partnership with provincial and territorial governments, Health Canada provides national leadership to develop health policy, enforce health regulations, promote disease prevention, and enhance healthy living for all Canadians. Health Canada ensures that health services are available and accessible to First Nations and Inuit communities. It also works closely with other federal departments, agencies, and health stakeholders to reduce health and safety risks to Canadians.

Although Health Canada branches, divisions, and units are frequently reorganized in an effort to streamline operations and reduce waste, the basic priorities have remained fairly stable over the past several years. In 2000, Health Canada undertook a realignment to ensure that the department has the appropriate organizational structure and fundamental systems, process, and infrastructure to deliver on its mission. As a result of the realignment, the major structural changes include the creation of the Health Products and Food Branch, the Healthy Environments and Consumer Safety Branch, and the Population and Public Health Branch. In addition, the former Medical Services Branch was changed to the First Nations and Inuit Health Branch to reflect its primary mission more accurately. The following section outlines some of the functions and activities carried out by each branch and its sub-divisions. Health Canada publishes the most up-to-date and accurate information on its organizational structure on its Web site (1).

Health Canada is made up of seven branches including a number of directorates and units. There are six regional offices throughout Canada: the Atlantic region, Quebec, Ontario and Nunavut, Manitoba and Saskatchewan, Alberta and Northwest Territories, and British Columbia and the Yukon.

The federal Minister of Health is responsible to parliament for administering some 20 health-related laws and associated regulations that govern the overall programs and policies of Health Canada as well as a few independent agencies, which will be described in the next section (2, 3).

The Deputy Minister and Associate Deputy Minister of Health, working with the Departmental Secretariat, support the Minister and manage departmental operations. Six Assistant Deputy Ministers located in Ottawa manage the department's program and administrative branches. Six Regional Directors General represent departmental interests across the country through regional offices. The offices and branches are under the jurisdiction of the Deputy Minister and Associate Deputy Minister of Health.

1.1.   BRANCHES OF HEALTH CANADA

Only those offices that are directly related to health activity are listed here. Those not listed have mainly administrative and management functions. As provinces and territories have prime responsibility for health matters, the federal government is restricted to acting as a clearinghouse for information in many instances and developing a national consensus or guidelines. The federal government develops and implements policies whenever there is a joint federal-provincial/territorial initiative, when both parties have signed agreements or accords, or when there are constitutional amendments. Most of the time the federal government exerts its influence through financial incentives or disincentives and, from time to time by providing moral leadership.

1.1.1. Corporate Services Branch

The Corporate Services Branch (CSB) provides financial planning and administration, human resources services, assets management, occupational health and safety services, and security operations.

1.1.2. First Nations and Inuit Health Branch

The First Nations and Inuit Health Branch (FNIHB) is responsible for providing health services to those Aboriginal peoples with whom the government of Canada had signed treaties and are living on reserves. The health status of Aboriginal peoples is describe in Chapter 6, which provides contextual framework for this section. The mandate of FNIHB is to assist First Nations and Inuit communities and people to address health inequalities and disease threats through health surveillance and population health interventions; to ensure the availability of, or access to, health services for First Nations and Inuit people; and to devolve the control and management of community-based health services to First Nations and Inuit communities and organizations (4).

There are three main programs. The Non-Insured Health Benefits Program (NIHB) provides registered Indians and recognized Inuit and Innu peoples with a range of medically necessary goods and services, which supplement benefits provided through other private or provincial and territorial programs. Non-insured health benefits include drugs, dental care, vision care, medical supplies and equipment, short-term mental health services, and transportation to access medical services. The Community Programs Directorate (CPD) works in partnership with First Nations and Inuit peoples to deliver a wide range of programs in key community health sectors. All CPD activities have the goal of maintaining and improving the health of First Nations and Inuit, and facilitating First Nations and Inuit control of health programs and resources. CPD is organized as follows: Children and Youth Division; Mental Health and Addiction Division; Chronic Disease Prevention Division; and Addiction programs (4). The Primary Health Care and Public Health Directorate (PHCPH) is responsible for primary healthcare delivery in partnership with First Nations and Inuit health authorities. All PHCPH activities strive to support knowledge and capacity building among First Nations and Inuit people, and to facilitate First Nations and Inuit control of health programs and resources. The PHCPH has the following divisions: the Primary Health Care Division, the Infectious Disease Control Division, the Environmental Health Division, and the Dental and Pharmacy Programs Division (4).

Nurse practitioners or physicians provide primary care in remote and isolated communities. In certain provinces and territories, several universities provide medical personnel and students on rotation. Since Aboriginal peoples live all over Canada, there is a network of 567 specially designed health facilities that operate in all provinces and territories (82 nursing stations, 189 health stations, 94 health offices, 202 health centres), five hospitals, 54 alcohol and drug abuse inpatient treatment centres, and 10 solvent abuse inpatient treatment centres for youth. Provincial departments of public health do not provide services on reserve. Unlike in the provincial and territorial healthcare systems, public health programs for reserve residents are not mandated by legislation. A comprehensive public health program attempts to provide dental care for children, immunization, school health services, health education, and prenatal, postnatal, and healthy baby clinics, and it provides care on reserves that other residents of Canada would receive from provincial and territorial governments, such as home care. Due to chronic shortage of qualified staff, many services are either not delivered or are inadequate.

As residents of a province or territory, First Nations people are entitled to the benefits of the cost-shared provincially operated plans for medical and hospital insurance on the same terms and conditions as other Canadians. As many of the First Nations communities are small and often located in remote and isolated areas, these insured benefits are supplemented by the FNIHB, which assists First Nations bands to arrange transportation and to obtain drugs and prostheses. The FNIHB is in the process of transferring control of health services to the First Nations.

The FNIHB's Program Policy, Transfer Secretariat, and Planning Directorate facilitates the transfer of authority for community-based health programs and services to First Nations and Inuit control. This involves the development of policies, health-funding arrangements, planning strategies that support that role, and activities leading to the negotiation and conclusion of self-government agreements with First Nations. At the time of writing, of the total 602 First Nations and Inuit communities, 286 communities have signed transfer agreements with the Program Policy, Transfer Secretariat, and Planning Directorate. The branch, which serves as a national clearinghouse, has also established programs on Aboriginal diabetes, prenatal nutrition, home and community care on reserves, injury prevention and control, and alcohol and drug abuse, and has also initiated a national First Nations telehealth project. (See Chapter 15 for details on telehealth.)

1.1.3. Health Policy and Communications Branch

The Health Policy and Communications Branch (HPCB) plays a lead role in health policy, communications, and consultations, which are described below.

The Canada Health Act Division is part of the Intergovernmental Affairs Directorate of Health Policy and Communications Branch. It administers the *Canada Health Act* and provides policy advice related to the Act and monitors a broad range of sources to assess provincial and territorial compliance with its criteria and conditions. It also informs the minister of possible noncompliance with the Act and recommends appropriate action. The division develops interpretations under the Act, provides support to legal counsel in court cases involving the Act, and maintains a centre of expertise on the Canadian health insurance system. As required by section 23 of the Act, the division produces an annual report for each fiscal year on the extent to which provincial and territorial healthcare insurance plans have satisfied the criteria and conditions for payment (5). These reports are excellent sources of detailed and up-to-date information on each provincial and territorial health insurance program.

The branch's other major responsibilities are intergovernmental and international affairs; media relations, marketing, and public communications; women's health; nursing policy; and increased links with other regional programs to balance the regional and national perspectives in Health Canada's communications activities. To carry out these responsibilities, the branch has initiated several major programs on communications, including launching Health Canada Online and Health Promotion Online, as well as on the Health Transition Fund, and international affairs. In addition, the branch is responsible for the Women's Health Bureau, which is guided by Health Canada's Women's Health Strategy. It has four main objectives: to ensure that Health Canada's policies and programs are responsive to gender differences and to women's health needs, to increase knowledge and understanding of women's health and women's health needs, to support the provision of effective health services to women, and to promote good health through preventive measures and the reduction of risk factors that imperil the health of women.

One of the major activities of the Women's Health Bureau is the Centres of Excellence for Women's Health Program. Based in Halifax, Montreal, Toronto, Winnipeg, and Vancouver, these multidisciplinary centres operate as partnerships among academics, community-based organizations, and policy makers. The Canadian Women's Health Network is responsible for disseminating the research findings of the centres and other information on women's health.

1.1.4. Health Products and Food Branch

The two main goals of the Health Products and Food Branch (HPFB) are to promote good nutrition and informed use of drugs, food, and natural health products and to maximize the safety and efficacy of drugs, food, natural health products, medical devices, and biologics and related biotechnology products in the Canadian marketplace and health system. Its three major programs are described below.

The Therapeutic Products Directorate (TPD) is responsible for the regulation of pharmaceutical drugs, medical devices, and other therapeutic products available to Canadians. This includes evaluating and monitoring their safety, effectiveness, and quality (6). By definition, Canada's *Food and Drugs Act* encompasses a range of products:

- therapeutic products, including pharmaceuticals, prescription and over-the-counter drugs;
- homeopathics, herbal remedies, and nutraceuticals;
- biological products, such as vaccines, blood and blood products, certain hormones and enzymes, tissues and organs;
- xenografts;
- medical devices, such as medical and dental implants, medical equipment and instruments, test kits for diagnosis, and contraceptive devices;
- disinfectants;
- low-risk products, such as sunscreens, antiperspirants, and toothpaste; and
- narcotic, controlled, and restricted drugs.

The TPD regulates both the manufacture and distribution of pharmaceutical drugs in Canada. Facilities that manufacture biological products to be sold in Canada, such as serums and vaccines, must be licensed according to the specifications of the *Food and Drugs Act* and Regulations, whether they are located in Canada or abroad.

Another major activity of HPFB is the Quality Assessment of Drugs Program, which includes inspection of manufacturing facilities, assessment of claims and clinical equivalency of competing brands, and provision of information to professionals and to the general public.

The Marketed Health Products Directorate (MHPD) is responsible for maintaining consistency in post-approval surveillance and assessment of signals and safety trends concerning all marketed health products. The MHPD works closely with other directorates in the Health Products and Food Branch and other branches.

The HPFB's Food Program is responsible for establishing policies and standards for the safety and nutritional quality of food sold in Canada, as well as the administration of those provisions of the *Food and Drugs Act* that relate to public health, safety, and nutrition. It is also responsible for assessing the effectiveness of the Canadian Food Inspection Agency's activities related to food safety (7, 8). Recently, the government passed regulations which make nutrition labelling mandatory on most food labels; updated requirements for nutritional content claims; and permitted for the first time in Canada diet-related health claims for foods (9).

The Natural Health Products Directorate ensures that Canadians have ready access to safe, effective, high-quality natural health products by maintaining proper labelling and implementing a regulatory framework that supports freedom of choice and cultural diversity. It was established in March 2002, and is based on the 53 recommendations contained in the Standing Committee on Health's report entitled "Natural Health Products: A New Vision" (10, 11).

The Biologics and Genetic Therapies Directorate (BGTD) is responsible for the regulation of biological and radiopharmaceutical drugs, including blood and blood products, viral and bacterial vaccines, genetic therapeutic products, tissues, organs, and xenografts. This includes evaluating and monitoring their safety, effectiveness, and quality.

1.1.5.   Information, Analysis, and Connectivity Branch

The mandate of the Information, Analysis, and Connectivity Branch (IACB) is to improve the analytical basis of decision making at all levels in Health Canada, to develop the long-range strategic framework and policies on the involvement of the federal government in health research policy, to develop the creative use of the information highway in the health sector, to establish an integrated information management and information technology policy and infrastructure, and to manage requests for access to information and manage the Government On-Line (GOL) Project Office.

The IACB created the Office of Health and the Information Highway (OHIH) in 1997 for all matters concerning the use of information and communications technologies in the health sector. The OHIH is concerned with knowledge development, partnerships and collaboration, and federal policy development. It coordinates, facilitates, and manages activities related to health "infostructure," both within Health Canada and with external stakeholders (for example provinces, territories, university health research facilities, Statistics Canada, etc.) (12). One project currently under development is the New Brunswick Wellness Network, a secure private network linking all hospitals and health centres in all eight health regions with a 100% fibre-optic infrastructure.

1.1.6. Population and Public Health Branch

The Population and Public Health Branch (PPHB) is primarily responsible for policies, programs, and systems relating to prevention, health promotion, disease surveillance, community action and disease control. Its several centres and programs are described below (13).

The Centre for Surveillance Coordination is devoted to strengthening Canada's capacity to identify and reduce risk factors that can cause injury, illness, and disease.

The Centre for Healthy Human Development (CHHD) is responsible for implementing policies and programs that enhance the conditions within which healthy development takes place. The CHHD is built on the concept of a comprehensive multidisciplinary approach (physicians, epidemiologists, social scientists, health promotion experts, etc.) tailored to the different stages of life.

The Centre for Chronic Disease Prevention and Control is mandated to reduce the burden of chronic disease in Canada through building an evidence base for detecting and assessing chronic disease threats.

The Centre for Infectious Disease Prevention and Control promotes improvement in population health status in the area of infectious diseases through public health action.

The Centre for Emergency Preparedness and Response (CEPR) was recently created to strengthen Health Canada's capacity to respond to global and domestic public health threats including natural disasters, accidental and deliberate emergencies, and international public health risks. The CEPR acts as the coordinating point for dealing with public health emergencies. Active 24 hours a day, 7 days a week, it also works closely with other internal experts in areas such as infectious disease, food, blood, nuclear emergencies, and chemicals.

Health Canada is also responsible for the National Emergency Stockpile System, Emergency Social Services, and the Federal Nuclear Emergency Plan, as well as providing emergency health care for First Nations and Inuit communities, the health of travellers to Canada, occupational health for federal government employees, and providing expert health advice when assessing potential threats.

The National Microbiology Laboratory was recently relocated to a new state-of-the-art facility in Winnipeg. It also consists of external national reference centres across Canada.

The Laboratory for Foodborne Zoonoses, a science-based organization in Guelph, Ontario, provides and integrates scientific information for the development, implementation, and evaluation of policies and programs that reduce risks to health associated with food-borne microorganisms across the food chain.

Quarantine and Migration Health (QMH) is responsible for protecting Canada from the importation of dangerous communicable diseases that might pose a threat to the public's health. In collaboration with the Occupational Health and Safety Agency of Health Canada, QMH is responsible for the *Quarantine Act* and Regulations, which control the importation of infectious diseases into Canada through the international movement of people, conveyances, and goods. As well, QMH plays the lead role in coordinating Canada's response to outbreaks of international disease, which may involve implementing contingency plans and other measures. QMH works closely with the Travel Medicine Program to monitor diseases occurring internationally that could have an impact on Canada and disseminate this information to both national and international public health authorities.

1.1.7.   Healthy Environments and Consumer Safety

The Healthy Environments and Consumer Safety (HECS) Branch is responsible for promoting safe living, working, and recreational environments. It emphasizes health in the work environment and delivering occupational health and safety services; assessing and reducing health risks posed by environmental factors; promoting initiatives to reduce and prevent the harm caused by tobacco and the abuse of alcohol and other controlled substances; and regulating tobacco and controlled substances. It also provides drug analytical services, regulates the safety of industrial and consumer products in the Canadian marketplace, and promotes their safe use (14).

The Drug Strategy and Controlled Substances program regulates controlled substances such as opiates, opiates derivatives, and hallucinogenic substances, and promotes initiatives that reduce or prevent the harm associated with these substances and alcohol. It also provides expert advice and drug analysis services to law enforcement agencies across the country.

The Occupational Health and Safety program establishes workplace health and safety policies and provides services to protect the health of the public sector, the travelling public, and dignitaries visiting Canada.

The Product Safety program regulates the safety of commercial and consumer chemicals and products, and promotes their safe use. The Safe Environments program promotes healthy and safe living, working, and recreational environments. It also assesses and reduces health risks posed by environmental factors. The Tobacco Control program regulates tobacco and promotes initiatives that reduce or prevent the harm associated with tobacco use (see below).

The Office of Sustainable Development is responsible for coordinating the implementation and monitoring of Health Canada's Sustainable Development Strategy and is also located within HECS (see Chapter 9).

1.2.   INDEPENDENT AGENCIES OF HEALTH CANADA

These agencies report to the Minister of Health at arm's length.

Canadian Institutes of Health Research

Canadian Institutes of Health Research (CIHR) constitute Canada's federal agency for health research, established in 2000 to replace the former Medical Research Council. CIHR's objective is to excel, according to internationally accepted standards of scientific excellence, in the creation of new knowledge and its translation into improved health for Canadians, more effective health services and products, and a strengthened healthcare system. This involves a multidisciplinary approach, organized through a framework of "virtual" institutes, each dedicated to a specific area, and linking and supporting researchers located in universities, hospitals, and other research centres across Canada. The institutes embrace four pillars of research: biomedical research, clinical science, health systems and services, and the social, cultural, and other factors that affect the health of populations. CIHR's 13 institutes are Aboriginals Peoples Health; Cancer Research; Circulatory and Respiratory Health; Gender and Health; Genetics, Heath Sciences, and Policy Research; Healthy Aging; Human Development, Child, and Young Health; Infection and Immunity; Musculoskeletal Health and Arthritis; Neurosciences, Mental Health, and Addiction; Nutrition, Metabolism, and Diabetes; and Population and Public Health (15). In 2001–02, CIHR's base budget was $477 million, out of which it funded 3,251 grants, 1,625 awards, 644 Career Awards, and approximately 4,000 trainees.

Patented Medicine Prices Review Board

The Patented Medicine Prices Review Board (PMPRB) is an independent quasi-judicial body, created in 1987 under the *Patent Act* to protect consumer interests in light of increased patent protection for pharmaceuticals. Its mandate is to ensure that the prices charged by manufacturers of patented medicines in Canada are not excessive, to report annually to Parliament on the price trends of all medicines in Canada, and on the ratio of research and development expenditures to sales by patentees. The PMPRB does not review the prices of non-patented medicines, but it does oversee the selection and utilization process of any medicines, patented or not, including which drug the doctor prescribes, the amount prescribed, how the product is used, and the coverage provided by third-party and provincial and territorial drug plans (16).

Hazardous Materials Information Review Commission

The Hazardous Materials Information Review Commission is an independent agency created in 1987 by proclamation of the *Hazardous Materials Information Review Act*, accountable to the Parliament of Canada through the minister of health. It is a small but important public sector institution charged with providing the protection mechanism for trade secrets within the Workplace Hazardous Materials Information System (WHMIS).

The WHMIS requires that manufacturers and suppliers provide employers with information on the hazards of materials produced, sold, or used in Canadian workplaces (17). Employers, in turn, provide that information to employees through product labels, worker education programs, and material safety data sheets (MSDS). A product's MSDS must fully disclose all hazardous ingredients in the product, its toxicological properties, and any safety precautions workers need to take when using the product and treatment required in the case of exposure. The WHMIS is a nation-wide system, which contributes to the reduction of illness and injury caused by using hazardous materials in the Canadian workplace (see Chapter 10).

1.3.   HEALTH CANADA OFFICES

Three offices — Office of the Chief Scientist, the Office of Cameron Visiting Chair, and the Pest Management Regulatory Agency — report to the Minister of Health through either associate deputy ministers or departmental secretariat.

Pest Management Regulatory Agency

The Pest Management Regulatory Agency (PMRA) is responsible for protecting human health and the environment by minimizing the risks associated with pest control products. All products used, sold, or imported into Canada to manage, destroy, attract, or repel pests are regulated by the PMRA. These pesticides include chemicals, devices, and even organisms. The use of pesticides is regulated by the *Pest Control Products Act* as well as provincial/territorial legislation. The agency's health activities are linked to those of other branches, with emphasis on monitoring disease trends to provide a signal of potential health effects from pesticide exposure, assessing the impact of pesticide use on the quality of the Canadian food supply, and regulating pesticides that are no longer registered but find their way into the environment as contaminants. The PMRA collaborates with Environment Canada, Agriculture and Agri-Food Canada, the Canadian Food Inspection Agency, and other organizations in environmental and pesticide research and monitoring, including sustainable pest management (18).

2.   RELEVANT SOCIAL PROGRAMS

Under the general government reorganization in June 1993, several social and income security programs that directly and indirectly affect health were transferred from Health and Welfare Canada to the Ministry of Human Resources Development. Additionally, the Child Tax Benefit Program (formerly the Family Allowance and Child Tax Credit) was transferred to the Department of Revenue, while medical assessment of immigrants was transferred to the Department of Citizenship and Immigration. The social programs described briefly below promote and strengthen the income security of Canadians, share the cost of provincial and territorial social assistance, welfare services, and rehabilitation programs, and assist in the development of social services to meet changing social needs.

Income Security Programs

The income security programs promote and preserve the social security and social welfare of Canadians through the administration of number of programs: Guaranteed Income Supplement, Home Adaptations for Seniors Independence, Canada Pension Plan Disability Benefits, Employability Assistance for People with Disabilities, Veteran Disability Pension, Canada Child Tax Benefit, and Maternity, Parental, and Sickness Benefits (19). Through a network of regional offices and client service centres, these programs provide financial assistance to people with disabilities, the elderly, single-parent families, orphans, unemployed, and low-income individuals. The programs complement existing social welfare, provincial and territorial, and local programs.

Social Service Programs

Social service programs consist of major federal-provincial cost-sharing programs that provide basic assistance for those whose budgetary needs exceed available resources (for whatever reason). They also provide consultation on social and welfare-related issues, including employability and vocational rehabilitation; alcohol and drug treatment and rehabilitation; services to people with physical and mental impairment; child welfare, child abuse, and family violence; family and community services; and voluntary action. Contributions are provided to help seniors maintain and improve their quality of life and independence, as well as to encourage senior to utilize their skills, talents, and experience within the community. The National Adoption Desk has also been incorporated into this division to coordinate the adoption of children from other countries into Canada.

3. OTHER RELEVANT PROGRAMS

Health Canada is involved in a number of other interdepartmental activities related to health. The tasks of these relevant advisory councils are given below.

Canadian Institute for Health Information

The Canadian Institute for Health Information (CIHI) grew out of a report by the National Task Force on Health Information, released in June 1991. This task force highlighted the need for a nationally coordinated approach to Canada's health information system. In September 1992, federal, provincial, and territorial ministers of health approved the creation of CIHI, which was launched in 1994 following the amalgamation of the Hospital Medical Records Institute and the Management and Information Systems Group. The following year, specific health information programs from Health Canada and activities from Statistics Canada joined. CIHI is a not-for-profit organization, funded primarily through bilateral funding agreements with federal and provincial and territorial ministries of health and individual healthcare institutions (20).

CIHI is governed by a board of 15 directors who are chosen from health sectors and regions of Canada to create a balance. The board provides strategic guidance to CIHI as well as to Statistics Canada's Health Statistics Division. In addition, it maintains strong links with the Conference of Deputy Ministers of Health, advising them on health information matters. CIHI has one of the best Web sites for data on Canadian health and healthcare system (20).

The Canadian Strategy on HIV/AIDS

Canada's response to the HIV/AIDS epidemic has evolved significantly over the past two decades. In 1990, the federal government established the National AIDS

Strategy (NAS) to help organize the various players, which now included professional associations, the medical community, researchers, and the private sector, into a more formal, interconnected approach. In 1993, the NAS was renewed for five years, with annual funding increased from $37.3 million to $42.2 million.

Following extensive stakeholder consultations in the summer of 1997, the Canadian Strategy on HIV/AIDS (CSHA) was launched in 1998. It receives permanent funding for an ongoing, coordinated national response and represents a shift from a disease-oriented approach under NAS to one that looks at the root causes, determinants of health, and other dimensions of the HIV epidemic (21). People living with HIV/AIDS and those at risk of HIV infection are the focus and centre of CSHA efforts.

Tobacco Control Strategy

Initiated in 1985, the National Strategy to Decrease Tobacco Use in Canada (22) coordinates federal, provincial, and local government efforts as well as programs and activities of health and non-governmental organizations that work to decrease smoking among Canadians. Health Canada administers the *Tobacco Act* (23), which restricts the sale of tobacco products to minors and prohibits the advertising and promotion of these products. Other legislation requires that warning messages be printed clearly on tobacco product labels. Apart from legislative activities, the strategy coordinates and facilitates health promotion programs, disseminates information through the National Tobacco Clearinghouse, operates programs for preventing and quitting smoking, engages in research, and funds local initiatives. New federal initiatives are listed in the *New Directions for Tobacco Control in Canada* (24).

The National Advisory Council on Aging

The National Advisory Council on Aging was created by Order-in-Council on May 1, 1980, to advise the Minister of Health Canada on issues related to the aging of the Canadian population and the quality of life of seniors (25). The council has members from all parts of the country as well as a mix of language, ethnic groups, and occupational backgrounds. It reviews the needs of seniors, recommends remedial action, acts as liaison with other groups, encourages public discussion, and disseminates information. In carrying out its responsibilities, the council works closely with the minister of state for seniors.

4.   PROVINCIAL AND TERRITORIAL HEALTH SYSTEMS

Constitutionally, the provincial and territorial governments have primary responsibility for all personal health matters, such as disease prevention, treatment, and maintenance of health — a right that provinces and territories increasingly cite in order to exercise greater freedom in health system restructuring and reform without perceived federal interference. This has become an increasingly contentious issue, although there appears to be a conciliatory gesture on parts of the federal government and all provinces and territories except Quebec, by being signatory to the Social Union Agreement in 1999 and by commiting to reform the healthcare system in 2000 (see Chapter 12).

The financing of services such as preventive health services, medical services, hospital services, and treatment services for tuberculosis and other chronic diseases, and rehabilitation and care for people who are chronically ill and disabled depends chiefly on provincial and municipal governments. Provincial and territorial administrations fund and regulate hospitals and some functions of voluntary community health associations, a number of healthcare professions, and teaching and research institutions. Methods of organizing, financing, and administering health ministries vary from province to province and information from the ministry of health in each province is accessible through the Government of Canada's Web site (26) or from the Web site of the provincial or territorial ministry of health. For instance, programs such as hospital insurance, medical care insurance, tuberculosis control, cancer control, and alcoholism may be administered directly by the province or territory. Alternatively, the same programs may be the responsibility of separate public agencies directly accountable to a provincial or territorial minister of health. In British Columbia, there are four ministers who are responsible for health: the minister of health planning, the minister of health services, the minister of state of intermediate, long-term, and home care, and the minister of mental health. In some provinces and territories, such as Quebec and Prince Edward Island, the ministry of health is amalgamated with the ministry of community and social services, an emerging trend across the country. Also, in an attempt to focus on health promotion, Alberta's ministry of health is known as the Ministry of Health and Wellness.

Other ministries can also finance some of the health-related services. For example, in some provinces and territories, the ministry of labour is responsible for occupational health, the ministry of community and social services is responsible for people with cognitive impairment, and the ministry of education is responsible for the management and treatment of children with physical disabilities. Voluntary associations such as the Victorian Order of Nurses and the Arthritis Society may provide specialized health services, which are often largely supported by government financing. This diversity stems from traditional and financial considerations. In many provinces and territories, one third to one half of the total budget is allocated to health services.

There are two likely explanations for these diversities. First, provincial governments differ in their views of health — that is, what is to be included in health, such as services for children with special needs or health surveillance in the workplace. Second, in order to reduce the power of a single ministry with such a large budget, the functions of the health ministries are distributed across different ministries; however, this results in the fragmentation and duplication of services. More recently, fiscal constraints and political and ideological shifts have also increased the amount of privatization of both financing and delivery of services within the health sector.

4.1.   LOCAL AND REGIONAL HEALTH AUTHORITIES

Beginning in the early 1990s, many provincial ministries of health have held extensive public consultations and reviews in an effort to improve the functioning of their health systems. A key component of these recent reforms are the devolution and decentralization of decision making for health to the regional and local levels. Based on the premise of increased community and consumer empowerment through increased participation in health, and on the belief that the health sector needed greater flexibility and responsiveness to local needs, regionalization has proceeded swiftly in every province except Ontario. However, within the health community, there is a growing suspicion that regionalization has been created to cut healthcare costs and to shift "blame" from the provincial government to the local level.

In the 1990s, most provinces and territories in Canada partially devolved their responsibility to sub-provincial regions. This resulted in the establishment of regional health authorities across Canada. One objective was to streamline the delivery system, making it less fragmented and more responsive to local needs. Some provinces and territories set additional goals to increase community-based services, improve public participation in health care, and encourage policies and programs to promote health.

Regionalization has taken different forms across the country. Typically, however, there is a provincially appointed (sometimes locally elected) board responsible for the delivery of healthcare services and programs to the region. The implications of regionalization for improving health effectiveness and efficiency and its broader social implications for community participation and understanding of health have yet to be fully documented; nonetheless, recent reports indicate that regionalization has been beneficial in many ways, such as in better integration of service delivery, reduced administrative costs, increased focus on illness prevention and public health, and greater flexibility in reallocating and consolidating clinical services between healthcare providers and institutions (27).

4.1.1.   Regional Health Authorities

Regional health authorities (RHAs) across Canada differ in size, structure, scope of responsibility, and number per province. The Canadian Centre for Analysis of Regionalization and Health defines **RHAs** as autonomous healthcare organizations responsible for health administration within a defined geographic region within a province or territory (28). They have appointed or elected boards of governance and manage the funding and delivering of community and institutional health services within their regions.

The following criteria determine whether an organization can be classified as an RHA. Within an identified region, RHAs (28):

- have autonomy and responsibility for the majority of health services in a region;
- have appointed/elected boards;
- are responsible for funding and delivery of community health services;
- are responsible for funding and delivery of institutional health services;
- have an increased focus on prevention;

- aim to integrate services; and
- aim to reduce duplication and overlap.

Every province except Ontario is divided into regions, ranging from five in British Columbia to 18 in Quebec, based partly on population size and natural geographic and administrative boundaries. Each region's health needs are managed by a regional or district health board composed of roughly 10 to 15 members. The process of choosing board members varies from province to province, but generally a board includes both elected and appointed officials who represent a wide variety of constituencies and interests. They are usually drawn from consumer or special-needs groups, hospitals and health services centres, professional groups, voluntary agencies, and elected officials. This mix of membership increases the board's accountability before its community and simultaneously ensures the inclusion of particular areas of expertise or the representation of particular cultural backgrounds that may not already be represented. Several provinces and territories, such as Alberta and Saskatchewan, have provided for direct links between regional boards and organizations of physicians to ensure that physicians have a voice in regional planning and resource allocation decisions. In the Northwest Territories, regional boards deal with both health and social services. Table 13.1 provides an overview of regionalization across Canada (29). In some cases, regionalization plans and implementation are still in various stages of implementation.

Functions of RHAs

The exact functions of regional health authorities across provinces and territories vary, but in general include (30):

- assessing health needs of the population in its region;
- developing policy and program priorities within the region and related allocation of resources;
- administering funding, including allocating funds to community and non-governmental organizations for primary care;
- planning and coordinating service delivery, including planning of capital projects;
- guaranteeing reasonable access to high-quality health services in a coordinated and integrated system of care;
- maintaining liaisons with community agencies and with the provincial and territorial ministry of health;
- managing and operating service delivery and financing of institutions, including hospitals, long-term care, and other health services centres;
- evaluating health system outputs and outcomes; and
- promoting public participation in the decision-making process.

Core Health Services

The following core services administered and funded by provincial and territorial regional health authorities, include (27, 30):

- public health (with the exception of New Brunswick);
- home care and community-based services (with the exception of Nova Scotia);

Table 13.1.   Provincial Overview of Regional Health Authorities

Province	# regional health authorities (or equivalent)	Date established	Population	Distinguishing features
British Columbia	5 RHAs, 15 Health Service Delivery Areas, 1 Provincial Health Service Authority	1997	320,000–1,300,000	
Alberta	17 RHAs (reduce to 5-7 by 2004)	1994	20,000–970,000	Two thirds elected, one third appointed board members
Saskatchewan	12 RHAs and 1 Northern Health Authority	1992, restructured in 2001/02	46,000–278,000	Moved from elected to appointed boards
Manitoba	12 RHAs (reduced to 11 by 2003)	1997, 1998	38,621–646,733	
Ontario	not regionalized 17 District Health Councils (advisory)	–	200,000–2,500,000	Health care administered and delivered by the province
Quebec	18 Régies régionales de la santé et des services sociaux	1989–1992	average 411,000	First province to establish regional structures
Nova Scotia	9 District Health Authorities (DHAs)	1996, 2001	34,000–395,000	4 regional health boards replaced by 9 DHAs in 2001
New Brunswick	8 RHAs	1992	31,293–200,000	First board elections slated for 2004
Prince Edward Island	5 RHAs (Provincial Health Services Authority and amalgamation of 2 RHAs)	1993, 1994	7,000–66,856	RHA responsible for primary health care services; PHSA responsible for secondary and acute care services
Newfoundland and Labrador	12 boards: 6 institutional, 4 health and community services boards, 2 integrated boards	1994	28,000–180,000.	Two parallel structures: institutional and community

Source: Canadian Centre for Analysis of Regionalization and Health. 2003. *Provincial overview of regional health authorities.* <*www.regionalization.org/provoverview/table_10_02.html*> *(March 2003).*

- mental health services (with the exception of New Brunswick and Alberta);
- long-term care institutions (with the exception of New Brunswick and Nova Scotia); and
- alcohol and substance abuse programs (with the exception of British Columbia and Alberta).

Hospitals are governed or funded by regional health authorities in all Canadian jurisdictions with regional structures. In Quebec, hospitals have individual boards but are funded by regional authorities. Hospitals in Manitoba have the option of maintaining individual boards.

There are some key services that continue to be administered and funded centrally by provincial and territorial governments and the most significant services are physicians services, with the exception of salaried physicians in Quebec and Manitoba; prescription drugs except for the Northwest Territories; and cancer services (30).

Funding Formulas

In order to increase the effectiveness of regional health authorities, which were usually only advisory in nature, most provinces and territories have passed legislation to restructure their ministries of health and devolve financial decision making and planning and prioritizing activities. With recent cuts at all level of government, one potential reason for restructuring was to transfer difficult funding decisions to the regional level during a time of downsizing so the provincial government does not have to bear the blame for unpopular decisions.

In general, recent provincial legislation has changed funding formulas to allow for the devolution of decision making. While the provincial and territorial ministries collect taxes to finance the healthcare system and develop regional funding envelopes, regional health boards allocate funds to service organizations based on their own needs assessments and policy priorities. For example, in Saskatchewan government funding to district boards is based on needs assessments and population counts. Each district can borrow the money but is not allowed to tax local communities. Other provinces and territories are also moving toward funding formulas based on population needs. In 2002, only Saskatchewan, Quebec, and New Brunswick had functioning budget formulas in place. British Columbia, Alberta, Manitoba, and Nova Scotia are in the preparatory/planning phases of implementing population-based funding. Funding for physician remuneration through provincial health insurance plans is, as a rule, maintained as a separate budget category within ministry (not regional board) budgets.

Different concerns over regionalization have been expressed from different perspectives. Concerns over regionalization generally include the notions that regional boards will create more government bureaucracy instead of increasing responsiveness to local needs, and that appointed rather than elected board members may cause the positive aspects of accountability to be lost. There are also concerns about regional boundaries and the maintenance of freedom of consumers to choose their healthcare provider regardless of region, and about funding envelopes and resource allocation mechanisms, especially with regard to specialized tertiary and quaternary care centres (e.g., does a region with highly specialized hospitals pay for the services of those hospitals that serve multiple regions?). In addition, in an era of fiscal restraint, many public health activists fear that public health and community services will lose in the funding allocation struggle as each board identifies which services it can and will fund.

4.2.   FUNCTIONAL ORGANIZATION OF PROVINCIAL MINISTRIES OF HEALTH

The role of the provincial and territorial ministries of health, in most cases, has been revised to meet the increased role of regional and local boards. In most cases, ministries have devolved service delivery responsibilities to regional boards while maintaining responsibility for overall health sector planning, corporate services, financing and the administration of funding envelopes, the administration of provincial and territorial insurance plans covering physician remuneration, evaluation and monitoring, and the management of computerized information systems.

The main exception to this trend is the Ontario Ministry of Health and Long-Term Care, where the organizational structure remains more or less unchanged and oriented toward financing individual hospitals and agencies rather than regional boards.

Since the administrative structures of provincial and territorial health ministries are constantly changing, no organizational chart of the ministries is included here; for up-to-date information, readers are advised to visit the Web site of each provincial and territorial ministry of health. However, the functional organization remains stable. Provincial and territorial health responsibilities fall into three areas: direct delivery of health services, financing of health services, and administrative services (see Table 13.2).

4.3.   SERVICE DELIVERY

Service delivery involves those services that, in most provinces and territories, fall under the jurisdiction of the ministry of health with regard to budget, policies, and control. For the most part, the actual delivery of health services is now the responsibility of regional health boards, with the function of the ministry of health at the provincial and territorial level limited to financing health services, administration, and planning (see below). Thus, regionalization represents the centralization of most services to regional levels from local bodies, and decentralization from the ministries of health.

Aboriginal and Northern Health Services

The health status of the Aboriginal population in Canada is far below the general population in all provinces and territories (see Chapter 6 and 18) and there are jurisdictional disputes between federal and provincial governments about their responsibilities toward this population. However, as more and more Aboriginal people migrate to urban areas, a number of provinces have begun to provide culturally appropriate care. In jurisdictions with sparsely settled northern areas, the provincial and territorial health departments provide both treatment and preventive health services.

Table 13.2. **Functions of Provincial and Territorial Health Systems**

Service delivery	Service financing (direct or via regional health board)	Administrative services
Services for tuberculosis and cancer patients Health services in remote areas Ambulance services Public health laboratories	Public health services[1] Homecare programs Mental health services Hospital and medical care Dental care Prescription drugs Services for allied health professionals Other services, e.g., health appliances and equipment Services for welfare recipients	Health services planning Health human resources planning, training, and regulation Standard setting for health institutions and public places Health research Health surveillance (communicable disease control) Emergency health services) Vital statistics

1. Most provinces except Ontario

Saskatchewan, Manitoba, and the Yukon have set up northern health services, and other provinces have similar services.

In British Columbia, the health needs of Aboriginal groups are now the responsibility of each regional health board. A special Aboriginal Policy Framework, which addresses issues particular to Aboriginal health, has been developed by the province's New Directions Development Division and delivered to regional boards for implementation. Regional boards are encouraged to include Aboriginal members. Since 1992–93, the provincial government has funded six regional Aboriginal Health Councils (AHCs) and tasked the Aboriginal Health Association of British Columbia (AHABC) with allocating and managing funding for addictions, mental health, and family violence programs in Aboriginal communities (31).

The Alberta Health and Wellness Department initiated the Aboriginal Health Strategy in 1996 to assist the regional health authorities and the Provincial Mental Health Board to consult with Aboriginal leaders and communities to provide health services in an appropriate, culturally sensitive way. The strategy's long-term goal is to reduce inequalities in health status between the Aboriginal and non-Aboriginal people in Alberta through a variety of ways, e.g., improving access to health careers by providing bursaries and developing an innovative primary care model for remote communities.

Manitoba's Aboriginal Health Strategy supports the overall goals and vision of health reform for Manitoba Health to improve the health status of Aboriginal people in partnership with Aboriginal communities (32). The province is responsible for providing clinical and community health services to communities with a majority non-Status Indian and Métis population (the federal government supplies such services to communities with a majority Status Indian population). The province's Community and Mental Health Services Division includes the Rural and Northern Operations branch, which provides services and ensures standards of care are implemented in hospitals, personal care homes, community health centres, funded agencies, and community-based health services. Regional offices provide a variety of community-based health and social services on behalf of the Health and Family Services departments. Health services include provision of health promotion, protection, and disease prevention programs; women's health programs; healthy child development programs; the homecare program, including assessment for personal care home placement; gerontology programs including support services to seniors; community mental health programs; and audiology and diabetes education programs (33). Most recently, Manitoba Health has become involved in the development of the community-based Aboriginal Health and Wellness Centre in Winnipeg.

Saskatchewan's Northern Health Services Branch, within the Strategic Services Division, provides primary care, public health nursing, mental health services, physician services, children's dental services, home care, public health inspection, nutrition counselling, speech and language pathology, and health education to residents of northern Saskatchewan. Community mental health nurses and mental health social workers maintain regular contact with all northern communities including First Nations band offices to ensure that northern residents with mental health problems receive assistance and counseling. As well, community health educators provide interpretive services to people who speak Cree and Dene.

Ontario has established the Aboriginal Health Office responsible for implementing the Aboriginal Health Policy Framework and, with the Ministry of Community Family and Children's Services, the Aboriginal Healing and Wellness Strategy. Ontario's Aboriginal Healing and Wellness Strategy is built on the philosophy that health must be addressed throughout the four life stages of an individual's life (infancy, youth, adulthood, and old age) in a holistic way (including physical, mental, emotional, spiritual, and cultural health) and within a continuum of care (including health promotion, prevention, treatment, and rehabilitation). Ten Aboriginal Healing and Wellness Centres across Ontario providing primary health care integrate western medical and traditional healing practices.

For northern Quebec, the Nunavik Regional Board of Health and Social Services and the First Nations of Quebec and Labrador Health and Social Service Commission are responsible for health and social services in their respective jurisdictions and are governed by Aboriginal boards (34). These boards control health and social service delivery in their jurisdiction. Quebec is a leader in area of transfer and control of health and social services to Aboriginal peoples.

Aboriginal Canada Portal is a very useful site that links to national Aboriginal organizations, 12 federal government departments with Aboriginal mandates, all provincial and territorial governments and organizations with Aboriginal responsibilities, as well as all related Aboriginal community information (34).

Public Health Laboratories

Public health laboratories assist with the identification and control of epidemic and endemic diseases. All provinces and territories maintain a central public health laboratory, and most have branch laboratories to assist local health departments and the medical profession in the protection of community health and the control of infectious diseases.

Occupational Health

Services designed to prevent accidents and occupational diseases and to maintain the health of employees are the common concern of provincial and territorial health departments, labour departments, workers' compensation boards, industrial management, and unions (see Chapter 10).

Emergency Health Services

All provinces and territories have emergency health services, which deal with the transportation of patients from their homes or institutions to service-providing institutions either in their community or farther away. This is accomplished by land, air, or water ambulance systems. In Saskatchewan, Manitoba, Quebec, and New Brunswick, regional health authorities are responsible for these services; in other provinces and territories, the municipalities or provincial and territorial departments are responsible for service provision and the provinces and territories set standards. All provinces and territories have emergency or disaster plans for such situations as ice storms, floods, forest fires, chemical spills, rail derailment, or threats of biological or nuclear warfare.

In most emergency situations, Health Canada works closely with the provinces and territories and local health officials. Cooperation can include working together on emergency preparedness, intelligence gathering, disease surveillance, detection and diagnosis, as well as on keeping the public informed during emergency situations, training first-responders (ambulance, fire, police, and emergency room staff), providing on-site field hospitals and pharmaceutical and medical supplies, protecting assets, decontaminating affected sites, and maintaining emergency equipment.

Health Canada also leads a provincial and territorial emergency response team that convenes during times of crisis. On the morning of September 11, 2001, for example, Health Canada's Centre for Emergency Preparedness and Response activated its Emergency Response Centre on a round-the-clock basis. Early links were established with provincial emergency response coordinators, the Office of Critical Infrastructure Protection and Emergency Response (OCIPEP), and the United States Department of Health and Human Services Office of Emergency Preparedness (13).

4.4. SERVICE FINANCING

As indicated above, all of the services listed in Table 13.2 are financed totally or partially by the provincial and territorial governments. As a result, provinces and territories exert pressure on professionals and institutions for setting standards for the services and controlling costs. Provinces and territories try to manage the system through their financial clout.

Health Insurance Programs

The basic principles of hospital and medical insurance stated by the federal government are described in Chapter 12, so only the relevant features of the provincial programs are described here. In some provinces and territories, the administration of the hospital insurance plan and the medical insurance plan is combined, whereas in others the two plans have separate administrative structures.

Health insurance coverage is automatic and compulsory across Canada, requiring only some form of registration. All provinces and territories, except Alberta and British Columbia, fund their health care only through general revenues or a levy on payrolls, or both. Alberta and British Columbia also have a component of premiums based on income. The Canada Health Act Annual Report, published by Health Canada, is an excellent source of details on the functioning of the health insurance plans in each province (35). Coverage for insured services is available to all Canadian residents on equal terms and conditions, and cannot be denied on grounds of age, income, or pre-existing conditions.

The federal government has established a Health Insurance Supplementary Fund (administered by the Canada Health Act Division) with provincial and territorial contributions to provide for payment of claims for hospital or medical services for residents of Canada who have lost coverage through no fault of their own. This might occur, for example, if someone changing residence was not recognized as eligible under the rules of any province. It would not apply if coverage was lost through the individual's own fault, as in non-payment of premiums. Contributions to the fund are made by all provinces and territories in proportion to population and are matched by the federal government. Those that charge premiums make some provision to cover those unable to pay (such as welfare recipients and those whose incomes are slightly above the poverty level) through full and partial subsidies. All provinces and territories also provide additional services for recipients of public assistance and for those over age 65. These commonly include prescription drugs and may also include dental services, eyeglasses, prostheses, homecare services, and nursing home care, depending on the province. Additionally, provinces and territories such as Ontario, Manitoba, Saskatchewan, Alberta, and British Columbia provide limited insurance coverage for the services of chiropractors, podiatrists, and optometrists. Usually there is a dollar limit on these services covered.

The Alberta Health Care Insurance Plan offers additional health insurance to residents who cannot obtain Alberta Blue Cross coverage through an employer on an individual basis at special rates. Two government-sponsored supplementary health programs are available from Alberta Blue Cross (36): Non-Group Coverage for Alberta residents under 65 years of age whose Alberta Health Care Plan premiums are paid, and who are not eligible to receive the Alberta Widows' Pension; and Coverage for Seniors for Albertans 65 years of age and older and their spouses and dependants, and all recipients of the Alberta Widows' Pension and their dependants. Benefits of each program include 70% of the cost of drugs, ambulance service charges, the services of a registered chartered psychologist, nursing care in the person's home, a portion of the cost of prosthetic and orthotic items, and private or semi-private room accommodation for insurable, differential charges in a public, general active-treatment hospital in Canada.

Drug Plans

Drugs continue to consume an increasing share of Canada's healthcare dollar, now accounting for the second largest category of health expenditures next to hospital services. In 2001, spending on drugs is expected to have reached $15.5 billion, representing 15.2% of total healthcare spending (37). The bill for prescription drugs is split almost equally between the public (49.2%) and private sectors (50.8%).

Most Canadians (88%) are covered by public or private drug plans: 62% have private insurance covering full or partial costs of drugs; 19% of Canadians are eligible for public drug insurance; and 7% have both private and public insurance; the remaining 12% have no coverage.

All provinces and territories have public prescription drug programs for recipients of social assistance, and all seniors (except in New Brunswick, and Newfoundland and Labrador — where eligibility in the government-sponsored drug plan is based on income) (27). Provincial governments in British Columbia, Saskatchewan, Manitoba, and Ontario have prescription drug plans targeted to the general population that provide a protective cap (in some cases based on family income) on the personal cost of drug expenses borne by individuals. Quebec mandates prescription drug coverage with an out-of-pocket cap no greater than $750 for all residents, whether under employer-sponsored programs or the provincial program. Alberta offers all residents a public, voluntary, premium based prescription drug insurance plan that provides significant coverage for drug expenses after a three-month waiting period. Prince Edward Island, the Yukon, and the Northwest Territories have programs for chronic disease and disabilities that provide prescription drugs for most chronic conditions. Most provinces and territories provide drugs for the treatment of venereal disease, tuberculosis, and other infections that pose a public health hazard, and for which treatment costs are very high (for example, cystic fibrosis or AIDS). The federal government assumes the full cost of providing prescription drugs for some Aboriginal populations and certain armed forces veterans.

The *Canada Health Act* includes drugs and biological and related preparations administered in the hospital within the definition of hospital services. However, prescription drug coverage in nursing homes or long-term care facilities differs across Canada. In British Columbia, Alberta, and Manitoba, costs are not shared with the resident. In Saskatchewan, Nova Scotia, Newfoundland and Labrador, Yukon, and the Northwest Territories, residents of nursing homes are eligible for government-sponsored drug plans in the same manner as other residents in the community. In New Brunswick and Ontario, low-income residents of nursing homes do not share the costs or pay reduced amounts. In Quebec and Prince Edward Island, residents of publicly owned or sponsored nursing homes and long-term care facilities receive drugs without charge, while those in private facilities are responsible for their drug costs.

Dental Plans

Most provinces and territories provide emergency basic dental health services to children, adults, and seniors on social assistance (38). A few provinces and territories, such as British Columbia, Quebec, and Newfoundland and Labrador, have special provision for children's dental programs, mainly in the area of preventive dentistry. The federal government provides basic dental services to Status Indians and Inuit with three delivery options: fee for service, contract session, or salaried staff.

Appliances and Equipment

Provinces and territories differ in the benefits provided for devices and equipment necessary or complementary to medical treatment,.

The Regional Health Authority's Home Care Program coordinates the Alberta Aids to Daily Living (AADL) program. AADL assists with the provision of program-approved medical equipment and supplies to residents living at home with a chronic or terminal illness or disability. Those over age 65 do not pay.

British Columbia's Community and Family Health Division runs the Medical Supply Services program, which provides support for specialized home maintenance care. The kidney dialysis service, for all home and community dialysis procedures, is the core operation of the program. Medical and nutritional supplies are also coordinated to address hemophilia, parenteral nutrition, and enteral nutrition. The At Home Program of the Services to the Handicapped Branch provides respite support, medical equipment, and supplies to families caring for children with severe disabilities. The Hearing Services Branch operates the British Columbia Hearing Aid Program to provide selection, fitting, repair, and sale of hearing devices at competitive prices.

Saskatchewan's Aids to Independent Living (SAIL) (39) provides benefits for people whose long-term disabilities or illnesses leave them unable to function fully, residents eligible for orthopedic services, special needs equipment, and home respiratory services, excluding those eligible under departments or agencies of the Government of Canada, the Workers' Compensation Board, Saskatchewan Government Insurance, or residents of general, rehabilitation, or extended care hospitals. People with specific disabling conditions may be eligible for benefits under the various Special Benefit Programs (Paraplegia Program, Cystic Fibrosis Program, End-Stage Renal Disease Program, Ostomy Program, and Aids to the Blind Program).

Within the Continuing Care Branch, Manitoba's Home Care Equipment and Supplies Branch provides a support service by acquiring, warehousing, distributing, maintaining, and repairing a range of medical supplies and equipment required in order to support the care and independent living of people with physical disabilities within their own communities. The equipment is purchased in bulk and provided on loan to eligible Manitoba residents under the authorization of a healthcare professional. People who are eligible include those who are physically disabled because of disease, traumatic injury, or the natural aging process, and need medical equipment to support their care and independence in the community.

The Operational Support Branch of the Ontario Ministry of Health and Long-Term Care administers the Assistive Devices Program (ADP) and the Home Oxygen Program

(HOP) (40). Both programs offer financial assistance to Ontario residents with long-term physical disabilities so they can obtain basic, competitively priced, and personalized assistive devices appropriate for individual needs and essential for independent living. These may allow them to avoid costly institutional settings and remain in a community living arrangement.

The Seniors Rehabilitation Equipment Program is run by the Community and Environmental Health Branch of the New Brunswick Public Health and Medical Services Division. Seniors may borrow, at no charge, standard and specialized equipment to assist in the activities of daily living. The equipment is loaned by the Canadian Red Cross Society and funded by the Department of Health and Community Services.

4.5. ADMINISTRATIVE SERVICES

Administrative services are those operational functions that government undertakes to plan, forecast, and evaluate necessary services.

Planning of Health Services

All provincial and territorial ministries of health have a group of civil servants who, with the help of outside consultants, do short- and long-range planning of health services. These groups may be loosely structured or have a defined status within the ministry, such as the division of strategic health planning within the Ministry of Health and Long-Term Care in Ontario.

Often the minister, recognizing the deficit in services, appoints a special committee composed of selected citizens and professionals who receive support from civil servants. The task of these committees is to recommend mechanisms for delivering health services to the population or sub-groups of the population. Recent reports are listed in references (see also Chapter 18) (41, 42).

The ministry of health in many provinces and territories actively assesses the future needs for health human resources. Most provinces and territories go through the cycle of over and undersupply of their health human resources. At the time of writing, all provinces and territories are faced with undersupply of health professionals (for example, doctors and nurses), and many have taken active steps to increase the number of students admitted into these professional schools or to facilitate licensing of foreign-trained professionals. Where there is a lack of human resources, subsidies have been provided to students entering that profession. Several provincial and territorial governments provide incentives for recruitment and retention of healthcare practitioners in rural areas.

Information Systems

In order to facilitate greater ease of informed decision making, there is increased interest in the development of integrated, system-wide information systems to be managed by provincial and territorial health ministries. Manitoba Health recently implemented the Drug Program Information Network (DPIN-ER) into 81 hospital emergency and admitting areas. DPIN-ER provides valuable drug history information to hospital medical professionals throughout the province (43).

Ontario's Ministry of Health and Long-Term Care has implemented Telehealth Ontario, a free advice telephone service for callers to speak directly with an experienced Registered Nurse, 24 hours a day, seven days a week.

The Saskatchewan Health Information Network (SHIN) is developing a province-wide health information network in a multi-year development initiative that will give healthcare providers immediate access to patient information and medical history, thereby decreasing costly duplication of services, increasing the quality of care by providing complete medical histories, avoiding dangerous drug interactions, and making it easier for providers to assess possibilities for patient treatment and support services in the community. In addition, planners at the provincial, regional, and district levels would have access to complete, accurate information about service utilization patterns and outcomes.

Recently, a number of provinces and territories have introduced unique identifier systems for individuals insured in their health plans. To avoid the fraudulent use of cards by non-registrants, the Northwest Territories, Ontario, Saskatchewan, and Quebec have introduced photo identification cards similar to the driver's licence, and other provinces and territories are in the process of adopting such a system.

Most provinces and territories emphasize the need for evidence-based decision making as a critical component in increasing the cost effectiveness of health services provision. Research institutes such as Ontario's Institute for Clinical Evaluation Sciences, Quebec's Conseil d'évaluation de la technologie de la santé and Manitoba's Centre for Health Policy play a critical role in health services research, clinical evaluation, and evidence-based policy recommendations.

Regulation of Health Professions

The established health professions, including medicine, nursing, chiropractors, dentistry, and pharmacy, are regulated by their respective licensing bodies, which are mandated by provincial and territorial legislation. Other health professionals and technicians are also usually regulated or certified (for details see Chapter 16).

Standard Setting for Health Institutions and Public Places

All acute, chronic, rehabilitation, extended care, and mental health hospitals are governed by specific legislation. Standards are set for nursing homes in many provinces and territories as well. There are definite standards and guidelines for public places such as restaurants, food-handling venues, industries, and factories. Legislation usually emanates from within the civil service or from concerned members of the legislature.

Health Research

Most provinces and territories have intramural health research to help long-range planning of health services. Wealthier provinces, such as Alberta, British Columbia, Quebec, and Ontario, earmark funds for extramural research. These research grants are usually peer-reviewed and span from basic research to demonstration grants for updating healthcare systems. In some provinces and territories, there has been a recent trend for the ministry of health to invite tenders for the areas to be researched.

Vital Statistics

Each province has a registrar general responsible for keeping records of vital events such as births, marriages, and deaths. This department usually provides statistical information pertaining to these vital events, which is mandatory in all provinces and territories. These data are provided to the federal government, which publishes national statistics. However, due to financial constraints, Statistics Canada recently announced that it would no longer publish nor require the collection of information on marriages. Statistics Canada asserts that, due to changing family structures in contemporary society, information on marriages is no longer relevant for health programs. Marriage statistics will continue to be collected through the Bureau of the Census.

5.   SUMMARY

This chapter dealt with the types of health services provided by the federal and provincial and territorial governments.

At the time of Confederation, the federal government had relatively little jurisdiction and involvement in the health care of Canadians. In 1919, the Department of Health was established and its responsibilities included "all matters relating to the promotion or preservation of health, social security and social welfare of the people of Canada over which the Parliament of Canada has jurisdiction." In 1945, Health and Welfare Canada was created with two primary tasks: to promote, preserve, and restore the health of Canadians, and to provide social security and social welfare to Canadians. In 1993, the Welfare Department of the ministry was separated. The federal ministry of health is now known as Health Canada and is composed of seven branches: the Corporate Services Branch, the First Nations and Inuit Health Branch, the Health Products and Food Branch, the Population and Public Health Branch, the Health Policy and Communications Branch, the Information, Analysis and Connectivity Branch, and the Healthy Environments and Consumer Safety Branch. Three branches are of particular relevance to public health: the Population and Public Health Branch (PPHB) is primarily responsible for policies, programs, and systems relating to prevention, health promotion, disease surveillance, community action, and disease control; the Health Policy and Communications Branch (HPCB) plays a lead role in health policy, communications and consultations. The Healthy Environments and Consumer Safety (HECS) Branch is responsible for promoting safe living, working, and recreational environments, including occupational health and regulating tobacco and controlled substances, and it provides drug analytical services, regulates the safety of industrial and consumer products in the Canadian marketplace, and promotes their safe use.

Health Canada has a number of other interdepartmental initiatives dealing with specific areas, such as the National Advisory Council on Aging, the Canadian Strategy on HIV/AIDS, and the Women's Health Bureau.

Income security and social services programs of the Ministry of Human Resources Development also influence health. They promote and strengthen the income security of Canadians, share in the cost of provincial and territorial social assistance, welfare services, and rehabilitation programs, and assist in the development of social services to meet changing social needs.

As noted in earlier chapters, provincial and territorial governments have primary responsibility for all personal health matters such as disease prevention, treatment, and maintenance of health. Activities such as preventive health services, hospital services, treatment services for tuberculosis and other chronic diseases, and rehabilitation and care of people who are chronically ill and disabled are all under the jurisdiction of the provincial and territorial governments.

The responsibilities of the provincial and territorial governments can be classified as service financing, service delivery, and administrative services.

In the 1990s, most provinces and territories in Canada partially devolved their service delivery responsibility to sub-provincial regions, resulting in the establishment of regional health authorities (RHAs) everywhere except in Ontario. The objective was to streamline the delivery system, making it less fragmented and more responsive to local needs. In some provinces and territories, additional goals were to increase community-based services, improve public participation in health care, and encourage policies and programs to promote health. RHAs are autonomous healthcare organizations responsible for health administration within a defined geographic region within a province or territory. They have appointed or elected boards of governance and are responsible for funding and delivering community and institutional health services within their regions.

RHAs fund and administer core services including public health; home care and community-based services; mental health services and long-term care institutions; and alcohol and substance abuse programs; and hospitals. While the provincial and territorial ministries collect taxes to finance the healthcare system and develop regional funding envelopes, regional health boards allocate funds to service organizations based on their own needs assessments and policy priorities. Health insurance claims covering physician remuneration and prescription drugs covered under the provincial plans remain, for the most part, under the administrative auspices of the province.

Service financing, involves those services that are paid for either totally or partially by either government-run health insurance programs (for example, hospital and medical services provided by a physician) or by subsidizing the cost for services, drugs, or appliances.

Health insurance coverage is automatic and compulsory in all provinces and territories, requiring only some form of registration. All, except Alberta and British Columbia, fund their health care only through general revenues or a levy on payrolls, or both. Alberta and British Columbia also have a component of premiums based on income.

Most Canadians (88%) are covered by public or private drug plans. All provinces and territories except New Brunswick and Newfoundland and Labrador have public prescription drug plans for seniors (in those two provinces, seniors' eligibility is based on income), and coverage for the general population differs among the provinces and territories.

Most provinces and territories provide emergency basic dental health services to children, adults, and seniors on social assistance. Appliances and equipment comprise devices and equipment necessary or complementary to medical treatment. Provinces and territories differ in the benefits provided.

Administrative services are those operational functions that government undertakes to plan, forecast and evaluate the necessary services.

6. REFERENCES

1. Health Canada. 2002. *Branches and organization.* <www.hc-sc.gc.ca/english/about/org.html> (November 2002).
2. Health Canada. 2002. *Acts and regulations.* <www.hc-sc.gc.ca/english/about/acts_regulations.html> (November 2002).
3. Health Canada. 2002. *Strategies and innovation.* <www.hc-sc.gc.ca/english/about/strategies.html> (November 2002).
4. Health Canada. 2002. *First Nations and Inuit telehealth: Future opportunities.* <www.hc-sc.gc.ca/fnihb/phcph/telehealth/introduction.htm> (November 2002).
5. Health Canada. 2002. *Canada Health Act annual report.* <www.hc-sc.gc.ca/medicare/AnnualReports.htm> (November 2002).
6. Health Canada. 2002. *Therapeutic Products Directorate: Who we are.* <www.hc-sc.gc.ca/hpb-dgps/therapeut/zfiles/english/fact-sht/fact_wwa_e.html> (November 2002).
7. Health Canada. 2002. *Health Canada Policy: Food Safety Assessment Program.* <www.hc-sc.gc.ca/food-aliment/fsa-esa/e_policy.html> (November 2002).
8. Health Canada. 2002. *Food program of Health Canada.* <www.hc-sc.gc.ca/food-aliment/dg/e_organization_chart.html> (November 2002).
9. Government of Canada. 2003. *Food and Drugs Acts; Nutiritonal labeling, Nutrient content claims and Health claims.* <www.canadagazette.gc.ca/partII/2003/20030101/htm/scrIl-e.htm> (March 2003).
10. Health Canada. 2002. *Natural Health Products Directorate.* <www.hc-sc.gc.ca/hpb/onhp/welcome_c.html> (November 2002).
11. Standing Committee on Health. 1998. *Natural Health Products: A new vision.* <www.parl.gc.ca/InfoComDoc/36/1/HEAL/Studies/Reports/healrp02-e.htm> (November 2002).
12. Health Canada, Office of Health and the Information Highway. 2002. *About OHIH.* <www.hc-sc.gc.ca/ohih-bsi/about_apropos/index_e.html> (November 2002).
13. Health Canada, Population and Public Health Branch. 2002. *PPHB centres.* <www.hc-sc.gc.ca/pphb-dgspsp/centres_e.html#cepr> (November 2002).
14. Health Canada. 2002. *Healthy environments and consumer safety.* <www.hc-sc.gc.ca/hecs-sesc/hecs/about_us.htm> (November 2002).
15. Government of Canada. 2003. *Canadian Institutes for Health Research.* <www.cihr-irsc.gc.ca> (March 2003).
16. Patented Medicine Prices Review Board. 2002. *About the PMPRB.* Ottawa. <ww.pmprb-cepmb.gc.ca/english/01_e/01ab_e.htm> (November 2002).
17. Health Canada. 2002. *Workplace hazardous materials information system.* <www.hc-sc.gc.ca/hecs-sesc/whmis/index.htm> (November 2002).
18. Pest Management Regulatory Agency. 2002. *About PMRA.* <www.hc-sc.gc.ca/pmra-arla/english/aboutpmra/about-e.html> (November 2002).
19. Canada. 2002. *Canada Benefits.* <canadabenefits.gc.ca/faechome.jsp?lang=en> (November 2002).
20. Canadian Institute for Health Information. 2002. *CIHI profile.* Ottawa. <secure.cihi.ca/cihiweb/dispPage.jsp?cw_page=profile_e> (November 2002).

21.   Health Canada. 2002. *Canada's report on HIV / AIDS 2001 — Current realities: Strengthening the response.* <www.hc-sc.gc.ca/hpb-dgps/therapeut/zfiles/english/fact-sht/fact_wwa_e.html> (November 2002).

22.   Health Canada. 1995. *Tobacco control: A blueprint to protect the health of Canadians.* <www.hc-sc.gc.ca/hecs-sesc/tobacco/research/archive/tobac_control.html> (November 2002).

23.   Canada. 1997. *Tobacco Act.* <laws.justice.gc.ca/en/T-11.5/index.html> (November 2002).

24.   Health Canada. 1999. *New directions for tobacco control in Canada.* <www.hc-sc.gc.ca/hecs-sesc/tobacco/policy/new_directions/index.html> (November 2002).

25.   Health Canada. 2002. *National Advisory Council on Aging.* <www.hc-sc.gc.ca/seniors-aines/seniors/english/naca/naca.htm#WhatIs> (November 2002).

26.   Canada. 2002. *Provincial and territorial government organizations.* <chp-pcs.gc.ca/CHP/index_e.jsp?pageid=10042> (November 2002).

27.   Kirby M, LeBreton M. 2002. *The health of Canadians: The federal role. Volume 6: Recommendations for reform.* Standing Senate Committee on Social Affairs, Science and Technology. <www.parl.gc.ca/37/2/parlbus/commbus/senate/com-e/soci-e/rep-e/repoct02vol6-e.htm> (November 2002).

28.   Canadian Centre for Analysis of Regionalization and Health. 2002. *What is regionalization?* Saskatoon. <www.regionalization.org/Regionalization.html> (November 2002).

29.   Canadian Centre for Analysis of Regionalization and Health. 2002. *Provincial overview table.* Saskatoon. <www.regionalization.org/ProvOverviewTable_10_02.html> (November 2002).

30.   Ontario Hospital Association. 2002. *Regional Health Authorities in Canada: Lessons for Ontario.* <www.oha.com/oha/reports.nsf/($Att)/pspr56wmkq/$FILE/Regional HealthAuthoritiesinCanada.pdf?OpenElement> (November 2002).

31.   British Columbia. 2001. *Aboriginal Health Division program summary 2000/2001.* Victoria. <www.healthservices.gov.bc.ca/aboriginal/pdf/programsummaries.pdf> (November 2002).

32.   Manitoba Health. 1997. *Aboriginal health strategy.* <www.gov.mb.ca/health/ann/199697/3a-m4.html> (November 2002).

33.   Manitoba Health. 1997. *Rural and northern operations.* <www.gov.mb.ca/health/ann/199697/3a-m7.html> (November 2002).

34.   Canada. 2002. *Aboriginal Canada portal.* <www.aboriginalcanada.gc.ca> (November 2002).

35.   Health Canada. 2002. *Canada Health Act annual report 2000–2001.* <www.hc-sc.gc.ca/medicare/AnnualReports.htm> (November 2002).

36.   Alberta Ministry of Health and Wellness. 2002. *Non-group prescription drug coverage.* <www.health.gov.ab.ca/coverage/benefits/drugs/non_group.html> (November 2002).

37.   Canadian Institute for Health Information. 2002. *Drug expenditure in Canada.* <secure.cihi.ca/cihiweb/dispPage.jsp?cw_page=AR_80_E> (January 2003).

38.   Main P. Dental public health programs in Canada 1995: Cross-Canada dental check-up. *Canadian Journal of Community Dentistry* 1995; 10(1):12-5.

39.   Saskatchewan Health. 2002. *Saskatchewan aids to independent living.* <www.health.gov.sk.ca/ps_sail.html#top> (November 2002).

40.   Ontario, Ministry of Health and Long-Term Care. 2002. *Assistive Devices Program (includes the home oxygen program).* <www.gov.on.ca/health/english/program/adp/adp_mn.html> (November 2002).

41.   Alberta, Premier's Advisory Council on Health. 2002. *A framework for reform: Report of the Premier's Advisory Council on Health.* <www.gov.ab.ca/home/health_first/documents_maz_report.cfm> (November 2002).

42.   Saskatchewan Commission on Medicare. 2001. *Caring for medicare: Sustaining a quality system.* <www.health.gov.sk.ca/info_center_pub_commission_on_medicare-bw.pdf> (November 2002).

43.   Canadian College of Health Service Executives. *Health systems updates 2000–2001,* 8th ed. Ottawa: Canadian College of Health Service Executives, 2002.

❧14❧

FUNDING, EXPENDITURES, AND RESOURCES

The healthcare industry is the fifth largest industry in Canada and hires about 10% of the workforce. Canadians spent more than $100 billion on health care in 2002, amounting to at least one third of total provincial government expenditures. Since the inception of national health insurance programs, constant concerns have been expressed about the financing and delivery of health care. This chapter describes the funding and allocation of health resources of the Canadian healthcare system, provides international comparisons and the strategies used by different levels of governments to ensure sustainability, accessibility, and availability of quality health services, and presents indicators that evaluate health system performance.

1. THE FINANCING OF HEALTH CARE

One of the most basic series of questions about the organization of any healthcare system relates to the financing of health services: where does the money for health care come from? Where should it come from? How is it collected? What services and what groups of people are covered?

As discussed in the previous two chapters, Canada does not have a single national healthcare system, but rather has ten provincial, three territorial, and federal systems (the federal system provides care to certain Aboriginal groups, the RCMP, the armed forces, etc.) — all operating under the same founding principles and guidelines. Thus, although every province autonomously makes its own health finance decisions, there are certain generalities that apply to all.

1.1. SOURCES OF FINANCING

The public and private sectors both finance Canada's health system (see Figure 14.1). Health expenditures by government and government agencies (i.e., the public sector) are financed by three levels of government — the federal, provincial and territorial, and municipal levels — and by workers' compensation boards and other social security schemes. Private sector expenditure has three distinct components:

Figure 14.1.   **Funding Structure of the Health System in Canada**

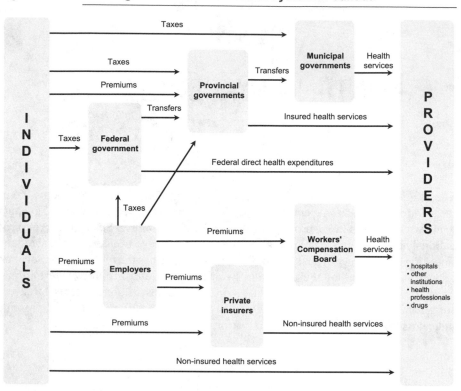

Source: Adapted from National Forum on Health. *The public and private financing of Canada's health system: A discussion paper.* Ottawa, 1995.

household out-of-pocket expenditure, private insurance expenditure, and non-consumption expenditure (1).

Money for financing is raised predominantly through provincial and federal taxes and is allocated, for the most part, from general provincial revenues. According to the *Canada Health Act,* each provincial health plan must cover all "medically necessary" health services delivered in hospital and by physicians. Provinces can choose to provide additional services, as described in Chapter 13. Personal expenditures include dental and other services, such as those delivered by alternative healthcare providers not covered by government insurance and payments for extra services such as private hospital rooms. Some provinces have recently shifted costs to the private sector for rehabilitative care as a result of motor vehicle collisions by charging personal automobile insurance policies for these fees. Non-insured health services and fees are covered either by private health insurance (voluntarily purchased on an individual basis or offered by an employee plan) or by the individuals. Treatment for work-related injuries and disease can be covered through the workers' compensation funds.

Table 14.1.   Distribution of Public Sector Healthcare Financing

Year	Provincial Government %	Federal Direct %	Municipal Government %	Social Security Funds %	Total Public Sector %	Private Sector %
1975	71.4	3.3	0.6	1.0	76.2	23.8
1999	64.9	3.8	0.9	1.2	70.8	29.2

Source: Canadian Institute for Health Information. *National health expenditure trends, 1975–2001.* Ottawa: Canadian Institute for Health Research, 2001.

Public sector revenue includes federal, provincial or territorial, and municipal government revenue generated from general taxes and borrowing as well as funds from social security funds such as workers' compensation funds and the Quebec Drug Insurance Fund. The individual pays the remainder either directly or through private health insurance (see Table 14.1). Public sector funding is much higher (70.8%) in Canada than in the United States (just under half of total at 45.7%) but, according to the Organisation for Economic Co-operation and Development (OECD), it is lower than some other developed nations where the average is 75%. Figures indicate that the public sector funding for health care in Canada has declined since 1983, when the total public sector share of health expenditures was 76.6%. The private share of healthcare expenditure has increased from 23.4% in 1983 to 29.2% in 2000 and is expected to increase slightly to 29.3% in 2002 (2).

In Canada, the bulk of total healthcare expenditures (64.9%) is financed from general revenue by provincial governments. Provincial government expenditure as a proportion of total expenditure gradually fell from 71.4% in 1995 to 64.9% in 1999. National health expenditures are based on the principle of responsibility for payment rather than the source of funds. Federal government transfers are therefore included in the provincial government sector. The federal government contributes to provincial revenue in the form of transfer payments, which are tax credits, and cash as agreed under the *Canada Health and Social Transfer Act* (see Chapter 12). Additionally, the federal government pays directly for 5.3% of the public sector expenditure on health care.

The provinces generate their share of the revenue for the health expenditures as follows (3).

- The public pays 72.5% of healthcare costs in the form of taxes.
- Only Alberta and British Columbia charge individual premiums to those who request medicare benefits; Alberta earmarks money from the premiums for health care.
- Quebec, Manitoba, and Newfoundland and Labrador levy payroll taxes on employers: Quebec charges a flat rate of 3.75% of every employer's payroll; Manitoba charges 2.25%; Newfoundland and Labrador charges 1.5%, with smaller employers exempted. Payroll taxes tend to be controversial as they do not spread the net as wide, and the

Table 14.2.   Provincial and Territorial Health Expenditures, 1999

Province	Population estimates, 1999*	Expenditure ($ 000,000)**	Total expenditure per capita*	Total health expenditure as a percent of GDP*	Public sector as a percent of total*	Life expectancy at birth, 1999
Newfoundland and Labrador	541,000	1,570	2,903	12.7	79.6	77.7
Prince Edward Island	138,000	373	2,712	12.0	69.3	78.4
Nova Scotia	940,000	2,749	2,926	12.0	71.5	78.7
New Brunswick	754,000	2,063	2,735	11.0	71.2	78.4
Quebec	7,350,000	19,915	2,710	9.5	72.4	78.5
Ontario	11,523,000	34,902	3,029	8.6	67.1	79.3
Manitoba	1,142,000	3,661	3,205	11.5	74.5	78.0
Saskatchewan	1,026,000	2,981	2,907	9.9	76.7	78.5
Alberta	2,960,000	8,630	2,916	7.4	71.5	79.2
British Columbia	4,028,000	12,231	3,036	10.1	73.4	80.0
Yukon	31,000	108	3,466	9.7	84.7	77.45
Northwest Territories	41,000	232	5,664	11.0	91.2	75.6
Nunavut	27,000	131	4,873	15.6	93.9	68.95
Canada	30,500,000	89,547	2,936	9.2	70.8	79.0

* Based on estimates form Demography Division, Statistics Canada (the figures have been rounded off).
** *Provincial and Territorial Government Health Expenditures Estimates, 1974/1975 to 2001/2002* Canadian Institute for Health Information published January 2002:32.

self-employed escape the tax altogether. Overall, however, payroll taxes do not generate a significant portion of health revenues and have recently been discontinued in Ontario.

In the past decade, premiums and payroll taxes have only paid for about one tenth of health spending in Alberta and British Columbia and one quarter in Quebec. General revenue is the predominant funding resource available for health care.

2. HEALTH EXPENDITURES

2.1. OVERALL EXPENDITURES

In 1999, Canada spent 9.2% of GDP, or $89.5 billion, on health care; that amount is estimated to be 9.8% of GDP, or $112.2 billion, in 2002 (1, 2). This figure is down slightly from its high point of 9.9% reached in 1992. This translates to $2,936 per person spent on health care. Table 14.2 summarizes recent levels of health expenditures throughout Canada. The total health expenditures per capita varies due to a variety of different factors, including age distribution, population density, geography, population health needs, and the organization and financing of healthcare delivery. The health expenditure per capita is highest in the territories because of their large geographical area and low population density. After adjusting for inflation, provincial and territorial government health expenditure grew at 6.6% in 1999–2000 and is expected to have increased by an additional 6.2% in 2000–01, and 6.4% in 2001–02 (4).

2.2. TRENDS IN HEALTH EXPENDITURES

Table 14.3 shows that after many years of steady increases, the percent of GDP spent on health care in Canada declined in the mid 1990s and is now slowly regaining its previous position. In 1999, Canada spent 9.2% of its GDP on health care, an increase from the 1996 level of 8.9% but lower than the 1992 level of 9.9%. The first significant rise was in the late 1960s, following the introduction of universal health insurance. By the early 1970s, the federal and provincial governments became alarmed by this rapid rise and set up a task force on the cost of health services, which delivered its report in 1970. Attempts to control the level of health expenditure met with temporary success in the 1970s. The proportion of GDP declined initially and then levelled off to 6.8% in 1979, although both the actual dollars and per capita dollars spent had risen. Since 1980, it has been rising again.

2.3. SUSTAINABILITY IN HEALTH CARE

In late 1980s and early 1990s, most experts believed that the fundamental financial problems in Canada's healthcare system were due neither to under funding nor to overspending, but rather to poorly distributed and misdirected spending and ineffectively managed resources (5-7). However, after the recession from 1990 to 1992, governments

Table 14.3.   Trends in Health Expenditures in Canada, 1975–1999

	1975	1980	1990	1992	1996	1999
Total health Expenditure (millions of dollars)*	12,200	22,308	61,047	69,764	74,689	89,546
Per capita expenditure (dollars)*	527	910	2,203	2,458	2,517	2,936
Percent of GDP	7.0	7.1	9.0	9.9	8.9	9.2

*(in current dollars)
Source: Canadian Institute for Health Information. *National Health Expenditure Trends, 1975-2001*. Ottawa: Canadian Institute for Health Information, 2001.

introduced fiscal restraint measures that affected public spending on health and social programs. Between 1975 and 1991, the average annual rate of growth in health expenditures by governments and government agencies was 11.0% (1). That growth fell to 0.5% from 1992 to 1996, with virtually no growth in 1995 and 1996. By 1997, public spending on health had increased by 4.2%. The ability to fund health programs had become a focal point for policy debates about provincial and territorial health spending in the 1990s. The debates have often focused on the relative importance of provincial revenues and federal transfers in funding the healthcare system (4).

Because the CHST feeds directly into provincial budgets and allows each province to allocate whatever proportion it deems necessary for health, Health Canada and Statistics Canada no longer report statistics on proportions of provincial health expenditures financed through federal transfers. The provincial governments claimed that the federal contribution had gone down substantially and received only small portions of health care cost; on the other hand the federal government claimed that they were paying their fair share but it was more from transfer of tax point than from cash contribution (8).

2.4.   THE FEDERAL GOVERNMENT'S RESPONSE

Thanks to an improved economy, a balanced budget, and public outcry, the 1999 federal budget allocated an additional $11.5 billion in cash payments ($2 billion each for fiscal years 1999–2000 and 2000–2001and $2.5 billion for the remaining three fiscal years) to the provinces on an equal per capita basis over five years, designated specifically for health care. At the same time, the federal government allocated $1.4 billion over four years for investment in health information, research, and prevention. The 2000 federal budget announced an additional $2.5 billion over four years to fund post-secondary education and health care. Furthermore, the health accord signed by the federal and provincial governments in 2000 further supplemented the CHST by gradually adding annual increases that will increase the transfer from $15.5 billion in 2000–01 to $21 billion by 2005–06 (9). The accord added an additional $2.3 billion in transfers from the federal government over five years beyond the CHST mechanism for health information technology, the Medical Equipment Fund, and the Health Transition Fund for Primary Care.

Recent federal reports had recommended enlarging the federal contribution to health care (10, 11). The federal government responded in 2003 by committing to provide $34.8 billion over five years (12). In that period, the Health Reform Fund will target $16 billion to primary health care, home care, and catastrophic drug coverage; $2.5 billion from the CHST will relieve existing pressures; the Diagnostic/Medical Equipment Fund will spend $1.5 billion to improve access to publicly funded diagnostic services; $600 million is committed to develop electronic health records; and $500 million is allocated to the Canada Foundation for Innovation (12) (see Chapter 18).

The 2003 Health Care Renewal Accord also promises to establish a new long-term Canada Health Transfer (CHT) by 2004, which will include the portion of the current CHST (both cash and tax points) that corresponds to the current proportion of health expenditures in provincial social spending supported by this federal transfer (12). The CHT will facilitate predictable annual increases in health transfers, thus accomplishing the federal government's goals of sustainability and accountability.

2.5. INTERNATIONAL COMPARISONS

Table 14.4 compares the percentage of GDP spent by selected countries on health care. Caution should be taken when making cross-country comparisons as countries include different types of expenditures when calculating total health expenditures (13). For example, Germany excludes expenditures for health research, military health, and prison health, as well as private household expenditures on patient transport and patient care when calculating its total health expenditure, whereas these expenditures are included in the Canadian determination. The trend indicates that the percentage spent increased until 1992, when it stabilized and began slowly decreasing. In 1999, based on OECD estimates, Canada spent 9.2% of its GDP on health care, the United Kingdom spent 7.1%, and the United States spent 13.0%.

Many other factors contribute to these international variations in healthcare expenditures. As described in Chapter 12, healthcare systems differ widely in their sources of funding, including the balance of private and public funding. They also vary in the degree and form of state planning, the remuneration of healthcare professionals (particularly physicians), and the nature of services provided. Thus, international comparisons are of questionable significance: they tell us *what* nations spent, but little, if anything, about *how* they spent it — the mix of services, possible duplication of facilities, physician-to-population ratios, healthcare needs, or system inefficiencies. There is no evidence that Americans, for example, are healthier because their country spends a higher share of GDP on health care.

Table 14.4.   International Comparison of Total Health Expenditures as a
Percentage of Gross Domestic Product

Country	1975	1980	1990	1995	1996	1997	1998	1999
Australia	7.0	7.0	7.9	8.2	8.3	8.3	8.6	8.5
Canada	7.1	7.1	9.0	9.3	9.1	9.0	9.3	9.2
France	6.8	7.4	8.6	9.6	9.5	9.4	9.3	9.4
Germany	8.8	8.8	8.7	10.2	10.6	10.5	10.3	10.3
Japan	5.6	6.5	6.1	7.2	7.1	7.4	7.5	7.4
United Kingdom	5.5	5.6	6.0	6.9	7.0	6.7	6.8	7.1
United States	7.8	8.7	11.9	13.2	13.2	13.0	12.9	13.0

Source: Organization for Economic Co-operation and Development. *OECD Health Data 2002: A comparative analysis of 30 countries*. Paris, 2002. December 2002 update. CD-ROM. (Figures reported by the Canadian Institute for Health Information differ slightly for Canada from those reported in the *OECD Health Data 2001*.)

One significant difference, however, between the healthcare system in the U.S. and in Canada is the administrative cost. In the U.S., which has voluntary medical and hospital insurance systems, 12.5% of spending goes to administrative overhead, whereas Canadian administrative costs are less than 3%. Furthermore, there are savings in Canadian hospital administrative costs because there is no need to list the price of every service, bandage, and pill on the patient's bill. The savings in accounting, nurses' time, and paperwork are large.

Moreover, there are savings in the more rational distribution of high technology such as MRI scanners, which U.S. hospitals acquire for competitive reasons and then frequently under-utilize. The Canadian single-payer system — the provincial government — pays for hospital and physicians, covering 70.8% (1999) of the total cost of health care in Canada. Provincial governments are directly responsible for the overall allocation and coordination of resources to the health services sector. This avoids the fragmentation of decision making and wasteful competition for resources that can occur when independent non-profit or fee-for-service providers seek financing from a variety of private and public sources. Although Canadians are faced with their own set of health system challenges, the single-payer financing system, together with universal coverage for all Canadians, has proven more effective than the U.S. market system of health in controlling overall health expenditures but less effective than the systems in some European countries (14).

3.   CATEGORIES OF HEALTH EXPENDITURES

The Canadian Institute for Health Information (CIHI) uses the following categories of health expenditures:

- hospitals;
- other institutions, including residential care types of facilities;
- physicians;
- other professionals, which includes expenditures for the services of privately practicing healthcare professionals, and which is divided into the following sub-categories:
  - dental services;
  - vision care services;
  - other, which includes chiropractors, massage therapists, orthoptists, osteopaths, physiotherapists, podiatrists, psychologists, private duty nurses, and naturopaths;
- drugs, further divided into the following sub-categories:
  - prescribed drugs;
  - non-prescribed drugs, including over-the-counter drugs and personal health supplies but not drugs dispensed in hospitals and most other institutions;
- capital, which includes expenditure on construction, capital equipment purchases for hospitals, and other health-related institutions;
- public health and administration; and
- other health-related spending, which includes expenditures on home care, medical transportation, hearing aids, other appliances and prostheses, prepayment administration, health research and miscellaneous health care, and is divided into the following sub-categories:
  - prepayment administration;
  - health research; and
  - other.

Table 14.5 summarizes the percentage distribution of total health expenditures by category of expenditure for 1999. The largest category of spending is hospitals, at 31.9%, followed by physicians and other professionals, who in total account for 25.7% of the total health expenditure (1).

3.1.   INSTITUTIONAL EXPENDITURES

Of the $37 billion (41.2% of total) spent on institutional care in 1999, $28.5 billion (31.9%) was spent on hospitals and $8.5 billion (9.5%) was spent on other institutions and allied special hospitals. For more than a decade, Canada's inpatient hospital sector has been shrinking. Fewer patients are hospitalized overnight each year, and those who are admitted stay, on average, for shorter periods.

On average, the per diem cost in acute care hospitals is usually two to three times higher than that in chronic or long-term care hospitals.

Table 14.5.   Distribution of Health Expenditures by Category of Expenditures, 1999

Category	%
Hospitals	31.9
Other institutions	9.5
Physicians	13.6
Other professionals	12.1
Drugs	14.9
Capital	3.3
Public health administration	6.1
Other health spending	8.5

Source: Canadian Institute for Health Information. *National health expenditure trends, 1975-2001*. Ottawa: Canadian Institute for Health Information, 2001: 84-85.

Almost all the funding for Canada's hospitals comes from provincial governments. The cost of running a hospital has risen roughly 8% per year over the past decade, although this rate of increase has significantly slowed since 1991. Due to increasing pressures across the country to control healthcare costs, public hospitals indicate negative (–2.4%) average annual growth in operating expenses since 1991–92. This has been largely due to hospital downsizing, restructuring, and re-engineering.

Wages, salaries, and benefits account for almost three quarters of the operating budgets of public hospitals, with 45% of this budgetary portion paying nurses. Canada has more than 231,512 working registered nurses (RNs). General duty RNs earn between $37,693 and $58,968 per year. Hospitals employ approximately 63% of the registered nurses (15).

Several factors have led to the increased costs:
- binding arbitration of unsettled labour disputes;
- increases in workers' compensation assessments, payroll health taxes, employment insurance, and Canada Pension Plan payments;
- new laws on environmental protection, pay equity, and occupational health and safety;
- new technology, drugs, and treatment methods (hospital drug costs alone have risen 10% to 14% per year);
- the cost of other supplies and services, which has risen faster than government financing; and
- more severe diseases treated as in-patients than before.

3.2.   INSTITUTIONAL RESOURCES

As already stated, the most expensive health resources are health-related institutions, because they rely heavily on technology and human resources. In 1999, some 512,000 people worked in hospitals across Canada (16). Statistics Canada classifies hospitals according to the services they provide, as follows.

- General hospitals provide acute care in the community, and may have units for long-term care. If a general hospital is affiliated with a university, it is called a teaching hospital.
- Allied special hospitals provide chronic care, such as rehabilitation or extended care, or deal with special age groups (e.g., pediatrics) or specific conditions (e.g., cancer);
- Minimal care or nursing homes are organized residential facilities where some residents receive nursing care from full-time registered or licensed practical nurses, medications are supervised, and assistance is provided for three or more activities of daily living (e.g., bathing, dressing, walking, eating).
- Mental institutions include mental hospitals dealing with chronic long-term mental illness, psychiatric hospitals, and psychiatric units in general hospitals dealing with short-term intensive psychiatric treatment, and special facilities for people who are emotionally or mentally challenged.

According to Statistics Canada, there has been a marked decline in the number of hospitals and hospital beds throughout Canada. In 1999, hospitals accounted for 31.9% of all healthcare expenditures in Canada, compared with 44.7% in 1975. In 2000–01, Canada had more than 569 general and allied hospitals, with 98,132 approved beds. In the previous five years, more than 275 hospitals closed, merged, or were converted to another type of facility. Since 1984–85, the number of approved hospital beds has decreased almost 40% and the number of hospital day programs has increased almost 100%. Researchers continue to monitor and evaluate the impact of hospital closures and health system reform on the health of Canadians (16, 17). In 2000–01, there were 2,227 beds for rehabilitation, 5,879 for extended care (patients with long-term beds), and 24 separate long-term psychiatric hospitals with 9,565 beds.

Public hospitals accounted for 92% of all hospitals and 98% of the beds (18). Of the public hospitals, 73% of the approved beds were in general hospitals, 10% were in extended care hospitals, and the rest were distributed among psychiatric, pediatric, and rehabilitation hospitals.

Although there is no standard definition of a long-term care centre in Canada, it usually includes homes for special care, nursing homes, homes for the aged, and community care facilities. Most general and chronic hospitals and the majority of nursing homes are publicly owned, and most mental institutions are owned by provincial governments.

For every 1,000 Canadians in 2000–01, there were 3.9 beds in institutions (3.3 beds for short-term care or shared short-/long-term care beds, and 0.3 beds exclusively for long-term care).

Interprovincial variations exist within each category, due mainly to the fact that the population is widely dispersed rather than to different morbidity patterns in the population. For mental institutions, the bed capacity in 2000–01 for Canada was 0.3 per 1,000 persons. The de-institutionalization of mental patients, which means a shift to community-based living, has resulted in a decline in bed capacity.

For special care facilities, the bed capacity was 8.6 per 1,000 population in Canada in 1993. In addition to providing care for people with special needs, these include nursing homes, and facilities with a minimum of four beds that provide nursing, custodial, or counselling services but not active treatment. Capacity rates vary widely among the provinces, from 11.9 beds per 1,000 population in Saskatchewan and 16.9 in Prince Edward Island to 5.4 in Quebec. Newfoundland, Yukon, and the Northwest Territories all have rates below the Canadian average, possibly because of the age structures of their population.

3.2.1.   Utilization of Institutional Resources

Canadians spent almost 21 million days as inpatients in acute care hospitals in 1999–2000, down 15.6% from 1994–95 (19). The average length of hospital stay for 2000–01 was 7.2 days. The average length of stay for hospital care was the shortest in Nunavut (3.3 days), while Manitoba had the longest average length of stay (9.5 days). Although provincial variations continue to exist, due to increasing pressures to use hospital resources more efficiently, the length of stay for inpatient care continues to decrease. By 1995, Ontario, for example, reached an average length of stay of 9.7 days for all types of care, with an average of 3.1 days if acute care cases only are considered. In 2000–01, the average length of stay in hospitals in Ontario was 6.5 days. The average length of stay for long-term care hospitalization (153 days) is much higher than for acute care, but this too shows the same decreasing trends.

Hospital separation rates per 1,000 population ("separations" include discharges plus deaths) are another indication of hospital utilization. These rates also varied among the provinces. In 2000–01, the national rate was 94 per 1,000. There was a definite downward trend in hospital separations per 1,000 population from 1974 through 1993 to 2000 (from 165 to 128 to 94). More than 9 million patient days were spent caring for people in psychiatric and general hospitals in 1999–2000, but many of these patient days were attributed to people with a very long duration of stay. Admission rates per 10,000 population for 1998–99 nationally was 62.0 with the highest admission rate in the Northwest Territories (116.5) and the lowest rate in Nova Scotia (51.3).

3.2.2.   Optimizing the Use of Institutional Resources

In recent years, a number of strategies have been employed to optimize the use of institutional resources that consume the largest proportion of health dollars.

Rationalization

The rationalization of health services may involve restructuring, realignment, downsizing, decentralization, and some institutional closures. These attempt to minimize the duplication of services, provide appropriate levels and types of care, consolidate strengths, and create innovative structures and functional arrangements that make better use of resources and contain costs. Many analysts maintain that the central problem of health services in Canada is that hospitals and other medical institutions have acted in the interests of the healthcare providers instead of the communities they serve.

Rationalization usually involves major transformations of the healthcare system. As described in Chapter 13, it has occurred in every province except for Ontario. Alberta provides a particularly good example for rationalization in the healthcare system. In 1993, the province released its first recommendations leading to health reform and regionalization (20). The key recommendation was to establish regional structures. Regional Health Authorities (RHAs) were established in Alberta in the following year, with the goal of ensuring a wellness-based, integrated, accessible, appropriate, and affordable health system.

An additional key component of system rationalization, especially in the transitional period, is the ongoing monitoring and evaluation of health system effects on the population. A survey of the Alberta general public indicated that 88% were very or somewhat satisfied with the healthcare services they received in 2001 (19).

Funding of Acute Care Hospitals

Approximately one third (34.2%) of all health expenditures in Canada relate to acute hospital care. Modes of hospital funding differ in different provinces and are described in Chapter 15. Although the implementation of global budgeting for funding acute care hospitals had some effect in controlling the costs in Canada in the 1970s and 1980s, it has been recommended that hospitals be funded on a case-mix basis — that is, by the type and severity of diseases treated at the hospital. This is similar to the concept of Diagnostic Related Groups (DRGs), which gained prominence in the 1980s in the U.S.: hospitals were reimbursed for the intensity of care needed according to the severity classification of illness. However, hospitals tended to classify patients into more severe diagnostic categories in order to gain more reimbursement (often referred to as "DRG creep") and cost containment could not be achieved. With regionalization, population-based funding method is becoming popular.

Ambulatory Care, Day Care, and Extended Care

The original federal-provincial funding arrangements specified in the *Hospital Insurance and Diagnostic Services Act of 1957* encouraged expansion and utilization of acute care hospitals, for which federal funds were provided. Ambulatory care, day care, day surgery, health centres, rehabilitation services, extended care facilities, and home care each cost less than acute care hospitals but their costs were not shared with the federal government. This imbalance was addressed by Established Programs Financing (EPF) in 1977 and the *Canada Health and Social Transfer Act* (CHST), which replaced EPF in 1996. EPF included a per capita grant for extended health care, designed to cover nursing homes and ambulatory care; the CHST allows provinces to make this funding decision on their own. The flexibility of the two funding formulas permits provinces to develop these services in anticipation of the growing needs associated with the aging society in Canada. Consequently, spending has shifted toward extended health care. According to Health Canada, the total federal cash contribution to extended health care increased from $20 per capita in 1977–78 to $51.21 per capita in 1995–96; for public health services, it increased from 3.6% of total health care cash transfers in 1975 to 5.0% in 1996.

Pre-admission and Discharge Planning

Hospital stays for surgery or for elective procedures can be shortened by outpatient laboratory tests and other work-up conducted prior to admission. After-care in a stepped-down environment where the patient is provided with less intense care and preparation-for-discharge care is effective in reducing hospital costs.

Home Care

Home care makes institutional beds available for acute care and costs considerably less than hospital care. Some researchers claim that home care of the elderly can result in savings of up to 75% of the costs of equivalent care in a hospital (21). The elderly are better able to adapt to a disability in their own home, and homecare patients tend to comply more readily with treatment requirements. Home care also results in psychological benefits experienced by the patient and his or her family. Furthermore, patients who are treated in hospitals often experience confusion, disorientation, anxiety, and personality conflicts, all of which can hinder healing. A homecare program can also be tailored to an individual's particular needs and home (see Chapter 15).

All provincial and territorial governments fund some homecare services, but what is covered varies throughout the country as this falls outside the scope of the *Canada Health Act*. In 1998–99, Canadian governments spent just under $3 billion on home care, up significantly over the last decade. Total provincial homecare spending increased by more than 350% between 1988–89 and 1998–99. With the downsizing, closure, and merger of acute hospitals, patients are discharged home much earlier. This has created pressure on home care and has shifted health care costs to consumers.

Homecare reformers are thus faced with two opposing trends. On the one hand, with decreasing lengths of stay in hospitals and increasing pressure to push care into the community and home, away from institutional care, ever increasing numbers of patients require care in the home. On the other hand, as fiscal constraints tighten, provinces may continue to de-list services such as home care that are not strictly required by the *Canada Health Act*. Recent federal reports have recommended post-acute home care and palliative home care to be covered under the *Canada Health Act* (10, 11). The 2003 Health Care Renewal Accord recognized home care as one of the priority area to receive substantial funding (12).

3.3.   HUMAN HEALTH RESOURCES EXPENDITURES

The largest components of human health resources are nursing and the expenditure figures for them are subsumed under institutional expenditure as the majority of them are on salaried positions. In 1999, the expenditure for professional services by physicians, dentists, and other specialists amounted to about $23 billion (25.7% of total spending); this does not include professionals employed by institutions, such as nurses, physiotherapists, occupational therapists, social workers, and some physicians. Of that figure, physicians' services alone constituted approximately 52.9%, amounting to $12.2 billion (1). In 1972, physicians' services totalled $0.6 billion. Relatively high fee increases in some provinces, especially in British Columbia, Ontario, and Alberta in the early 1980s, caused significant changes in these figures. Physicians now receive about 13.6¢ of every healthcare dollar in the form of fees; however, how they decide to treat patients significantly influences how the rest of that dollar is spent. For example, it is estimated that every doctor in Ontario costs the system about $500,000, one half in direct billings and the other half in drugs prescribed, laboratory tests ordered, and hospital admissions authorized.

In 2000, there were more than 57,800 physicians in clinical practice across Canada (19). In 1998–99, the average payment per full-time fee-for-service physician in Canada was $244,135 (22). According to CIHI 2000–01 estimates, about 11% of the total clinical payments to physicians in the 10 provinces comes from some alternative form of payment (other than fee for service). Most doctors in private practice are paid on a fee-for-service basis, although the percentage varies across Canada. In Alberta, 98% of doctors are paid only on a fee-for-service basis compared to a low of 40% in Manitoba (19). Government employees, community health centre staff, and most of the interns and residents in hospitals are salaried doctors.

Slightly less than 12.1¢ of each healthcare dollar is spent on the services of dentists and other healthcare professionals such as chiropractors, optometrists, and physiotherapists.

3.3.1 Human Health Resources

Human health resources consist of those individuals who provide direct healthcare services (such as nurses, physicians, dentists, chiropractors, respiratory technicians, and alternative healthcare providers), and those who provide ancillary and support services (such as maintenance and repair, housekeeping, food services, and administrative services).

About 1 in 10 employed Canadians work in health and social services (19). It is estimated that 827,700 persons were employed in health occupations in 2000. This represents a 13.7% increase over a 10-year period. About 65% of those directly provide health services, and 35% are in ancillary jobs. Health human resources emerged as the number one issue from an extensive consultation process with health experts in 2001 (23).

3.3.2. Trends in Human Health Resources

The most up-to-date data on healthcare personnel in Canada are kept on 20 health occupations providing direct health services to Canadians (24). According to CIHI, about 536,900 individuals provided direct health services to Canadians in 2000, an increase of 5.6% from 1991. Of these, 43.3% (232,412) are Registered Nurses (RNs), 13.6% (72,905) are Licensed Practical Nurses (LPNs), 10.8% (57,803) are physicians, 4.6% (24,518) are pharmacists, and 3.9% (21,061) are dentists. Table 14.6 shows number

Table 14.6.   Number and Ratio of Active Health Human Resources, 2000

Health Occupation	Total	Ratio to Population	Ratio in 1976
Chiropractors	5,633	1 : 5,468	1 : 13,623
Dentists	17,287	1 : 1,786	1 : 2,463
Dental hygenists	14,525	1 : 2,073	1 : 11,962
Dieticians and nutritionists	6,892	1 : 4,499	1 : 8,726
Health records administrators	1,119	1 : 27,599	1 : 11,269
Health services executives	2,716	1 : 11,367	1 : 19,331
Midwives*	355	-	-
Nursing:			
Registered	232,412	1 : 133	1 : 168
Licensed nursing assistant	72,905	1 : 423	1 : 323
Occupational therapists	9,485	1 : 3,255	1 : 15,388
Optometrists	3,780	1 : 8,149	1 : 13,128
Pharmacists	24,518	1 : 1,259	1 : 1,658
Physicians	64,454	1 : 478	1 : 557
Physiotherapists	15,640	1 : 1,967	1 : 16,449
Psychologists	13,226	1 : 2,334	N/A
Social workers	17,874	1:1,727	N/A
Technologists:			
Laboratory	17,723	1 : 1,742	1 : 1,415
Radiation	14,499	1 : 2,122	1 : 2,890
Respiratory	6,204	1 : 4,976	1 : 17,692

* Only licensed in four provinces. N/A: Not available.
Source: Canadian Institute for Health Information. *Health personnel in Canada, 1991-2000*. Ottawa: Canadian Institute for Health Information, 2002. <www.cihi.ca> (November 2002).

and ratio of health professionals to Canadians for 2000. Since 1991, the number of RNs employed in nursing in Canada remained relatively unchanged, decreasing 0.6% to a total in 2000 of 232,412. There was a 2.9% reduction of LPNs (including nursing assistants in some areas of Canada) from 1995 to 1996. In 2000, there were approximately 10,000 fewer LPNs in Canada than in 1991, a reduction of 13.1%. Since World War II, the traditional healthcare professions of physicians, nurses, and dentists have expanded to include some 32 regulated health professions and more than 150 categories of healthcare occupations (see Chapter 16). Most are extensions of established healthcare professions (e.g., nursing assistants, LPNs, technicians, nurse practitioners, dental hygienists, dental technicians). Others have developed from some special body of knowledge (e.g., clinical psychologists). As these new occupations evolve, many of their practitioners try to achieve independent status as self-regulatory professions. Most provincial governments now regulate and license a number of the health professions (see Chapter 16).

Human health resources are unevenly distributed and mainly concentrated in large urban centres and in wealthy provinces such as Ontario, Quebec, and British Columbia. Over the past few decades, they have significantly increased in number, thus reducing their ratio to the population in most categories This trend is now reversed as is the case with physicians and LPNs (19). The two largest categories of health professionals are described below.

3.3.3. Nurses

Nursing is the largest health profession and accounts for more than half of all healthcare providers in Canada. There are three regulated nursing groups: Registered Nurses (RNs), Licensed Practical Nurses (LPNs), and Registered Psychiatric Nurses (RPNs). In 2000, 232,412 RNs were employed in nursing across the country. On average there were 754 RNs per 100,000 Canadian. But this ratio varies across the country, with a high of 1,027 RNs per 100,000 in the Northwest Territories and a low of 333 in Nunavut.

Most RNs work in hospitals, although the number employed in community health is gradually increasing. Information about LPNs and RPNs is more limited. However, in 2000 there were 72,905 LPNs and 5,000 RPNs working in Canada. RPNs are licensed only in British Columbia, Alberta, Saskatchewan, and Manitoba (25).

3.3.4. Physicians

After nursing, medicine represents the second largest regulated healthcare profession. In 2000, there were more than 57,800 physicians in clinical and non-clinical practice in Canada. The total number of active civilian physicians in Canada increased from 52,726 in 1991 to 57,800 in 2000, an increase of 9.6% (24). During this period, the number of specialist grew more (7.4%) than did the number of family doctors (3.2%). Growth patterns differed across the country. Between 1996 and 2000, Alberta is estimated to have had the largest growth (12.2%) in the total number of physicians. There was also substantial growth in Nova Scotia (8.8%), Saskatchewan (6.5%), British Columbia (5.9%), and Manitoba (5.8%). In Ontario, Quebec, New Brunswick, and Prince Edward Island, the increases were smaller. And, although physician numbers were stable in Newfoundland and Labrador, they fell by 12.8% in the Yukon and by 11.4% in the Northwest Territories and Nunavut (25). Since 2000, specialists have accounted for just under half of all physicians (49.6%). The physician-to-population ratio in 2000 was 1 to 534; according to the World Health Organization, the optimum ratio is 1 to 655. The physician-to-population ratio varies across Canada with a ratio of 1 to 1,298 in the Northwest Territories and a ratio of 1 to 468 in Quebec (24).

3.3.5.   Utilization of Physician Services

The most detailed information is available for physicians because physicians are generally paid directly through provincial health insurance per item. Physicians represent the third largest category of total health expenditures in 1999 at $12.2 billion, representing 13.6% of the total health expenditures or $399 per capita. In 1998–99, 81% of the Canadian population aged 12 and older reported contact in the 12 previous months with a physician (25). Expenditures for physicians' services grew at above average rates through the mid 1980s, and peaked at 15.7% of total expenditure in 1987. Expenditure grew at below average rates during the 1990s, leading to a decline in the share of total expenditure. Since 1975, the public sector expenditure on physicians has remained above 98% of total physician expenditure. Households account for almost all private spending for physician services. Insurance of supplementary charges to patients for medically necessary services was discouraged prior to the *Canada Health Act*, and such charges are not permitted under the Act. The category of other professionals accounted for $10.9 billion, or 12.1% of total expenditures, in 1999 and remains the highest percentage of private spending of all major expenditure categories. The private share declined until 1981, reaching a low of 81.7% and gradually increased to almost 90% in 1999. This category includes dentist and denturists, optometrists and opticians, chiropractors, physiotherapists, and private duty nurses. More than 60% of expenditure for other professionals is for dental care (1). The per capita costs for physician and other professional services have steadily increased since 1975.

Ontario's physician billing data according to the Ontario Health Insurance Plan (OHIP) illustrate some of the factors that result in rising expenditures. First, there was an overall increase in total physician billings from $1.06 billion in 1980–81 to $4.1 billion in 1994–95, Only $3.8 billion of this amount was actually paid to physicians due to government policies that clawed back earnings that exceeded a specified amount in any given year. Nevertheless, this figure amounts to a 258.1% increase in OHIP billings over 15 years (or an average increase of 10.1% annually). Part of the increase is due to physician factors, such as an increase in the number of physicians working in Ontario, while a smaller portion is due to an increase in the province's population. From 1980–81 to 1994–95, the number of physicians billing OHIP increased by 56.3% (or 3.3% annually). In that same period, the number of people living in Ontario increased by 25.1% (1.6% annually). However, it is important to remember that within the increase in Ontario's overall population, there was a 51.6% increase in the number of people age 65 and over — that group of people who require more frequent and more costly medical care. Thus, the combination of increased numbers of physicians (increased supply) and increased numbers of people, especially of the elderly (increased demand), has greatly increased utilization. One can speculate about the extent to which this increase is also caused by increased needs or expectations of the consumer versus physician-generated factors, such as extra recalls and procedures. Also of great importance is whether better health resulted from this increase.

3.3.6. Optimizing Human Health Resources: Physicians

There are a number of ways to optimize the work of human health resources and thereby decrease the cost and or improve the quality of care. As physicians are one of the larger components of health care and their services are publicly funded, attention has been paid to control their number and remuneration, which had emerged in the early 1990s as major issues of concern to provincial governments (27).

Supply of Physicians

During the late 1990s, there was a growing consensus that Canada was facing a physician shortage. As a result, most provinces increased medical school admissions and stepped up efforts to license international medical students. This perceived shortage was in sharp contrast to the perceived surplus of physicians earlier in the decade. In 1991, the Barer-Stoddard Report prepared for the Federal/Provincial/Territorial Conference of Deputy Ministers of Health on physician resource planning was released (5, 28-33). This report drew on the input and views of major stakeholders, and was based on the assumption that cost control in the healthcare system is intimately linked to the supply, mix, and distribution of physicians and their remuneration. Although physicians generate most healthcare costs either directly or indirectly, the public interest may not be met by this distribution of resources (34). The Barer-Stoddard Report recommended an immediate 10% reduction in the number of medical undergraduate students in Canadian universities. The deputy ministers agreed with this analysis. By 1993, a number of provinces had limited the number of medical students, enforcing compliance of graduates of foreign medical schools with visa requirements, and attempting to reduce physician-generated costs by reducing the number of physicians. The response of organized medicine was, in part, mixed. The Royal College of Physicians and Surgeons of Canada expressed concerns about the reduction in undergraduate medical students and the adjustment of specialty ratios; nonetheless, it recommended a moratorium on the recognition of new specialties. The implementation of the 10% reduction in medical school admissions has been blamed for the physician shortage of the late 1990s. However, one analyst concluded that "policy-makers need to monitor, on a regular basis, the impact of a broader range of policies which may affect physician supply and demand, when conducting physician human resource planning" (35). The key messages of this report indicated that

- the real physician-population ratio declined by 5.1% between 1993 and 2000;
- much of the decline can be traced to a sharp drop in Canadian postgraduates entering practice from 1994 to 2000, because of longer training requirements;
- other factors, such as fewer international medical graduates entering practice, increased retirements, migration abroad, and the 10% reduction in medical school enrollment in 1993;

Physician Remuneration

Several strategies relate to physicians' remuneration. Whether there is a surplus or shortage of physicians, lobbying efforts on the part of medical associations, the performance of the economy, and the public attitudes toward compensation of physicians, governments have responded by introducing different measures for remunerating physicians.

Two strategies to reduce the open-ended provincial spending on physicians is to cap individual incomes at a certain level (as occurred in Ontario in 1992) and to cap or limit overall provincial payments for medical fees. This latter strategy may be accompanied by utilization adjustment, or the deduction from physician payments for increases in the use of medical services beyond specified levels for a period. In some provinces, when physician billing exceeds the limits, the provincial government institutes a claw-back policy. In Ontario, organized medicine collaborated with government to limit billings and to impose penalties, and in British Columbia similar initiatives resulted in a protest from organized medicine and a number of doctors, particularly in the rural areas, withdrew their services temporarily.

Other recommendations include restricting the billing privileges and prorating payments for new physicians. Joint management committees of organized medicine and government have been struck in some provinces, principally in Ontario, where the Ontario Medical Association agreed to the limits on physicians' billings on condition that the association was recognized as the exclusive bargaining agent for physicians in the province. However, given that this is a contentious subject, there may be confrontations as well as partnership strategies to find solutions.

In addition to the costs related to the number of physicians, there is the issue of physician remuneration itself (36). This issue has become increasingly contentious in recent years. Physicians want to receive what they consider fair compensation for their services, which may lead to practices such as opting out, extra billing, or balanced billing. All involve a payment by the patient to the physician in addition to the amount paid by the provincial health plan. Under the *Canada Health Act*, provinces that allow extra billing are penalized financially, and by 1987 all provinces had banned the practice. However, questions of fair compensation remain. Recently, both Alberta and British Columbia allowed some form of private payment to physicians for the services which are not insured and are provided with the insured services — in British Columbia, it is in the form of extra billing, and in Alberta it is in the form of private diagnostic clinics (37). Both provinces discontinued these practices when the federal government, citing the terms of the *Canada Health Act*, took dollar-for-dollar deductions from those provinces' transfer payments for health. The issue of extra-billing may arise again; however, the CHST, which guaranteed a federal payment of $15.5 billion in 2000–01, maintains the federal government's influence over the fulfilment of the requirements of the Act by provincial health insurance programs.

It has also been argued that the present fee-for-service system does not adequately compensate preventive services and encourages rapid patient turnover, excessive patient recalls, and the performance of unnecessary procedures. Although a restructuring of fee schedules might correct this problem, those holding this view usually favour salaries for physicians as a better way to align services with patient needs. Another alternative is payment by capitation. Some combination of these mechanisms is also feasible and is used in the primary care reform model in Ontario and other jurisdictions.

A growing trend is to adopt a team approach to health care, particularly in ambulatory settings such as community health centres, with the effective utilization of nurses, dietitians, social workers, and other professionals. These professionals might provide primary care in their field of expertise or work as part of a more comprehensive approach to health care, particularly in its preventive aspects, than is now provided in many primary care settings. There have been alternative models recommended, such as the health services organization model or the health maintenance organization (HMO) model (see Chapter 15). Quality of care might be improved or services could be reduced, as has happened in some HMOs in the U.S. Clearly, for economic benefit to occur, these alternative approaches must reduce the need for, and use of, physicians' services, and not simply add to them. Alternative healthcare delivery models should explore the use of healthcare professionals other than physicians, such as using midwives for normal home and hospital deliveries.

Practice Guidelines

Today, when there is a constant explosion of scientific and clinical information, clinical guidelines are designed so that the evidence-based approaches to medical decision making are used. Guidelines are not enforced; rather, they are recommendations that may change professional norms, but they are explicit, so they can provide standards for optimum care and for evaluating the quality of care. Thus, they have the potential to enhance quality of care (38), cost containment, and more appropriate use of resources.

However, the existence of guidelines does not ensure their implementation. Some people see them as an intrusion into the professionalism of healthcare providers. If they are marketed effectively, guidelines can change behaviour. They also require practical assistance, such as the availability of alternative tests or procedures. For example, guidelines for the utilization of Caesarean sections were developed by the obstetric profession in Canada in response to major variations in rates different provinces for Caesarean sections in and vaginal birth after Caesarean section (VBAC). The rate of VBACs in Canada is now 35% and the rate of Caesarean sections is lower (19.2%) than previous average of 25%. This is considered a more appropriate utilization of surgery and likely contributes to cost containment.

Increasing public interest in the outcome of medical care, the need for cost containment, and the suspicion that some medical care may be unnecessary or inappropriate are all likely to result in a shift toward the supervision of quality of care and the identification of optimal practice patterns. It is considered that "sensible, flexible guidelines produced by the appropriate panels will help improve practice" (39). Recently, government and organized medicine have become interested in the cost-containment potential of guidelines. For example, the Institute for Clinical Evaluative Sciences (ICES) was established by Ontario's Ministry of Health and the Ontario Medical Association partly to undertake research into practice styles, that is, the individual characteristic approaches of physicians to investigating and managing problems based on factors other than rational scientific evidence.

3.4. DRUGS

Retail sales of prescribed and non-prescribed drugs together represent the second largest single category of health expenditures in 1999. The drug category does not include drugs dispensed in hospitals and generally in other institutions. In 1999, $13.3 billion was spent on drugs, an increase of 7.7% over 1998. The expenditure on drugs has increased more rapidly than total health expenditure. As a result, the share of total health expenditure allocated to drugs increased from a low of 8.4% in the late 1970s to 14.9% in 1999. Prescribed and non-prescribed drugs accounted for 11.3% and 3.6% of the total health expenditure respectively; within the total drug expenditures category, 75.8% of expenditure on drugs were for prescription drugs and the remaining 24.8% were for non-prescription drugs (which included over-the-counter drugs and personal health supplies). The public sector funds only prescribed drugs and accounts for 66.8% of the total expenditure on prescribed and non-prescribed drugs. Private sector funding accounts for 33.2% of the total expenditure and funds both prescribed and non-prescribed drugs. The share of prescribed drugs financed from private sources had increased steadily from 1992 to 1998, reaching 58.5%. In 1999, the share fell to 56.3% and in 2001 was expected to fall to 50.8%, thus reflecting an increased share of public sector financing (1). With the recent federal commitment of increasing financing to provinces for coverage of catastrophic drugs, it is anticipated that there will be a further rise in the share of public sector financing for drug expenditures.

Ninety percent of Canadians have insurance coverage for prescription drugs from one source or another (see Chapter 13). However, 10% of these individuals are underinsured (40).

Optimizing Drug Coverage

The Romanow Commission (11) supported the development of a national drug agency to evaluate and approve new prescription drugs, provide ongoing evaluation of existing drugs, negotiate and contain drug prices, and provide comprehensive, objective, and accurate information to healthcare providers and the public. The commission also recommended a review of drug patent protection to ensure an appropriate balance between protection of intellectual property, the need to contain costs, and to improve access on non-patented prescription drugs.

4. ENHANCING HEALTH SYSTEM PERFORMANCE

The ultimate aim of the health expenditures and resources utilization is to produce good health and quality of life. As seen in Chapter 3, indicators to measure health are a difficult task. The public demands accountability from governments, providers, and institutions. Hence it is important to assess the performance of the health care system using several indicators to account for accessibility, quality, safety, efficiency, and effectiveness of health care. As a matter of fact, recent accords between federal and provincial governments stipulate that health system reforms be monitored by using sets of agreed-upon indicators and providing annual reports to public (12, 41). This section describes a number of performance indicators and some of the proposed solutions within the healthcare system to enhance the performance.

4.1.   SELECTED HEALTH INDICATORS AND IMPROVEMENT OF DELIVERY

In recent years, CIHI, Statistics Canada, and various professional groups have developed a framework to measure the Health Indicators (see Chapter 3). This framework has four large categories: health status, the determinants of health, health system performance, and community and health system characteristics. The categories of health system performance includes acceptability, accessibility, appropriateness, competence, continuity, effectiveness, efficiency, and safety. The category of community and health system characteristics relevant to the discussion of health indicators are as follows: health expenditures; the number of doctors, nurses, and other health professionals; the number and types of available hospitals; the types of available specialized services such as coronary artery bypass graft or hip and knee replacement; and contact with health professionals, mental health professionals, dental professionals, and alternate healthcare providers (26).

The following section describes health system performance indicators. At present, indicators are being developed for acceptability, competence, and continuity. The data presented here are derived from CIHI information, which also provides individual provincial and regional data (42).

Accessibility

Accessibility is defined as the ability of patients to obtain care or service at the right place and the right time, based on need (see Chapter 3). The proxy indicators for accessibility are the proportion of the population that receives influenza immunization (65 years and over), Pap smears (women aged 18 to 69 years), screening mammography (women aged 50 to 69 years), and childhood immunization. Data for Canadian population for these indicators are described in Chapter 4. According to the Health Services Access Survey 2001, just under 4.3 million (18%) of Canadians who needed routine care, health information, or immediate care for minor health problems encountered a difficulty of some kind. About 1.4 million (23%) of those requiring specialist visits, non-emergency surgery, and diagnostic tests also encountered difficulties, with the most frequently cited reason being waiting time (43).

Optimizing Delivery Systems

There are many entry points into the healthcare system (see Figure 14.2). With provincial and private health insurance plans (which cover dental, drug, and private nursing), there are relatively few financial barriers at these entry points. The services of psychologists, social workers, dentists, denturists, and nurse practitioners in private practice are less commonly covered, making these entry points more costly to the consumer, if not to government budgets. Most people, however, receive their primary

Figure 14.2.   Points of Entry into the Healthcare System

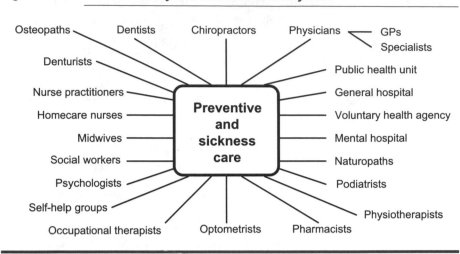

care through general or family practitioners and use specialized resources upon referral by those practitioners, who play a gatekeeper role.

It should be noted that the current healthcare system is heavily oriented to treating illness. At present in most provinces, regional health authorities are mandated to coordinate institutional sectors of health services as described in Chapter 13. Nonetheless, services between primary and specialized care are poorly developed in most parts of the country. People have direct access to primary or secondary care, depending on their proximity to and knowledge of resources and their attitudes toward the system. Many healthcare planners prefer that there be a linear and seamless progression by the individual to primary care to secondary care to tertiary care, as required (see Figure 14.3). However, this progression would be difficult to achieve in the current healthcare system unless its organization and payment system are drastically restructured, which is why several provinces are considering the creation of integrated service delivery systems. The one major step toward it is primary care reform.

Integrated delivery systems (IDS) are defined as "a network of organizations that provides or arranges to provide a coordinated continuum of services to a defined population and is willing to be held clinically and fiscally accountable for the outcomes and the health status of the population it services" (44). The continuum of primary and specialized services provided in such arrangements most often includes primary care, health promotion and disease prevention programs, secondary care with links to tertiary care facilities, rehabilitation, palliative care, long-term care, home care, and community support services. IDS can provide these services or purchase services through contracts with outside care providers — whichever is the most cost-effective use of existing resources. The system of payment for IDS varies, but most often requires a roster of a particular population group with physician remuneration for services based on a capitation formula. As illustrated in Figure 14.3, the physical site of service delivery

Figure 14.3. Patient Progress through Healthcare System

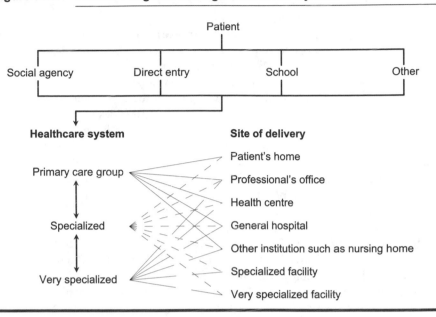

Source: Ontario Health Planning Task Force. *Ontario Health Planning Task Force Report*. Toronto: Government of Ontario, 1974.

may be the same for primary, specialized, and very specialized care. Certainly, most of these services, as well as their coordination, management, and financing, would occur in some single location. Health Canada has stated that the *Canada Health Act* does not preclude rostering individuals in a plan as long as the individual can choose to leave the group at a specified time (45). This interpretation paves the way for reform in primary health care. The Health Transition Fund has been funding 41 provincial and national pilot and evaluation projects on integrated services delivery since 2000, and evaluations of these projects support IDS (45).

Appropriateness

Appropriateness is defined as a care or service provided that is relevant to the patient's needs and is based on established standards (see Chapter 3). In Canada in 2000, 18.7% of births were Caesarean deliveries, which is one of the indicators for appropriateness. The rate varies from a low of 15.6% in Saskatchewan to a high of 23.6% in Newfoundland. Teaching hospitals and those with evidence-based guidelines in place had lower Caesarean rates (17). In 2001, the vaginal birth after Caesarian rate (the other indicator) in Canada was 35%, in New Brunswick 17%, and Saskatchewan 44%.

Optimizing Quality Assurance and Total Quality Management Programs

Quality assurance (QA) is a management system to assure the quality of health care provided by workers and received by patients. Care should be correctly given, reliable, and empathetic. QA constantly improves standards and the frequency of attaining them. The Canadian Council on Health Service Accreditation (CCHSA), a national agency that accredits healthcare facilities of all descriptions across Canada, defines the following **five-stage process for quality assurance** as the establishment of functional goals, the implementation of procedures to achieve those goals, the regular assessment of performance relative to the goals, the proposal of solutions to close the gap between performance and goal, and the documentation and reporting of this assessment activity.

For QA to work, institutions must encourage both the continuous assessment of quality and the communication of problems, and attainment of desired changes through the management structure (46). A number of approaches have been developed specifically for the hospital sector, such as the Medical Audit Committee, which compares care for a specific disease with the standards set for that disease. Another example is the Tissue Committee, which reviews all tissue removed during surgery and compares it to the pre-operative diagnosis. The third example is the Health Record Committee, which reviews selected patient records for completeness. CIHI also provides large sets of data for comparisons between institutions of similar size.

Although institutions have QA programs, there is rarely an organized review of the community-based practices of healthcare professionals. Licensing or regulating bodies usually deal with patient complaints; however, recent legislation in a number of provinces now requires quality of care provided by their constituents to be monitored. Increasingly, healthcare professionals and institutions are required to be accountable to the public and the government for the resources they use and how they practise.

Total quality management (TQM) is a management philosophy for improving quality while controlling costs. In TQM, management focuses on the system rather than the individual, so decisions are made to support quality and remove barriers to quality inherent in the bureaucratic, hierarchical system. Participation and teamwork are vital. Because TQM is based on a continuous feed-forward process called continuous quality improvement (CQI), it differs from quality assurance, which tends to depend on retrospective recognition of exceptions to patterns of care. However, TQM has not yet been widely implemented in the healthcare system in Canada, although there have been several initiatives for implementing it. TQM complements QA by providing a management system for rectifying identified difficulties, an aspect which is frequently missing from QA activities. QA tends to emphasize data collection. QA also focuses on individuals, often in relation to their peers, and is thus less powerful than TQM, which examines issues affecting the performance of the organization as a whole.

Optimizing Technology Assessment

Technology (some of it very expensive) has made tremendous advances in health care in recent times. Technology assessment has been developed to examine the efficacy and safety of a technology, its appropriate clinical use, the relative risks and benefits, and the ethical and social implications. However, no systematic process for the identification and acquisition of new technology exists in Canada. Interprovincial differences in priorities and disparities in wealth make it difficult to establish uniform approaches to health technology. Health Canada's Health Products and Food Branch administers the *Food and Drugs Act*, which regulates a limited number of medical devices as well as medications. These devices include implantables, condoms, AIDS tests, menstrual tampons, and contact lenses. The Act does not cover devices used externally or most other technology that is introduced independently by the provinces. The Canadian Coordinating Office for Health Care Technology Assessment is a non-profit organization funded by federal, provincial, and territorial governments to undertake technology assessments on request from provinces, Health Canada, and other sources (47).

A fundamental concept, which provides the rationale for technology assessment, is the diffusion of technology. As new technology emerges, it is usually taken up enthusiastically, followed by a period of reassessment during which limitations or adverse effects come to light. The technology then becomes incorporated into the practices of healthcare professionals and institutionalized, even if the initial glowing promise is (usually) not fully realized. Unless this cycle is interrupted, such as by an assessment of the cost effectiveness, enormously expensive technology can become the standard of practice without evidence of its efficiency.

The Technology Assessment Iterative Loop (48) provides a model for informed decision making as a result of technology assessment. It sets out seven steps: identify technologies with the greatest potential for reducing the burden of illness by primary, secondary, or tertiary prevention or by levels of care; establish efficacy, i.e., therapeutic potential under ideal circumstances; establish procedures for screening and diagnosis, i.e., accurate detection of those in need; determine community effectiveness (see also Chapter 3); assess efficiency (see also Chapter 3); develop procedures for synthesis and implementation; and monitor and reassess the process.

Technology assessment may use cost-utility ratios, whereby the social value of the technology is incorporated into the assessment for comparison of competing technologies. The incremental costs of technologies are compared in order to achieve, for example, an additional quality-adjusted life year (QALY) (49). It has been recommended that the use of health technology be based on defined population needs.

Effectiveness

Effectiveness is defined as the care or service, intervention, or action achieving the desired results (see Chapter 3). Some examples are listed below. Successful programs for immunization will eliminate or reduce cases of vaccine preventable diseases such as whooping cough or measles (see Table 5.3 in Chapter 5). Similarly, successful screening programs for cervical cancer or hypertension will reduce age-standardized death rates for cervical cancer and hypertensive diseases (see Chapter 7).

For acute myocardial and stroke mortality, the 30-day inpatient hospital mortality rate reflects the care these patients receive in hospital and their quality of life after discharge. For the year 1999–2000, 12.6% and 19.2% of patients died in hospital within 30 days (19). In this situation, bench marks are not yet developed but regional and provincial variation provides useful information.

Readmission rates can be influenced by the quality of care a patient receives while hospitalized. Although not all readmissions are avoidable or preventable, higher rates for certain conditions reflect the quality of care. The readmission rates of patients to hospital within 28 days due to acute myocardial infarct and asthma reflects such concerns and their rates were 7.3% and 6.4% respectively.

The indicator for pneumonia and influenza hospitalization reflects the burden of illness due to these two illnesses, a portion of which may be preventable through influenza and pneumococcal immunization programs. High rates of preventable pneumonia and influenza in people aged 65 and over may suggest a problem with access to immunization. In 2000, the age-standardized rate of acute care inpatient hospitalization for both illnesses was 1,241 per 100,000 population aged 65 and older (19).

With regard to ambulatory/outpatient care, patients with certain conditions do not require hospitalization. Although not all admissions for such ambulatory care sensitive conditions are avoidable, it is assumed that appropriate prior ambulatory care could prevent the onset of this type of illness or condition (e.g., complications of diabetes), control an acute episodic illness or condition, or manage a chronic disease or condition. The appropriate level of utilization is not known; however, a disproportionately high rate is presumed to reflect problems in obtaining access to primary care. The age-standardized rate for acute care hospitalization for inpatients with conditions where appropriate ambulatory care prevents or reduces the need for admission to hospital was 447 per 100,000 population.

For volume and surgical outcomes, researchers have found that hospitals with a high volume tended to have lower risk-adjusted mortality rates. For the year 1999–2000, high-volume procedures for knee replacement (21,649) and hip replacement (19,853) were examined: 70% of knee replacements were done in hospitals that performed 100 cases or more a year, and almost 7% were done in hospitals doing fewer than 50 cases a year. The situation was similar for hip replacements (19).

Optimizing Utilization Review and Management

Utilization review compares the volume and intensity of how services are used. Large differences exist in the rates of use of medical services among geographic regions or practitioners, yet there are no discernible differences in health outcomes. However, establishing ideal rates is problematic. Big variations in the rates of medical or hospital services among geographic regions are called small-area variations (SAV), which are adjusted for age, sex, and other variables. SAV findings question the assumption that all the services in the regions with higher rates are medically necessary (50). Statistics Canada and CIHI have produced a detailed report on health indicators for provinces and their regions, which provides useful data to compare SAV(51).

Utilization review and management monitor the use of services, analyze variations, and assess interventions in order to reduce the inappropriate use of services and to provide feedback and education (52). They may be hospital-based or community-based.

5.   RATIONING IN HEALTH CARE

When resources for health care and services are finite and limited, rationing is one option that may result in equitably distributed health care. Medical savings accounts

(MSAs) have been suggested as a possible improvement to Canada's healthcare funding. The Senate Standing Committee on Social Affairs, Science, and Technology indicated that a system of MSAs might be appropriate in a limited sphere, such as paying for long-term-care facilities, where there are already significant private out-of-pocket charges (53). However, MSAs should not be applied in the broader healthcare field involving already insured services. The Alberta Advisory Council on Health Care recommended further studies on MSAs (54).

MSAs attempt to reduce healthcare costs by transferring responsibility for expenditures to patients while providing them with state-supported base amounts to cover some of the costs. They offer an alternative form of health coverage that involves a combination of catastrophic health insurance with a savings account used to pay for non-catastrophic medical expenses. Money is put aside either by an employer, by an individual, or, in the model proposed for Canada, by government in the form of public funds already earmarked for health in a savings account. Until the high deductible of the catastrophic plan is met, the individual must pay for health services either out of pocket or with money from the savings account. This approach is intended to reduce demand for health services by making individuals financially responsible for their pattern of consumption.

Governments would take funds already earmarked for health care for deposit into an MSA for every individual to purchase healthcare services. Amounts in individual accounts would be determined by estimating the average expenditure based on demographic experience. Canadians would then use the money to pay for health services until they have exhausted their account. In most models, the individual would be responsible for all costs over the amount in their account to some predetermined maximum. This is often called a "corridor." The government would then pick up the cost of the amount over the corridor, or a portion of the MSA could be used to purchase catastrophic insurance as protection against excessive costs for individual's health needs. According to proponents, if an individual does not use the maximum in the account, it could be saved for future healthcare needs or used to purchase other services e.g., health fitness memberships, smoking cessation programs, or, in some models, vacations.

Supporters of MSAs usually point to Singapore. Measures such as population health, life expectancy, and infant mortality in Singapore are comparable to Canada, yet Canada spends a larger percentage of GDP on health care. But as noted earlier, cross-country comparisons can be misleading. The determination of total health expenditure can differ and what gets included in total health expenditure can also differ.

A study investigating the effectiveness of MSAs in Manitoba concluded that such a system will not save money but will instead, under most formulations, lead to increased spending on the healthiest members of the population (55). Between 1997 and 1999, physician and hospital costs attributed to individual Manitoba residents averaged $730 each year. About 40% of the entire population of Manitoba used less than $100 each, and 80% used less than $600. The highest-using 1% of the Manitoba population accounted for 26% of all spending on hospital and physician care, whereas the lowest-using 50% accounted for 4%. When examined by age category, the results were similar.

If the entitlement under an MSA scheme was set at the current average cost of $730 per year, then total spending by the Manitoba government on health care for this healthy group would increase (by $505 million) rather than decrease. If the threshold above which the insurer would pay costs was set at $1,000 per year, then the sickest 20% of Manitoba residents would become personally responsible for just over $60 million of current healthcare costs. The net result is a 54% increase in spending on hospital and physician costs that can be allocated to individuals. The World Health Organization recently concluded that MSAs are neither a panacea nor a catastrophe for the healthcare system, and must be evaluated in the context of the entire health financing system (56).

6.   SUMMARY

Canada has a predominantly publicly financed health system with universal coverage for all permanent residents, without regard to their ability to pay for care. In 1999, Canada spent $87.2 billion on health care (9.2% of the GDP), which translates to $2,936 per person. Most money for health care is raised through provincial and federal taxes and is allocated, for the most part, from general provincial budgets. Public sector funding accounted for 70.8% of health expenditures and the remaining 29.2% came from private sector. Treatment for work-related injuries and disease is covered through worker's compensation funds.

Health expenditures are categorized into eight major categories: hospitals, other institutions, physicians, other health professionals, drugs, public heath and administration, capital, and other health spending. In 1999, the largest category of healthcare spending was institutional care, at 31.9% or $37 billion, of which $28.5 billion was spent on hospitals and $8.5 billion was spent on other institutions and allied special hospitals; about one quarter was spent on professional services, and $13.3 billion or 14.9% on drugs. These rapidly rising costs in health care, particularly in the acute care sector, as well as expanding high-cost technology are straining Canada's resources.

Institutions are the most expensive element of health care as they rely on both technology and human resources. In 2000–2001, Canada had more than 569 general and allied hospitals, with 98,132 approved beds. In the previous five years, more than 275 hospitals closed, merged, or were converted to another type of facility. In 2000-2001, there were 2,227 beds for rehabilitation, 5,879 extended care (patients with long-term beds) and 24 separate long-term psychiatric hospitals with 9,565 beds. For every 1,000 Canadians in 2000-2001, there were 3.9 beds in institutions (3.3 beds for short-term care or shared short-/long-term care beds, and 0.3 beds exclusively for long-term care). Canadians spent almost 21 million days as inpatients in acute care hospitals in 1999–2000, down 15.6% from 1994–95. The average length of hospital stay for 2000–01 was 7.2 days.

To improve the utilization of institutional resources the following strategies are considered:

- rationalization of healthcare services involving restructuring, realignment, closures, and mergers of institutions;

- increased ambulatory care, day care, and extended care;
- pre-admission planning and discharge planning, which shorten hospital stays.

The largest components of human health resources are nurses and the expenditure figures for them are subsumed under institutional expenditure as the majority of them are salaried. In 1999, the expenditure for professional services by physicians, dentists, and other specialists amounted to about $23 billion (25.7% of total spending); physicians' services alone constituted approximately 52.9%, amounting to $12.2 billion. Physicians now receive about 13.6¢ of every healthcare dollar in the form of fees.

The healthcare industry is the third largest industry in the country, employing about 827,700 Canadians, of whom 80% work in health institutions. There are more than 150 categories of health occupations. They have been developed either as extensions of established healthcare professions or alongside some special body of knowledge. Human health resources are unevenly distributed, because the main concentration is in large urban centres and traditionally wealthy provinces.

The following are current approaches to increasing efficient utilization human health resources (specifically physicians):

- management of physician human resources, including linking cost control in the healthcare system to the supply, mix, and distribution of physician human resources and their remuneration;
- management of physician remuneration, particularly the rights of physicians to receive what they regard as fair compensation for their services and team approach to health care;
- caps on physician incomes;
- clinical practice guidelines, which use clinical judgement and decision making to enhance the quality of care and facilitate cost containment and appropriate utilization of resources.

The health system performance measurements include the categories of acceptability, accessibility, appropriateness, competence, continuity, effectiveness, efficiency, and safety to evaluate the system.

- Approaches suggested to improve health system performance include:
  - technology assessment, a process that examines the efficacy and safety of a technology, its appropriate clinical use, its relative risks and benefits, and its ethical and social implications;
  - quality assurance, a process for establishing functional goals, implementing procedures to achieve these goals, regularly assessing performance, closing the gap between performance and goal, and documenting and reporting;
  - utilization review and management, which involves monitoring the use of services, analyzing variations, assessing interventions to reduce inappropriate use of services, collecting feedback, and providing education, based on total quality management; and
  - healthcare rationing to distribute health care equitably when resources and services are finite and limited. Medical savings accounts have been suggested by some as a possible improvement to Canada's healthcare funding.

7.   REFERENCES

1.   Canadian Institute for Health Information. *National health expenditure trends, 1975-2001.* Ottawa: Canadian Institute for Health Information, 2001.
2.   Canadian Institute for Health Information. 2002. *National health expenditure trends, 1975-2002.* <secure.cihi.ca/cihiweb/dispPage.jsp?cw_page=AR_31_E> (January 2003).
3.   Health Canada. *Canada Health Act: Annual report.* Ottawa, 1994.
4.   Canadian Institute for Health Information. *Provincial and territorial government health expenditure estimates.* Ottawa: Canadian Institute for Health Information, 2002.
5.   Barer M, Stoddard G. Toward integrated medical resource policies for Canada: 1. Background, process, and perceived problems. *Canadian Medical Association Journal* 1992; 146(3): 337-51.
6.   Armstrong P, Armstrong H. *Wasting away: The undermining of Canadian health care.* Toronto: Oxford University Press, 1996.
7.   Deber R, Williams P, Duvlako K, *et al. Report to the Task Force on the Funding and Delivery of Medical Care in Ontario: The public-private mix in health care.* Toronto: University of Toronto, 1995.
8.   Deber R. 2000. *Getting what we pay for: Myths and realities about financing Canada's health care system.* <www.m-thac.org/cgi-bin/WebObjects/mthac.woa/wa/DetailDirect/literature?id=1000001> (February 2003).
9.   First Ministers' Meeting. 2000. *New federal investments to accompany the agreements on health renewal and early childhood development (September 11, 2000).* <www.scics.gc.ca/cinfo00/80003807_e.html> (January 2003).
10.   Kirby M, LeBreton M. 2002. *The health of Canadians: The federal role. Volume 6: Recommendations for reform.* Standing Senate Committee on Social Affairs, Science and Technology. <www.parl.gc.ca/37/2/parlbus/commbus/senate/com-e/soci-e/rep-e/repoct02vol6-e.htm> (November 2002).
11.   Romanow R. *Building on values: The future of health care in Canada.* Ottawa: Commission on the Future of Health Care in Canada; Government of Canada, 2002.
12.   Health Canada. 2003. *First ministers' accord on health care renewal.* <www.hc-sc.gc.ca/english/hca2003/accord.html> (February 2003).
13.   Deber R, Swan B. Canadian health expenditures: Where do we really stand internationally? *Canadian Medical Association Journal* 1999; 160(12):1730-34.
14.   Deber R. Health care reform: Lessons from Canada. *American Journal of Public Health* 2003; 93(1):20-4.
15.   Canadian Institute for Health Information. *Supply and distribution of registered nurses in Canada, 2001.* Ottawa: Canadian Institute for Health Information, 2001.
16.   Canadian College of Health Services Executives. *Health systems update 2000-2001*, 8th ed. Ottawa: Canadian College of Health Services Executives, 2001.
17.   Canadian Institute for Health Information. *Health care in Canada 2001.* Ottawa: Canadian Institute for Health Information, 2001.
18.   Statistics Canada. *Hospital statistics: Preliminary annual report, 1993-1994.* Ottawa: Government of Canada, 1996.
19.   Canadian Institute for Health Information. *Health care in Canada 2002.* Ottawa: Canadian Institute for Health Information, 2002.
20.   Alberta Health Planning Secretariat. *Starting points: Recommendations for creating a more accountable and affordable health system.* Edmonton, 1993.
21.   Lesemann F, Martin C. *Home-based care, the elderly, the family, and the welfare state: An international comparison.* Ottawa: University of Ottawa Press, 1993.
22.   Canadian Institute for Health Information. *Average payment per physician report: Canada, 1996/97-1998/99.* Ottawa: Canadian Institute for Health Information, 2000.

23. Gagnon D, Menard M. *Listening for directions: A national consultation on health services and policy issues*. Ottawa: Canadian Health Services Research Foundation, 2002.

24. Canadian Institute for Health Information. *Health personnel in Canada, 1991-2000*. Ottawa: Canadian Institute for Health Information, 2002. <www.cihi.ca> (November 2002).

25. Canadian Institute for Health Information. 2001. *Canada's health care providers*. Ottawa. <secure.cihi.ca/cihiweb/dispPage.jsp?cw_page=AR_35_E> (January 2003).

26. Canadian Institute for Health Information. 2002. *Health indicators: Definitions and data sources*. <secure.cihi.ca/indicators/en/definitions.shtml> (January 2003).

27. Barer ML, Lomas J, Sanmartin C. Re-minding our Ps and Qs: Medical cost controls in Canada. *Health Affairs* 1996; 15(2):216-34.

28. Barer M, Stoddard G. Toward integrated medical resource policies for Canada: 3. Analytic framework for policy development. *Canadian Medical Association Journal* 1992; 146(7):1169-74.

29. Barer M, Stoddard G. Toward integrated medical resource policies for Canada: 2. Promoting change — general themes. *Canadian Medical Association Journal* 1992; 146(6):697-700.

30. Barer M, Stoddard G. Toward integrated medical resource policies for Canada: 6. Remuneration of physicians and global expenditure policy. *Canadian Medical Association Journal* 1992; 147(1):33-8.

31. Barer M, Stoddard G. Toward integrated medical resource policies for Canada: 4. Graduates of foreign medical schools. *Canadian Medical Association Journal* 1992; 146(9):1549-54.

32. Barer M, Stoddard G. Toward integrated medical resource policies for Canada: 7. Undergraduate medical training. *Canadian Medical Association Journal* 1992; 147(3):305-12.

33. Barer M, Stoddard G. Toward integrated medical resource policies for Canada: 5. The roles and funding of academic medical centres. *Canadian Medical Association Journal* 1992; 146(11):1919-24.

34. Lomas J, Barer M. And who shall represent the public interest? The legacy of Canadian health manpower policy. In Evans R, Stoddard G, editors. *Medicare at maturity*. Calgary: University of Calgary Press; 1986.

35. Chan B. *From perceived surplus to perceived shortage: What happened to Canada's physician workforce in the 1990s?* Ottawa: Canadian Institute for Health Information, 2002.

36. Hall EM. *Canada's national-provincial health program for the 1980s: A commitment for renewal*. Ottawa: Health and Welfare Canada, Special Commissioner, 1980.

37. Flood C, Archibald T. The illegality of private health care in Canada. *Canadian Medical Association Journal* 2001; 164(6):825-30.

38. Health Services Research Group. Standards, guidelines, and clinical policies. *Canadian Medical Association Journal* 1992; 146(6):833-7.

39. Linton A, Peachy D. Guidelines for medical practice: 1. The reasons why. *Canadian Medical Association Journal* 1990; 143(6):485-90.

40. Canadian Institute for Health Information. 2002. *Drug expenditure in Canada*. <secure.cihi.ca/cihiweb/dispPage.jsp?cw_page=AR_80_E> (January 2003).

41. Federal-Provincial-Territorial Council on Social Policy Renewal. 2002. *Social union framework agreement: Review*. <socialunion.gc.ca/menu_e.html> (September 2002).

42. Canadian Institute for Health Information. 2002. *Data tables*. <secure.cihi.ca/indicators/en/tables.shtml#performance> (January 2003).

43. Chen J, Hou C, Sanmartin C, et al. Unmet health care needs. *Canadian Social Trends* 2002; 67:18-22.

44. Shortell SM. *Health care management: Organization, design, and behavior*, 3rd ed. Albany, NY: Delmar Publishers, 1994.

45. Leatt P. 2002. *Integrated service delivery*. <www.hc-sc.gc.ca/htf-fass/english/integrated_en.pdf> (January 2003).

46. Wilson CRM. *Hospital-wide quality assurance: Models for implementation and development*. Toronto: W.B. Saunders, 1987.

47.   Canadian Coordinating Office for Health Technology Assessment. 2002. *About CCOHTA: FAQs*. <www.ccohta.ca/entry_e.html> (January 2003).

48.   Feeney D, Guyatt G, Tugwell P. *Health care technology: Effectiveness, efficiency, and public policy*. Montreal: Institute for Research on Public Policy, 1986.

49.   Goel V, Deber R, Detsky A. Non-ionic contrast media: Economic analysis and health policy development. *Canadian Medical Association Journal* 1989; 140(4):389-95.

50.   Health Services Research Group. Small area variations: What are they and what do they mean? *Canadian Medical Association Journal* 1992; 146(4):467-70.

51.   Statistics Canada. How healthy are Canadians? 2002 annual report. *Health Reports* 2002; 13(suppl). <www.statcan.ca/english/IPS/Data/82-003-SIE2002001.htm> (January 2003).

52.   Anderson G, Sheps S, Cardiff K. Hospital-based utilization management: A cross-Canada survey. *Canadian Medical Association Journal* 1990; 143(10):1025-30.

53.   Kirby M, LeBreton M. 2002. *The health of Canadians: The federal role. Volume 4: Issues and options*. Standing Senate Committee on Social Affairs, Science and Technology. <www.parl.gc.ca/37/1/parlbus/commbus/senate/com-E/SOCI-E/rep-e/repintsep01-e.htm> (January 2003).

54.   Mazankowski D. 2001. *A framework for reform: Report of the Premier's Advisory Council on Health*. <www.premiersadvisory.com/reform/council.html> (January 2003).

55.   Forget E, Deber R, Roos L. Medical savings accounts: will they reduce costs? *Canadian Medical Association Journal* 2002; 167(2):143-7.

56.   Hanvoravongchai P. *Medical savings accounts: Lessons learned from international experience*. Geneva: World Health Organization, 2002. EIP/HSF/PHF Discussion Paper No. 52.

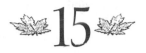

COMMUNITY HEALTH SERVICES

1. OVERVIEW OF COMMUNITY HEALTH SERVICES

When illness, suffering, or symptoms occur, an individual usually relies on informal support, sometimes for prolonged periods (see Chapter 5, Figure 5.1). When this support is exhausted, the individual turns to local community-based health services, which can include primary care, secondary care, hospital care, home care, public health services, and private nursing homes. Community health services may also deal with specific groups of people, e.g., Aboriginal peoples, battered women, and people with Alzheimer's disease.

Government health insurance plans cover basic hospital and medical services in all the provinces and territories, but there are extreme variations in the coverage of extended health services, whether in the home or in the community, paid by provincial or private insurance or by the individual. Affluent provinces provide a larger range of services financed through public revenue (see Chapter 13).

This chapter discusses basic health services; however, many other services related to health promotion, disease prevention, and health maintenance are described, as are support services (such as social, educational, and vocational services) for those who are chronically or acutely ill.

1.1. PRIMARY HEALTHCARE SERVICES

At this point, it is appropriate to define the commonly used term **primary health** *care*. Sometimes called first-contact care, this includes services provided at the first contact between the patient and the healthcare professional. Physicians, dentists, chiropractors, pharmacists, nurse practitioners, midwives, optometrists, dietitians, and others generally provide primary health care. Services include treatment, promotion and maintenance of health, follow-up care, and the complete continuing care of the individual (including referral when required). Therefore, primary healthcare providers perform three essential functions beyond treating the patients (1):

- *Guardian.* The primary care provider and patient and his or her family enter into a relationship in which continuity is implicit. As a result of the increasing complexity of the Canadian healthcare system, there is an increasing need for someone (perhaps a team) to accept responsibility for the ongoing care of the person or family.

- *Gatekeeper.* The primary care provider has a dual role as a guide or information resource and as the appropriate source for referral elsewhere in the healthcare system.
- *Chronicler.* The primary care provider acts as a chronicler or recorder of the patient's health-related interactions with the system and its providers.

1.2. SECONDARY, TERTIARY, AND QUATERNARY HEALTH CARE

People with specialized training usually deliver **secondary health care**. Patients normally enter secondary care after referral from primary care providers because their health problems require specialized skills and facilities not available in the primary care sector. Such problems include serious cardiovascular disorders, unintentional injuries, burns, fractures, cancers, behavioural disorders, and pediatric, medical, and obstetric problems, which usually require specialized care provided by specialists in a community or general hospital. Unusual inherited disorders, certain forms of cancer, complicated pregnancies, rare and complicated cardiovascular disorders, catastrophic trauma, and complex immunological disorders need treatment by further referral to **tertiary healthcare centres**, which have very specialized facilities and professional skills and are usually found only in university teaching hospitals. Extremely complex situations, such as heart, lung, kidney, liver, bone marrow transplant, and unusual procedures such as separation of Siamese twins require services of **quaternary health care** that is always associated with the teaching hospitals.

2. PROVISION OF MEDICAL SERVICES

The major component of primary health care in Canada is primary medical care, usually provided in the community by general or family practitioners and, to a lesser extent, by nurse practitioners, pediatricians, internists, obstetricians, gynecologists, and midwives. This is not the case in the United States, where specialists provide primary medical care predominantly. A small proportion of the Canadian population seeks their primary medical care through community health centres, walk-in clinics, or hospital emergency rooms. More than 90% of the Canadian population can identify their primary medical care provider. The major part of secondary medical care is also provided in the community setting, and tertiary medical care is mainly provided by physicians and others practising in the hospital setting, usually in teaching centres.

2.1.   PHYSICIAN REMUNERATION

As discussed in Chapter 14, Canadian physicians receive remuneration for their services by different methods, namely fee-for-service basis, by sessional payment, or by salary. The majority bill for most of their services through provincial health insurance plans (i.e., **fee-for-service**). The mix varies across Canada. In Alberta, 98% of physicians in 1998–99 were paid only on a fee-for-service basis, compared to 40% in Manitoba. According to 2000–01 estimates from the Canadian Institute for Health Information, about 11% of the total clinical payments to physicians in the ten provinces come from some form of payment other than fee-for-service. Those who receive **sessional payments** receive a lump sum for the time they make their services available; for example, a psychiatrist working a half-day in a mental health clinic receives a flat rate for this service. However, there is a lot of variation in physician-payment modalities. In 2002, 58% of Canadian physicians received at least 90% of their income from fee-for-services, 8% received at least 90% from a salary, and the remaining 34% did not receive 90% of their income from any single source (2). Provider organizations, such as health services organizations (HSOs) in Ontario and the managed care organizations in the U.S., follow the capitation system used by funding organizations. In the **capitation system**, an organization receives a fixed amount per patient for all services rendered and, in turn, purchases physicians' services by salary or fee-for-service. Some consider the capitation or the salary system to be conducive to a holistic approach to health care, so the physician is more likely to pay attention to all determinants of health and practise disease prevention and health promotion. It is used for primary care physicians in the United Kingdom and usually in health maintenance organizations (HMOs) in the U.S. and in Ontario HSOs. Traditionally, salaries and sessional payments are more often used in rural regions or under-served areas of the provinces. However, the capitation system is currently drawing increased interest as part of primary healthcare reforms and endeavours to control health expenditures on physician services.

In the 1990s, several provinces undertook initiatives that supported the expanded role for non-physician primary care providers, such as integrating midwifery services into the healthcare system. Midwifery practice is now legal in several provinces and publicly financed in Ontario, Quebec, Manitoba, and British Columbia (see Chapter 16).

Support for the role of nurse practitioners (NPs) in primary care has been slower to develop. NPs are generally found in remote rural communities. Nurse-run outpost clinics in Newfoundland and Labrador have been a reality for many years, and there are NP-physician collaborations operating in many parts of the province (3). Such collaborations are also under way in other provinces, such as Saskatchewan. Because of the shortage of physicians in southern and urban areas, there is an increased demand for primary care provided by NPs (3).

2.2.   ORGANIZATION OF PRIMARY CARE

Office Practice

Most physicians in Canada practise medicine as solo practitioners (24%), in shared practices, or in group practices either in hospital or in the community (61.7%). The remainder have a variety of arrangements (2). Generally, a shared practice is distinguished from a group practice by the extent of patient sharing among the participating physicians. *Shared practices* are usually limited to two or more physicians who have completely separate practices but share office space, rent, and secretarial services. *Group practices* usually involve income distribution, formal contracts, shared patient records, shared practitioner responsibilities, and possible provision of care in one another's absence (4). Most group practices (80%) consist of physicians in the same discipline, such as family practitioners, while a smaller proportion consists of specialists from different disciplines. Most practitioners have their offices in the community. In urban centres with medical schools, practices of full-time teachers, called geographic full-time practitioners, are located in the university hospitals. With the implementation of primary care reforms larger number of family physicians will join in the organized group practices.

Walk-In-Clinics

There has been a growing interest in walk-in clinics since they first began operating in 1984. Although there is no universally accepted definition of a **walk-in-clinic**, it is usually a freestanding group practice that offers extended hours for services (weekend and evening hours) and does not require an appointment. Walk-in-clinics are usually located in urban or suburban centres with large proportions of young families.

Although they are convenient for consumers, in the medical community there is a concern that walk-in-clinics may provide lower quality care due to lack of physician and care continuity, or because they are more often staffed by recent medical school graduates or physicians who might have less than adequate training (5, 6). There is also some anecdotal evidence that people who see physicians at walk-in-clinics after hours see their family practitioner for the same problem the next day. Proposed primary care reforms in most provinces will require family practitioners to provide services 24 hours a day and 7 days a week. This would require in future either elimination of freestanding walk-in-clinics or development of new models of care.

Community Health Centres

A community health centre (CHC) has a voluntary board composed of members from the community. It receives an annual budget from the provincial government for specific health programs, and it provides a wide range of services such as medical, dental, social, and nursing by a multidisciplinary staff all under one roof. All the professionals, including physicians, are on salary. In all provinces except Quebec, many of these centres are located in under-served areas or serve groups that are often not well served, such as the poor, the elderly, Aboriginal peoples, and immigrant groups (7).

In Quebec, these centres are part of the regionalized health and social service system, and are called **centres locaux des services communautaires** (local community service centres, or CLSCs), of which there are approximately 146. CLSCs integrate health and social services and emphasize prevention, health promotion, and provision of other personal services, including occupational health services, at one location; they are also required to provide services for extended hours in the evenings and on weekends. CLSCs are considered either alternative, competing models of primary care or complementary to private practice (see Chapter 17) (8).

Outside Quebec, CHC programs are most extensive in Ontario. CHC programs were initiated in the late 1970s as a complementary program to health services organizations. As of April 2002, there were 56 CHCs in Ontario, which provide primary care for approximately 2% of the province's population. CHCs have also been established in Nova Scotia (four), New Brunswick (four), Manitoba (14), Saskatchewan (five), Alberta (two), and British Columbia (four).

Health Services Organizations in Ontario

Health services organizations, which have existed in Ontario since the late 1970s (8), are a form of group practice with two or more physicians. Instead of fee-for-service, physicians receive remuneration on a fixed per capita rate. These payments are based on the current provincial average costs of physician utilization under fee-for-service for different age and sex groups. Patients enroll voluntarily to receive services from the group for a defined period. The HSO is penalized financially when patients on its roster receive outside services for which the HSO has received funding. Unlike health maintenance organizations in the U.S., this penalty is incurred by the HSO; in the U.S., it is the patient who must pay.

Program expansion halted in the early 1990s in response to a growing government perception that the program had failed to achieve its intended objective of reducing healthcare costs while maintaining or improving healthcare quality. At present, there are 63 HSOs in Ontario, with a total rostered population of 2.7% of the provincial population (8).

2.3. NEW MODEL OF PRIMARY HEALTH CARE

Since the mid 1990s, primary care reform has been characterized by pilot and demonstration projects. Federal funding has supported this primary care reform and the variety of innovations initiated.

In September 2000, Canada's premiers and the Prime Minister agreed that improvements to primary health care are crucial to the renewal of health services. The federal government established the $800 million, four-year Primary Health Care Transition Fund (PHCTF) to accelerate the transition to new primary care models (9). The main objectives of the PHCTF are to assist provinces and territories to bring about permanent and sustainable changes within provincial and territorial healthcare systems. These changes could include an increased number of community-based primary healthcare organizations that provide comprehensive services to defined population; more interdisciplinary teams with enhanced roles for registered nurses, pharmacists, and other providers; better links to hospitals, specialist, and other community services; an increased emphasis on health promotion, disease and injury prevention, and management of chronic diseases; and expanded access to essential services around the clock. The PHCTF also has a $240 million national component to support common approaches to primary healthcare reform and initiatives that include First Nations, Inuit, and Métis health; official language minorities; multi-provincial initiatives; and national partnerships with nurses, doctors, rural physicians, and other public health stakeholders.

Accordingly, Alberta, Manitoba, Saskatchewan, and Ontario have either pilot projects or actual reform. Ontario has also announced plans to enroll 80% of the province's family doctors into teams or health networks by 2004; however, as of early 2003, only a very small number of practitioners have enrolled. Saskatchewan has set a target of 25% of doctors practising in non-fee-for-service group practices within four years and 100% within a decade. Quebec's 2000 Health Review recommended that doctor's practices and the CLSCs be considered the foundation of primary health care delivery, with the CLSC focusing on the social dimension and group practices on the delivery of medical services(10). Realizing the resistance of primary care physicians to joining the reform, the 2003 First Ministers Health Accord committed more funds toward the reform with a stated goal that 50% of the population will have access to an appropriate health care providers, 24 hours a day, 7 days a week, within next eitht years (11).

3.   SERVICES OF OTHER HEALTHCARE PROFESSIONALS

Among the many other healthcare professionals who provide primary health care in their specialty are those described here.

Nurses

Some nurses work together with a physician and provide primary health care with a physician's supervision, while others work independently in community health centres or occupational health services, or in remote areas where no physicians are available. They are generally paid by salary. Despite increasing recognition of nurse practitioners in Canada, not every province recognizes the specialty. NPs are trained to provide primary care and are allowed to dispense certain drugs. Currently, new or amended provincial and territorial legislation allows for an expanded role for registered nurses as NPs in Newfoundland and Labrador, Nova Scotia, New Brunswick, Ontario, Manitoba, Saskatchewan, Alberta and Yukon. Other areas are working on implementing similar legislation (see Chapter 16).

Dentists

Primary dental services are provided mainly in the offices of dentists with the support of dental hygienists. In 2000, Canada had 17,287 licensed dentists and 14,893 licensed dental hygienists (12). To some extent, local public health units or government-sponsored clinics also provide primary dental health services, usually to particular at-risk groups such as seniors or immigrant children. More specialized dental care can be provided by dental surgeons in hospital. Dentists are paid mainly by fee-for-service through private insurance or by the individual. The extent of funding from provincial health insurance plans varies across Canada for routine dental care. In some provinces, routine dental care is covered for children and seniors. Services provided by dental surgeons in hospital are covered by all provincial insurance plans (13). However many of the procedures performed by dental surgeons are performed outside of the hospital setting and therefore are not paid for by the provincial insurance plans.

Chiropractors

Chiropractors usually specialize in the manipulation of joints and muscles in order to correct musculoskeletal and other disorders. Chiropractic services are mainly provided in offices and, to a limited extent, in clinics organized by workers' compensation boards. Chiropractors are usually paid on a fee-for-service basis, through private insurance or out-of-pocket by individuals, and partially by provincial government health insurance plans in British Columbia, Alberta, Saskatchewan, Manitoba, and Ontario (13). In 2000 there were 5,633 licensed chiropractors in Canada (14).

Podiatrists

The podiatrist usually deals with foot problems. Like chiropractors, most work in private offices, although some work in either public health units or general hospitals. Their payment mechanism is also similar to that of chiropractors. The provincial insurance plans of British Columbia, Alberta, Saskatchewan, and Ontario cover part of the cost of services provided by podiatrists (13).

Optometrists

Optometrists handle refractory errors and minor ailments of the eye. They usually work in private offices or with optical dispensing outlets. Most optometrists are paid on a fee-for-service basis with a variety of payment mechanisms, depending on who is receiving services. Newfoundland and Labrador and Prince Edward Island are the only provinces in Canada that do not cover any services provided by optometrists. Other provinces, such as British Columbia, Saskatchewan, Manitoba, and Ontario, cover some costs through their provincial insurance plans. Alberta and Nova Scotia cover optometrists' services to children and the elderly, and Quebec covers services to the poor and to certain groups. The balance of the costs is covered by private insurance companies or directly by consumers (13). In 2000, 3,780 registered optometrists practised in Canada (14).

Midwives

Midwives deal with normal pregnancy, labour, delivery, and post-partum care. As of 2000, midwives were officially recognized as primary healthcare professionals and are regulated in Quebec, Ontario, Alberta, British Columbia, and Manitoba. Saskatchewan is developing appropriate regulatory legislation. Midwives usually work in small group practices and are generally paid a yearly salary or on a per-case basis. Their main source of income used to be charges to individual users of their services, but now

Ontario, Quebec, Manitoba, and British Columbia publicly fund midwifery services. In 2000, there were 358 active midwives in Canada (14).

Pharmacists

By law, pharmacists' practice includes dispensing prescription medications. Canada's 24,518 licensed pharmacists are distributed among three major employment groups. Approximately four out of very five pharmacists (80%) work in community pharmacies, another 15% in hospital or institutional pharmacies, and the remainder work in situations that may not legally require licensed pharmacists, such as associations, pharmaceutical companies, and consulting firms. Pharmacists working in privately owned and operated drug stores receive a dispensing fee for filled prescriptions as part of their remuneration. Non-owner and institution-based pharmacists such as those working in hospitals are usually paid by salary.

Others

Hospitals, home care, and public health units usually employ physiotherapists, occupational therapists, speech pathologists, audiologists, social workers, nutritionists, and clinical psychologists. A number of them are in private practice and the costs of their services are covered by individuals or by private health insurance.

Alternative Healthcare Providers

Significant numbers of Canadians (approximately 11%) seek services from alternative healthcare providers (15). **Alternative healthcare providers** include massage therapists, acupuncturists, homeopaths or naturopaths, Feldenkrais or Alexander teachers, relaxation therapists, biofeedback teachers, rolfers, herbalists, reflexologists, spiritual healers, and religious healers. These practitioners usually work in solo practices and are paid by those individuals seeking such services (16).

As one can see, there is a range of primary health care services provided by different professionals. The entry point into the primary healthcare system depends upon various factors, such as the employment, economic status and education of consumers, their health beliefs, the type of health insurance, and the availability and accessibility of services and professionals.

4.   HEALTHCARE INSTITUTIONS

Major institutions include allied special hospitals, chronic care hospitals, and nursing homes. In Quebec, the organization and activities of healthcare institutions is regulated by the *Act Respecting Health Services and Social Services and Amending Various Legislation* (passed in 1991). According to this act, Quebec differentiates between a centre and an institution. A centre is a place where health and social services are dispensed and can include general and specialized hospitals, psychiatric hospitals, local community service centres, residential and long-term care centres, and certain categories of rehabilitative care centres. An institution (*établissement*) is an organization responsible for service activities pertaining to the mission of one or more centres and is, in effect, an umbrella organization that ensures the provision of a continuous spectrum of accessible and high-quality health or social services, as well as the reduction of the health and welfare problems of its particular population group. An institution is frequently responsible for the management of several centres with differing missions, thus allowing for better integration and coordination of care, while centres are directly involved in service delivery (17). Many provinces have adopted similar structures through their regional health authorities (see Chapter 13).

4.1. HOSPITALS AND ACUTE CARE FACILITIES

4.1.1. Historical Evolution of Modern Hospitals

The earliest hospitals in Canada were established by religious orders. For example, the first hospital in Canada, Hôtel Dieu de Précieux Sang, was established in Quebec City in 1639 by the Catholic Church. Prior to 1850, hospitals were perceived as dirty, infested, crowded, and unpleasant places, staffed by heartless and ignorant attendants, to which people would go only as a last resort. At the time, the overall mortality rate was high (20%). Florence Nightingale, Joseph Lister, and others revolutionized hospital care by introducing antisepsis, asepsis, good food, and proper nursing. This reduced mortality from 20% to 2%. By the beginning of the 20th century, people were choosing to go to hospitals to be cured. Canadian hospitals became acceptable and were no longer viewed as "a well of sorrow and charity" but as a workplace for the production of health. The access that private practitioners gained to hospitals, without becoming employees of the hospitals, became one of the distinctive features of medical practice in North America. In Europe and most other areas of the world, when patients enter a hospital, their doctors typically relinquish responsibility to the hospital staff. In North America, private doctors often continue to follow their patients into the hospital and continue to attend them. This arrangement complicates hospital administration, since many of the people making vital decisions are not the institution's employees.

Hospitals' modern role in health care emerged following World War II. There was a concentration of curative medical technology developed during the war, primarily because of the advent of modern antibiotics and technology. Until the widespread introduction of antibiotics in the 1940s, hospitals and physicians mainly cared for the ill — with antibiotics they could in fact cure many diseases and infections. With emerging technology, physicians were able to improve their ability to diagnose a condition. The combined impact of these developments in medical science also had its influence on hospitals: hospitals adopted (and often still use) hierarchical organizational structures originally established by the British army. During the next few decades, the consolidation of hospital dominance occurred through the development of the Canadian healthcare model, including the *Federal Grants-in-Aid* (1948), the *Hospital Insurance and Diagnostic Services Act* (1957), the *Medical Care Act* (1966), and the *Canada Health*

Act (1984). All these steps resulted in the institutionalization and expansion of the Canadian hospital system (18).

Today, hospitals are the major centre for healthcare activities. They primarily take care of sick people by providing inpatient services, services for many ambulatory patients in outpatient clinics and emergency rooms, and rehabilitation services. In certain cases, they also provide limited public health and homecare services. Some large hospitals act as teaching resources for the education of physicians, nurses, and other allied healthcare professionals. Many teaching hospitals are also engaged in research activities. In recent years, there has been a trend to broaden the hospital's role to include disease prevention and health promotion.

4.1.2. Funding of Hospitals

Traditionally, provincial and territorial governments pay most hospital costs. Payment methods include (19):

- *Line-by-line funding*, which used to be the most popular method of hospital financing in Canada. It involves negotiated amounts for specific line items (or inputs) such as inpatient nursing services or medical/surgical supplies. The total budget allocation for an individual hospital, then, is simply the sum of the line items. British Columbia and New Brunswick still rely on line-by-line budgeting (combined with a population-based method).
- *Ministerial discretion*, based on decisions made by the provincial minister of health in response to specific requests by the hospital concerned. This method is used as the primary funding approach in Manitoba, Nova Scotia, Prince Edward Island, and Newfoundland and Labrador.
- *Population-based*, which uses demographic information such as age, gender, socioeconomic status, and mortality rates to forecast the demand for hospital services. Matching the predicted demand for certain health services with the estimated cost of providing these services yields a spending forecast for individual hospitals (or for regional health authorities). At present, Alberta and Saskatchewan use population-based funding as their primary method; Newfoundland and Labrador, Nova Scotia, Ontario, and Quebec are considering it.
- *Global budget*, which adjusts previous spending (such as the previous year's base allocation) to derive a proposed funding level for the upcoming year. The focus is on the total hospital budget rather than on individual service activities, or cost centres within the hospital. Adjustment can be made to the base amount using a multiplier (such as the rate of inflation) or a lump-sum amount to establish the funding level for future periods. Quebec introduced global budgets as its primary funding approach in 1994, while Ontario has used this method since 1969.
- *Service-based funding*, often referred to as a "case-mix-based approach." This method uses the volume and type of cases treated (such as volume of dialysis, bypass surgery, knee or hip replacement, etc.) by a hospital to determine funding. It requires the classification of patients into clinically meaningful groups that use

similar levels of hospital resources and the attachment of a weight to each group to estimate relative resource use. These weights usually reflect the average cost of treating the patients in each group; they are used to construct individual hospital case-mix indices that measure average patient resource intensity, usually relative to a national norm. Ontario used a service-based funding method in the summer of 2001 to distribute $95 million of additional lump-sum funding to hospitals.

Although these payment methods remain in place, the procedures for funding and governing hospitals have changed with the advent of *regionalized health authorities* (RHAs) in all provinces except Ontario. Provincial governments transfer a lump sum of money to RHAs in funding envelopes that cover the costs of providing a "basket of healthcare services" to their population, with the exception of money needed to cover physicians' services and drug expenses for the elderly and for those with low incomes. The regional authorities decide how much money is allocated to institutional care and how hospitals in their region are reimbursed. In New Brunswick, the eight regional hospital corporations receive a global budget that they administer to cover hospital costs in their region and the costs of physician services. Generally, provincial ministries of health make special arrangements for the financing of highly specialized tertiary and quaternary hospitals, which provide services to the entire provincial population regardless of region of residence. However, in most provinces and territories, the planning and provision of mental health services is under their control (as opposed to regional control), including psychiatric hospitals. In recent times, some provinces such as Alberta are devolving mental health service planning and provision to the regional health authorities.

4.1.3. Organization of Hospitals

A voluntary board of trustees governs hospitals, under legislation such as Ontario's *Public Hospitals Act*. There are various forms of hospital boards, which are constantly evolving; some are being phased out. Generally speaking, most board members are not professionals in the healthcare field and are either elected or appointed. Recently, physicians practising in the hospital and other hospital employees have also been represented on some hospital boards. In addition, some hospital administrators now also sit on hospital boards as voting members, sometimes holding office. Under provincial legislation, the board is responsible for the governance of the hospital, subject to compliance with the terms of the legislation. The board acts as the agent for the public in assuring proper financial operations and quality of care.

As the healthcare system has been regionalized (discussed in Chapter 13), the functions of most hospital boards have been taken over by *regional health boards* (RHBs) and the legislation has been amended accordingly. Ontario is the only province where RHBs have not replaced hospital boards. Almost all hospitals have a chief executive officer (CEO), president, or administrator in charge of daily operations and executing policies formulated by the regional or hospital board, and to whom all personnel report. One or more assistant administrators may support the administrator, each controlling a functional area (e.g., medical director and directors of nursing, plant and engineering, finances, and human resources). In Quebec, where healthcare institutions can oversee the work of several different health centres, the CEO and the senior management staff are responsible for the administration and operation of all of the centres operated by the institution. The CEO and the board are assisted by a management staff (including a director of professional services), a council of physicians, dentists, and pharmacists, a council of nurses, and a multidisciplinary council. Many hospitals have a Joint Conference Committee (JCC) — a tripartite body composed of representatives from medicine, the administration, and the board. Its purpose is to resolve workplace-related issues for physicians, much the way a union-management or co-determination committee functions. It is usually chaired by the president of the medical staff, who is usually selected by the physicians who have privileges at that institution. The president of the medical staff often sits on the board, and represents the viewpoint of the physicians who practise in that hospital.

Legislation requires that the board establish a *professional advisory committee* (PAC) or a *medical advisory committee* (MAC). In many hospitals, the PAC is responsible for advising on capital purchases of medical equipment, regulation of the professional staff, and similar matters. It is usually chaired by the chief of staff and consists of chiefs of different medical disciplines, chiefs of other healthcare professional services, and a member from the board.

The work of a hospital is usually organized according to either functions or divisions (20). A functionally organized hospital is divided into departments according to the number of functions performed. This usually involves vertically hierarchical reporting and decision making, and is well suited to small organizations with few goals and uncomplicated environments, such as a small community hospital or nursing home. The traditional functional organization of a hospital is illustrated in Figure 15.1, which is an organizational chart that covers the whole range of services a hospital may provide, although not all hospitals provide all the services listed. A hospital's size and teaching status determine the complexity of services available. Larger hospitals with multiple stakeholder interactions — frequently teaching hospitals and academic health centres — usually provide the widest range of services and are organized by division or programs. This type of organization involves the creation of smaller, semi-autonomous units organized according to traditional medical specialties. Each sub-unit has its own management team composed of medical, nursing, and administrative representatives, and usually has complete authority for the operation of the unit. Although divisional structures are much better at dealing with the multiple tasks required of an academic teaching hospital, and usually increase turnaround time for decision making, they run into problems of coordination, competitiveness among units, and, at times, goals incompatible with the goals and objectives of the larger corporate structure.

Organizational measures undertaken to integrate all hospital units (regardless of functional or divisional organization) include matrix designs that create dual reporting structures by function and by medical division (e.g., a nurse working in a cardiac unit is responsible to both the director of the cardiac unit and to the director of nursing), and parallel structures such as special problem-solving teams or task forces.

Figure 15.1. The Functional Organization of a Hospital

Regional board

Hospital

President

Medical affairs	Nursing	Diagnostic and therapeutic services	Educational programs	Administration and support services
Clinical departments:	Nursing	Organized outpatient services	Medical education	General administration
Medicine	Nursery	ECG, EEG, laboratory	Nursing education	Medical records, hospital library, laundry and housekeeping services
Surgery	Surgical suite	Radiology	Laboratory technicians	
Obstetrics and gynecology	Inpatient units	Special clinics	Radiological technicians	Plant operation and maintenance
Pediatrics	Emergency	Nuclear medicine	Other formal education programs	Dietetics
General practice	Central supply	Pharmacy		Ancillary operations
Psychiatry		Social work		Other
Radiology		Day care program		
Anesthesia		Home care program		
Ophthalmology		Respiratory therapy		
ENT		Poison control centre		
		Public health services		

More recently, in an effort to improve quality of care, responsiveness to patient needs, and accountability, many hospitals have adopted an organizational structure of program management. Program management is "a Canadian health care term that is synonymous with product line management in the private sector and in hospitals in the United States" (21). In this structure, the hospital is a portfolio of separate businesses with decision making pushed down the organization to teams of managers who are fully responsible for their programs. In a large urban centre, programs have 100 to 150 beds each and can be defined according to population group (e.g., gender, ethnicity, age, geography), by disease or health problem (e.g., AIDS, cancer, heart disease), by patient need (e.g., rehabilitation, continuing care), by type of service (e.g., outpatients, home care), or by medical specialty (e.g., medicine, surgery). Most important, programs are multidisciplinary, self-contained units that are each unique or special in some way, with the capacity to become centres of excellence. This method of organizing hospitals has developed in the last few years and is currently being evaluated for effectiveness.

There is a movement (especially in provinces such as Alberta) to facilitate the creation of hyper-specialized hospitals that will function as "focused factories." Examples include the Shouldice Hospital in Toronto (for hernia treatment) and the Gimble Eye Centre (cataracts and corrective eye surgery) in Calgary. These hospitals are based on the notion that very high volume and high frequency procedures, such as hernia surgery, cataract surgery, coronary bypass surgery, and cancer radiation, are associated with better outcomes when done in a specialized hospital. In the future there will likely be more of these types of hospitals because they can improve quality outcomes (they work at very high volumes under highly standardized routines and protocols) and have the potential to reduce waiting lists because they address health needs that occur with high frequency. In Quebec, university networks of hospitals have also changed as hospitals have merged, creating unified teaching facilities (such as the Centre hospitalier de l'Université de Montréal and the McGill University Health Centre). Four integrated university health networks are planned in order to consolidate teaching, research, and service efforts (see Chapter 17).

In recent years, communities have been concerned about the organization, governance, accountability, and functions of public hospitals. Many provinces have chosen regionalization as a response. As indicated above, the regionalization of responsibilities for health care has been undertaken to improve accountability and responsiveness to community needs. For the most part, regional health boards or regional institutional boards (in the case of New Brunswick and Newfoundland and Labrador) have replaced individual hospital boards. Because RHB members are usually elected and include representatives from local communities, RHBs will likely address some of these community concerns. Indeed, regionalization and devolution are particularly popular across Canada because they address these very issues. There is a great deal of interest in the effectiveness of regionalized governance structures (22); however, systematic evaluation has so far been limited but does indicate that they are successful (19).

4.1.4. Organization of Staff in Hospitals

Physicians play a pivotal role in terms of hospital utilization (20). They admit patients and determine what tests and treatments are needed and how long patients stay. In most Canadian hospitals, physicians are not employees but users of hospital facilities on behalf of their patients. This arrangement complicates hospital administration, since many of the people making vital decisions are not the institution's employees.

However, some radiologists, pathologists, and a few other specialists such as emergency room physicians are employed directly by the institution. In the last decade, Canadian hospitals have witnessed the emergence of the "hospitalist" as a new occupational category. Hospitalists are physicians (usually with a specialization in internal medicine) who are employees of the hospital (most often on salary) and who manage the medical care for hospital inpatients who do not otherwise have a primary care physician. Hospitalists will become more common in the future.

Typically, a physician requests the privilege of admitting patients to a general hospital, and expects to be responsible not only for their care but also for patients referred by other doctors. It is usually a subcommittee of the MAC that screens physicians' credentials, competencies, and resources consumption and advises the board, which has the final authority for approval. Admitting privileges are granted according to an impact analysis, which considers the potential number of patients who would be attracted to the hospital by the physician's specialized skills, the effect on hospital resources caused by the physician's activities, the ability of the physician's reputation to enhance the hospital's prestige, and the number of physicians already providing the same or similar services The board may reject the application or grant full or partial privileges, perhaps with some conditions (e.g , a general practitioner may not be allowed to do major surgery). Physicians usually complete a probationary period of an average of 12 months before receiving full hospital privileges; appointments are usually made for one year. Once physicians become members of the medical staff, they undertake certain responsibilities to the hospital, in addition to the right and responsibility of looking after any patients they admit. Medical staff members may be required to provide service in the emergency room in rotation, serve on committees, maintain and give final approval to hospital medical records, and attend staff meetings; they must abide by the rules and regulations passed by the medical advisory committee or hospital board.

The medical staff is expected to be self-governing and self-disciplining through peer review and a wide variety of devices that have developed between medical staff and boards and, in some cases, governments. The most common devices are organizational. For example, it is assumed that every hospital should have a chief of staff, usually a respected senior doctor, for each medical and surgical discipline. This individual is elected by his or her peers and is responsible for ensuring the quality of care delivered. Formerly, the chief of staff exercised influence by example or persuasion, but recent legislation in some jurisdictions gives the office the authority to relieve a physician of a case if it is obvious that the physician is not giving adequate or proper care to the patients.

In addition, it is common practice for hospitals to set up a series of committees charged with responsibility for monitoring the hospital's functioning. Some of these are the admission and discharge (or utilization) committee, the medical records committee, and the tissue committee. Sophisticated data processors can automatically examine performance in terms of established norms (e.g., the number of cases admitted with a diagnosis of pneumonia with appropriate bacteriological work done or the number of antibiotic sensitivity tests conducted). For most provinces, the Canadian Institute for Health Information does this type of analysis for monitoring on a collective basis.

4.1.5. Current Challenges and Realities

By the 1990s, hospitals had emerged as the cornerstone of medicare as well as many local economies. They are major employers and engines of economic growth, and are the key to physicians' incomes. They also compete for equipment, areas of specialization, and "star" physicians. Yet there is still almost no direct public accountability with respect to how hospitals spend their funding, although they have also become very expensive organizations.

Hospital restructuring in Canadian provinces has followed different routes. For instance, in provinces that have regionalized, such as New Brunswick, restructuring has been achieved through vertical integration (increasing the scope of operations through mergers — merging acute care, long-term care, public health, community care, and so on into one regional authority). In Alberta, restructuring has been achieved through horizontal integration (increasing the scale of operations through mergers and amalgamations of hospitals, which keep their autonomy). To date it is unclear how vertical or horizontal integration strategies affect the quality of patient care. The current trend is toward bigger institutions that address higher acuity needs in large urban centres. As a result of this, capacity to deliver emergency care in emergency departments and non-acute care in hospitals has lessened with resultant impact on homecare services.

In spite of cutbacks, hospitals remain the largest component of health budgets in all provinces. Significant health system restructuring is not possible without hospital restructuring, but because there is little new money to invest in health, restructuring requires reallocating dollars. It is not clear if hospitals will remain sheltered by medicare if they move beyond acute care, for example into continuing care or community-based care.

In addition, the debate about the efficiency and efficacy of a parallel system of private hospitals has resurfaced. Some clear examples of private sector health legislation in Canada are Alberta's Bill 11, which empowers regional health authorities to sub-contract surgical procedures to private providers under certain conditions, the *Ontario Private Hospital Act* (1990), Ontario's *Independent Facilities Act* (1990), and Saskatchewan's *Health Facilities Act*.

Public accountability requires transparency in terms of the quality of health care delivered by hospitals. In recent years, the Ontario Hospital Association, in collaboration with the provincial government, has produced a report card for each hospital, which looks at four important areas of hospital performance: patient satisfaction, patient care, hospital finances, and the hospital's ability to keep pace with change. Hospitals do not receive a single overall score in each area. Instead, researchers and healthcare experts choose 39 different indicators of performance. There are 8 indicators for patient satisfaction, 12 for patient care, 9 for hospital finances, and 10 for keeping pace with change. This report card includes hospital-by-hospital results for 16 of the 39 indicators, chosen for their accessibility and to provide a balanced picture of performance (23).

5. PUBLIC HEALTH SERVICES

No common definition of public health is in use in Canada. Sometimes it is used interchangeably with population health. Sometimes it refers to the publicly funded healthcare system, rather than the privately funded system. **Public health** has been defined as "one of the efforts organized by society to protect, promote, and restore the peoples' health. It is the combination of sciences, skills, and beliefs that is directed to the maintenance and improvement of the health of all the people through collective or social actions. The programs, services and institutions involved emphasize the prevention of disease and health needs of the population as a whole. Public health activities change with changing technology and social values, but the goals remain the same; to reduce the amount of disease, premature death, and disease-produced discomfort and disability in the population" (24).

5.1. LOCAL PUBLIC HEALTH UNITS/DEPARTMENTS

Public health is considered primarily a provincial and territorial responsibility under the constitution; however, responsibility for health protection is less clear, with responsibilities shared among federal and provincial and territorial governments. In Canada, government and non-government agencies as well as the private sector provide public health. Public health units/departments are primary providers of publicly funded statutory and non-statutory programs and activities for disease prevention, health protection, and health promotion at the local or regional level in all provinces and territories. These activities fall within the five core functions: population health assessment, health surveillance, health promotion, disease and injury prevention, and health protection.

Public health activities in all provinces and territories are governed by public health legislation and accompanying regulations and a variety of other acts specific to different functions, such as health protection and promotion, regional health authorities, occupational health and safety, and tobacco sales. Some jurisdictions also have public health standards to which regional or local public health bodies must adhere. At the ministry level, all provincial governments maintain central departments responsible for public health matters and have a chief medical health officer or equivalent. Most, but not all, have statutory powers related to communicable disease control; other responsibilities include acting as a consultant or advisor to regional or local medical health officers, providing policy advice on population health promotion, and acting as spokespersons on public health issues. They are part of the government hierarchy, depending upon provincial structure.

Currently, public health services are, for the most part, the responsibility of regional or district health authorities. Provinces are divided geographically into health units. Because metropolitan areas have a high population density, they have their own health units. Health units are semi-autonomous, community-based delivery structures that form liaisons with local hospitals, medical practitioners, and voluntary health agencies and have their own buildings and staff, except in Quebec. The province of Quebec has been divided into 18 regional boards of health and social services (Régies régionales de la santé et des services sociaux), each with a director of public health responsible for the assessment of the health needs of the population and the development of the most effective preventive interventions, surveillance, and control of communicable and non-communicable diseases; the director of public health also deals with real or perceived public health emergencies and health promotion and disease prevention, working closely with the CLSCs and other regional health and social services agencies. Most health units are now under the direction of regional health boards that determine the overall direction of programs and policies, as well as the amount of public funding. The major portion of funding for local health units comes from the provincial government (through regional funding) with some funding from local governments. However, in Alberta, total funding comes from the provincial government, and in Ontario, approximately 50% of the total funding of public health services comes from the provincial governments in the form of grants with the remainder from the local municipalities. With these financial arrangements, local governments retain autonomy in policy and program planning while following provincial guidelines. The lack of uniformity in services provided across the province is compensated by assessment and fulfilment of local needs.

5.1.1. Functions of Local Public Health Units

Public health programs and services vary greatly in geographic area and population size served. Population count could range from hundreds to more than 2 million, and catchment areas can vary from 15 to 1.5 million square kilometres. Programs also serve a variety of communities (most serve a combination of urban and rural populations). As already mentioned, the mandate of the local health units stems from the public health acts or regulations passed by the provincial legislature. For example, Ontario's Mandatory Health Programs and Services Guidelines outlines standards for public health services in general and lists the goals and objectives for specific programs. Local governments also pass health-related bylaws if the province so authorizes (e.g., bylaws regulating noise levels or smoking in public places). The extent of services provided depends on the province's public health act and the number of qualified personnel employed by each agency in relation to the population. Many rural agencies do not have enough personnel to employ a full complement of public health staff. In addition to mandated activities, regional health authorities have expanded into many new health fields outside their traditional role, especially in urban areas. Foremost among these are health promotion, mental health, services for people who are aged, disabled, and issues related to the physical environment.

Communicable Disease Control

The control of communicable disease continues to be a basic function of health units. Their duties include disease surveillance, the provision of consultation services to local physicians and hospitals, the supply of immunizing agents, health education, and special epidemiological surveys and studies. Health units are granted authority to control communicable disease by legislation and regulations; they are also responsible for the investigation and management of outbreaks such as food poisoning in nursing homes, measles in schools, and diarrhea in daycare centres. Most local health units operate sexually transmitted disease (STD) clinics, either by themselves or in conjunction with the local hospital; these clinics provide free diagnostic and treatment services at convenient hours. In some areas, these units pay private physicians to give free and anonymous treatment; also with their help local health units are involved in case finding of STDs and other communicable diseases, follow-up of contacts, and health education programs for STDs. Local public health units provide the contraceptive and family planning services as well.

Women's Health and Maternal and Child Health

In recent years, maternal and child health divisions in public health units in many provinces have been renamed and their functions expanded to focus more on family and women's health. The divisions may have different names in different provinces, but they all have similar functions. Public health nurses employed by local health units carry out preventive health programs such as education and immunization of infants and children in clinics. The maternal and child health services may include classes for expectant parents, postnatal visits to all or high-risk new parents, advice on parenting, and visits to daycare centres. Immunization of children is a statutory program in public health units in Alberta and Prince Edward Island, whereas private physicians and health units in other provinces share immunization responsibilities. Alberta also has comprehensive preschool surveillance programs (to monitor growth and development), which cover about 90% of children. In many provinces, health units provide healthcare services for school children; however, in others, the local education authority or private practitioners may provide this service. The type of school health services varies considerably across Canada, and the provision of services by larger city departments may differ from that found in a rural health unit. Vision screening tests and immunization programs have become standard practice in most local areas, while audiometric screening is discretionary in some areas. The public health nurse provides continuity for the health surveillance of school children, and maintains contact with the parents and family doctor.

Health Promotion

Public health units increasingly emphasize health promotion, community development, and health advocacy. Health promotion as a separate discipline has been receiving growing recognition. Strategies include educational methods to improve knowledge and skills, encouragement of public participation in health practices conducive to healthy living, and public policies that create environments that support health. Many local health departments employ health promotion specialists. Their responsibility includes continually assessing the health needs of their community, coordinating local health promotion services, and consulting with personnel in the voluntary and civic organizations interested in health. Public health nursing is involved in implementing and planning health promotion strategies. Community development workers may help communities mobilize against a public health problem; for example, they can provide information on second-hand smoke and its effects on health, enabling citizens to bring about the necessary environmental changes through political or legislative processes. Nutrition consultants prepare reference and educational materials for professional healthcare personnel and for the public. Examples of health promotion programs include the heart health programs in most provinces, and the City of Toronto programs aimed at groups such as recent immigrants, refugees, visible minorities, and the homeless. Health promotion programs provide education in schools on smoking, alcohol, drugs, AIDS, sex, and nutrition. The extent of the diffusion of the innovative approach of health promotion in public health units has, however, not been evaluated. Academic health promotion units in many provinces have developed affiliations with public health units to promote basic research in the discipline of health promotion and its application.

Dental Health

Public health initiatives such as fluoridation of municipal water supplies and improved dental hygiene have successfully reduced dental caries in Canadian children. Public health now focuses on provision of dental treatment to underprivileged groups and the elderly. Dental health divisions of provincial ministries, in collaboration with local health units, have sponsored the provision of dental care for children in remote areas. There are travelling clinics staffed by provincial dental teams in Manitoba, Nova Scotia, Ontario, and Prince Edward Island that visit rural and remote areas. These clinics deliver a considerable amount of emergency care for all age groups. A program to subsidize dental expenses in communities that do not have a resident dentist has been developed in British Columbia; in rural Alberta, dentists who volunteer to supply services on a private practice basis for short periods are provided with dental equipment, office facilities, and living accommodation. In some provinces, the dental health division of the provincial health department administers school dental programs. This responsibility may be delegated either to the department of education or to the board of health, particularly in cities.

In all of these models, dentists or dental hygienists are employed to carry out functions such as case finding, education, prevention, and treatment. Such services are generally provided to preschool children or up to grade one or two. Treatment services are offered primarily to children from lower income groups.

Environmental Health

Public health inspectors hired by local health units protect the public from physical, chemical, and biological hazards. This is carried out through the inspection of food-handling premises such as restaurants, butcher shops, and bakeries. Public health inspectors are responsible for community sanitation such as the maintenance of sanitary supplies of potable water, milk, and food, disposal of wastes, and the quality of recreational water. They also respond to public complaints and emergency situations such as spills of toxic chemicals. In some of the larger cities, indoor air pollution monitoring is carried out by public health units. A number of health units have hired environmental specialists to conduct environmental risk assessments and provide consultation for their staff.

Population Health Assessment

Population health refers to the health of a population as measured by health status indicators, described in Chapter 3. The belief that social, economic, and environmental conditions have a great deal of influence over health has been integral to public health since the beginnings in the 18th century. Epidemiologists assess the health indicators for populations and sub-populations that are necessary for the linked functions of effective public health practice, health promotion, disease and injury prevention, and health protection.

Health Surveillance

Health surveillance is the tracking and forecasting of any health event or health determinant through the collection of data and its integration, analysis and interpretation into surveillance products, and the dissemination of those surveillance products to those who need to know (25). Similar to population health assessment, health surveillance capacity is an integral part of public health, as it provides essential knowledge for the planning of effective interventions. It too is carried out by epidemiologists.

6.   HOME CARE

Home care in Canada is often defined as "an array of services enabling Canadians, incapacitated in whole or in part, to live at home, often with the effect of preventing, delaying, or substituting for long-term care or acute care alternatives" (26). Homecare services comprise medical and support services provided in the home setting to meet the needs of individuals and their families and volunteer caregivers. Generally, a homecare program substitutes for services provided by hospitals and long-term care facilities, serves as a maintenance function so clients can remain in their current environment rather than moving to a new and often more costly venue, and serves as a prevention function by providing patient services and monitoring at additional short-run but lower-run costs (27).

Publicly funded homecare programs exist in every province and territory in Canada. Nationally, home care accounts for 3.3% of the total public healthcare expenditures. Because home care is not included in the *Canada Health Act 1984*, its services are not insured in the same way as hospital and physician services. Homecare policies and their delivery vary across the country (28).

Most current health reform aims to strengthen and expand community-based and home-based care. This shift away from hospital-based care is motivated in part by fiscal constraints (home care is purportedly less expensive than institutional care) and in part by the belief that services provided in the home effectively meet the needs and preferences of patients, especially among the elderly. Only a small percentage of provincial health budgets are allocated to home care, but most provinces have increased these budgets in recent years.

6.1.   HISTORY

Until early in the 20th century, the rich were cared for at home and the poor, homeless, or indigent were treated in hospitals. With the emergence of provincial and national health insurance plans and the resulting expansion in the institutional sector, homecare functions were transferred to hospitals and nursing homes. However, this pattern has gradually been reversing in the past 20 years. In most provinces, provision of homecare services began with smaller, urban programs run by agencies such as the Victorian Order of Nurses (26). As a result of rising hospital costs and pressure on hospital facilities, homecare programs were developed, mainly to relieve hospitals of the care of patients who only needed additional nursing services or physiotherapy. Some provinces developed comprehensive, government-oriented homecare plans in the 1970s. In 1977, as a part of the Extended Program Financing services, legislation provided the first concrete financial support for homecare programs (see Chapter 12). By the late 1990s, all provinces and territories had government homecare directorates or divisions, although there is no common approach to funding and delivery. For example, Veterans Affairs Canada offers homecare services to clients with wartime or special duty area service when the service is not available to them through provincial and territorial programs. Health Canada's Territorial region, created in 1998, is responsible for the delivery of various community-based programs to Aboriginal people in the three territories.

It still remains unclear whether the development and strengthening of homecare programs is an effective cost-saving measure for provincial budgets, or whether it is currently an added cost to health systems, and a transfer of cost to patients and their families. In 2000, more than 1 million Canadians were enrolled in homecare programs across Canada. Greater demand for home care has resulted over the years due to a number of different factors, including:

- improved technology that allows for the delivery of services in the community (e.g., home-based dialysis);
- increase in outpatient surgery, earlier hospital discharges, and reduction in long-term and acute care hospital beds;
- patients' desire to have care delivered closer to home be it in the community or in the home;
- increasing average life expectancy, particularly among the baby boomers;

- decreased availability of informal care-giving by family members due to changing family structure, and work patterns (19, 27).

6.2. TYPES OF HOME CARE

Different basic forms of home care are described below.

Maintenance and Preventive

Home support services (such as homemaker, transportation, and meals-on-wheels programs) provide autonomy and mobility for those with assessed functional deficits. These services are not primarily medical, and may be provided along with medical treatment. Although many people can remain at home without the help of these services for some time, early use of the services can prevent health decline and institutionalization.

Long-Term Care Substitution or Chronic Care Services

Long-term care substitution or chronic care services are provided to people with significant functional deficits, usually resulting from one or more medical conditions, who require these services in order to remain in their homes. Chronic care services are designed for people with stable conditions, or designed to delay deterioration and thus institutionalization.

Acute Care Substitution

Acute home care is usually provided after hospitalization to people who are unable to travel to outpatient facilities, and is provided on a short-term basis according to need. It is designed to reduce the length of hospital stay and to assist the recovery process. People usually receive acute home care from two or three days to a maximum of 90 days.

Extra-Mural Hospital or Hospital without Walls

Founded in 1981, this New Brunswick program was Canada's first government-funded home-hospital program. The mandate of the Extra-Mural Program (EMP) is to provide a broad range of home healthcare services to all residents for the purpose of promoting, maintaining, and restoring health within the context of their daily lives, and to provide palliative services. It is administered free of charge to a case-load equivalent to that of a 200-bed hospital. Services include a range of palliative and acute care services such as nursing, physiotherapy, intravenous medication, nutritional counselling, respiratory care oxygen therapy, and sick room equipment. Meals-on-wheels, homemaking, and other support services can be purchased by the patient, who must be formally admitted by an attending physician who directs the medical care plan and authorizes discharge. Nursing services are available 24 hours a day, seven days a week, while all other disciplines deliver services Monday to Friday. To be eligible, the patient must be acutely but not critically ill, and must require one or more professional services such as nursing, occupational therapy, or physiotherapy. Thirty service delivery sites provide the delivery of EMP services to clients across the entire province.

Palliative Home Care

Palliative home care is provided to terminally ill patients such as those with AIDS or cancer. Palliative care is provided by a multidisciplinary team at home and is described in greater detail below.

6.3.   FUNDING AND DELIVERY

Two features characterize most homecare programs: centralization of control of services within the program and ongoing coordination of services to meet the changing needs of the patient. In all provinces except Nova Scotia and Ontario, the regional health authorities are responsible for administration of home care programs. In 1998, the Ontario Ministry of Health and Long-term Care consolidated 38 homecare programs and 36 placement coordination services when it established 43 Community Care Access Centres (CCACs) across the province. CCACs are to provide a single point of access to the long-term care system including both home care and facility-based care. There is also a substantial private sector component to home care with services financed directly by the patient or family.

At present, spending on homecare programs accounts for approximately 3.3% of total public spending in the Canadian health system. Most provincial homecare programs are funded by the government, but some charge user fees, often based on the ability to pay (28). For example, in British Columbia, all public homecare programs are fully or partially funded by the Home and Community Branch of the Ministry of Health Services. Homecare services such as case management, home nursing care, and community rehabilitation are provided to those who qualify at no charge, while the homemaker services charge people according to income testing.

All provinces offer a similar range of basic services (29): client assessment, case coordination, case management, nursing services, and home support, including personal care, homemaking, Meals-on-Wheels, and respite services. Other services, such as rehabilitation services (e.g., physiotherapy, occupational therapy), oxygen therapy, respirology, and specialized nursing services are in development as part of home care in some provinces. Seven provinces have contracts for oxygen therapy services (British Columbia, Alberta, Saskatchewan, Manitoba, Ontario, New Brunswick, Nova Scotia). Social work, speech therapy, and dietician services are offered as part of some homecare programs. There is a greater emphasis placed on applying a multidisciplinary approach to care in some jurisdictions. Overall service delivery models are undergoing review and/or change in some provinces (including British Columbia, Ontario, and Quebec).

There are four basic models of provincial and territorial homecare programs, presented below (29). In each case, single-entry functions include assessment, case management, and discharge planning; and professional services include nursing, occupational therapy, and physiotherapy.

- Single-entry functions are delivered by public employees or staffs of publicly funded community agencies, while professional services and home support are contracted.
- Single-entry functions plus some professional services are delivered by public employees. However, some nursing services and home support services are contracted out either province-wide or in certain regions (as in Nova Scotia, and in most of Manitoba, where therapy services are contracted by agency and, in Winnipeg, where most nursing services and a small portion of home support services are contracted).
- Single-entry functions plus all professional services are delivered by public employees (as in New Brunswick, Newfoundland and Labrador, British Columbia, Alberta). Home support services are contracted out by agency or client in most instances.
- Single-entry functions and professional and home support services are mainly delivered by public employees (as in Saskatchewan, Quebec, Prince Edward Island, Yukon, Northwest Territories).

In 2003, the First Ministers' Accord on Health Care Renewal agreed to provide preliminary coverage for a basket of services that, when provided at home, are more appropriate and less expensive than acute hospital care and include acute community mental health care and end-of-life care (11). This will supplement homecare programs and make home care a core service.

7. PALLIATIVE CARE

According to a recent Senate report, more than 220,000 Canadians die each year; 75% of those deaths occur in people over 65 years of age, 75% take place in hospital and long-term care facilities, and each one potentially affects the well-being of an average of five other people. An estimated 5% of dying Canadians receive integrated and interdisciplinary palliative care; most recipients of palliative care are those with cancer, even though cancer accounts for only 25% of total deaths (30). As many as 90% of Canadians would prefer to die at home, close to their families, living as normally as possible.

Palliative care is a relatively new field in Canada, having emerged in 1974, and the demand is increasing (31). In recent years many provinces have responded to the need of palliative care programs in their jurisdiction; however, there is a dearth of palliative care programs, particularly in rural settings and Aboriginal communities, for children, and for those responding to the needs of cultural communities.

Palliative care or end-of-life care, also called comfort care, is a special kind of health care for individuals and families living with a life-threatening illness that is usually at an advanced stage. The goal for palliative care is comfort and dignity for the person living with the illness as well as the best quality of life for both this person and his or her family. An important objective of palliative care is relief of pain and other symptoms. Palliative care is planned to meet the physical needs as well as the psychological, social, cultural, emotional, and spiritual needs of each person and the family (32). The goal is not to cure, but to provide comfort and maintain the highest possible quality of life for as long as life remains. The focus is on compassionate specialized care for the living.

Terminal care refers to care delivered at the end of life and reflects only a portion of all of palliative care. Palliative care may be delivered in hospice and homecare settings or in hospitals.

Hospices are residential facilities — separate buildings or apartments where palliative care is provided in a home-like setting. Some people move into hospices to receive palliative care on a 24-hour basis. Because medical needs vary depending on the disease that is leading toward death, specialized palliative care programs exist for common conditions such as cancer and AIDS. Specialized care giving is also needed if organic changes in the brain lead to coma and dementia.

Palliative care is well suited to an interdisciplinary team, often supplemented by volunteers, that provides support for the whole person and those who are sharing the person's journey. Palliative care should involve psychological support, assistance in interpersonal skills, coordinated service delivery, symptom control, bereavement counselling, independent living, counselling in legal and financial issues, and counselling in matters of spirituality, lifestyle, culture, and religion (33, 34). It can be given in the home or in an institutional setting. Acute care facilities, which are geared to diagnosis and treatment, do not usually have the environment, skills, and flexibility needed to provide support to terminally ill patients and their families unless specialized facilities are available, such as designated palliative care beds and a palliative care team (35). As stated in the homecare section, palliative homecare is finally recognized as part of the core services.

8.   SERVICES FOR MENTAL ILLNESS

Mental health services, broadly defined, comprise a mix of health, social, vocational, recreational, volunteer, occupational therapy, and educational services, as well as housing and income support. They include activities and objectives ranging from mental health promotion and the prevention of mental health problems to the treatment of acute psychiatric disorders and the support and rehabilitation of persons with severe and persistent psychiatric disorders and disabilities. The morbidity, mortality, and economic burden associated with mental illness are described in Chapter 5 and 7. In Canada, the provincial and territorial governments have primary jurisdiction in the planning and delivery of mental health services. Most provinces have a separate branch or department dealing with mental health and are either part of the ministry of health or community services or an independent ministry. For detailed programs and services provided by the provinces, readers are advised to visit provincial government Web sites.

Among provincially operated health services, mental health services represent one of the largest administrative areas in terms of expenditure and employees. In every province, at least 88% (nationally, 96%) of the revenue for mental institutions comes from the provincial government or the provincial insurance plan. For the past four decades, the provision of mental health services has gradually shifted from institutions to community-based services. Depending on the nature and the severity of illness, services are now provided by mental institutions, psychiatric units of general hospitals, special hospitals, private hospitals, clinics, mental healthcare centres, prisons, halfway houses, sheltered workshops, and private practitioners such as psychiatrists, family physicians, clinical psychologists, and social workers. Interested readers are advised to refer to *Mental Health Care in Canada*, which provides an excellent review and looks at the challenges in the mental health service delivery system (36).

Community mental health facilities are now extended beyond mental institutions to provide greater continuity of care, to deal with incipient breakdown, and to rehabilitate patients in the community. Psychiatric units in general hospitals contribute by integrating psychiatry with other medical care and making it available in the community. Hospital psychiatric units admit approximately 86% of total admissions to all kinds of mental institutions (37). Inpatient services in psychiatric units are paid for by all provincial hospital insurance plans. Some provinces have small regional psychiatric hospitals that facilitate patient access to treatment and complete integration of medical services. There are daycare centres across the country that allow patients to be hospitalized during the day and return home at night, as well as community mental health clinics (some provincially operated, others municipally) and psychiatric outpatient services.

Specialized rehabilitation services, which assist former patients to function optimally, are operated by mental hospitals and community agencies. They include sheltered workshops that pay for work and provide training, and halfway houses where patients can live and continue to receive treatment while settling in jobs. At present, there is a large gap in available community services for mental health patients because of shortages of affordable housing, jobs, recreational facilities, and mental health workers.

Facilities for people who are mentally challenged include day training schools or classes, summer camps, and sheltered workshops, as well as residential care in institutions and community group homes. These provide social, academic, and vocational training; some offer academic education, some support self-care, some teach manual skills, and some help find job placements in the community. Children with personality or behaviour disorders are treated at hospital units, community clinics, child guidance clinics, and other outpatient facilities.

At least 2% to 5% of adult Canadians are addicted to licit and illicit drugs, alcohol, and gambling. Substance abuse and addiction are treated in hospitals, outpatient clinics, hostels, long-term residences, or special facilities. Official and voluntary agencies conduct public education programs, treatment, rehabilitation, and research, including Alcoholics Anonymous, the Alcoholism Foundation of British Columbia, Quebec's l'Office de la prévention et du traitement de l'alcoolisme et des autres toxicomanies, the Addictions Foundation of Manitoba, and the Nova Scotia Alcoholism Research Foundation. The Narcotic Addiction Foundation of British Columbia and the Addiction

Research Foundation of Ontario, supported primarily by provincial funds, have established community treatment programs. However, there are not enough available services for addiction.

9.   SERVICES FOR CANCER PATIENTS

More than one in three Canadians will get cancer in his or her lifetime; most will be diagnosed in their middle and later years. Between 1972 and 2001, the number of new cancer cases diagnosed in Canada every year has more than doubled (38). According to the National Cancer Institute of Canada, in 2001 there were an estimated 134,000 new cases of cancer and 65,000 deaths from cancer in Canada. Special provincial agencies for cancer control, usually run by the health ministry or a separate cancer institute, carry out cancer detection and treatment, public education, and professional training and research, in cooperation with local public health services, physicians, and voluntary Canadian Cancer Society branches (e.g., the Alberta Cancer Board, the British Columbia Cancer Agency). Although the provisions are not uniform, cancer programs in all provinces provide a range of free diagnostic and treatment services both to outpatients and to inpatients. Hospital insurance benefits for cancer patients include diagnostic radiology, laboratory tests, and radiotherapy. A number of provinces, including British Columbia, Ontario, Quebec, New Brunswick, and Nova Scotia, have organized screening programs for breast cancer for women.

The lack of uniform provision of services, however, results in differences in community cancer services between provinces and between communities. This can result in a lack of coordination of treatment and less than optimal dissemination of cancer treatment knowledge and information in the major centres.

10.   SERVICES FOR PERSONS WITH SPECIAL NEEDS

Social and support services are available in the community for people with special, multidisciplinary needs (such as seniors, or people with mental or physical challenges) and vary depending on the location of the community and the nature and type of disability. Overall, rural communities have sparse services, whereas metropolitan areas offer a full range of services. People with rare or very severe disabilities have fewer resources available for their care in the community. Medical and institutional care, such as long-term care in hospitals, extended care, rehabilitation care, and nursing home care, as well as many assistive devices for daily living, are available through either government insurance or subsidies and have been described in Chapter 13. Most communities have homecare programs available for those with multiple needs. In addition, the provinces are increasingly establishing "one-stop" access centres (such as multiple service agencies) to evaluate, assess, coordinate, and provide (or contract for the provision of) a wide range of health, social, and support services to seniors or people with disabilities. There are two types of voluntary agencies that deal specifically with people with mental or physical challenges: agencies that exclusively deal with people with a specific disease or problem (e.g., the Multiple Sclerosis Society), and agencies that deal with specific groups with a disability (e.g., the Easter Seal Society, which deals with children with physical disabilities). Depending on the special needs of each individual, many voluntary agencies also provide a range of services, such as Meals-on-Wheels, visiting homemaker services, travelling clinics, provision of appliances and equipment, and wheelchairs. At the social services level, there are income maintenance programs, recreational programs, vocational rehabilitation services, special transportation services, and independent living accommodations available for individuals (see Chapter 13).

11. VOLUNTARY AGENCIES

Voluntary organizations play an important part in shaping our health, welfare, and educational systems. These are non-profit organizations led by boards of volunteers rather than under the direct control of the government. Their primary or major objectives are the promotion of health, the prevention of illness or disability, and the identification, treatment, or rehabilitation of people with a disease or disability. Voluntary organizations differ in the nature of their membership: some are organized by citizens to provide service to others and are designated as citizen-member organizations; more recently, groups have been organized by patients and their relatives and their friends to provide services for themselves, and hence are designated patient-member organizations.

The citizen-member organization is the familiar form of philanthropy. Its members are interested in community service and thus are motivated to give time, thought, and money to accomplish an objective to promote the welfare of their community. Patient-member organizations are motivated by mutual aid. Those who have a disease for which there is now no known cure or have a disability that causes them to be different from, and even shunned by, other people often become isolated and withdrawn or seek the company of fellow sufferers. They are faced with anxieties and frustration from which they find some relief by uniting to fight their common enemy, the disease. The patients may be able to help themselves in specific ways (e.g., by organizing better treatment facilities) or they may hope to help other sufferers, including their families if the disease is hereditary. They gain support from the knowledge that they are not alone in facing their problems. Recently, some groups such as AIDS groups have taken an advocacy role.

Voluntary organizations are financed to a considerable extent, if not wholly, by fundraising. The organization may conduct its own campaign for funds, or be a member of a federated fund. Many of the agencies also receive public grants.

Objectives and Activities

Generally, the objectives and activities of many voluntary organizations include (39):
- *education:* public education and dissemination of information to lay and professional people;

- *advocacy:* social action, sometimes specified, sometimes implied;
- *research:* collection of statistics, investigation of reported cures, surveys of resources and needs, encouragement and support for basic and clinical research;
- *direct patient services:* supply of diagnostic and treatment clinics, special equipment (e.g., wheelchairs, crutches, colostomy bags, hoists, inhalation tents, prosthetic appliances), transportation and accommodation for patient and family, home treatment, therapies, vocational assessment and workshops; some take on official functions (e.g., the Children's Aid Society) and provide many services needed by society, including eye banks and first aid;
- *prevention:* the prevention and eradication of the disease or disability;
- *coordination of key players:* the coordination of public and private agencies with similar interests; and
- *fundraising.*

Role in Relation to Government

Voluntary agencies continually identify new areas of need and provide for those needs to the limit of their capacity. This capacity relates directly to the agency's ability to raise money and, in some cases, needs are only barely met. Nevertheless, the organizations often are able to impress upon the public's mind the importance of the services they provide and occasionally change the public's sensitivity to needs. In the past, with increasing affluence and heightened social conscience, governments recognized that many of these initiatives were universally needed for the care of citizens and hence funded or took over the responsibilities of many volunteer organizations' services. However, in recent years, this trend has reversed and there is increased reliance on the voluntary sector. In practice, the functions of voluntary organizations and the government in the healthcare field intermingle to such an extent that at times there is little differentiation in function, which may create tension between the government and voluntary organizations.

Scope of Work

Examples of national voluntary organizations are presented here.

The Canadian Red Cross Society was established to furnish volunteer aid to the sick and wounded of armies in time of war, in accordance with the Geneva Convention, and in times of peace or war to carry on and assist in the improvement of health, the prevention of disease, and the mitigation of suffering throughout the world. Activities include veterans' services, international relief, emergency services, water safety services, Red Cross Youth, and Red Cross Corps. (As of 1997, the Canadian Red Cross is no longer involved in the provision of blood transfusion services in Canada.)

The Canadian Cancer Society was established in 1938 to coordinate individuals and agencies to reduce the mortality from cancer in Canada, to disseminate information on cancer, and to research activities about cancer.

Local volunteer groups include local chapters of larger organizations, as well as volunteer organizations that meet special needs in the community. These include volunteer groups working in hospitals, nursing homes, and crisis centres.

Voluntary agencies have adapted to the changing needs of society. For example, what was once known as the Canadian Tuberculosis Association has changed its name and mandate, with the decreasing incidence of tuberculosis, to the Canadian Tuberculosis and Respiratory Disease Association; its Ontario chapter calls itself the Ontario Lung Association and focuses on all lung diseases. Voluntary health organizations fulfil an important role in shaping the healthcare system and in recent years have taken up the burden of many of the services previously provided by the governments.

12. SELF-HELP GROUPS

People join together in groups for companionship, mutual assistance, and the exchange of problem-solving skills. The most obvious example of the self-help concept is the family, a small group where socialization, identification, and support originate. Self-help efforts are also evident in collective enterprises such as food or housing cooperatives, tenants' associations, and civil rights groups. But groups also exist for those who have a common personal concern, such as a physical disability or an addiction. Self-help groups can be defined as small, autonomous, open groups that meet regularly (40). Members share common experiences and meet each other as equals. The primary activity of these groups is personal mutual aid, a form of social support that focuses on sharing experiences, information, and ways of coping. In addition to personal change, members often engage in activities directed to social change. Group activities are voluntary and usually free. In some cases, there is already a national or international body of self-help groups focused on a given concern, and this may offer consultative and public relations support to new self-help groups or associations. Alcoholics Anonymous, established in 1935, has been the model for the development of other self-help groups (e.g., Narcotics Anonymous, Schizophrenics Anonymous).

Self-help groups usually attract members who are between 30 and 50 years of age, from the middle class or a common educational level or socioeconomic status. For many people with many types of difficulties, such groups can be very effective for coping with personal pressures. The major activities of these groups include group meetings, sponsorship of new members, educational activities for their members and the general public, and advocating for change. Apart from these general services, activities are as diverse as the groups themselves. They include home or hospital visits to the sufferer, hot lines, newsletters and brochures, public conferences, fairs, advocacy, recreational activities, and material aid (e.g., sitter services, transportation, exchange of goods). There are a number of support groups that help persons with specific health conditions, such as AIDS, breast cancer, and prostate cancer.

13. TELEHEALTH

Telehealth can refer to an array of technical applications, tools, and processes but is generally defined as the use of information and communications technology to deliver health care, health education, and health information over large and small distances. There are many different types of telehealth applications. **Telemedicine** is the delivery of medical services at a distance. Canada has the world's longest-running telemedicine service at the Memorial University of Newfoundland. **Health information networks and inter-institutional networks** (also known as health infostructure) enable institutions and individuals to exchange electronic health records and share information systems and databases to collect or deliver health information at a distance. **Tele-education** and multimedia applications can be used for professional and patient education and research. Other examples of telehealth applications include call centres (known as telecare or teletriage), telemonitoring, and telehomecare. The overall Canadian strategy is to use the tools of telecommunications and information technology to enhance the delivery of health care, and to share health information and expertise.

Telehealth networks in rural, northern, and remote communities are designed to overcome the challenges faced in delivering healthcare services to these communities. For example, the Yukon government is in partnership with the British Columbia and Alberta governments to establish a telehealth information and services network in six Yukon communities. All sites are to be equipped with video-conferencing workstations and technology that allows for the transmission of medical images over a secure network to specialists in urban centres. In addition these technologies will be used to deliver telehealth services and programs such as tele-mental health, tele-learning, and X-ray emergency support (41). Most provinces, including Quebec, New Brunswick, Nova Scotia, and Ontario, have programs for telehealth to serve its rural and remote communities.

The federal government funded the National First Nations Telehealth Research Project from 1998 to 2000 to test and evaluate telehealth's ability to improve both access to high-quality health care and the cost-effective delivery of health services in the First Nations communities (42). It was found to benefit communities by improving access to quality health services, reducing transportation costs, helping to overcome patient isolation, and enhancing the community's capacity building by providing employment and training opportunities. Benefits to healthcare providers included professional support, reduced professional isolation, continuing education and training, and improved standards of care. Telehealth also helps patients to find their way around the healthcare system and to get the health information they need.

14. SUMMARY

Health care is delivered at the local level through a variety of services, including primary care, secondary care, hospital care, home care, public health services, mental health care, and public and private nursing homes. The funding sources for these services are diverse. Although basic hospital and medical services in every province and territory are provided through government health insurance plans, what is provided either through public or private insurance varies.

Primary health care is service provided at the first contact between the patient and the healthcare professional and is usually provided by general or family practitioners in their offices on a fee-for-service basis. Most physicians bill provincial health insurance plans for their services. Apart from the physician, there are a number of other healthcare professionals who provide primary health care (including dentists, nurses, chiropractors, optometrists, podiatrists, and physiotherapists). Walk-in clinics that offer primary care are becoming increasingly popular.

Specialized practitioners using specialized resources usually deliver secondary care. Patients usually receive secondary care after referral from a primary care provider. Tertiary care requires very specialized facilities and professional skills.

Today, hospitals are the major centre for healthcare services. They provide inpatient services, services for ambulatory patients in outpatient clinics, emergency rooms, and rehabilitation services. Hospitals are classified on the basis of the kind of the service they provide, and are paid by the provincial government. In most provinces a regional board governs them. Hospitals usually have a chief executive officer, president, or administrator who is in charge of day-to-day operations and executes policies formulated by the regional board. Most physicians are considered users of hospitals via hospital privileges rather than as employees of the hospital.

With the advent of *regionalized health authorities* (RHAs) in all provinces except Ontario, provincial governments transfer a lump sum of money to RHAs to cover the costs of providing health care to their population, with the exception of money needed to cover physicians' services. The regional authorities decide how much money is allocated to institutional care and how hospitals in their region are reimbursed. Payment methods to hospital include line-by-line funding, ministerial discretion, population-based funding, a global budget, and service-based funding, often referred to as a "case-mix-based approach."

Health units are semi-autonomous in nature and form liaisons with local hospitals, medical practitioners, and voluntary health agencies. Their functions depend on the mandate set out by the provincial public health act and funding, and include the control of communicable disease, maternal and child health services, health promotion, dental health, and environmental health.

Recently, there has been increasing emphasis on home care. The services delivered by the homecare programs range from nursing services to an array of health and social services. There are four basic models for home care: the maintenance and preventive model, the long-term care substitution model, the acute care substitution model, and palliative care model. Most provincial homecare programs are funded by the provincial or territorial government; some charge user fees, often based on the ability to pay.

Mental health activities represent one of the largest administrative areas in terms of expenditure and employees. Community mental health facilities are reaching beyond mental health institutions to provide greater continuity of care, deal with incipient breakdown, and rehabilitate patients in the community. Currently, funding is not adequate to meet the needs of de-institutionalized patients.

The availability of social and support services in the community for people with disabilities depends on the location of the community and the nature and type of disability. Most communities have homecare programs available for people with disabilities.

Voluntary organizations have played and continue to play an important part in shaping our health, welfare, and educational systems. These non-profit organizations operate under boards of volunteers, with the primary or major objectives being the promotion of health, the prevention of illness or disability, and the identification, treatment, or rehabilitation of people with disease or disability.

Self-help groups are small, autonomous, open groups that meet regularly. As a result of personal crisis or chronic problems, members share common experiences and meet each other as equals. The primary activity of these groups is personal mutual aid, a form of social support that focuses on the sharing of experiences, information, and ways of coping.

Telehealth involves the use of communications technology to improve access, offer support and enhance the efficiency and effectiveness of many dimensions of health care, health education, and health information. There are many different types of telehealth applications.

15.   REFERENCES

1.   Tonkin R. Primary health care. *Canadian Journal of Public Health* 1976; 67(4):289-94.
2.   Martin S. More hours, more tired, more to do: Results from the CMA's 2002 Physician Resource Questionnaire. *Canadian Medical Association Journal* 2002; 167(5):521-2.
3.   Milne C. Parcelling out primary care. *Medical Post* 2001, March 6. <www.medicalpost.com/mdlink/english/members/medpost/data/3709/41A.HTM> (November 2002).
4.   Vayda E. Physicians in health care management: 5. Payment of physicians and organization of medical services. *Canadian Medical Association Journal* 1995; 150(10):1583-8.
5.   Barnsley J, Williams A, Kaczorowski J, *et al.* Who provides walk-in services? Survey of primary care practices in Ontario. *Canadian Family Physician* 2002; 48:519-26.
6.   Williams A, Barnsley J, Vayda E, *et al.* Comparing the characteristics and attitudes of physicians in different primary care settings: The Ontario walk-in-clinic study. *Family Practice* 2002; 19(6):647-57.
7.   Shah C, Moloughney B. 2001. *A strategic review of the community health centre program.* <www.gov.on.ca/MOH/english/pub/ministry/chc_stratreview/chc_review.html> (March 2003).
8.   Hutchinson A, Abelson J, Lavis J. Primary care in Canada: So much innovation, so little change. *Health Affairs* 2001; 20(3).
9.   Health Canada. 2002. *Primary Health Care Transition Fund: Frequently asked questions.* <www.hc-sc.gc.ca/phctf-fassp/english/faq.html> (October 2002).
10.   Chodos H. *Quebec's Health Review (The Clair Commission).* Ottawa: Parliamentary Research Branch, 2001. Report No. PRB 00-37E. <dsp-psd.pwgsc.gc.ca/Collection-R/LoPBdP/BP/prb0037-e.htm> (November 2002).
11.   Health Canada. 2003. *First Ministers' Accord on Health Care Renewal.* <www.hc-sc.gc.ca/english/hca2003/accord.html> (February 2003).
12.   Canadian Institute for Health Information. *Health care in Canada, 2000: A first annual report.* Ottawa: Canadian Institute for Health Information, 2000. <www.cihi.ca> (November 2002).

13. Health Canada. 2002. *Canada Health Act annual report.* <www.hc-sc.gc.ca/medicare/ AnnualReports.htm> (November 2002).

14. Canadian Institute for Health Information. *Health personnel in Canada, 1991-2000.* Ottawa: Canadian Institute for Health Information, 2002. <www.cihi.ca> (November 2002).

15. Statistics Canada. 2002. *Contact with alternative health care providers, by age group and sex, household population aged 12 and over, Canada, 2000/01.* <www.statcan.ca/english/ freepub/82-221-XIE/00502/tables/html/4265.htm> (November 2002).

16. Millar WJ. Uses of alternative health care practitioners by Canadians. *Canadian Journal of Public Health* 1997; 88(3):154-8.

17. Collège des médecins du Québec. *ALDO-Quebec: Legislative, ethical, and organizational aspects of medical practice in Quebec.* Montreal: Collège des médecins du Québec, 1995.

18. Gamble P, Health Services Management Program, Ryerson University, 2002 (Personal Communication).

19. Kirby M, LeBreton M. 2002. *The health of Canadians: The federal role. Volume 6: Recommendations for reform.* Standing Senate Committee on Social Affairs, Science and Technology. <www.parl.gc.ca/37/2/parlbus/commbus/senate/com-e/soci-e/rep-e/ repoct02vol6-e.htm> (November 2002).

20. Leatt P, Vayda E, Williams JI, *et al. Medical staff organization in Canadian hospitals.* Ottawa: Canadian Hospital Association Press, 1987.

21. Leatt P, Lemieux-Charles L, Aird C, *et al. Strategic Alliances in Health Care.* Ottawa: Canadian College of Health Services Executives, 1996.

22. Gray C. CMA-cosponsored conference raises many questions about future of regionalized health care. *Canadian Medical Association Journal* 1995; 153(5):642-5.

23. Ontario Hospital Association, Government of Ontario, Canadian Institute for Health Information, *et al.* 2002. *Hospital report 2001: Acute care.* <secure.cihi.ca/hreports/research/ HospitalReport2001.pdf> (November 2002).

24. Last J. *A dictionary of epidemiology,* 4th edition. Oxford University Press, 2001.

25. Health Canada. 2002. *Network of health surveillance in Canada.* <www.hc-sc.gc.ca/pphb-dgspsp/csc-ccs/network_e.html> (November 2002).

26. Health Promotion and Services Branch. *Report on home care.* Ottawa: Ministry of Supply and Services, Health and Welfare Canada, 1990.

27. Canadian Home Care Association, Canadian Association for Community Care. 2002. *Sustaining Canada's health care system: The role of home and community care.* <www.cdnhomecare.on.ca/doc/What's%20New/finalengCACC5pginsert.pdf> (November 2002).

28. Canadian Home Care Association. 2002. *Home care information: Public home care programs.* <www.cdnhomecare.on.ca/info.php?id=4> (November 2002).

29. Health Canada. 2002. *Provincial and territorial home care programs: A synthesis for Canada.* <www.hc-sc.gc.ca/homecare/english/syn_2.html> (November 2002).

30. Carstairs S, Beaudoin G. 2000. *Quality end-of-life care: The right of every Canadian (final report).* <www.parl.gc.ca/36/2/parlbus/commbus/senate/com-e/upda-e/rep-e/repfinjun00-e.htm#PART%20I> (November 2002).

31. Vincent L, Dawson H, Trentowsky S, *et al.* Survey underscores challenge of planning palliative care services for cancer patients. *Ontario Medical Review* 1990; 57(10):17-22.

32. Health Canada. 2002. *Palliative Care: Info Sheet for Seniors.* <www.hc-sc.gc.ca/seniors-aines/pubs/palliative_care/pall_e.htm> (November 2002).

33. Health Services Directorate. *Palliative care service guidelines: Report of the Subcommittee on Institutional Program Guidelines.* Ottawa: Health Services and Promotion Branch, Health and Welfare Canada, 1989.

34. Royal Victoria Hospital. *The RVH manual on palliative hospital care.* Montreal: Royal Victoria Hospital, 1980.

35. Mount B. The problem of caring for the dying in a general hospital: The palliative care unit as a possible solution. *Canadian Medical Association Journal* 1976; 115(2):119-21.

36.   Bachrach L, Goering P, Wasylenki D. *Mental health care in Canada*. San Francisco: Jossey-Bass Publishers, 1994.
37.   Health Canada. 2002. *A report on mental illnesses in Canada*. Ottawa. <www.hc-sc.gc.ca/pphb-dgspsp/publicat/miic-mmac/pdf/men_ill_e.pdf> (October 2002).
38.   National Cancer Institute of Canada. 2001. *Canadian cancer statistics, 2001*. Toronto. <66.59.133.166/stats/maine.htm> (November 2002).
39.   Govan E. *Royal Commission on Health Services, Voluntary Health Organizations in Canada*. Ottawa: Ontario Queen's Printer, 1966.
40.   Romeder J. *The self-help way: Mutual aid and health*. Ottawa: Canadian Council on Social Development, 1989.
41.   Health Canada. 2002. *Yukon telehealth*. <www.hc-sc.gc.ca/ohih-bsi/about_apropos/chipp-ppics/proj/yktele_e.html> (November 2002).
42.   Health Canada. 2002. *First Nations and Inuit telehealth: Future opportunities*. <www.hc-sc.gc.ca/fnihb/phcph/telehealth/introduction.htm> (November 2002).

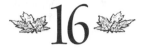

THE REGULATION AND HEALTH OF HEALTHCARE PROFESSIONALS

Canada's healthcare team includes a wide range of regulated and unregulated, and informal and volunteer caregivers. The largest group of unregulated healthcare providers consists of family members, friends, and community volunteers. According to Statistics Canada, 2.1 million adult Canadians provide support for one or more seniors in 1996. The Canadian Institute for Health Information (CIHI) has found that there are now more than 1.5 million people — approximately 10% of the total Canadian workforce — working in healthcare and social services (1).

More than 30 health professions are now regulated under legislation in at least one province or territory. Most healthcare providers work in hospitals, but this is changing as the sites of care move from the hospital into the community to include community clinics and client homes.

This chapter presents a synopsis of those regulated occupations directly involved with patient care. Before describing the various healthcare professions, para-professions, and allied occupations, it defines professionalism and offers a brief history of the modern medical profession, followed by a discussion of how different healthcare professions are regulated and future of regulatory trends. It also describes the health of healthcare workers.

1. PROFESSIONALISM

The concept of professionalism is very difficult to define. Most writers list traits or characteristics normally attributed to the established professions, and the significance assigned to those traits varies widely. According to Webster's Third International Dictionary the meaning of the word "profession" is "a calling requiring specialized knowledge and often long and intensive preparation including instruction in skills and methods as well as in the scientific, historical or scholarly principles underlying such skills and methods, maintaining by force of organization or concerted opinion, high standards of achievement and conduct, and committing its members to continued study and to a kind of work which has for its prime purpose the rendering of a public service." Most definitions emphasize the public service or altruistic aspect of professionalism.

This type of description is an idealized one (2) and, if one considers the influence wielded by the established professions, the above definition undoubtedly represents the image projected by the professions themselves. The following are characteristics commonly attributed to an established profession.

Specialized Knowledge and Skill

There is a specific body of detailed knowledge and complex skills, common and unique to the members of the profession, which require a lengthy period of training to acquire. Professionals' extensive education and the importance of their role in society entitle them to the confidence of their clients and to a position of prestige.

Autonomy

Professions are self-regulating, which means they are governed by organizations made up of members of the profession. The professional association sets standards for the practice of the profession, determines who is qualified to practise (licensing authority), and enforces uniformity of practice. A code of ethics is defined. The professional organization disciplines those who fail to meet the prescribed standard or who violate the code of ethics. Members are free to practice independently in the manner of their choice (within the aforementioned prescribed limits) and judgement in the best interests of their patients and are relatively free of bureaucratic control. Even those members who choose to be employed by institutions or corporations rather than practise privately are generally free to create their own roles (3).

Service Orientation

Professionals deal directly with their clients, and their prime concern is to provide good service rather than to pursue self-gain. This does not necessarily imply altruism, but simply that personal gain is secondary to service. The professional must be free of outside influence to be able to make unbiased decisions with only the client's welfare in mind.

Responsibility

The professional helps clients make informed decisions and also makes decisions on their behalf. In the case of medicine, these decisions may involve life or death. The clients trust the professional, and divulge confidential and privileged information. The professional must maintain an impersonal and objective approach.

Recognition

Members of established professions are recognized by the public as being "professional" and are accorded a certain degree of respect. In most cases, government also extends this recognition, so that the established professions are accorded formal status by statute.

However, non-professionals sometimes take exception to these characteristics of professions. The requirement of difficult and lengthy training, for example, is seen as an obstacle for entry into the profession that restricts membership to an elite group. Self-regulation, particularly with regard to licensing authority, is a means of establishing a monopoly (4). Licensed members of a profession practise under a protective cloak of presumed competence whether or not they actually are competent. Incompetence or unethical behaviour is rarely punished, and members of the profession are reluctant to criticize one another. Uniform norms of practice inhibit innovation.

Many people deny that there is any reliable evidence that professionals are more service oriented than are non-professionals. There is a strong movement, particularly in the way people deal with the medical profession, toward accepting greater responsibility for oneself and surrendering less control to the professional. Many question the power and prestige traditionally enjoyed by the established professions, especially the dominant role played by medicine.

The truth must lie somewhere between these opposite views of professionalism There is no question that established professions occupy positions of power and prestige in society. But social structure is dynamic. The medical profession in particular has not always enjoyed the pre-eminence that it does today, as is discussed in the next section. Furthermore, significant changes in both the status and the regulation of the professions are currently taking place.

2.   EVOLUTION OF THE MEDICAL PROFESSION

The practice of medicine is ancient, as evidenced by the trephined skulls of prehistoric humans, and the recorded histories of Babylon, Egypt, India, and China. However, the profession of medicine as it exists in the western world today is relatively recent. Western medicine had its beginnings in ancient Greece with Hippocrates and Aristotle, and with the founding of a Greek medical school in Alexandria in 300 B.C., which continued to operate during the heyday of the Roman Empire. After the fall of Rome, although the knowledge of the Greeks was preserved and translated by monks, little progress was made until the late Middle Ages. The practice of medicine was a trade learned by apprenticeship, with much the same status as other trades.

The first medical school in Europe was founded at Salerno, Italy, in the 11th century. In 1221, the Holy Roman Emperor, Frederick II, decreed that no one could practise medicine unless he had attended the school at Salerno. This seems to have been one of the earliest attempts at regulation. Later in the Middle Ages, medical faculties were established at universities in the major cities of western Europe. The first medical faculty at a university in the United Kingdom was founded in Edinburgh in 1726, and the first medical school in the United States opened in Philadelphia in 1766.

With the establishment of medical faculties at the medieval universities of western Europe, medicine joined the more traditional professions of law and theology as one of the "learned professions," and thus achieved some status. Although the mainstream of the medical profession was now formally trained at universities and medical schools, there was still little scientific basis to the art of medicine. The rapid expansion of scientific knowledge and the tremendous growth of universities that occurred in the late 1800s and early 1900s dramatically changed the practice of medicine. The scientific basis of medicine was established by the great discoveries of men such as Pasteur, Lister, and Koch. Medicine became ever more closely connected with science, particularly following the Flexner report on medical education in the United States and Canada published in 1910. Professional schools changed from institutions that had no prerequisites for admission to those that required high school graduation and then university training in the basic sciences. Professional courses lengthened from a few months of lectures to years of disciplined study. Concurrently, the effectiveness of treatment dramatically improved.

The physician became someone to be trusted and sought out in time of suffering, rather than one to be feared and avoided. At the same time, the great body of knowledge required to practise medicine increased the educational gulf between practitioners and patients, giving the profession an aura of mystique. All these factors combined to enhance the prestige of the profession. The profession also achieved considerable influence with governments, so that by the early 20th century, all western countries (except the then newly founded Soviet Union, which purposefully sought to decrease physician autonomy and equalize the status and prestige of all healthcare workers) had enacted legislation to make the medical profession self-regulating with powers of licensure and discipline. This act indicates that the state recognized its own responsibility with regard to the regulation of the medical profession, but delegated this responsibility to the profession. Once the statutes were in place, most states adopted a policy of non-interference and, in a sense, abdicated responsibility. There were no government representatives on the governing councils of the professional associations. The medical profession achieved virtual autonomy.

The last two decades have seen the beginnings of a reversal in the evolution of medical dominance described above (5). The scientific knowledge upon which medicine is based and the effectiveness of medical treatment have both continued to grow. Nevertheless, the authority of the profession, particularly the monopoly over service delivery and the degree of autonomy enjoyed for at least the last half century, has been increasingly questioned. There are several reasons for this. First, the increasing democratization of western societies has resulted in less deference to all forms of authority. Second, the great increase in the general level of education, especially among the large numbers of individuals employed in scientific disciplines and social sciences, has removed the mystique once associated with the profession. Third, consumer demand has achieved the recognition of alternative forms of health services delivery even when the state was not yet prepared to sanction them (e.g., the legal recognition of midwifery). Fourth, there is a growing perception that the profession is more interested in preserving its self-interest (dominance), which has created barriers to health reform.

In Canada, the most important de-professionalizing factor has undoubtedly been the establishment of government-sponsored universal medical insurance. Because the state pays for physician services, it has an obligation to its citizens to ensure that they receive good value for their tax money. The responsibility for regulating the practice of medicine, once delegated to the profession by the state, is now in the process of being taken back. Although the profession still enjoys considerable autonomy, it is becoming more accountable to government and consumers. However, others argue that medicare has institutionalized physician dominance as physicians make up the major professional group that is covered by medicare, again creating a barrier for entry into medicare for other professionals.

3. EVOLUTION OF OTHER HEALTHCARE PROFESSIONS

An industrializing society has been described as a professionalizing society. The rapid proliferation of knowledge in all fields of science and technology has, in recent decades, brought about the establishment of many new professions, some of which are in the healthcare field. In seeking professional status, these groups usually follow the model set by the older established professions. They develop complex technologies, establish lengthy periods of training, impose strict registration requirements, develop codes of ethics, and seek statutory recognition.

However, although many groups have been accorded professional status, it could be argued that few of them could be described in terms of the dictionary definition quoted earlier. The word "profession" seems to have become more narrowly associated with specialized knowledge, and there appears to be less emphasis on the characteristics of autonomy, service orientation, and responsibility. Most of the health-related non-physician groups have followed the same pattern established by medicine, but only dentistry has achieved a similar degree of autonomy. With the exception of nursing and midwifery, all have a much shorter history than medicine. For example, the world's first school of dentistry was established in Baltimore in 1840.

Medicine is the dominant profession in the health field. In achieving professional status, the mainstream of medicine eliminated, absorbed, or controlled competing disciplines. Pharmacy and nursing, for example, achieved professional status by becoming subordinate to medicine (6). Osteopathy, naturopathy, and homeopathy have remained separate entities, on the fringe of medicine and, in most communities, in restricted forms of practice. Optometrists and chiropractors have an autonomous status, but also are subject to many restrictions (e.g., practitioners cannot prescribe drugs or perform surgery). Most of the other healthcare professions and allied technical trades have developed as auxiliaries to medicine and are a product of the expansion of the scientific basis of medicine and the resulting need for division of labour. This is true, for example, of physiotherapy, laboratory technology, and radiation technology.

Canada's Health Care Providers lists 187 health programs offered in Canadian universities, colleges, and selected complementary health institutions; Table 16.1 provides a review of the status of licensing requirements in different provinces for the major healthcare providers) (1). Similarly, federal publications are available for certifying bodies, professional associations, and accrediting agencies for various healthcare occupations in Canada (7, 8). The next section of this chapter provides examples of how some of these professions are regulated in Quebec and Ontario.

Table 16.1.   Who is Regulated Where?

	NF	PE	NS	NB	QC	ON	MB	SK	AB	BC	YT	NT	NU
Dental hygienist	●	●	●	●	●	●	◆	●	●	●	●	●	●
Dentist	●	●	●	●	●	●	●	●	●	●	●	●	●
Licensed practical nursing assistants	●	●	●	●	●	●	●	●	●	●	●	●	●
Physicians	●	●	●	●	●	●	●	●	●	●	●	●	●
Optometrists	●	●	●	●	●	●	●	●	●	●	●	●	●
Pharmacists	●	●	●	●	●	●	●	●	●	●	●	●	●
Registered Nurses	●	●	●	●	●	●	●	●	●	●	●	●	●
Chiropractors	●	●	●	●	●	●	●	●	●	●	●		
Denturists	●		●	●	●	●	●	●	●	●	●	●	●
Psychologists	●	●	●	●	●	●	●	●	●	●		●	●
Ophthalmic dispensers, opticians	●	●	●	●	●	●	●	●	●	●			
Physical therapists, physiotherapists	●	●	●	●	●	●	●	●	●	●			
Occupational therapists	●	●	●	●	●	●	●	●	●	●			
Dental technicians, techonologists	●	●	●	●	●	●		●	●	●			
Dietians, nutritionists	●	●	●	●	●	✳	●	●	●				
Social workers	●	●	●	●	●	□	●	●	●	✪			
Chiropodists, podiatrists					●	●	●	●	●	●			
Medical radiation, radiological technologists		●	●	●	●		●	●					
Medical laboratory technologist					●	●	●		●	●			
Naturopathic physicians						●	●	●	○	●			
Respiratory therapists					●	●	●		●	◆			
Speech language pathologists & audiologists					●	●	●	●	●	○			
Midwives						●	●	●	○	●			

Notes:
●   regulated
○   legislation forthcoming
✪   regulated under *Social Workers Act*
□   self-regulated under Ministry of Community and Social Services
◆   not self-regulating
✳   Dietitians - yes; Nutritionists - no

Source: Adapted from *Health Policy & Communications Branch,* Health Canada, February 2000. © Reproduced with the permission of the Minister of Public Works and Government Services Canada, 2003.

More than 30 health professions are currently regulated in at least one province or territory. The table summarizes the status of regulation as of February 2000. Some changes have already occurred since then. For example, British Columbia recently became the first province to regulate Chinese medicine practitioners, who will be governed by the College of Acupuncturists of British Columbia.

4. REGULATION OF HEALTHCARE PROFESSIONS

The *Constitution Act of 1867* gave provincial governments the responsibility for health care, and as a result the legislation that regulates the activities of the various healthcare occupations is provincial. It follows then that there are 13 different groups of legislation (ten provincial and three territorial). Although they are generally similar, there are important differences. As already stated, the medical profession (and some other healthcare professions) in Canada had achieved autonomy prior to the introduction of universal medical insurance. Since then, most provinces have enacted, or intend to enact, legislation to ensure greater public control of the professions.

Until recently, most healthcare professions that required a license to practice defined their own distinct scope of practice. Scopes of practice set out the services that members of an occupation perform and the methods they use. The *Scopes of Practice*, published by the Canadian Medical Association, outlines the general principles and criteria, which have been endorsed both by the Canadian Public Health Association and the Canadian Nurses Association (9). There has been a move toward **task-based** regulatory models or a system of controlled acts. Under this approach, only tasks judged to carry serious risks of harm if performed incorrectly require a license. In 1993, Ontario became the first province to adopt a system of controlled acts. British Columbia and Alberta have adopted a similar framework (1, 10).

4.1. PROFESSIONAL CODE OF QUEBEC

Quebec's *Professional Code*, enacted in 1973, places the regulation of all professions under one act (11). A total of 45 professions are listed by the Office des professions du Québec, with 22 of them in the healthcare field (12). The Code is unique in that it defines what a profession is and establishes formal criteria by which an occupation gains statutory recognition as a profession. Each recognized profession is governed by a professional order (previously called a professional corporation). The order is charged with the traditional functions of a licensing agency. It determines the qualifications necessary to enter practice, including setting the length of training, examines candidates' credentials, maintains a register of members of the profession, defines the scope of practice, regulates specialists' certificates, determines what acts may be delegated, collaborates with educational institutions, and handles disciplinary matters within the profession. Under each governing legislation, acts are given exclusively to a profession, which could delegate an act to other professions; these are known as **delegated acts**.

In addition, because the order is first and foremost concerned with the protection of the public, it is responsible for the ongoing supervision of the practice of its profession and is given broad powers to supervise the practices of individual members. This is a significant innovation. Traditionally, professional regulatory bodies have only disciplined members whose unethical, improper behaviour, or incompetence has been reported by third parties. The Code requires each professional order to maintain ongoing surveillance of the quality of individual practices and take corrective measures, such as requiring refresher training. In addition, it ensures that the administration of any given profession is not conducted exclusively by the members of that profession. Non-members are appointed by the Office des professions and are there to represent the government and to protect the interests of the public. The disciplinary committee of each order handles disciplinary matters. The committee is informed of and investigates every complaint made against a member. It consists of at least three members and is chaired by a lawyer with at least ten years of practice and is appointed by the government. Professionals conducting the inquiry of their order into any complaint, as well as those testifying before a discipline committee hearing, are immune from prosecution.

There are two types of professions in Quebec: exclusive professions and those with reserved titles. In **exclusive professions** (*professions d'exercice exclusif*), only members who belong to recognized orders may use the title and perform professional acts exclusive to them by law (for example, nurses or doctors). In professions with **reserved titles** (*professions à titre réservé*), members belonging to the order have the exclusive use of the title, although they do not have the exclusive right to perform professional acts (for example, social workers or psychologists) (13). The Code also establishes two overall supervisory and regulatory bodies. The Office des professions du Québec is a governmental agency composed of five members appointed by the Lieutenant Governor-in-Council (the provincial Cabinet). It is responsible for ensuring that each order properly carries out its duty to protect the public. It monitors the performance of each order and takes corrective action when necessary. For example, it may require an order to issue a new regulation or revise an old one, and, if the order fails to do so, the board may act in its place. The Office reports directly to Cabinet. The second body is the Conseil interprofessionnel du Québec, made up of representatives from each of the professions covered by the Code. It coordinates the activities of the professional orders and deals with general issues encountered by all professional orders. It has no power to regulate, but can, of course, make recommendations to the Office des professions du Québec (14).

4.2.   REGULATED HEALTH PROFESSIONS ACT OF ONTARIO (1991)

Ontario's Regulated Health Professions Act (RHPA) was passed in 1991 but was not proclaimed until December 31, 1993, to allow the newly recognized professions time to organize themselves (15). The RHPA replaced the *Health Disciplines Act* of 1974, which had regulated only the professions of medicine, nursing, dentistry, pharmacy, and optometry. It increased the number of professions under its jurisdiction, including seven not previously covered. At present, there are 23 different professions regulated by 21 colleges under the RHPA (16).

The RHPA has been amended twice since passage (17) — first in 1993 to include regulations and sanctions for sexual abuse by healthcare professionals (discussed later in this chapter), and then in 1996 by the Omnibus legislation (Ontario Act 26) to allow the RHPA to comply with changes to the *Ontario Drug Benefit Act* and the *Prescription Drug Cost Regulation Act*. Like Quebec's *Professional Code*, the RHPA was enacted to obtain greater public accountability in the regulation of the healthcare professions. Many consider the RHPA to be progressive legislation. A "template from which many future legislative efforts in healthcare will evolve" (18), the RHPA increases equity within the healthcare professions by reducing the role of the physician as gatekeeper and increasing direct patient access to a wider variety of professionals. It allows for the growth of emerging healthcare professions, which can apply for regulation to raise their status. It allows for flexibility in reform and for the delegation of acts among healthcare professionals. Regulation is a separate issue from funding, however; although 23 healthcare professions are officially recognized and regulated in the RHPA, they are not all funded by the provincial health insurance plan (see Chapter 14).

The most progressive aspect of the legislation is that professionals are licensed to perform various **controlled acts** or tasks that are judged to carry serious risk of harm if performed incorrectly.

Only five of the professions — medicine, chiropractic, optometry, dentistry, and psychology — are licensed to diagnose, and the title "doctor" is also limited to these professionals. Other professionals are licensed only to assess and not diagnose. Neither diagnosis nor assessment is defined in the legislation, and interpretations are left for courts to determine. There are 13 controlled acts in total:

- communicating a diagnosis;
- performing a procedure on tissue below the dermis, below the surface of a mucous membrane, below the surface of the cornea, or below the surfaces of teeth, including scaling of teeth;
- setting or casting a fracture of a bone or dislocation of a joint;
- moving the joints of the spine beyond usual range of motion;
- administering a substance by injection or inhalation;
- applying or ordering a form of energy prescribed by regulations under the Act;
- putting an instrument, hand, or finger into a specified list of body orifices;
- prescribing, dispensing, selling, or compounding a drug as defined in the *Drug and Pharmacies Regulation Act*;
- prescribing or dispensing for vision or eye problems, contact lenses, or eyeglasses;
- prescribing a hearing aid;
- fitting or dispensing dental devices;
- managing labour or delivering a baby; and
- administering an allergy challenge test.

None of the regulated healthcare professions is authorized to perform all of these controlled acts (although physicians are authorized to perform 12 out of the 13, only fitting or dispensing dental devices falls outside their practice; some of them are not authorized to perform any of them, such as dieticians, speech and language pathologists, occupational therapists). However, sometimes these controlled acts can be delegated to others or performed under the supervision of a licensed individual. Furthermore, the same controlled act can come under the purview of more than one profession. For example, physicians, physiotherapists, and chiropractors are all authorized to manipulate the joints of the spine. These multiple authorizations were legislated in order to help break the monopoly that medicine had over healthcare services and allow people a greater range of healthcare providers when making decisions concerning their personal health. Traditional Aboriginal healers and Aboriginal midwives are exempt from the RHPA. Uncontrolled acts are open to all, including unregulated workers.

In addition to the controlled acts, the RHPA also specifies the **scope of practice** for a profession. Section 30(1) says: "No person, other than a member treating or advising within the scope of practice of his or her profession, shall treat or advise a person with respect to his or her health in circumstances in which it is reasonably foreseeable that serious physical harm may result from the treatment or advice or from an omission from them" (15). The Act also outlines the generic terms for authorized acts or, in other words, the activities a regulated healthcare professional may undertake once ordered to do so by a physician. One exception is people who perform acts that maintain the activities of daily living, such as insulin injections or colostomy changes. In its present form, the Act does not prohibit such "controlled acts" from being carried out by someone who does not fall under the jurisdiction of the RHPA, such as an acupuncturist.

The RHPA is structured so that individual acts regarding each profession's scope of practice and licensed acts follow a general section on legal and procedural provisions, which pertain to all the professions included in the Act. This allows for legislation to be coordinated instead of the previous patchwork of legislation. It gives the minister of health broad powers to supervise the regulation of all 23 disciplines, increasing their accountability and protecting the interests of the public. The emphasis is on the public good, rather than professional interests.

Each healthcare profession must constitute a college that is responsible for regulating the practice of its profession and governing its members in accordance with the RHPA (16). The college must maintain standards of entry, qualification, and practice, and must establish and maintain standards of competence and ethics among its members. Each college must have a governing council that excludes members of healthcare professions. The Lieutenant Governor in Council appoints public members to the council. Meetings of council, except in prescribed circumstances, are open to the public. In addition, a standard system of committees and a uniform method of handling licensing, hearings, and discipline are established for all colleges.

The statutory committee structure for each of the 23 professions included in the legislation is identical. There must be an executive committee, a registration committee, a complaints committee, a discipline committee, a fitness to practice committee, a continuing competence committee, a quality assurance committee, and a patient relations committee. The actual membership of each committee and quorum, however, differ; these are described under the specific profession.

The Health Disciplines Board established under the *Health Disciplines Act* continues as the Health Professions Board, an independent, appointed body of 12 to 20 members, none of whom is a healthcare professional, indicating greater participation by lay members in regulatory affairs. The Board acts as an appeals agency for decisions made by the complaints committees and the registration committees of each college. It does not hear appeals from the disciplinary committees; these are made directly to the Supreme Court of Ontario. The disciplinary committee chairperson can assign a panel of three to five members for a hearing, one of whom must be a member of the public.

The minister of health is the designated member of Cabinet who is responsible for administering the RHPA. The minister's duties are to ensure that the regulatory system works, and to focus both on the professions (making sure that they are regulated and coordinated in the public interest and that standards of practice are kept) and on consumers (ensuring freedom of choice of healthcare provider and that consumers are treated fairly and sensitively). To this end, the minister may conduct investigations into the operations of institutions or practices, may require reports to be submitted by the colleges, reviews proposed changes in college regulations, and may request that a college make, amend, or revoke regulations. If the college fails to do so, the minister may act in the college's place (through Cabinet). In practice, however, these powers are rarely exercised. In Quebec, these functions are carried out by the Office des professions du Québec, rather than directly by Cabinet.

At this point, a distinction should be made between licensing and certification. Certain healthcare professionals are required to be **licensed**; that is, they must hold a licence in order to practise their profession, and all others are prohibited from such practice. Other professions and occupations are **certified**. In some instances, certification is controlled by government regulations, in which case individuals are prohibited from using the relevant title or claiming to be qualified in the occupation unless they are appropriately certified and registered, such as a personal support worker. They are not necessarily prohibited from performing some functions of the occupation. In some occupations, certification (or registration) is granted by voluntary organizations. This type of certification has no legal status, but employers frequently hire only those who are certified by their national or provincial associations; an example is social workers, who are certified by the College of Social Workers.

Health Professions Regulatory Advisory Council

The Health Professions Regulatory Advisory Council (HPRAC) is an independent council, separate from both the Minister of Health and the professional colleges and created by the RHPA in order to facilitate ongoing policy development concerning the healthcare professions. Specifically, the duties of the HPRAC include: advising the minister of health on matters relating to regulating new healthcare professionals or deregulating existing ones, including changes in scope of practice and licensed acts; suggesting amendments to the Act and related regulations; and providing advice and policy guidance on any matter referred to it by the minister of health. Additionally, the HPRAC exercises supervisory functions, ensuring that the healthcare professionals (through their colleges) maintain good patient relations and effective quality assurance programs. The HPRAC is made up of five to seven lay people appointed by the Lieutenant Governor in Council, and excludes registered healthcare professionals and Ontario public servants.

The HPRAC also has a number of statutory evaluation responsibilities. It is required to report to the minister of health five years following proclamation of the RHPA on the effectiveness of each college with regard to complaints and discipline procedures, professional misconduct of a sexual nature, patient relations programs, and quality assurance programs.

These reviews have recently been completed for the first time and the HPRAC's comprehensive review of the RHPA, which was completed March 2001, concluded that the RHPA requires an adjustment in favour of greater transparency and accountability. The report was also in favour of supporting greater awareness by the public. It contained 67 recommendations that were made (19).

4.3.   MAJOR HEALTHCARE PROFESSIONS

Several of the major healthcare professions are described here, as well as their regulatory organizations in Ontario. Health human resources and issues related to their utilization, type, and the location of their practices and payment mechanisms are described in Chapter 14 and 15.

Medicine

Physicians are required to be licensed in all provinces. Although each provincial college has its unique requirements for licensors, a certain standard of uniformity has been established. All provinces require the physician to pass the national examination of the Medical Council of Canada plus examination by the Royal College of Physicians and Surgeons of Canada for specialists and, for family practice, by the College of Family Physicians of Canada (20). The example of Ontario is used here, as most provinces have similar structures.

In Ontario, the licensing agency is the College of Physicians and Surgeons of Ontario and is made up of the following bodies, as detailed in the province's *Regulated Health Professions Act*:

- *Council of the College*. The overall governing body and board of directors of the College is made up of four members appointed by the medical faculties of four universities in Ontario, four to six lay members appointed by the Lieutenant Governor in Council, and 12 to 16 members elected by the membership at large. The inclusion of large numbers of lay members in Council and on other committees indicates the public's desire for greater participation in the regulatory affairs of professional bodies. The Council's most important functions are the preparation of regulations for the profession as authorized by the Act and subject to approval by the Minister, and the appointment of members to the Executive Committee, Registration Committee, Complaints Committee, Discipline Committee, Fitness to Practice Committee, and Continuing Competence Committee. All these committees, with the exception of the Fitness to Practice Committee, have lay members.

- *Executive Committee.* This committee is drawn from the Council and acts for it between Council meetings. Actions taken by the Executive Committee are subject to ratification at the next Council meeting.
- *Registration Committee.* This committee determines eligibility for licensure. The Registrar of the College, who is appointed by the Council, performs this function on a daily basis, but refers any doubtful applications for licensure to the Registration Committee.
- *Complaints Committee.* This body investigates complaints made by members of the public or the College about the conduct of any member of the College. Anyone can complain, regardless of whether or not the complainant was the patient involved in alleged poor treatment (in practice, however, complaints are most often made by patients or their families). The procedures followed ensure that the member against whom the complaint has been made is given a fair hearing. The Committee may refer its findings to the Discipline Committee or the Executive Committee, or may direct that the matter not be referred further.
- *Discipline Committee.* The Discipline Committee considers allegations of professional misconduct or incompetence referred to it by the Council, the Executive Committee, or the Complaints Committee. If it determines that the allegations are correct and that a member of the College is guilty of professional misconduct or incompetence, it may take the following actions: revoke the license of the member, suspend the license for a stated period, impose restrictions on the license, reprimand the member, impose a fine to the maximum of $5,000, direct that any penalty above be suspended for a period of time, or any combination of these.
- *Fitness to Practice Committee.* If the Registrar of the College has evidence that a member may be incapacitated, the Registrar reports this to the Executive Committee, who in turn may appoint a board of inquiry. The board of inquiry investigates the matter and reports back to the Executive Committee. If appropriate, the Executive Committee refers the matter to the Fitness to Practice Committee, which will hold a formal hearing. If the member is found to be incapacitated, the Fitness to Practice Committee may revoke the member's licence, suspend the licence for a stated period, or attach limits to the licence.
- *Continuing Competence Committee.* This committee is a new statutory committee under the RHPA. Its purposes are to maintain and enhance the competence and standards of practice of members in the care of patients, and in record keeping in relation to members' practices. The program established by the Committee may involve member participation in continuing education and remediation programs, written or oral tests of clinical knowledge, skill, or judgement, and other modalities.
- *Medical Review Committee.* This committee was established under the *Health Insurance Act.* It is a committee of the College of Physicians and Surgeons composed of six members nominated by the College but appointed by the minister of health, plus two lay members also appointed by the minister. It reviews billing matters referred to it by the provincial health insurance plan. Such referrals occur if a physician appears to have billed for services not rendered, for services that

were not medically necessary, for services not provided in accordance with accepted professional standards, or where the nature of services provided is misinterpreted. After reviewing the matter, the Committee may recommend that the health insurance plan refuse payment, reduce the amount of the payment, or require reimbursement from the physician. Thus, it is a potent regulatory agency and functions in addition to the regular committees of the College as established by the RHPA.

Dentistry

Dentists are required to be licensed in every province (21). Graduates of approved Canadian dental schools are not required to write a licensing examination. They may apply for a certificate from the National Dental Examining Board (NDEB). Graduates of other institutions must pass an NDEB examination to obtain the certificate, which is recognized in all provinces. Provincial licensing agencies certify specialists. In Ontario, the dental profession is now regulated in a manner similar to physicians under the RHPA.

Nursing

Nurses perform many functions depending on their location, their employer, and their appointment. At present, there are 12 nursing specialties (22). Hospital nurses may perform general bedside nursing care or may work in very specialized units such as intensive care, coronary care, renal dialysis, or neurosurgical units. Public health nurses deal with the community in such matters as immunization and health education. Many nurses hold administrative positions within hospitals or other institutions. Nurses who work in frontier communities frequently perform many of the functions normally performed by physicians (these positions are generally held by nurse practitioners). In addition, physicians, chiropractors, private care institutions, and corporations may privately employ nurses.

Registered nurses and registered nursing assistants (now referred to as registered practical nurses, or RPNs) in Ontario are required to be certified and licensed by the College. Generally, this means that they have passed an examination prepared by the Canadian Nurses' Association (a national body). If their certification has expired or they have been unemployed for a certain period, they may be required to take refresher training before being re-certified. Quebec has a distinct and separate regulatory body for nurses called the Ordre des infirmiers et infirmières du Québec. In Ontario, nurses are regulated by the RHPA as described above. In other provinces, regulation is delegated to the voluntary professional organizations. The increase in the status and importance of nursing in recent years is indicated by the fact that three provincial ministries of health (British Columbia, Alberta, and Manitoba) now have special ministerial positions for provincial nursing officers or provincial nursing advisory councils.

Recently, nurse practitioner (NP) programs have received increased attention. Currently, new or amended provincial/territorial legislation allows for an expanded role for registered nurses as nurse practitioners in eight jurisdictions (see Chapter 15).

Availble data from Newfoundland and Labrador, Ontario, Alberta, and the Yukon indicate that there are at least 620 NPs in Canada (23).

Although medicine, dentistry, and nursing are three healthcare professions traditionally considered most important to the delivery of health services, chiropractic and midwifery are two healthcare professions in which consumer demand for alternative delivery modalities helped create pressure for official recognition.

Chiropractic

The practice of chiropractic is defined as "the assessment of conditions related to the spine, nervous system and joints, and the diagnosis, prevention and treatment, primarily by adjustment of ... the spine and joints" (18). In order to receive the legitimacy and official recognition of being one of the regulated healthcare professions, the practice of chiropractic moved much closer to mainstream medicine. Originally, in its historic development, it was seen as a direct alternative to medicine and was associated more closely with naturopathy. This association, as well as the broader scope of practice associated with earlier years of chiropractic, has been downplayed in recent years as chiropractors have become regulated and have come to comprise part of the primary healthcare delivery team (5).

Because chiropractors are considered one of the primary care providers in Ontario, they do not require referrals from other physicians. This status, together with their position as one of the five healthcare professionals authorized to diagnose, has been allowed because of the current general-diagnosis training of chiropractors is similar to that of physicians in medical schools. Chiropractors are licensed in all provinces (24). In Ontario, the College of Chiropractors of Ontario regulates chiropractors.

Midwifery

The practice of midwifery is defined as "the assessment and monitoring of women during pregnancy, labour, and the post-partum period and of their newborn babies, the provision of care during normal pregnancy, labour and post-partum period and the conducting of spontaneous normal vaginal deliveries" (17). Although community midwives have been practising throughout Canada (especially in rural and northern regions) for more than a century, they have received little official recognition from the state. This has slowly started to change, largely due to ongoing consumer pressure to receive non-medical labour and delivery care. Midwives are officially recognized as primary healthcare professionals and are regulated in Quebec, Ontario, Alberta and British Columbia, and appropriate regulatory legislation is in various stages of development in Manitoba and Saskatchewan. Ontario, Quebec, Manitoba, and British Columbia publicly fund midwifery services (1).

5.   SEXUAL ABUSE OF PATIENTS

Sexual abuse of patients by members of healthcare professions, in particular the medical profession, emerged as a prominent and distressing concern in some provinces, particularly Ontario, Alberta, and British Columbia in the early 1990s. Sexual abuse represents a transgression of the trust placed in a healthcare professional. Due to the position of power of the healthcare professional in relation to the patient, any suggestive or sexual behaviour or language in a clinical setting is deemed inappropriate.

In Ontario, a task force on the sexual abuse of patients, which was an independent body commissioned by the College of Physicians and Surgeons, made a series of recommendations following the review of evidence from patients reporting sexual improprieties on the part of medical practitioners. These recommendations were reviewed and published by the Council of the College of Physicians and Surgeons in 1992 (25), which recommended that the RHPA be amended to include a new section regarding actions of professional misconduct of a sexual nature with different levels of offence and penalties, such as fines or revocation of licence for the more severe offences. The legislative amendments have included a requirement that any healthcare professional with reasonable grounds to believe a colleague had committed any of the sexual offences must report this offence. Sexual abuse in the RHPA is now defined as sexual intercourse or other forms of physical sexual relations between the practitioner and the patient, touching of a sexual nature of the patient by the practitioner, or behaviour or remarks of a sexual nature toward the patient. However, the legislation also states that the words "sexual nature" do not include touching, behaviour, or remarks of a clinical nature appropriate to the service provided. The RHPA includes procedures for awarding financial compensation to patients who have been sexually abused by healthcare professionals to cover costs of counselling and treatment for sexual abuse; financial compensation is not foreseen by the RHPA for any other patient complaints.

6.   THE HEALTH OF HEALTHCARE WORKERS

The health of healthcare workers receives relatively little attention, except for the vast array of results produced by the Nurses' Health Study from Harvard University (26), which are related more appropriately to the overall lives of nurses than to work-related issues. The relation of work and health was described in Chapters 1 and 10. The nature of jobs for healthcare workers include caring for people under stress, lifting patients, giving needles, stitching wounds, and working in a changing environment that can expose workers to specific health risks. (Much of the information in this section comes from *Canada's Health Care Providers* (1).)

In the 1998–99 National Population Health Survey (NPHS), the majority (95%) of healthcare workers rated their health as good or excellent. However, they were more likely to miss work due to illness or disability. On average, they lost twice as many days as workers did in general. Different types of work are associated with different types of job-related health risks. Nurses, nursing aides, orderlies, physiotherapists, and laboratory workers are at high risk for back problems and other soft-tissue sprains and strains. Job strain (high demand and low control in the workplace) creating stress and burnout is more common among those who are at the lower end of the hierarchy, for example nursing aides, orderlies, and attendants; strain and burnout is less common among nurses and least common among physicians. However, in recent years, physicians have been experiencing increased amounts of stress in their job related to structural issues in health care. National data on physician suicide in Canada do not formally exist; unpublished data from British Columbia, however, report the rate of suicide at 21.9 per 100 000 population among physicians compared to 13.9 per 100 000 for the general population.

Healthcare workers are also exposed to infectious diseases such as tuberculosis, HIV due to needlestick injury, hepatitis B and C, and Norwalk-like viruses (see Chapter 10). They are also exposed to numerous irritants and chemicals, such as nitrous oxide and latex allergies. In recent years, nurses have reported experiencing violence in forms of verbal abuse or physical abuse. This is much more prevalent in long-term care facilities.

Larger hospitals have employee health services and assistance programs to deal with issues related to the health of their employees. Recently professional associations in collaboration with regulatory bodies have developed anonymous treatment facilities dealing with healthcare workers having mental health or addiction problems. The bloodpborne occupational diseases, and the universal precautions needed to be taken in handling the body fluids by the healthcare workers are described in Chapter 10.

7. TRENDS AND ISSUES

It was mentioned earlier in this chapter that a recent process of de-professionalization has begun. Legislation aimed at obtaining greater public control of the self-regulating professions has been enacted. This process is certain to continue. This section presents some of the issues involved and trends that may be expected.

Because governments now pay most medical bills, they are likely to become more interested in the value they receive for taxpayers' money, not only in terms of quantity but also of quality. This could mean greater government involvement in the design of medical school curricula, in the licensing procedures of provincial colleges, and in the monitoring of individual practices. The result could be periodic re-examination for re-licensure, enforced continuing education, and similar measures for ensuring the competence of licensed physicians and other healthcare providers. Professions have responded by introducing codes of ethical conduct, clearly stating their legal responsibilities, spelling out detailed knowledge of informed consent, and increasing awareness about the overall healthcare system, and the role their own discipline plays in a larger context, and introduction of mandatory continuing education requirements (1, 9). The Medical Council of Canada's *Objectives of the Considerations of the Legal, Ethical and Organizational Aspects of the Practice of Medicine*, which lists needed competencies in these areas, and the Canadian Nurses Association Code of Ethics for Registered Nurses point to the future direction in health sciences education (22, 27).

The medical profession is certain to see increased government regulation as a threat to its freedom and autonomy. The recent introduction of Quebec's Bill 114, which forced doctors to work in understaffed emergency rooms, is an example of increased control by the government on the practice of medicine (28). Bill 114 was withdrawn, but Bill 142 was introduced in November 2002; it in essence requires a detailed regional plan for the staffing requirement for each region that considers the need of population, hospitals, emergency rooms, CLSCs, long-term care facilities, and so on, for both general practitioners and specialists (29). Once these plans are approved, practitioners can be assigned to where shortages are envisioned as part of their conditions to participate in health insurance plans. The profession has reacted by becoming more politicized, by lobbying governments and enlisting the aid of the public. Union-like activities (e.g., withholding of services) will probably become more common. The profession is also likely to react by improving its own regulation and becoming more socially accountable to communities in which they practice (30, 31). Stricter requirements for re-licensure, continuing education, peer review, and evaluation of individual practices may be imposed to forestall government action in these areas. Some degree of confrontation seems inevitable, but it is to be hoped that those issues described will be resolved in a manner that will lead to better health care for Canadians and, in the long run, a stronger, if less autonomous, profession.

Ontario's RHPA also throws some light on the future direction of the regulation of healthcare professionals (32). It states that "the sole purpose of professional regulation is to advance and protect the public interest. The public is the intended beneficiary of regulation, not the members of the professions. Thus, the purpose of granting self-regulation to a profession is not to enhance its status or increase the earning power of its members by giving the profession a monopoly over the delivery of particular health services."

Another major change is that an increasing number of healthcare occupations are demanding to be considered as professions and to participate in health insurance programs. This will create tension among the different healthcare providers. Definitions of healthcare professions will become restrictive, and professionals will be equated with individuals with specialized knowledge and skill but not necessarily those with responsibility, autonomy, or service orientation. Many more new problems will undoubtedly arise as both governments and consumers seek a greater voice in healthcare. One thing is certain: the 1990s have brought many changes and the next decade will bring more.

8.   SUMMARY

This chapter examined the definition of professionalism, discussed the historical background of the modern medical professions, and listed and described the various healthcare professions, para-professions, and allied occupations, and discussed their regulation and future trends in regulation.

The concept of professionalism is very difficult to define; hence most definitions consist of lists of characteristics commonly attributed to an established profession. These characteristics include specialized knowledge and skill, autonomy, service orientation, responsibility, and external recognition.

Medicine is the dominant profession in the healthcare field. In achieving this dominance, the mainstream of medicine eliminated, absorbed, or controlled competing disciplines. Other healthcare professions have followed the same pattern established by medicine, but only dentistry has achieved a similar degree of autonomy.

Most provinces have enacted, or intend to enact, legislation to ensure greater public control of the professions. The earliest and most significant changes occurred in the provinces of Quebec and Ontario.

Quebec's *Professional Code* defines what a profession is and establishes formal criteria by which an occupation gains statutory recognition as a profession. Furthermore, each profession is governed by a professional order. This order maintains surveillance of the quality of individual practices, and is empowered to take corrective measures. The Code also establishes two overall supervisory and regulatory bodies: the Office des professions du Québec and the Conseil interprofessionnel du Québec.

In Ontario, the *Regulated Health Professions Act* (RHPA) was enacted in 1991. One of the major aspects of the new legislation is the expansion of the number of professions under its jurisdiction to 23. The RHPA was enacted to obtain greater public accountability in the regulation of the healthcare professions, and is regarded as increasing equity among the healthcare professions, reducing the role of the physician as the gatekeeper, and increasing direct access for the consumer to a wider variety of professionals. The most revolutionary aspect of the legislation is that the professions are not defined by the scope of practice but professionals are licensed to perform various procedures, or controlled acts, that are potentially dangerous.

The RHPA gives the minister of health broad powers to supervise the regulation of the 23 disciplines included, and increases the accountability and protection of the interests of the public. The emphasis is on the public good, rather than professional interests.

Each healthcare profession is required to constitute a college that is responsible for regulating the practice of the profession and to govern its members in accordance with the RHPA.

Physicians are required to be licensed in all provinces by the College of Physicians and Surgeons. This licensing agency is made up of the council of the college, the executive committee, the registration committee, the complaints committee, the discipline committee, and the fitness to practice committee, the continuing competence committee, and the medical review committee. Dentists, like physicians, are required to be licensed in every province. As well, in Ontario, the dental profession is regulated in a manner similar to physicians under the RHPA. Nurses perform many functions depending on their location, their employer, and their appointment. Registered nurses in Ontario must be licensed by their college. Chiropractic and midwifery are two healthcare professions where consumer demand for alternative healthcare delivery modalities helped to create pressure for official recognition.

Different types of work in health care are associated with different types of job-related health risks. Nurses, nursing aides, orderlies, physiotherapists, and laboratory workers are at high risk for back problems and other soft tissue sprains and strains. Job strain, creating stress, and burnout are more common among those who are at the lower end of the hierarchy, such as nursing aides, orderlies, and attendants; for nurses, it is less common, and for physicians it is the least common. Healthcare workers are also exposed to infectious diseases such as tuberculosis, HIV due to needlestick injury, hepatitis B and C, and Norwalk-like viruses, as well as exposed to numerous irritants and chemicals such as nitrous oxide and latex allergies. In recent years nurses have reported experiencing violence in forms of verbal abuse or physical abuse, which is much more prevalent in long-term care facilities.

A recent process of de-professionalization has begun. Legislation aimed at obtaining greater public control of the self-regulating professions has been enacted and this process is certain to continue. The medical profession is certain to see increased government regulation as a threat to its freedom and autonomy. Reaction by the profession is likely to take two forms: the profession will become more politicized and may attempt to improve its own regulation.

9.   REFERENCES

1.   Canadian Institute for Health Information. 2001. *Canada's health care providers*. Ottawa. <secure.cihi.ca/cihiweb/dispPage.jsp?cw_page=AR_35_E> (January 2003).
2.   Bohnen L. *The sociology of the professions in Canada: Four aspects of professionalism in Canada*. Ottawa: Consumer Research Council of Canada, 1977.
3.   Bucher R, Stelling J. Characteristics of professional organizations. *Journal of Health and Social Behaviour* 1969; 10(1):3-15.
4.   Freidson E. *The profession of medicine*. New York: Dodds, Mead, and Co., 1970.
5.   Coburn D. State authority, medical dominance, and trends in the regulation of the health professionals: The Ontario case. *Social Science and Medicine* 1993; 37(2):129-38.
6.   Torrance G. Socio-historical overview: The development of the Canadian health system. In Coburn D, D'Arcy C, New P, editors. *Health and Canadian society*. Toronto: Fitzhenry and Whiteside Ltd.; 1981.
7.   Health and Welfare Canada. *Directory of national certification bodies: National professional associations and national accreditation agencies for various health occupations in Canada*. Ottawa: Health and Welfare Canada, Health Human Resources Division, 1990.
8.   Casey J. *Status report and analysis of health professional regulations in Canada*. Edmonton, 1999. Prepared for the Federal/Provincial/Territorial Advisory Committee on Health Human Resources.
9.   Canadian Medical Association. 2002. *Scopes of practice*. <www.cma.ca/cma/common/displayPage.do?pageId=/staticContent/HTML/N0/l2/where_we_stand/2002/01-21.htm> (February 2003).
10.   British Columbia, Ministry of Health Planning. 2002. *Proposal to amend the Health Professions Act: Improving governance and accountability*. <www.healthplanning.gov.bc.ca/leg> (February 2003).
11.   Government of Quebec. 1973. *Professional Code*. Updated to December 19, 2001. <www.canlii.org/qc/sta/c26/whole.html> (October 2002).
12.   Office des professions du Québec. 2002. *Système professionnel québécois: Conseil interprofessionnel du Québec*. <www.opq.gouv.qc.ca/03systeme/conseil_interprofessionnel.htm> (October 2002).
13.   Canadian Council of Human Resources Association. 2002. *It should be noted that the situation in Québec differs from that in the rest of Canada*. <www.chrpcanada.com/en/quebec_situation.asp> (October 2002).

14. Collège des médecins du Québec. *ALDO-Quebec: Legislative, ethical, and organizational aspects of medical practice in Quebec*. Montreal: Collège des médecins du Québec, 1995.

15. Government of Ontario. 1991. *Regulated Health Professions Act*. <192.75.156.68/DBLaws/Statutes/English/91r18_e.htm> (October 2002).

16. Government of Ontario. 2001. *Health profession colleges – Ontario*. <www.gov.on.ca/health/english/program/pro/procol_dt.html> (October 2002).

17. Bohnen L. *Regulated Health Professions Act: A practical guide*. Aurora: Canada Law Book, 1994.

18. Pooley D. Regulated Health Professions Act, 1991: The new benchmark for future health care legislation. *Journal of Canadian Chiropractic Association* 1992; 36(3):161-4.

19. Health Professions Regulatory Advisory Council. *Adjusting Balance: A Review of the Regulated Health Professions Act*. Toronto: Ontario Ministry of Health and Long-Term Care, 2001.

20. Medical Council of Canada. 2002. *MCC function and structure*. <www.mcc.ca/about.html> (October 2002).

21. National Dental Examination Board of Canada. 2002. <www.ndeb.ca> (October 2002).

22. Canadian Nurses Association. 2002. *Code of ethics for registered nurses*. Ottawa. <www.cna-nurses.ca/pages/ethics/ethicsframe.htm> (October 2002).

23. Canadian Institute for Health Information. 2002. *Supply and distribution of registered nurses in Canada, 2001 Report: Part 3*.
<secure.cihi.ca/cihiweb/dispPage.jsp?cw_page=AR20_2001sum_e_3> (October 2002).

24. Chiropractic in Canada. 2002. *Provincial Licensing Offices*. <www.ccachiro.org> (October 2002).

25. Task Force on Sexual Abuse of Patients. *The final report of the Task Force on Sexual Abuse of Patients*. Toronto: College of Physicians and Surgeons of Ontario, 1991.

26. Nurses' Health Study. 2003. *Publications*. <www.channing.harvard.edu/nhs/pub.html> (February 2003).

27. Medical Council of Canada. 1999. *Objectives of the considerations of the legal, ethical and organizational aspects of the practice of medicine*. <www.mcc.ca/pdf/cleo_e.html> (October 2002).

28. Borsellino M. Bill 114: How to rally MDs united in opposition. *Medical Post* 2002, September 3.

29. Quebec, Assemblée Nationale. 2002. *An act to amend the Act respecting health services and social services as regards the medical activities, the distribution, and undertaking of physicians*. (February 2003).

30. Can Med 2000 Project. *Skills for the new millennium: Report of the Societal Needs Working Group*. Ottawa: Royal College of Physicians and Surgeons of Canada, 1996.

31. Health Canada. *Social accountability: A vision for medical schools*. Ottawa: Minister of Public Works and Government Services Canada, 2001.

32. Government of Ontario. *Regulated Health Professions Act (Ontario), 1993*. Government of Ontario, 1993.

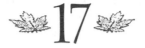

17

Quebec's Healthcare System: Origins, Organization, and Future

The province of Quebec is the largest province in Canada and the second most populous, with 7 million inhabitants. Its high level of quality care and a well-developed public health infrastructure contribute to one of the best population health statuses in the world. This chapter provides a brief overview of the Quebec healthcare system from its origins, its current organization, and its governance mechanisms to its envisaged future.

1. THE DEVELOPMENT OF QUEBEC'S HEALTHCARE SYSTEM

As stated earlier, the *Constitution Act of 1867* gave exclusive jurisdiction to provinces in personal healthcare matters. In Quebec, communities and religious charitable hospitals provided care for indigent and poor populations since the 18th century, thus creating the foundation for what has become the province's healthcare system (1, 2). The involvement of the provincial government in the healthcare system, limited at first to complementing the work of charitable institutions, reflected a world-wide interest in controlling epidemic diseases through sanitation (3). This resulted in the establishment of quarantine measures, followed by hospitals for immigrants and municipal health bureaus. Most healthcare and public health interventions were provided by private religious hospitals and municipal administrations, respectively (4), but taking care of the ill and infirm remained the responsibility of family members and parish and religious organizations. Quebec's healthcare system remained poorly developed until the middle of the 19th century.

In the 20th century, the development of the professional practice of medicine and the specialization of hospitals led to the gradual emergence of organized health care. Despite the government's reluctance to its involvement in sanitation, the 1921 adoption

Contributors: *Jean-Frédéric Lévesque and Pierre Bergeron*

of the *Loi établissant le service d'assistance publique* (*Act to Establish Public Assistance*) marked a departure in the way health services were perceived. From being a charitable intervention, they were now seen as a legitimate service provided by the state. Following this the provincial government, municipalities, and religious hospitals participated in financing the care of indigent populations.

Around the same time, the *Loi des unités sanitaires* (*Sanitary Units Act*) stimulated the creation of permanent sanitary (public health) units — where physicians, nurses, and sanitation inspectors worked — responsible for the surveillance and protection of the population's health in their territory. The province's first department of health was created in 1936 to provide support to sanitary units and to advise the public administration on medical and technical matters (2). Despite these developments, emphasis on public health services dwindled during this period compared to the increasing interest in clinical medicine.

The 1940s and 1950s saw an increasing preoccupation with the organization of curative services. Quebec's interventions in health care did not in fact change during that period: the organization of the healthcare system remained locally regulated and linked to private initiatives. Despite resistance from many provinces, various federal spending initiatives on provincial matters contributed to the establishment of a state-operated formal healthcare system in Quebec. Federal grants also resulted in a significant increase in the number of hospitals in the province, with a relative lack of control from the provincial government. From 1932 to 1970, the number of hospitals in Quebec increased from 79 to 187, doubling the ratio of beds to 6 per 1,000 residents (5). The government of Quebec adopted the *Loi des hôpitaux* (*Hospitals Act*) in 1962, after joining the federal hospitalization insurance program in 1961. This law created corporations, independent from religious communities, that administered hospitals.

The period between 1970 and 1990 can be seen as a time of increased state involvement in health care. The report of the Commission d'enquête sur la santé et le bien-être social (Commission of Inquiry into Health and Social Well-being) recommended a planned, coordinated, and integrated health system with regard to institutions, programs, and provision of care (6). Consequently, the provincial government joined in the federal-provincial program for insuring medical services (passing the *Loi sur l'assurance-maladie*, or *Health Insurance Act*, in 1970) and enacted the *Loi sur les services de santé et les services sociaux*, or *Act Respecting Health Services and Social Services*, in 1971). The Ministère des Affaires sociales (Ministry of Social Affairs) was created to insure a wide range of services, oversee the system, and encourage public participation in the administration of health institutions. This reform also created 12 consultative regional boards (Conseils régionaux de la santé et des services sociaux, or CRSSS) and local community services centres known as CLSCs (Centres locaux de services communautaires) responsible for providing health and social services. Despite central administrative and technical regulations, physicians retained their professional autonomy and hospitals remained relatively autonomous (1).

Subsequently, public health functions became integrated into the healthcare system at the ministerial, regional, hospital, and local levels (7). After 1974, 32 community health departments were created to integrate most public health functions into hospital structures. These were responsible for epidemiological studies, control of infectious diseases, and environmental threats, health promotion, and prevention programs as well as administrative functions, while CLSCs remained responsible for providing individual preventive and social services.

This model remained predominant until the beginning of the 1990s. Since the middle of the 1980s, however, the Quebec government had begun to scrutinize its publicly funded healthcare system, as had governments elsewhere in Canada and Europe. This reexamination stemmed mostly from increased public spending for health care, the gradual questioning of the level of public spending, and the realization that the health of the population does not seem directly linked to the level of healthcare spending.

The 1991 *Loi sur les services de santé et les services sociaux* (*Health and Social Services Act*) reaffirmed the social goals of the 1970s but also introduced many changes aimed at tightening the management of the system and its focus on the citizen. This move complied with the recommendations of the Commission d'enquête sur les services de santé et les services sociaux (Commission of Inquiry into Health Care and Social Services) (8) and other ministerial reports. The CRSSS were transformed into administrative regional boards (Régies régionales de la santé et des services sociaux, or RRSSS) in 1991 and mandated to regulate the healthcare system at the regional level. A set of health goals to be attained by 2002 was articulated. Public health institutions were integrated into the regional boards in order to identify health needs, priorities, and solutions for an entire region, in addition to fulfilling their traditional mandates of health protection, health promotion, and disease prevention.

To address the government's need to reduce its deficit and balance its budget in the mid 1990s, drastic reductions in public spending on health care stimulated a set of measures aimed at restructuring the institutional network (closing of some facilities, amalgamation of others) and making ambulatory care more available (see Chapter 18). There was also a program to encourage physicians and nurses to retire. Since this move away from a hospital-based healthcare system, recent governmental studies have examined the role of private funding in the healthcare system (9) and potential solutions to various problems plaguing the healthcare delivery system (10). The 2000 Clair Commission recommended strengthening the primary care network with an integrated approach to care and increased management in order to create a flexible organizational system and an interdisciplinary approach to health care. It also suggested regulations that distinguish between political issues (objectives and social goals) and administrative issues (management).

Recent legislation aimed at tightening management accountability has reversed some of the decentralization of the administration of the healthcare system, and has reinstated regional boards as administrative units. The results of this trend toward administrative regulation and accountability are hospital report cards, formal contracts between regional boards and healthcare institutions and providers, and the planning of public health activities (Programme national de santé publique).

This section has briefly outlined the principal origins of the public healthcare system in Quebec. The next section describes the organization of the public healthcare system and its various institutions and mandates.

2.   ORGANIZATION OF THE HEALTHCARE SYSTEM IN QUEBEC

2.1.   SERVICES FINANCED BY THE PUBLIC SYSTEM

Quebec's healthcare system is designed to address the needs of the general population and vulnerable groups as it integrates health services and social services under one ministry. Furthermore, the health care in the province is organized at three levels. The central level (the Ministère de la Santé et des Services sociaux and affiliated organizations) establishes the program priorities and defines necessary budgetary parameters. The regional level (regional boards) organizes and coordinates services and allocates budgets. The local level (institutions, centres, and private providers) provides basic healthcare services. Specialized services, organized regionally and across the province, complete the service network (11).

The Quebec healthcare system is publicly financed (approximately 70% public versus 30% private funding) and publicly regulated despite a large proportion of services provided by fee-for-service practitioners in private clinics. Expenditures for the health and social services system amount to about $16.2 billion, or $2,079 per capita, accounting for 34.5% of government spending for 2000–01 (40% excluding debt servicing), an increase since the 1994 level of $13.1 billion. Approximately $205 million is allocated for central functions and provincial programs, $11.8 billion for regional and local programs (provision of health care and public health and social services), and $3.9 billion mainly for the remuneration of physicians and drug costs. Despite strong measures to control the increase in healthcare costs, spending has increased at a rate of around 5% per year since the cutbacks of the 1990s (12).

Three main plans provide financing in Quebec: hospital care, health insurance, and the drug plan. The Régime d'assurance-hospitalisation du Québec (Hospital Insurance Plan) is administered by Quebec's ministry of health and social services. It is designed to finance hospital-related services as in other provinces and fulfils the requirments of *Canada Health Act* (11).

The health insurance plan is administered by the Régie de l'assurance-maladie du Québec (RAMQ), a public authority appointed by the provincial government and accountable to the Minister of Health. It finances necessary medical services and fulfils the requirements of *Canada Health Act*. It also covers dental care for young children and dental care and optometry services for recipients of employment assistance and welfare benefits. All residents of Quebec must register with the RAMQ to be eligible for the health insurance programs.

The third universal plan is the Régime d'assurance-médicaments du Québec (Prescription Drug Plan), created by the 1997 *Loi sur l'assurance-médicaments*. This legislation responded to the significant increase in spending for outpatient medications, which rose from 5.8% in 1980 to 16.9% in 2000 as a proportion of total healthcare spending (13). These increasing costs put a sizeable proportion of the population, namely those who do not receive governmental assistance or who could not afford private insurance coverage, at a disadvantage.

The prescription drug plan provides complete coverage of the population in a partnership between the government and private insurers. By law, the entire population is covered, either by a private insurance plan or by a public plan administered by the RAMQ. Those who do not have access to a private plan, or are aged 65 and over, or receive income assistance (welfare) are covered by the public insurance plan. Some exceptional medications are also universally covered (for example, drugs used to treat tuberculosis and sexually transmitted diseases). Under the public plan, participants pay a lump sum via taxation (currently fixed at $385 per year). In addition, when they purchase prescription drugs, they pay a deductible (about $8) and a co-insurance amount (about 25%), up to a monthly maximum. Children and people unable to work are exempt from this payment. The maximum annual contribution is set at approximately $800.

The public drug insurance plan currently covers around 3 million or 43% of the Quebec population. Without it, approximately 1.7 million people would not be covered (14). The rest of the population (57%) have private insurance plans. The public and private plans have seen annual rises in total costs of 16.6% and 18.3% respectively during the first years of universal implementation. These seem to stem from the increase in number of people covered, an increase in the average number of prescriptions per person, an increase in the average unit costs of medications, and the introduction of medications for diseases previously not treatable. The cost of the plan rose from $715 million in 1997 to $1.4 billion in 2002 (13).

2.2. ORGANIZATION OF THE PUBLIC SYSTEM

2.2.1. Ministry of Health and Social Services and Regional Health Boards

In Quebec, the Minister of Health and Social Services is responsible for developing and instituting policies on health and social services and for regulating and financing the provincial and regional components of the healthcare system (12). The ministry determines the objectives, directions, and priorities for health and social services; establishes the necessary mechanisms to carry them out; and evaluated their attainment. Furthermore, the ministry establishes frameworks for managing human resources, coordinates interventions between regions as well as public health programs, and assures the health protection of the population (15).

Various organizations come under the jurisdiction of the ministry. Six have administrative responsibilities. Of these, as already mentioned, the RAMQ administers the health insurance plan according to the *Health Insurance Act*. It also administers the public drug insurance plan. The Office des personnes handicapées du Québec (Quebec Office for People with Disabilities) oversees the services provided to disabled persons and promotes their interests. The Institut national de santé publique du Québec (National Public Health Institute of Quebec) supports central and regional public health authorities and manages public health laboratories. The Corporation Héma-Québec manages the provincial blood bank system (16).

Eight organizations fulfil recommendation and consultation mandates. The Conseil de la santé et du bien-être (Council for Health and Well-being) was created in 1993 to advise the Minister of Health on improving the health and well-being of the population. The Conseil médical du Québec (Medical Council of Quebec), established in 1991, advises the minister on medical services, taking into account the needs of the public, trends in costs of medical services, and the public's capacity to pay. Six other organizations counsel the minister on issues such as mental health, illegal drug abuse, cancer, and prescription drugs (16).

At the regional level, 16 RRSSS and two regional health councils plan, organize, and coordinate programs and services, as well as allocate resources in the regions. Their mission is to adapt health and social services to the needs and situations of the various groups of their territory.

In addition, the Agence d'évaluation des technologies et modes d'intervention en santé (AETMIS, or the Health Technology and Intervention Evaluation Agency) is an independent organization that reports to Quebec's Minister of Finance, Economy, and Research. Its mission is to support, by means of assessing technology and medical interventions, decision makers in the healthcare sector.

2.2.2. Organization of the Healthcare and Social Services Network

More than 480 public and private institutions provide health care and social services in Quebec. There are 118 acute care and psychiatric hospitals with approximately 22,000 acute and psychiatric care beds (see Chapter 15 for organization and governance of institutions in Quebec). Hospitals are publicly funded (17).

University networks of hospitals have changed in Quebec as hospitals have merged, creating unified teaching facilities (such as the Centre hospitalier de l'Université de Montréal and the McGill University Health Centre). Four integrated university health networks are planned in order to consolidate teaching, research, and service efforts (18).

There are 91 rehabilitation centres and 317 residential and long-term care centres (Centres hospitaliers de soins de longue durée) that offer alternative living environments and services to adults with loss of functional or psychosocial autonomy. In addition, there are 20 child and youth protection centres that provide psychosocial services and child placement and family mediation services (17).

One distinctive feature of Quebec's healthcare and social services system is its 147 CLSCs, which have existed for 30 years. They have always faced obstacles in being accepted by private medical clinics and gaining recognition from the population as the first point of contact to the healthcare system. Private medical clinics, emergency departments and hospitals remain the principal entry points to the system for medical services, and CLSCs still have difficulty recruiting physicians to provide medical services outside normal working hours (19). CLSCs are now mandated to provide basic health and social services of a preventive and curative nature, as well as rehabilitation and reintegration services, by multidisciplinary teams to a geographically determined population. CLSCs receive individuals, evaluate their care requirements, and either arrange for the provision of services such as day programs or home care or refer individuals to the appropriate agency. Info-santé CLSC, a telephone service staffed by nurses and launched in 1996, also provides counselling, emergency information, and advice 24 hours a day, 7 days a week. Intermediate-care nursing homes, adult residential care, and homecare services are also available through a coordinated regional system and based on a single assessment tool.

In addition, more than 3,500 community (voluntary) organizations, as partners of the ministry of health, regional boards, and institutions, provide services such as prevention, assistance and support, promotion, advocacy for patients' rights, health promotion and social development, and services for specific groups (17).

Quebec also has more than 800 private practice clinics, which provide the majority of personal primary and secondary medical care services on a fee-for-service basis. The provincial health insurance plan pays these practitioners.

2.2.3. Organization of Public Health Services

Public health services are highly organized in Quebec. At the central level, there is the ministry of health's Direction générale de la santé publique (Public Health Branch), which plans public health services. It also sets up, coordinates, and evaluates the public health program. This program specifies the public health interventions based on the core functions of surveillance, promotion, prevention, and protection, and it identifies specific health and action targets. The ministry finances and plans universal preventive and screening programs (such as screening for breast cancer and immunization for influenza) implemented in the regions.

Also at the central level, the Institut national de santé publique du Québec was founded in 1998 to improve the coordination, development, and use of expertise in public health through specialized advice and assistance, laboratory services, research, information, training, and international cooperation.

At the regional level, the 18 public health departments of the regional boards are responsible for the coordination and provision of public health services and the implementation of the public health program. At the local level, CLSCs and community groups, in partnership with the public health departments, provide most of the direct public health services to the population.

In the area of occupational health, the public health departments protect and promote the health of workers in close partnership with the Commission de santé et sécurité au travail (Workers' Health and Safety Commission), the organization in charge of regulating health protection standards and compensating workers for work-related illness and injuries in Quebec.

2.3. HUMAN RESOURCES AND REGULATION

Healthcare human resources represent 10% of Quebec's labour force. Approximately 14,000 doctors are distributed evenly between general practitioners and specialists. Most physicians practice within the provincial health insurance plan, despite two other permitted options. Professionals who have withdrawn from the plan but adhere to the provincial fee schedule are paid directly by patients after they receive payment from the RAMQ. Physicians who choose not to accept the government fee schedule are paid directly by their patients. In 2000–01, fee-for-service accounted for 73% of physician costs, while 10% of costs went to salary and mixed remuneration (14). There is no extra-billing by physicians in Quebec.

Despite various incentives to attract physicians to remote regions and disincentives for young medical doctors to start their careers in urban centres, the distribution of healthcare professionals across the province remains unbalanced. Regional plans of physician requirements (Plans régionaux d'effectifs médicaux) are being elaborated based on growth projections, imbalances to be corrected, and the needs of hospital catchment areas. In each region, a Commission médicale régionale (Regional Medical Commission) advises the regional board on organization and distribution of medical services and medical staffing and a Département régional de médecine générale (regional general medicine department) defines, evaluates, and completes a regional organization plan for general services and a regional medical staffing plan. Regional boards must submit plans to restrict recruitment of physicians accordingly. After cuts in the number of admissions to medical school during the 1990s, the number of admissions has increased from 406 in 1998 to 666 in 2003 (20).

There are more nurses than any other health professionals in Quebe, with more than 62,000 registered in their professional organization. Nonetheless, recent trends suggest an acute shortage of nurses. Indeed, institutions often face shortages and difficulties in recruiting and retaining nursing staff (21). This situation is expected to continue unless teaching programs can increase the number of graduates over the next 15 years (22).

Since the midwife profession was recognized by law in 1999, approximately 60 midwives have registered. As independent health workers, they have signed contracts with seven CLSCs, becoming members of their perinatal teams. There are six Maisons des naissances (birthing centres), which are CLSC service points, and regulations and agreements are being developed to facilitate the practice of midwives in hospitals and at home.

The regulation of healthcare professionals in Quebec is described in Chapter 16. The recent *Loi modifiant le Code des professions et d'autres dispositions législatives dans le domaine de la santé* (*Act Changing the Code of Professions and Other Legislation in the Health Sector*) attempted to change the way healthcare personnel work together in the healthcare system by redefining the responsibilities of physicians, nurses, and other healthcare professionals.

The number of nurses and physicians who have recently retired also affects access to health care for many hospital services (23). It is just one element of the relative shortage of health professionals that lies ahead, considering the aging workforce, the decrease in the number of professionals enrolled in training programs during the 1990s, and the fact that young professionals tend not to work as many hours or in the same areas as their predecessors.

As in other parts of Canada, the regulation of health professionals has traditionally proved to be difficult in Quebec. Strong professional associations, corporations, and federations have been very active in preserving the independent professional status of their members. The fact that medical doctors in Quebec remain independent workers providing services in institutions by which they are not employed (yet have control over the organization of medical services inside these organizations) is a good illustration of the compromises that must be made in the formal organization of the healthcare system. It is still the professional organizations that have the ultimate responsibility to assess the quality of services provided by physicians and other health professionals in Quebec and that set the boundaries of each profession.

Any overview of human resources regulation would be incomplete without mentioning the existence of the many patients' interests groups and employee unions that shape the responses of a sizeable portion of the population to proposed modifications to the healthcare system and the way it is managed.

3.   A HEALTH SYSTEM IN TRANSFORMATION

This chapter has tried to present a general overview of the Quebec healthcare system, its origin and present configuration. Recent developments suggest that the province's healthcare system will continue to evolve in accordance with previous reforms and changes. Quebec and Prince Edward Island remain the only provinces where health care and social services are united under one administrative organization. Despite recent changes, this integration has been preserved and does not seem to be threatened by recent commissions and reforms (24).

Increased accountability of decision makers at various levels, from government officials and regional planners to local providers, seems an actual impetus for change. A recent law modified the governance of institutions by changing the composition of administrative boards, which will ensure better representation from the community and professional groups while maintaining the presence of elected representatives (24). In addition, the idea of increasing the population's involvement in governance is supported by the creation of a system of public consultations called Forums de la population administered by the regional boards.

Results-based governance is also sought with clear management agreements being demanded from regional boards, local institutions, and service providers. The recent publication of performance reports for hospitals (*Bulletins de santé*) by the Ministère de la Santé et des Services sociaux attests to this desire to increase institutional accountability toward the general public (see Chapter 15). Accordingly, the public health program requires that regional public health departments develop regional public health action plans on a three-year basis in partnership with CLSCs. These changes confirm the ministry's mandate and they clearly establish priorities, preferred modes of interventions, objectives, and evaluation frameworks. The program seeks to maintain consistency among its public health services among all regions and to ensure better control of the actions of regional organizations.

After a decade of hospital mergers, closures, and restructuring — which mostly affected the availability of hospital care rather than its core organization — the ministry is now directing its efforts toward reforming the primary care infrastructure, as is the case in other provinces and territories. The Clair Commission pointed out problems in the implementation of basic primary medical care at CLSCs (mainly because of professional opposition) and the fact that the position of the hospital in the system resulted in an emphasis on specialized care and a weak primary care system(10). However in recent months, Quebec is moving forward with the implementation of the Family Medicine Groups that were recommended by the Clair Commission.

Generally speaking, the problems facing Quebec's healthcare system relate to organization (e.g., access, continuity) rather than to quality of care (e.g., technical skill, interpersonal relations, diagnostic accuracy, efficacy of care). This can partially explain the very high level of satisfaction among users but the lack of confidence expressed by non-users. Despite a number of substantial innovations being implemented, major challenges remain in the progression toward a more organized healthcare system.

Other major challenge for the healthcare system is the need to modify the remuneration system for doctors and the budget allocation for hospitals (16). While doctors are now mostly paid on a fee-for-service basis and the hospitals by a central budget, there is a move to pay hospitals for the actual services they provide and doctors for the total amount of care needed by a population; this trend could generate strong opposition by interest groups. Furthermore, reversing the pyramid of care by investing more into primary care in order to reduce the need for hospitalization and decrease the number of emergency department visits will prove difficult in a system already overwhelmed by demands and waiting lists. Federal initiatives and funding suggested by the Romanow Commission could again be the occasion for federal-provincial conflict but could also be the impetus for changes in all provincial healthcare systems(25).

4.   SUMMARY

The province of Quebec, the largest province in Canada, is the second most populous, with 7 million inhabitants. In both the pre- and post-confederation eras, communities and religious, charitable hospitals provided care for indigent and poor populations, creating the foundation for what has become the province's healthcare system. The province's first department of health was created in 1936 to provide support to sanitary units and to advise the public administration on medical and technical matters. The Ministère des Affaires sociales (Ministry of Social Affairs) was created to insure a wide range of services, oversee the system, and encourage public participation in the administration of health institutions. This reform also created 12 consultative regional boards (Conseils régionaux de la santé et des services sociaux, or CRSSS) and local community services centres known as CLSCs (Centres locaux de services communautaires) responsible for providing health and social services. Despite central administrative and technical regulations, physicians retained their professional autonomy and hospitals remained relatively autonomous. The 1991 Loi sur les services de santé et les services sociaux (Health and Social Services Act) 'transformed the CRSSS into administrative regional boards (Régies régionales de la santé et des services sociaux, or RRSSS) to regulate the healthcare system at the regional level. Public health institutions were also integrated into the regional boards in order to identify health needs, priorities, and solutions for an entire region, in addition to fulfilling their traditional mandates of health protection, health promotion, and disease prevention.

Quebec's healthcare system is designed to address the needs of the general population and vulnerable groups as it integrates health and social services under one ministry called the Ministère de la Santé et des Services sociaux (the Ministry of Health and Social Services). Health care in the province is organized at three levels. The central, ministerial level establishes the program priorities and defines necessary budgetary parameters. At the regional level, 16 RRSSS and two regional health councils plan, organize, and coordinate programs and services, as well as allocate resources in the regions. The local level (institutions, centres, and private providers) provides basic healthcare services. Specialized services, organized regionally and across the province, complete the service network.

More than 480 public and private institutions provide health care and social services in Quebec. There are 118 acute care and psychiatric hospitals with approximately 22,000 acute and psychiatric care beds; these are publicly funded. The 147 CLSCs are mandated to provide basic health and social services of a preventive and curative nature, as well as rehabilitation and reintegration services, by multidisciplinary teams to a geographically determined population. Quebec also has more than 800 private practice clinics, which provide the majority of primary and secondary care services on a fee-for-service and are paid by the provincial health insurance plan.

Public health services are highly organized in Quebec. At the ministerial level, there is the Direction générale de la santé publique (Public Health Branch), which plans public health services. Also at the central level, the Institut national de santé publique du Québec (National Public Health Institute of Quebec) generates relevant public health knowledge and provides expertise to support central and regional organizations. At the regional level, the 18 public health departments of the regional boards are responsible for the coordination and provision of public health services and the implementation of the public health program. At the local level, CLSCs and community groups, in partnership with the public health departments, provide most of the direct public health services to the population.

The Quebec healthcare system is publicly financed (approximately 70% public versus 30% private funding) and publicly regulated. Expenditures for health and social services system amounts to about $16.2 billion, or $2,079 per capita, accounting for 34.5% of government spending for 2000–01. Three main plans provide financing in Quebec: hospital care, health insurance (both of these are similar to other provinces), and the drug plan, which provides complete coverage of the population in a partnership between the government and private insurers.

Healthcare human resources represent 10% of Quebec's labour force. Approximately 14,000 doctors are distributed evenly between general practitioners and specialists. Most physicians practice within the provincial health insurance plan. There are approximately 62,000 nurses registered in their professional organization.

Quebec's healthcare system is going through transformation. Increased accountability of decision makers at various levels, from government officials and regional planners to local providers, is driving the change. Results-based governance is also sought, with clear management agreements being demanded from regional boards, local institutions, and service providers. Generally speaking, the problems facing Quebec's healthcare system relate to organization (e.g., access, continuity, universal access) rather than to quality of care. Quebec is also in the midst of primary care reform similar to that of other provinces.

5. REFERENCES

1. Bergeron P, Gagnon F. La prise en charge étatique de la santé au Québec: émergence et transformations. In Lemieux V, Bergeron P, Bégin C, Bélanger G, editors. *Le système de santé au Québec: organisation, acteurs et enjeux*. Sainte-Foy: Les Presses de l'Université Laval; in press.

2. Desrosiers G, Gaumer B. *Des unités sanitaires aux DSC et CLSC. Des réalisations de la santé publique aux perspectives de la santé communautaire*. Research report no. 16 for the Commission d'enquête sur les services de santé et les services sociaux. Quebec: Les Publications du Québec, 1987.

3. Rosen G. *A history of public health*. Baltimore: Johns Hopkins University Press, 1993.

4. Gow JI. L'administration québécoise de 1867 à 1900: un État en formation. *Revue canadienne de science politique* 1979; 7(3):555-620.

5. Renaud M. Les réformes québécoise de la santé ou les aventures d'un état narcissique. In Bozzini L, *et al.*, editors. *Médecine et société les années 80*. Montreal: Albert St-Martin, 1981.

6. Commission d'enquête sur la santé et le bien-être social [Commission Castonguay-Nepveu]. *Rapport de la Commission d'enquête sur la santé et le bien-être social*: Volume 4: La Santé, Book 2: Le régime de santé. Gouvernement du Québec, 1980.

7. Comité d'étude sur la prévention sanitaire [Comité MacDonald]. *Rapport du comité d'étude sur la prévention sanitaire*. Quebec, 1971. December 24.

8. Commission d'enquête sur les services de santé et les services sociaux [Commission Rochon]. *Rapport de la Commission d'enquête sur les services de santé et les services sociaux*. Quebec: Les Publications du Québec, 1988.

9. Ministère de la santé et des services sociaux. *La complémentarité du secteur privé dans la poursuite des objectifs fondamentaux du système public de santé au Québec: constats et recommandations sur les pistes [Rapport Arpin]*, 1999.

10. Commission d'étude sur les services de santé et les services sociaux du Québec [Commission Clair]. *Les solutions émergentes*. Quebec: Ministère de la Santé et des Services sociaux, 2000. Volume 1: Rapport et recommandations.

11. Ministère de la Santé et des Services sociaux. 2001. *In brief: The health and social services system in Quebec*. Quebec. <www.msss.gouv.qc.ca/intl/en/en_bref/index.shtml> (January 2003).

12. Ministère de la Santé et des Services sociaux. *Organisation des services: état de situation et perspectives*. Quebec, 2001.

13. Ministère de la Santé et des Services sociaux. *L'assurance-médicamments: un acquis social à préserver*: Régie de l'assurance-maladie du Québec, 2002.

14. Ministère de la Santé et des Services sociaux. *Rapport annuel de gestion 2001-2002*. Quebec, 2002. <www.msss.gouv.qc.ca/f/documentation/index.htm> (January 2003).

15. Ministère de la Santé et des Services sociaux. *Plan stratégique 2001-2004*. Quebec, 2001. <www.msss.gouv.qc.ca/f/documentation/index.htm> (January 2003).

16. Ministère de la Santé et des Services sociaux. *La budgétisation et la performance financière des centres hospitaliers*, 2002. Summary of report of the Comité sur la réévaluation du mode de budgétisation des centres hospitaliers de soins généraux et spécialisés, January.

17. Ministère de la Santé et des Services sociaux. *Rapport annuel 2000-2001*, 2001. <www.msss.gouv.qc.ca/f/documentation/index.htm> (January 2003).

18. Comité sur la vision du réseau d'hôpitaux universitaires [Comité Carignan]. *Vers un réseau universitaire intégré en santé*, 2002. June.

19. Turgeon J, Anctil H. Le Ministère et le réseau public. In Lemieux V, Bergeron P, Bégin C, Bélanger G, editors. *Le système de santé au Québec: organisation, acteurs et enjeux*. Sainte-Foy: Les Presses de l'Université Laval; 1994.

20. Ministère de la Santé et des Services sociaux. *Plan de la santé et des services sociaux: pour faire des bons choix*. Quebec, 2002. <www.msss.gouv.qc.ca/f/documentation/index.htm> (January 2003).

21. Dallaire C, O'Neill M, Lessard C, *et al*. La profession infirmière au Québec: des défis majeurs qui persistent. In Lemieux V, Bergeron P, Bégin C, Bélanger G, editors. *Le système de santé au Québec: organisation, acteurs et enjeux*. Sainte-Foy: Les Presses de l'Université Laval; in press.

22. Ministère de la Santé et des Services sociaux. *Rapport du forum sur la planification de la main-d'oeuvre*. Quebec, 2000.

23. Direction de la santé publique de Montréal-Centre. *Rapport annuel 2000 sur la santé de la population: impact de la reconfiguration du réseau montréalais sur la santé*, 2000. <www.santepub-mtl.qc.ca/Publication/autres/impact2000.html> (January 2003).

24. Turgeon J, Anctil H, Gauthier J. L'évolution du Ministère et du réseau: continuité ou rupture? In Lemieux V, Bergeron P, Bégin C, Bélanger G, editors. *Le système de santé au Québec: organisation, acteurs et enjeux*. Sainte-Foy: Les Presses de l'Université Laval; in press.

25. Romanow R. *Building on values: The future of health care in Canada*. Ottawa: Commission on the Future of Health Care in Canada; Government of Canada, 2002.

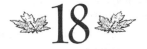

FROM REPORTS
TO REFORMS TO REPORTS

The current national healthcare system in Canada is a mixture of community-based services, home care, and extended care services, imposed onto a pre-existing system of hospitals and medical care. Furthermore, because most healthcare matters are the exclusive jurisdiction of the provinces (and not the federal government), there are regional variations. Also, variable fiscal capabilities and ideologies amongst provinces have influenced the type and extent of health services financed by provinces. As seen earlier, only those services, which fell under the terms and conditions of the *Canada Health Act,* were to an extent uniform across the country. These have led to ten separate provincial and three territorial healthcare systems. Although these are referred to as "the healthcare system," their primary focus and funding mechanisms deal with illness rather than health.

From an international perspective, in the last two decades the healthcare systems in industrialized nations, including Canada, have been under considerable stress, leading to a universal re-examination of how to provide the most effective health care while limiting rising costs. These stressors include:

- continually increasing costs to look after the sick and infirm;
- questions about the appropriate role of government in society;
- the need for evidence-based care, resulting in conflicts between government and healthcare professionals;
- the rise of consumerism;
- changing demographics, with greater numbers of the elderly and increased demand for expensive, high-technology medical care;
- evidence of health-related inequities among people living in poverty;
- the need for disease prevention and health promotion; and
- the inappropriate use of resources by both patients and providers.

Since the late 1980s and into the mid 1990s, every province in Canada, as well as the federal government, had appointed various task forces, commissions, boards of inquiry, and working groups to conduct their own fundamental reviews of the healthcare system. All the subsequent reports as a result of these reviews have been summarized (1, 2), and reform efforts have also been summarized in several key publications (3).

A review of the provincial commissions on healthcare reform during that period revealed several issues common across Canada (2, 4-10). Specifically, the committees studied the questions of rising healthcare costs, a lack of responsiveness in the system, and health services efficacy in improving health status. Proposed solutions also converged: regionalize decision-making structures and decentralize decision-making authority, reform the healthcare system to prioritize primary care and the broad determinants of health, reform health human resources policies, and improve evaluation and research to allow for more effective decision making. As a result of these reports, all provinces except Ontario regionalized their healthcare systems; reduced the capacity of acute care facilities by merging, closing, or downsizing the hospital sector; reduced the number of healthcare professionals by promoting early retirement, reclassifying jobs, or eliminating positions, and, in the case of physicians, reducing enrollment in medical schools by 10% and denying practice entry for international medical graduates.

The federal government also reduced its transfer payments to provincial governments in 1994–96 (see Chapter 14). All these factors strained an already overworked system. Provincial governments responded by limiting or delisting certain services and even attempting to privatize certain services, thus transferring the costs from the public sector to the private sector or to the consumer. This led to a public outcry about the accessibility of health care and the possibility of two-tiered medical care. The provinces responded by appointing more task forces and commissions. The following is a list of provincial commissions and their final reports from 1996 to 2001:

- *Caring for Medicare: Sustaining a Quality System,* by the Commission on Medicare, Province of Saskatchewan, 2000–2001 (11). A one-member commission identified key challenges facing the people of Saskatchewan in reforming and improving medicare, recommended an action plan for delivery of health services, and made recommendations to ensure the long-term stewardship of a publicly funded, publicly administered medicare system.
- *A Framework for Reform,* by the Premier's Advisory Council on Health, Province of Alberta, 2000–2001(12). A 12-member council analyzed the challenges facing Alberta's health system.
- *Les solutions émergentes,* by the Commission d'étude sur les services de santé et les services sociaux, Province of Quebec, 2000 (13). A nine-member commission held a public discussion on the issues facing the health and social services system and proposed solutions for the future. Health and social services are under the jurisdiction of one government department in Quebec; thus, the commission considered child and family services as well as health care.
- *Health Renewal,* by the Premier's Health Quality Council, Province of New Brunswick, 2000–2002 (14). A 14-member council developed an action plan to move to a system of regional health authorities, oversee the implementation of a healthcare report card and other quality reporting measures, and assist in developing a patient charter of rights and responsibilities.

- *Looking Back, Looking Forward,* by the Ontario Health Services Restructuring Commission, Province of Ontario, 1996–2000 (15). A 12-member commission made decisions about hospital restructuring, advised the Minister of Health on reinvesting in health services, and recommended restructuring other components of the healthcare system to improve quality of care, outcomes, and efficiency, and help create an integrated health services system.

There have also, been several federal commissions during this period to assess the health of Canada's healthcare system.

- *Canada Health Action: Building on the Legacy,* by the National Forum on Health, Government of Canada, 1994–1997 (16). A 24-member forum was established by the Prime Minister in 1994 to inform Canadians and advise the federal government.
- *The Health of Canadians — The Federal Role. Volume Six: Recommendations for Reform,* by the Standing Senate Committee on Social Affairs, Science, and Technology, Government of Canada, 2001–2002 (Kirby Commission) (17). An 11-member committee of the Senate of Canada examined the principles on which Canada's publicly funded healthcare system is based, the history of the healthcare system in Canada, the pressures and constraints of current healthcare system, the role of the federal government in the healthcare system, and healthcare systems in foreign jurisdictions. The committee issued five volumes as interim reports and a final report in October 2002.
- *The Shape the Future of Health Care,* by the Commission on the Future of Health in Canada, Government of Canada, 2001–2002 (Romanow Commission) (18). A one-member royal commission appointed by the Prime Minister to inquire into and undertake dialogue with Canadians on the future of Canada's public healthcare system. The final report was released in November 2002.

All provinces as well as the federal government face similar challenges, and the recommendations and solutions proposed by the various commissions and councils have many similarities; the few differences depend upon the political ideology of the ruling party in the various jurisdictions (19-21).

This chapter outlines several key themes addressed in these reports as well as some of the ongoing and emerging issues that were not adequately dealt with. Both the Kirby and Romanow reports are national in scope, and are frequently mentioned; however, similar themes emerged in many of the provincial reports. The chapter concludes with a discussion of possible resolutions for some of the issues raised in the health accord agreed to by the federal and provincial governments in 2003.

1. THEMES OF RECENT REPORTS

1.1. OVERALL VALUES AND GUIDING PRINCIPLES

1.1.1. Fundamental Values of Canadians

The 1997 National Forum on Health identified, through public consultations, the fundamental values of Canadians toward their healthcare system: equity and access;

compassion; dignity and respect for all individuals; quality, efficiency, and effectiveness; personal responsibility for appropriate use of health resources; and public participation in health system decision making (16). The Romanow Commission has echoed similar sentiments from Canadians, including the notion that the healthcare system is premised on equity, fairness, and solidarity(18). It stated that "Canadians consider equal and timely access to medically necessary health care services on a basis of need as a right of citizenship, not a matter of privilege of status or wealth." Concerns over access to services have been particularly pronounced and some people have argued that a patient bill of rights needs to be developed to ensure timely access to services (22). The Kirby Commission had recommended addressing timely access through a national healthcare guarantee. The Romanow Commission recommended a Canadian health covenant as a common declaration of Canadians' and their governments' commitment to a universally accessible, publicly funded healthcare system, rather than establishing new rights that would be subject to legal interpretation and decisions by the courts. The covenant outlines the responsibilities and entitlements for each of the following constituencies: individual Canadians, healthcare providers, and governments (see Table 18.1). The covenant also identifies several specific values that overlap and expand on those identified by the National Forum on Health.

While the National Forum on Health emphasized personal responsibility for appropriate use of health resources, the Romanow Commission stresses mutual responsibility, acknowledging the balance between personal responsibility for health and mutual responsibility for the healthcare system. This includes the financial responsibility to contribute to the system within each individual's means. The commission also identified the values placed on the system's being a public resource, on patient-centred care, and on transparency and accountability.

1.1.2. Governance and Accountability

Despite the common use of the word "system," Canada has no one national healthcare system. Instead, there are separate systems in each province and territory, and even within each jurisdiction, services may not be organized and delivered in similar ways. Both reports recommended the formation of a national council with federal, provincial, and territorial representation. The Kirby Commission argued that the role of system evaluator should be separate from the role of insurer and should be a national undertaking, not federal. It envisioned a national healthcare council, chaired by a national healthcare commissioner, responsible for producing an annual report on the state of the system and the health status of Canadians. In addition, the council would advise the federal government on how to allocate new money raised to reform and renew the healthcare system.

The Romanow Commission recommended a health council built on the existing infrastructure of the Canadian Institute for Health Information (CIHI) and the Canadian Coordinating Office for Health Technology Assessment (CCOHTA). The commission's report provided more detailed information on the activities of the council (e.g., establishing indicators and benchmarks; drawing comparisons with other countries; reporting on efforts to improve quality, access, and outcomes; coordinating activities in health technology

Table 18.1.   A Proposed Health Covenant for Canadians

Healthcare should adhere to following fundamental principles:
Mutual Responsibility
It is a Public Resource
It must be Patient-Centred
Equitable
Universal, Accessible and Portable System
Respectful, and ethical system
Transparency and Accountability
Public Input
Quality, Efficiency and Effectiveness

Individual Canadians are responsible for:
their own well-being and health maintenance; use system prudently and support public financing;
Individual Canadians are entitled to:
health sevices based on health needs, not ability to pay; access to timely, high quality care; ability to make informed decisions; voice their concerns; and to be treated with respect and dignity.

Healthcare providers are responsible for:
highest priority on patient welfare; collaboration with government and others in improving quality of care and patient safety; confidentiality of patient information; open communications with patients; prudent use of health care resources; upholding all professional standards.
Healthcare providers are entitled to:
treated with dignity and respect; and have meaningful role in making decisions related to the operation of system.

Government are responsible for:
develop and administer health care system on principles of social justice and equity; provide adequate, stable and predictable funding in a transparent manner; work collaboratively with all stakeholders to foster innovation and responsive and sustainable system; regular review of performance and operation of system and reporting to public so Canadians can make informed decisiions and contributions to the system; transperancy and accountabilty in decision making; deveoping flexible system for local needs; public input in decision making process on the future of health system and development of healthy public policies.
Govenments are entitled to:
have their jurisdictional roles and responsibilities recognized and respected in charting new directions for the health care system in future.

Source: Adapted from R. Romanow. *Building on values: The future of health care in Canada*. Ottawa: Commission on the Future of Health Care in Canada; Government of Canada, 2002: 50–51.

assessment; etc.). The council would also provide ongoing advice and coordination on major structural issues (e.g., primary healthcare reform, health workforce strategies, dispute resolution under the *Canada Health Act*).

1.1.3.   Quality, Access, and Waiting Times

As indicated above, timely access to services is a major concern for the Canadian public. The Kirby Commission recommended that national standard definitions be developed for maximum needs-based waiting times for each type of major procedure and treatment. When the maximum time is reached, the government would be responsible for paying for the patient to seek the procedure or treatment immediately in another jurisdiction. The Romanow Commission focused on governments taking action to manage wait lists more effectively and providing funds to improve access to necessary diagnostic services and establish frameworks for measuring the extent of the problem.

1.1.4. Public Participation in Decision Making

Citizens have long been involved in organizing the delivery of health services to their peers. Over the last century, citizens have become more involved in the healthcare system through voluntary health agencies and, lately, through consumer advocacy movements. In recent years, consumers have expressed concerns about inconvenience, the availability of health services, difficulties in communication between practitioners and consumers, paternalism on the part of providers, lack of individual input into care plans, and inadequacy of health care for certain groups in society. Many people feel that the system is designed for the convenience of the healthcare practitioner rather than the patient. Many would prefer to take a more active part in decisions regarding their own health care, be better equipped to give informed consent, and develop a more personal relationship with their practitioners than the harried atmosphere that office visits or hospital consultations allows.

Consumer participation can be facilitated by sharing knowledge about the causation of diseases, participating in the formulation of healthcare policies, creating citizens' voluntary groups, and through membership on hospital boards or committees and boards that are involved in the regulation of health professions.

Consumer involvement in health care encounters obstacles at two levels: at the level of the individual consultation with the healthcare provider, and at the level of community involvement in health policy formation and system planning. At the individual level, health care — particularly medical care — is dominated by technology and professional super-specialization. How can an individual know whether the care received is good? The supply is restricted by the professional bodies through their licensing requirements, creating a monopoly, and the suppliers of health services can generate the demand for their own services (e.g., a physician or nurse practitioner can ask a patient to come back once or ten times for treatment of high blood pressure). In this context, the individual tends to do what the professional dictates. Health care is episodic and crisis oriented and even if the consumer is dissatisfied once the crisis is over, the problems encountered by consumers become less important than other aspects of their life, and hence complaints are rarely made to providers.

At the systemic level, public participation studies have consistently shown that only the more affluent and the higher educated consumers are likely to participate in policy formation debates (23). Alternatively, only those individuals with a vested interest in a particular issue find the necessary time and energy for political activism. Conversely, healthcare professional associations are better organized and better funded for political activism, and frequently have privileged access to state policy makers through well-established government committees. In light of these barriers, consumers and small consumer organizations frequently do not have the voice in policy debates that is required for truly effective involvement.

The increasing focus on consumers is evidenced by the recommendations of a healthcare guarantee and a healthcare covenant from the Kirby and Romanow reports. The increasing focus on sustainability, timely access, accountability, and transparency guarantees that consumers' perspective and involvement will continue to grow in decision making about the healthcare system.

1.1.5. International Agreements

The Romanow Commission expressed concern about protecting the healthcare system from potential interference by international trade agreements. It recommended that any future reforms should be implemented under the protection of the definition of public services and reinforced Canada's position that it has the right to regulate healthcare policy that is not subject to claims for compensation by foreign-based companies. In addition, alliances should be made with other countries, especially those that are members of the World Trade Organization, to ensure that future international agreements make explicit allowance for maintaining and expanding publicly insured, financed, and delivered health care.

1.2. FINANCING

1.2.1. Privatization and Public Goods

The Kirby Commission examined the implications of private healthcare insurance and private service delivery. A particular concern was that unless timely access to the publicly funded system could be assured, there would be increasing pressure to loosen restrictions and create a parallel system of private insurance and delivery. The committee concluded that when parallel private systems compete with publicly funded coverage, a number of problems develop including risk selection and "cream skimming" (i.e., the private system deals with low-risk patients and activities with a high financial return), no reduction in waiting lists in the public sector, queue jumping, and preferential treatment. It also observed that based on data from 22 countries, increases in private spending on health care were associated over time with decreases in public healthcare funding.

In addressing the same issue, the Romanow Commission noted that data from the United States indicates that the non-profit sector tends to result in better quality outcomes than the for-profit sector in areas such as nursing home care and managed care organizations and hospitals. For-profit hospitals have also been observed to have a significant increase in the risk of death, and tend to employ less highly skilled individuals than non-profit facilities. Similar to the Kirby Commission, the Romanow report observed that for-profit facilities tend to select specific services and use the public system as a back-up in case a poor outcome occurs. Similar to the Kirby conclusions, the Romanow report argued that governments should choose to ensure that the public system has sufficient capacity and is universally accessible, instead of subsidizing private facilities with public dollars.

1.2.2.   Funding and Financing

Federal health transfers payments are currently combined with other payments under the Canadian Health and Social Transfer. To improve transparency and accountability, both reports recommended a new, separate healthcare transfer fund. The Kirby report explicitly stated that system sustainability depended on new funds, but that these should only be used to finance reforms and be audited annually by the Auditor General. It also recommended that a healthcare insurance premium be implemented to raise the necessary federal revenue to implement the report's recommendations. The Romanow report stressed the need to set funding levels for five years forward to facilitate adequate planning and that a series of targeted funds be established: rural and remote access (including telehealth), diagnostic services, primary health care, home care, and catastrophic drugs.

1.3.   SCOPE OF SERVICES TO BE COVERED

At present, in Canada, the health insurance programs cover hospitalization in acute care facilities and medically necessary services provided by physicians. Both commissions recommended going beyond this coverage to include other services.

1.3.1.   Canada Health Act

Both the Kirby and Romanow reports recommended expanding the range of services covered by the *Canada Health Act* to include home care, palliative care, and prescription drugs, but differed in their emphasis. The increased accountability mechanisms discussed above would also be built into the Act. The coverage of specific services varies among provinces that have, over time, selectively removed conditions from the list of benefits. The Kirby Commission suggested the creation of a committee to review and make recommendations on the set of services to be covered. The Romanow Commission focused on clarifying coverage of diagnostic services. Further recommendations were made to clarify the principle of public administration and to develop an effective dispute resolution process.

1.3.2.   Drugs

The costs of drugs have been increasing faster than all other components of health care, are now second only to hospital costs, and have exceeded the costs of physician services. Since there are existing problems in timely access for services already covered by the *Canada Health Act*, the addition of a large and increasing cost item is problematic financially. Nevertheless, both reports suggested increased efforts to address drug costs including the development of a national formulary. The Kirby Commission recommended introducing a program to protect against catastrophic prescription drug expenses. Federal contributions would start once specific thresholds are set for absolute individual cost and percentage of family income spent on prescription costs. The Romanow Commission's approach would be to use a drug transfer fund to reduce disparities in coverage across the country by covering a portion of provincial and territorial drug plans. It also supported the development of a national drug agency to evaluate and approve new prescription drugs, provide ongoing evaluation of existing drugs, negotiate and contain drug prices, and provide comprehensive, objective, and accurate information to healthcare providers and the public. The commission also recommended a review of drug patent protection to ensure an appropriate balance between protection of intellectual property, the need to contain costs, and to improve access on non-patented prescription drugs.

1.3.3. Home and Community Care

Publicly funded homecare services vary considerably across the country. Both reports recommended coverage of post-hospital homecare services. The Kirby report specifically suggested that financing for this service flow through hospitals, as a hospital substitution strategy. The Romanow Commission emphasized the immediate need to consider home care for mental health as medically necessary under the *Canada Health Act*. With respect to palliative care services, the Kirby report recommended a national palliative homecare program that would be jointly funded (50:50) with provinces and territories. It also suggested examining the feasibility of changes to Employment Insurance, the Canada Labour Code, and tax measures to assist family members who choose to care for a dying relative at home. The Romanow report also recommended developing proposals for direct support to informal caregivers to allow them to spend time from work to provide homecare assistance.

1.3.4. Long-Term Care

Long-term-care (LTC) is required when an individual's health deficiencies impede independent functioning and help is required from formal service providers. The people who use such services are usually the elderly, people with disabilities, or people with a chronic or prolonged illness. There are also significant numbers of young people with disabilities in long-term institutions, or supported by family and friends whom they may outlive and so become dependent on the publicly provided system.

There is no identifiable Canadian policy, terminology, information system, or set of standards of care for LTC. The *Canada Health Act* does not cover it and each province has developed its own range of services and policies. As mentioned above, the Kirby and Romanow reports addressed the issue of acute post-hospital homecare services, which to a large degree is a hospital substitution strategy.

In some provinces, LTC is placed in the health portfolio and in others it is in social services. Even within a province, jurisdictional roles frequently change. The issue is further complicated by the fact that LTC can be provided by either the public or private sectors, and delivered in institutions as well as community- and home-based services. As a result, it is very difficult to gather information systematically concerning the provision of LTC. Furthermore, informal care by families and especially women, provide most LTC — approximately 80%. Significant changes to the structure and coherence of family units are reflected in the ability of family members to provide care.

Internationally and in most Canadian provinces there is an emphasis on community care (as opposed to institutional care) to encourage independence in the community for as long as possible. For the majority of the elderly, this can be achieved through the provision of instrumental support services (such as home maintenance). Personal healthcare services (such as bathing) may also be required for people who are elderly or disabled, and may be provided in the community, although more usually in an institutional setting. A spectrum of care settings is desirable, with staged residential care that allows for some supervision and support as an option between community independence and institutionalization. The predictors of institutionalization are advanced age, lack of spouse in the household, hospital admission in the previous two years, cognitive impairment, and difficulty with taking care of personal care needs. Of these, cognitive impairment is a determining factor for many elderly. It has been estimated that up to 65% of the very elderly suffer cognitive impairment, and provisions must be met for the necessary care.

The issue of referral and access to LTC has become a major concern and has been addressed by a number of provincial strategies and reform initiatives. The issue is whether homecare and chronic care beds should require a medical referral. Most LTC reform reports recommend that personal choice and consumer input in terms of preference be involved in placement decisions. Cultural sensitivity and appropriateness are also stressed. Of particular concern is the quality of life of residents in LTC institutions.

Many provincial commissions have recommended a shift away from institutionalization of extended care patients, as well as a reduction of extended care or chronic care beds in acute care hospitals to no more than 10% of the hospital's total beds. However, in order for de-institutionalization to be successful, more home support is needed. And while home-supported LTC placements seem preferable to institutionalized care in many respects, few provincial health plans can afford to cover the costs for families taking care of relatives at home. Some critics consider de-institutionalization of long-term care an attempt to shift healthcare costs out of government budgets and onto the private sector via the family.

In summary, the trend in LTC is to maximize independence in the community for people who are elderly, disabled, or chronically ill through the transfer of resources from the institutional sector to the community. Although LTC is deemed a high priority in every provincial health reform strategy, there is no national policy, and provinces are at different stages in adoption and development of more appropriate models of service delivery. There is need for leadership at top levels of governments in planning and policy for long-term care.

1.3.5. Mental Health Services

Mental health services, broadly defined, comprise a mix of health, social, vocational, recreational, volunteer, occupational therapy, and educational services, as well as housing and income support. They include a range of activities and objectives ranging from mental health promotion and the prevention of mental health problems to the treatment of acute psychiatric disorders and the support and rehabilitation of persons with severe and persistent psychiatric disorders and disabilities.

In the 1960s and 1970s, de-institutionalization policies promoted the integration and rehabilitation of inpatients in the community through a community mental health program. In 1961, the report of the Canadian Mental Health Association (24) and the

1964 Report of the Royal Commission on Health Services (25) both reflected a commitment to the philosophy of de-institutionalization. There was a call for the integration of psychiatric services into the physical and personnel resources of the rest of medicine, regionalized treatment services, decentralized management of psychiatric services, and close cooperation and coordination among the psychiatric services in hospitals, clinics, and community agencies.

Between 1960 and 1976, the numbers of beds in Canadian mental hospitals decreased by more than 32,000 and the bed capacity of psychiatric units in general hospitals increased to almost 6,000, from under 1,000. In addition to the removal of resources for specialized psychiatric care, there was inadequate follow-up in the community and lack of support for the mechanics of everyday living. The plight of the chronically disturbed ex-psychiatric patient frequently became homelessness or ghetto-type living, exacerbated by symptoms, despondency, suicidal tendencies, and alienation from the community. The effects of these well-intentioned but ultimately unproductive policies continue to reverberate.

In the 1990s, there has been a universal re-examination of mental health services, as well as an ongoing strong financial commitment to mental health reform in virtually every province and territory. With the advent of regionalization everywhere except Ontario, the funding and delivery of mental health services in some provinces is now the responsibility of regional health boards, whereas in others it is still managed by provincial or territorial government. Most provinces and territories have a central mental health advisory committee or council to help develop broader policies and strategic plans. In Ontario, the Ministry of Health continues to hold most responsibilities for mental health programs, with municipalities and local regions scheduled to take over this function in the near future.

All provinces and territories have now developed community mental health programs that include case management, rehabilitation, housing programs, and other support services. With an emphasis on multidisciplinary care and flexible service delivery, community mental health programs have come a long way in striving to meet the individualized needs of those who are mentally ill.

Community mental health facilities now extend beyond mental institutions to provide greater continuity of care, to deal with incipient breakdown, and to rehabilitate patients in the community. Psychiatric units in general hospitals contribute by integrating psychiatry with other medical care and making it available in the community. Psychiatric units in general hospitals admit approximately 86% of total admissions to all kinds of mental institutions (26). Inpatient services in psychiatric units are paid for by all provincial hospital insurance plans. Some provinces have small regional psychiatric hospitals that facilitate patient access to treatment and complete integration of medical services. There are daycare centres across the country that allow patients to be hospitalized during the day and return home at night, as well as community mental health clinics (some provincially operated, others municipally) and psychiatric outpatient services. Specialized rehabilitation services assist former patients to function optimally and are operated by mental hospitals and community agencies. They include sheltered workshops that pay for work and provide training, and halfway houses where patients can live and continue to receive treatment while settling in a job. At present, there is a large gap in available community services for mental health patients because of shortages of affordable housing, jobs, recreational facilities, and mental health workers.

Facilities for people who are mentally challenged include day training schools or classes, summer camps, and sheltered workshops, as well as residential care in institutions and community group homes. These facilities provide social, academic, and vocational training; some offer academic education, some support self-care, some teach manual skills, and some help find job placements in the community. Children with personality or behaviour disorders are treated at hospital units, community clinics, child guidance clinics, and other outpatient facilities.

Despite improvements, certain problems persist, such as fragmentation of care, poor accountability, ineffective case management, high readmission rates, and insufficient links between hospitals and the community (27). Recognizing these needs, the Romanow Commission recommended two types of homecare services for people with mental health problems. The first is case management, with a case manager who would work directly with the individual and with other healthcare providers and community agencies to monitor the individual's health and ensure the appropriate supports are in place. This would ensure both continuity and co-ordination of care. The second is home intervention to assist and support patients when they have occasional acute periods of disruptive behaviour that pose a threat to themselves or to others and could trigger unnecessary hospitalization.

1.4.   RESTRUCTURING OR IMPROVING THE DELIVERY SYSTEM

1.4.1.   Primary Health Care

Both reports stress the need to reform primary care delivery and suggest providing financial support to provinces and territories that implement reform. Similar to previous reports on primary care reform, the Kirby Commission recommended that multidisciplinary primary care teams should provide a range of services around the clock, use the most appropriate type of health professional, adopt alternative methods of payment, integrate health promotion and illness prevention, and assume a greater degree of responsibility for all health and wellness needs of the population they serve. The Romanow Commission recommended using targeted transfer funds to fast-track primary care reforms based on continuity of care, early detection and action, better information on needs and outcomes, and new and stronger incentives. It also recommended a national summit to mobilize concerted action, assess results, and address barriers to implementation.

1.4.2.   Health Information

Health care is an information-intense business, yet Canada's healthcare system is predominantly paper based. The Romanow and Kirby reports supported the development of electronic health records, which should be done in partnership with provinces and territories to avoid unnecessary duplication and systemic incompatibilities. Both reports stressed the importance of standards for handling information, including personal ownership by individual Canadians and protection of privacy. The Kirby Commission stressed the need for research on Canadian attitudes to the use of electronic health information, and Romanow emphasized the use of new technologies to link Canadians to health information that is properly researched, trustworthy, and credible in order to support more widespread efforts to promote health.

1.4.3. Organization and Integration of Services

The Kirby Commission's interest in infrastructure extended to recommending service-based funding of community hospitals, particularly in large urban centres. It further recommended giving regional health authorities (RHAs) in larger urban centres control over the costs of physician services and prescription drug spending. The intent was to allow RHAs to be able to choose providers on the basis of quality and costs and to reward the best providers with increased volume. Evaluation of the impact of internal market reforms was also recommended.

1.4.4. Medical Errors

Medical errors have been identified as a significant cause of morbidity and mortality in the U.S. healthcare system. The U.S. Institute of Medicine indicated that as many as 44,000 to 98,000 people die in hospitals each year as the result of medical errors in the United States (28). This would place such errors as the eighth leading cause of death, higher than motor vehicle collisions, breast cancer, or AIDS. Errors can also occur outside hospitals in physicians' offices, nursing homes, pharmacies, urgent care centres, and in the home. Consequently, multiple interventions have been proposed to reduce medical errors and improve patient outcomes.

In Canada, the National Steering Committee on Patient Safety recommended establishing an institute that would deal with issues related to patient safety (29). A study to examine the extent of medical errors in hospitals has also been launched, with the goal of developing a national strategy for patient safety by coming up with specific standards and a better flow of information through the development of databases(30). Research teams from British Columbia, Ontario, Alberta, Quebec, and the Maritimes will complete the study by 2004.

1.5. POPULATION HEALTH

1.5.1. The Determinants of Health

As described in Chapter 1, the healthcare sector is but one component of the many determinants of population health. General trends within the health and political sectors reflect growing national consensus for greater system-wide integration of policies to develop "healthy public policies". There is a clear need to coordinate government policies more effectively across all sectors of society. For example, in the 1997 federal election the issue of child poverty featured prominently in candidates' discussions. In addition, Parliament had passed an unanimous resolution in 1989 to eliminate child poverty in Canada by the year 2000. Governments had also made a commitment to reform child tax benefits and increase money for the support of children by the end of the twentieth century. The final report of the National Forum on Health also emphasized the importance of integrating broad social policy in order to improve the health of Canadians: "We believe that the social and economic determinants of health merit particular attention. We are particularly concerned about the impact of poverty, unemployment, and cuts in social supports on the health of individuals, groups, and communities" (16). Chapter 6 deals with some of the federal initiatives in the sections on health of children living in poverty, health of Aboriginal peoples, and seniors.

All the recent federal and provincial reports have identified several high-risk groups with health needs particularly affected by social, employment, housing, and education issues. There is a dire need for increased inter-sectoral coordination of policy to begin addressing issues related to determinants of health other than those in the health sector. The framework for addressing these issues are outlined in the Ottawa Charter on Health Promotion (see Chapter 1), but there seems to be insufficient collective will to move forward.

1.5.2.   Health Promotion and Disease Prevention

Conventional wisdom has long recognized that an ounce of prevention is worth a pound of cure, and the healthcare system is no exception. A vital step toward increasing the cost effectiveness of the Canadian healthcare system and improving its general effectiveness and quality is to focus on preventing ill health and disease before they start. All the provincial reports, as well as the final recommendations of the National Forum on Health and the Kirby and Romanow Commissions, pointed to the need for a greater emphasis on health promotion and illness prevention.

Currently, less than 5% of all healthcare dollars is spent in activities related to disease prevention and health promotion. A reduction in healthcare costs could be achieved through health promotion and disease prevention strategies. It has been recommended that a greater proportion of healthcare expenditures should be spent on these programs. The common recommendation was for a shift from curative to preventive health and a corresponding increase in funding for research and development into health promotion and preventive medicine, typically to 1% of the annual healthcare expenditures. Regional health boards are also mandated to focus, as a priority, on health promotion and disease prevention. Of the two major reports, the Kirby Commission addressed population and public health in greater detail, recommending increased funding including the development of a national strategy for preventing chronic disease. The Romanow Commission recommended a national immunization strategy as well as a federal, provincial, and territorial strategy for increasing physical activity in Canada.

1.5.3.   Literacy

Although literacy was not the subject of any of the reports, it deserves consideration. The high prevalence of problems with reading both simple and more complex sentences in the Canadian population has already been highlighted in Chapter 4. One out of every four Canadians is functionally illiterate. This has serious implications in terms of people's ability to participate fully in society, especially in terms of obtaining access to information, using community services, and complying with medication and other health-related instructions. It is unlikely that remediation and upgrading reading programs will reach all those who could benefit. Therefore, increased awareness and the development of strategies to address illiteracy at the level of the patient and at the level of the community, especially in community-based health education and communication programs, are needed.

The essential component of literacy awareness in health care is the critical analysis of printed material that is developed or distributed according to its readability. It is estimated that 50% of patients cannot read or have difficulty with instructions at the grade 5 level. Changes to written material can increase its readability for its intended audience. They include keeping sentences to 20 words or less (although varying the length), using simple concepts, using words that can be pictured, using active verbs, using material related to the patient's experience, and avoiding unnecessary words (31). Pictorial cues and the use of audiovisual media and stories using photographs or drawings can improve communication if there is a literacy problem (32).

It is estimated that 30% to 80% of patients do not use their medication properly. It has been shown that adherence can be improved, for example with verbal reinforcement of instructions by a pharmacist. More effective reinforcement comes via brochures or written instructions, if these are understood. However, one study of patient education aids assessed the average reading level of the educational material around the grade 11 level, which was considered to be far too high for the average patient (33).

1.6. ISSUES RELATED TO INFRASTRUCTURE

1.6.1. Health Human Resources

The training, recruitment, retention, and distribution of healthcare professionals are critical ongoing issues in the Canadian healthcare system. Both reports recommended systematic data collection and analysis of workforce data and the development of a comprehensive plan to address workforce issues. The reports differed in their suggestions for funding mechanisms as well as for the direct involvement of the federal government in funding health provider education programs. An independent review of the scope of practice rules and other regulations was recommended to enable services to be delivered by the most appropriately qualified professionals.

1.6.2. Healthcare Infrastructure

The Kirby Commission was particularly concerned about increasing federal funding for specific infrastructure elements including the expansion of hospitals in high population growth areas, academic health sciences centres, and the purchase and assessment of healthcare technology. The latter was a focus of the Romanow Commission, which urged streamlining technology assessment.

1.7.   ISSUES RELATED TO SPECIAL POPULATIONS

1.7.1.   Aboriginal Health

Aboriginal populations have substantially lower health status than the average Canadian (see Chapters 6 and 13). To address these inequalities, the Romanow Commission made several recommendations including the pooling of current funding for Aboriginal health services by the various levels of government into consolidated budgets in each province or territory and be used to integrate Aboriginal health services, improve access, and provide adequate, stable and predictable funding. The Kirby Commission recommended funding medical and nursing school positions for Aboriginal students, and increasing health research to improve Aboriginal health. It also identified Aboriginal health as a thematic issue for future study.

1.7.2.   Multicultural Health

Multicultural health is used to refer to health care provided in a culturally and racially sensitive manner. A multicultural healthcare facility "reflects the contributions and interests of diverse cultural and social groups in its mission, operations and products or services" (34). In order for health care to become truly multicultural, healthcare providers must be aware of the cultural and ethnic determinants of health, the differing beliefs about health and medicine among ethnic communities, and the barriers faced by members of ethnic minorities in gaining access to health care. A multicultural profile of the Canadian population is described in Chapter 4.

Determinants of Health in Multicultural Communities

In general, mortality and morbidity rates are higher among members of specific cultural groups. Contributing factors include assimilation into the culture of the host country in terms of diet and lifestyle, the degree to which the ethnic traditions are maintained, and the extent of support systems in the community of origin; these have a significant bearing on the incidence and prevalence of diseases such as elevated blood pressure and coronary heart disease.

Problems arising from environmental factors include the mental health problems experienced by many immigrants and refugees, especially those from visible minorities. Immigrants and refugees experience stress associated with migration, separation from family members and communities, loss of homes and possessions, possible inability to speak the language of their new community, difficulty in finding suitable employment, negative public attitudes toward newcomers, ethnocentrism and racism, and pressures of assimilation, all of which affect family relations. These experiences can lead to feelings of alienation, loss of self-esteem, and emotional disorders, placing immigrants to Canada at considerable risk for mental illness (35).

Inaccessibility of Health Care

Personal factors that contribute to the inaccessibility of healthcare services for members of ethnic minorities include their own cultural beliefs concerning health care and healthcare practitioners, language barriers, lack of knowledge about access to health services, and a fear of discrimination. Healthcare providers may be hindered by a lack of information about ethnic communities and health, lack of cross-cultural training and ethnically representative staffing, and an unwillingness to deliver health services in a culturally sensitive manner. Differing beliefs about health issues can significantly affect the approach to health care for members of some ethnic groups. For example, in many cultures birth control and open discussions of sex and sexuality are unacceptable. Reliance on herbal medicine or alternative treatments (e.g., acupuncture) can further complicate patient care. Although many cultural communities accept western medicinal practices, many prefer their own forms of treatment and delivery, or to discuss their problems with someone, regardless of training, of the same ethnicity.

Language Barriers

Demographic profiles indicate that approximately 1% of Canadians are unable to conduct a conversation in either official language. These people may be clustered in large urban areas (e.g., Toronto and Vancouver), or scattered sporadically across rural areas such as northern Canada. Without proper translation and interpretation services, this language barrier can affect members of ethnic minorities at every stage of the healthcare continuum. Educational materials provided only in French and English fail to inform members of linguistic minorities about health promotion, disease prevention, early recognition of certain health problems, and the availability of healthcare services and resources.

Ineffective translation and interpretation services prevent many people from seeking health care, and may create problems for those who do. Fortunately, many hospitals and community healthcare centres in cities with large immigrant populations such as Toronto and Vancouver are beginning to recognize this difficulty and are altering staffing patterns to include bilingual healthcare professionals for at least some of the more numerous ethnic clients being served (e.g., Cantonese speakers).

Racism and Ethnocentrism

Members of visible minorities and ethnic groups often experience racist or discriminatory treatment from healthcare practitioners. This behaviour may come in the form of negative comments or attitudes toward immigrants and refugees, a lack of respect or ignorance of the different health beliefs of ethnic communities, or stereotyping. The effects of this kind of treatment are twofold: the patient receives improper or inappropriate treatment and may therefore develop further health problems, and as a result of the poor treatment the patient and others from that community are discouraged from seeking future treatment. Difficulties are often not due to the traditional health beliefs and practices of ethnic communities. For example, for mental health services, the main perceived barrier is that therapists do not provide treatment that is culturally and linguistically appropriate (36).

Assimilation versus Accessibility

The reluctance of many healthcare professionals to develop multicultural structures and policies may be based on the belief that ethnic minorities should simply assimilate to the Canadian health culture, and that the healthcare system should not be responsible for ensuring the accessibility of services to members of cultural communities. This view is not only ethnocentric and unrealistic, but also ignores the health implications of forced assimilation. For example, individuals who identify strongly with their own ethnic communities have lower risk of suicide than those who did not consider themselves to be part of a cohesive ethnic community (36).

Organizational Barriers

Factors preventing healthcare organizations from successfully addressing multicultural health needs include an unwillingness to become culturally sensitive, a tendency to adopt superficial solutions such as using support staff as translators, a lack of demographic and health data on ethnic communities, insufficient financial and human resources, a lack of training and skills development, an absence of monitoring and evaluative mechanisms, rigid, hierarchical, and competitive organizational climates not conducive to change, and a lack of commitment from senior management (36).

Human Resources and Education

Once a commitment to multicultural health has been made, significant changes to the organization must occur, starting with the staff. Healthcare practitioners usually receive no education concerning the health profiles and needs of ethnic minority groups. Therefore, extensive cross-cultural training must be provided to and made mandatory for health services workers and students. Emphasis should be placed on the fact that what may be seen by the healthcare provider as an accessibility or educational problem may often be interpreted by the consumer as evidence of racism or ethnocentrism. As well as ensuring that properly trained translators and interpreters are provided, healthcare facilities and educational organizations should also promote the education and hiring of healthcare providers who are members of ethnic minorities.

The education and training of health services providers must be accompanied by a change in hiring practices. As well as ensuring that properly trained translators and interpreters are provided, healthcare facilities and educational organizations should also promote the education and hiring of healthcare providers who are members of ethnic minorities. This kind of affirmative action policy will reduce the need for translators and interpreters, and ensure understanding of the particular health problems of the community, as well as making the healthcare facility more welcome for members of the ethnic communities.

With the changing demography of Canada's population, this neglected aspect of health care will need increased attention in the future. The Romanow Commission mentioned the need to recognize francophones and other cultural minorities in only one recommendation.

1.8.   SCIENTIFIC ADVANCES

1.8.1.   Research and Innovation

The Kirby and Romanow reports both contained several recommendations for improving research and innovation in the healthcare system. These included improving dissemination of research knowledge to providers, developing a formal ethical governance system, and increasing research funding. Specific targets of funding included research on vulnerable populations, rural and remote health issues, interprofessional collaboration and learning, health promotion, and pharmaceutical policy.

1.8.2. Genomics and Biotech Advances

Many view the sequencing of the human genome as the beginning of a new paradigm in medicine. A draft of the entire human genome sequence was announced in June 2000, with analyses published in February 2001 (37). There are high expectations of the impact of such knowledge on the understanding of disease mechanisms, early detection, genetic therapies, and tailoring drug therapies to genotypes. The human genome contains 3 billion chemical base pairs. Despite the sequencing efforts, it remains unclear precisely how many genes the genome contains (38).

Further research will aim to understand the structure and function of the human genome and its role in health and disease. It will likely be possible to identify gene associations for many common illnesses in the next five to seven years, but that this will require sophisticated clinical investigation and improvements in technology to handle the vast amounts of data to be analyzed (39). Early detection will only be useful if it permits an intervention that improves the health outcome that would otherwise have occurred. Since most common illnesses such as heart disease and cancer are likely influenced by many genes as well as environmental factors, practitioners will be faced with explaining complex statistical risk information to inform patients of potential preventive options.

A major component of the Human Genome Project is the analysis of the ethical, legal, and social implications of this newfound genetic knowledge, and the subsequent development of policy options for public consideration. It is summarized by a recent publication of the Government of Ontario (40). For example, increased knowledge of individuals' disease susceptibilities raises several types of ethical issues, including the need to protect the privacy of individuals and to outlaw the use of predictive genetic information in the workplace and in obtaining health information. The U.S. National Human Genome Research Institute's Ethical, Legal, and Social Implications Program was established in 1990 as an integral part of the Human Genome Project to foster basic and applied research, and support education and outreach.

1.8.3. Cloning and Stem Cell Research

Stem cell research, which involves generating new cells from embryonic and adult tissue, has engaged ethical debate and government policy decisions around the world. Stem cells have the ability to develop into many different kinds of cells, offering a potential treatment for a wide range of medical conditions including stroke, multiple sclerosis, diabetes, and Parkinson's. Since the best source of stem cells is a human embryo, the research is swamped by a number of ethical concerns. In Canada, the *Assisted Human Reproduction Act* was introduced on May 9, 2002 (41). If passed, this bill would allow surrogacy, sperm donation, the use of eggs and other reproductive material, the use of embryos to assist conception and stem cells research. It would not allow human cloning, stem cell cloning, the growing of human embryos for research, sex selection, changes made to human DNA, and buying or selling embryos, sperm, eggs, or other human reproductive material.

1.8.4.   Pharmacogenetics

The vision for pharmacogenetics is to be able to provide tailored drug therapy based on genetically determined variations in effectiveness and side effects. Many drug-metabolizing enzymes result in large variations in function between individuals and likely contribute to the occurrence of adverse drug reactions (ADRs). Pharmacogenetics may identify the genotype of individuals at high risk. However, the results from ADR studies are not expected for another five years (42), and genetically tailored treatments will likely take as long as 10 to 12 years more. The medical and economic benefits that will be offered by pharmacogenetic targeted interventions must be weighed against the cost of genotyping all individuals in order to direct an intervention at possibly only a few (43). A relatively simple example of pharmacogenetics exists today. Women with the factor V Leiden mutation who are put on oral contraceptives have a 20- to 150-fold increased risk of thromboembolism (44). A total of 7,000 individuals would need to be screened in order to identify 350 carriers. All these carriers would be denied oral contraceptives in order to prevent one thromboembolic event.

A number of different challenges in this area exist for both physicians and patients including decisions about when and whom to test, how to use the results, issues of patient privacy, patient consent procedures, and the issue of legal protection for patients against unauthorized disclosure. Prescribing drugs according to genotype could reduce demand for particular drugs, thus lessening the stream of revenue and the profits available to invest in research and development for the pharmaceutical industry. In addition, regulatory policies would be required to oversee the validity and utility of genetic tests and laboratories' performance of the test (45).

2.   FIRST MINISTERS' ACCORD ON HEALTH CARE RENEWAL, 2003

Following the release of the Romanow Commission's report, the federal and provincial governments engaged in intense negotiations on how to reform the healthcare system and how to fund these reforms. Many provincial governments took the position that there should be increased federal funding, but without any limitations imposed on how the money was spent. This ran counter not only to the federal position, but also to the themes of greater system collaboration, accountability, and strategic investment described in the Romanow and Kirby reports.

On February 5, 2003, the First Ministers' Accord on Health Care Renewal was signed, with the federal government agreeing to provide $34.8 billion over five years (46). The first ministers consider the accord a covenant that will help ensure Canadians have timely access to health services that are high in quality, effective, patient-centred, and safe, and that the healthcare system is sustainable and affordable. While the accord reaffirms the five principles of public health insurance and commits to enhancing transparency and accountability, it is not as comprehensive and detailed as was recommended by the Romanow Commission.

The accord does address the high-profile themes of home care, drug costs, and primary care. Provinces and territories will provide first-dollar coverage for a basket of minimum services for short-term acute home care, including acute community mental health and end-of-life care. The minimum services that will be provided are still to be determined. The federal government agreed to make legislative changes to support family caregivers which were announced in the 2003 federal budget. Individuals who meet the eligibility requirements for Employment Insurance (EI) special benefits are entitled to a six-week EI benefit for compassionate family care leave to care for a gravely ill or dying child, parent, or spouse. Eligible family members will be able to share the benefit. The federal government will also propose changes to the Canada Labour Code so that permanent employees will have their jobs protected during their leave. This particular benefit is estimated to cost $86 million in 2003–04 and $221 million in 2004–05 and each year thereafter.

The first ministers also agreed that by the end of 2005–06, Canadians would have reasonable access to catastrophic drug coverage. There was also agreement on various other actions to improve the cost-effectiveness of drug use. The first ministers agreed to accelerate primary care initiatives immediately, with the goal of ensuring that at least 50% of their residents have round-the-clock access to an appropriate healthcare provider as soon as possible and the target be reached within eight years. Each jurisdiction is to develop its own multi-year targets.

The progresses on these three initiatives are to be provided annually by each first minister. Both the Kirby and Romanow reports had recommended some form of national accountability for monitoring the healthcare system. The accord states that each jurisdiction will report to its constituents and use common indicators on the themes of quality, access, system efficiency, and effectiveness. In addition, a health council will monitor and report annually on the implementation of the accord, particularly on the provisions for accountability and transparency. The council will include representatives from both levels of government, experts, and the public, and will report through federal, provincial, and territorial ministers of health. The council, however, falls far short of the role envisioned by both Kirby and Romanow.

Other initiatives in the accord include the development of a diagnostic/medical equipment fund to support specialized staff training and equipment to improve access to diagnostic services. Additional support will also be provided to Infoway to implement of electronic health records and further development of telehealth applications. The first ministers also directed their health ministers to work on improving patient safety, addressing health human resources, technology assessment, innovation and research, and coordinating approaches to address disparities in health status. Specifically, the health ministers were directed to pursue a national immunization strategy. The health challenges faced by Aboriginal Canadians were also identified and the federal government will enhance funding and work collaboratively with other governments to achieve better integration of health services. The 2003 federal budget committed $1.3 billion over the next five years to First Nations and Inuit health programs, including new investments for on-reserve nursing and capital development. This will include $32 million for a national on-reserve immunization strategy. The accord also states that the health ministers are to work with Aboriginal peoples on an Aboriginal health-reporting framework so that progress on key health outcomes can be monitored.

3.   FROM HERE TO THERE

The chapters in the last section of this book have addressed the evolution of the Canadian healthcare system into today's system. Canadian health care was, and continues to be, a matter of intense personal pride for Canadians: a modern-day social success story that helps define the Canadian national identity. But since the early 1970s, Canada, together with all other industrialized nations of the world, has faced a series of systemic stressors that have led to the re-examination of the healthcare system — its goals, its organization, and the way it functions. As a result, the current system is in flux as each province and territory in Canada as well as the federal government strives to find that particular combination of health policies and reforms that will best meet the health needs of its population. This chapter has highlighted some of the common themes found in all Canadian healthcare reforms and the underlying values each is trying to address. The roads to reform are many, but the ultimate destination is the same — improving the health of Canadians.

As Canada moves into the 21st century, many of the issues discussed in this chapter continue to dominate the policy agenda. Questions concerning cost effectiveness and cost control continue to play a lead role in all discussions. As a result, the possibility of creating more effective and cost-efficient models of health services delivery will need to be constantly re-evaluated. The implementation of primary care reforms will result in alternative payment systems for providers, some form of rostering of patients, and better integration with other healthcare system components. As the effects of the social sector on health continue to be understood, pressure will likely build to improve the coordination of government policies, in particular for the most vulnerable population in Canada (children, women, people who are poor or homeless, Aboriginal peoples, and ethnic and cultural minorities). One component of this increased emphasis on the needs of special groups is the need for broader citizen representation and more widespread public participation in health care, both at the individual level and the systemic level. Currently, regionalization of health services and the accompanying devolution of policy making to the local level attempt to broaden the spectrum of public participation in health care and to democratize the policy-making process. These models are not without their problems, however, and it is possible that federal, provincial, and territorial reformers will continue to tinker with various organizational models as their health systems are fine-tuned.

What remains clearest in all of this debate about health care and healthcare reform in Canada is that concerns with cost containment and system effectiveness must not overshadow the fundamental Canadian beliefs in compassion, respect for others, and the value placed on human dignity. It is the combination of all these fundamental values that will shape reform in the years to come and the quest for that unique Canadian combination that embodies those traits and beliefs that guide us through this century.

4.   SUMMARY

Canada aims to achieve equitable access to health care for all Canadians. So far, equal access to medical care has been largely achieved by the universal system of hospital and medical insurance. However, over the last two decades several trends have placed significant stress on healthcare systems throughout the industrialized world, including Canada; this phenomenon has led to a universal re-examination of how to provide the highest quality and most effective health care while decreasing health system costs. These stressors include continually increasing costs to look after the sick and infirm, questions concerning the appropriate role of the state in society, in particular resulting in conflicts between government and healthcare professionals, the rise of consumerism, changing demographic patterns leading to increased numbers of the elderly and increased demand for expensive, high-technology medical care, evidence of health inequities among particular high-risk population groups, and awareness of the need for disease prevention and health promotion. Since the late 1980s and early 1990s, every province in Canada, as well as the federal government, has undertaken a fundamental review of current health systems via task forces, commissions, boards of inquiry, and working groups to address these problems.

As a result of these reports, in the early nineties of the last century, a number of changes were implemented by provinces, including regionalization, the merging, downsizing, and closing of hospital, the delisting of services from publicly financed programs, and reducing health human resources. The federal government also reduced the cash portion of funding in the Canada Health and Social Transfer. All these changes resulted in inaccessibility of services that provoked public outcry. Provincial and federal governments appointed several commissions in late 1990s and early in the 21st century. Two recent reports which were national in scope were those of the Kirby Commission and Romanow Commission, known after the chairs of these commissions. Their reports dealt with a number of issues and recommended several reforms. The issues addressed were: fundamental values of Canadians, financing, scopes of services to be covered under the *Canada Health Act*, restructuring or improving the delivery system, population health, health infrastructure, and the health of special populations.

In 2003, the federal government responded to the recommendations in these reports and signed an accord with the provinces and territories to increase funding to remedy issues related to accessibility and targeted funding for primary care reform, home care, catastrophic drug plans, and diagnostic equipment. It also reaffirmed the principle of a publicly funded healthcare system with increased accountability and transparency.

As Canada faces the 21st century, many of the issues discussed in this chapter continue to dominate the policy agenda. Questions about cost effectiveness and cost control continue to dominate all discussions. As a result, the possibility of creating more effective and cost-efficient models of health services delivery will be constantly re-evaluated. What remains most clear in all of this debate about health care and healthcare reform in Canada, however, is that concerns about cost containment and system effectiveness must not overshadow the fundamental Canadian belief in compassion, respect for others, and human dignity. The combination of all these fundamental values will shape reform in the years to come, and will guide us through this century.

5.   REFERENCES

1.   Mhatre S, Deber R. From equal access to health care to equitable access to health: A review of Canadian provincial health commissions and reports. *International Journal of Health Services* 1992; 22(4):645-66.
2.   Angus DE. *Review of significant health care commissions and task forces in Canada since 1983-84*. Ottawa: Canadian Hospital Association, Canadian Medical Association, and Canadian Nurses Association, 1991.
3.   Health Canada. *Provincial health system reform in Canada*. Ottawa: Ministry of Supply and Services Canada, 1995.
4.   Government of Newfoundland and Labrador. *Report from the Royal Commission on Hospital and Nursing Home Costs to the Government of Newfoundland and Labrador*. St. John's: Government of Newfoundland and Labrador, 1984.
5.   Government of Newfoundland and Labrador. *A green paper on our health care system expenditures and funding*. St. John's: Government of Newfoundland and Labrador, 1986.
6.   Government of Nova Scotia. *Towards a new strategy: The report of the Nova Scotia Royal Commission on Health Care*. Halifax: Government of Nova Scotia, 1989.
7.   Ministère de la Santé et des Services sociaux. *A reform centered on the citizen*. Ste. Foy: Government of Quebec, 1990.
8.   Ministère de la Santé et des Services sociaux. *Improving health and wellbeing in Quebec: Orientations*. Ste. Foy: Government of Quebec, 1989.
9.   Ontario Minister's Advisory Group on Health Promotion. *Health promotion matters in Ontario: A report of the Minister's Advisory Group on Health Promotion*. Toronto: Advisory Group, 1987.
10.   Premier's Commission on Future Health Care for Albertans. *The rainbow report: Our vision of health*. Edmonton: Government of Alberta, 1989.
11.   Saskatchewan Commission on Medicare. 2001. *Caring for medicare: Sustaining a quality system*. <www.health.gov.sk.ca/info_center_pub_commission_on_medicare-bw.pdf> (November 2002).
12.   Mazankowski D. 2001. *A framework for reform: Report of the Premier's Advisory Council on Health*. <www.premiersadvisory.com/reform/council.html> (January 2003).
13.   Commission d'étude sur les services de santé et les services sociaux du Québec [Commission Clair]. *Les solutions émergentes*. Quebec: Ministère de la Santé et des Services sociaux, 2000. Volume 1: Rapport et recommandations.

14. New Brunswick. Premier's Health Quality Council. *Health renewal: Report from the Premier's Health Quality Council.* Saint John: Premier's Health Quality Council, 2002. <www.gnb.ca/op_cpm/highlights-e.pdf>> (September 2002).

15. Health Services Restructuring Commission. 2000. *Looking back, looking forward: A legacy report.* <192.75.156.24/HSRC.pdf> (February 2003).

16. National Forum on Health. *Canada health action: Building on the legacy.* Ottawa: Minister of Public Works and Government Services, 1997.

17. Kirby M, LeBreton M. 2002. *The health of Canadians: The federal role. Volume 6: Recommendations for reform.* Standing Senate Committee on Social Affairs, Science and Technology. <www.parl.gc.ca/37/2/parlbus/commbus/senate/com-e/soci-e/rep-e/repoct02vol6-e.htm> (November 2002).

18. Romanow R. *Building on values: The future of health care in Canada.* Ottawa: Commission on the Future of Health Care in Canada; Government of Canada, 2002. <www.healthcarecommission.ca> March 2003)

19. Canadian Medical Association. *Thematic overview of recommendations made by the Senate Committee on Health Care and the Romanow Commission.* Ottawa: Canadian Medical Association, 2002.

20. Fooks C, Lewis S. *Romanow and beyond: A primer on health reforms issues in Canada.* Ottawa: Canadian Policy Research Network, 2002. Discussion Paper No. H/05.

21. Canadian Healthcare Association. 2002. *CHA summary of key recommendations and government responses: Recent provincial and territorial health system reports.* <www.cha.ca/documents/Comprehensive_Grid.pdf> (October 2002).

22. Flood C, Epps T. *A patient's bill of rights: A cure for Canadians' concerns about medicare?* Toronto: Institute for Research on Public Policy, 2002. Volume 3: 12.

23. Alford R. *Health care politics: Ideological and interest group barriers to reform.* Chicago: The University of Chicago Press, 1975.

24. Committee on Psychiatric Services. *More for the mind.* Toronto: Canadian Mental Health Association, 1961.

25. Hall E. *Royal Commission on Health Services.* Ottawa: Queen's Printer, 1964.

26. Statistics Canada. 2003. *Hospitalizations for mental disorders.* <www.statcan.ca/english/Pgdb/health56a.htm> (March 2003).

27. Wasylenki D, Goering P, Lancee W, *et al.* Psychiatric aftercare in a metropolitan setting. *Canadian Journal of Psychiatry* 1985; 30(5):329-36.

28. Kohn L, Corrigan J, Donaldson M. *To err is human: Building a safer health system.* Washington DC: National Academy Press, 2000.

29. National Steering Committee on Patient Safety. *Building a safer system: A national integrated strategy for improving patient safety in Canadian health care.* Ottawa: Royal College of Physicians and Surgeons of Canada and Saskatchewan Health, 2002.

30. Baker R, Norton P. 2002. *A systemic review and analysis of leading practices in Canada with reference to initiatives elsewhere.* <www.hc-sc.gc.ca/english/care/report/index.html> (March 2003).

31. Berg A, Hammitt K. Assessing the psychiatric patient's ability to meet the literacy demands of hospitalization. *Hospital Community Psychiatry* 1980; 31(4):266-8.

32. Dunn M, Buckwalter K, Weistein L, *et al.* Innovations in family and community health. *Family Community Health* 1985; 8(3):76-87.

33. Mallet L, Spurull WJ. Readability evaluation of nine patient drug education sources. *American Pharmacy* 1988; NS28(11):33-6.

34. Doyle R, Rahi K. *Organizational change toward multiculturalism.* Toronto: Social Planning Council of Metropolitan Toronto, 1990.

35. Ministry of Supply and Services. *After the door has been opened: Mental health issues affecting immigrants and refugees in Canada.* Ottawa: Government of Canada, 1988.

36.   Tator C. Strategy for fostering participation and equity in the human services delivery. In Doyle R, Rahi K, editors. *Organization Change toward Multiculturalism*. Toronto: Access Action Council, 1990.

37.   U.S. Department of Energy. 2003. *Human genome project information*. <www.ornl.gov/hgmis> (February 2003).

38.   Guttmacher A, Collins F. Genomics medicine: A primer. *New England Journal of Medicine* 2002; 347(19):1512-20.

39.   Collins F, McKusick V. Implications of the Human Genome Project for medical science. *Journal of American Medical Association* 2001; 285(5):540-44.

40.   Government of Ontario. *Genetics, testing, and gene patenting: Charting new territory in health care*. Toronto: Government of Ontario, 2002.

41.   Health Canada. 2002. *Assisted human reproduction*. <www.hc-sc.gc.ca/english/protection/reproduction/index.htm> (February 2003).

42.   Roses A. Pharmacogenetics' place in modern medical science and practice. *Life Science* 2002; 70(13):1471-80.

43.   Khoury M, Morris J. *Pharmacogenetics and public health: The promise of targeted disease prevention*. Atlanta: Centers for Disease Control, 2002.

44.   Guzey C, Spigset O. Genotyping of drug targets: A method to predict adverse drug reactions? *Drug Safety* 2002; 25(8):553-60.

45.   Thiel K. 1999. *Pharmacogenomic medicine*. <www.biospace.com/articles/081999_print.cfm> (February 2003).

46.   Health Canada. 2003. *First ministers' accord on health care renewal*. <www.hc-sc.gc.ca/english/hca2003/accord.html> (February 2003).

APPENDIX

A

QUICK TABLES OF CURRENT RECOMMENDATIONS

The Canadian Task Force on Preventive Health Care (CTFPHC) was established in 1977 (as the Canadian Task Force on Periodic Examination) to provide evidence-based clinical prevention manoeuvres for primary care practices. The tables below list recommendations by strength of evidence (A, B and C) organized by patient category (see Chapter 11). They are reproduced here with permission of the Canadian Task Force on Preventive Health Care.

For more details not provided here, including lists of procedures deemed to be excluded from periodic health examination (D and E recommendations), readers are advised to visit the CTFPHC's Web site at <www.ctfphc.org>.

1. **Prenatal and Perinatal Quick Table: All Relevant Recommendations**

Condition	Manoeuvre	Population
A Recommendations (Do's)		
Congenital hypothyroidism	Thyroid-stimulating hormone (TSH) test	Neonates
Dental caries	Community fluoridation, fluoride toothpaste, or supplement	General population
Hemoglobinopathies	Hemoglobin electrophoresis	High-risk neonates
Household and recreational injury	Public education / legislation on poison control	General population
Vehicle-related injury	Legislation, restraint use, and control of drinking and driving	General population
Ophthalmia neonatorum	Ocular prophylaxis	Newborns
Phenylketonuria	Serum phenylalanine screening	Newborns

1.   Prenatal and Perinatal Quick Table: All Relevant Recommendations (cont'd)

Condition	Manoeuvre	Population
B Recommendations (Do's)		
Adverse consequences, children of alcoholics	Children of Alcoholics Screening Test (CAST)	General population
Household and recreational injury	Legislation, window and stair guards, smoke detectors	General population
Household and recreational injury	Public education / legislation, fire burn and water (tub and swimming) safety	General population
MVA injury	Counselling on restraint use and avoidance of drinking and driving	General population
Problem drinking	Case finding and counselling	General population
C Recommendations (Inconclusive)		
Child maltreatment	Sexual abuse, abduction prevention programs	General population
Dental caries	Counselling, diet or baby bottle	General and high-risk population
Iron deficiency anemia	Routine hemoglobin	General population
Lead exposure	Universal screening (Blood lead level or questionnaire)	General population

2.   Pediatric Quick Table: All Relevant Recommendations

Condition	Manoeuvre	Population
A Recommendations (Do's)		
All-cause morbidity and mortality	Day care or preschool programs	Disadvantaged children
Amblyopia	Eye exam	Infants

2. Pediatric Quick Table: All Relevant Recommendations (cont'd)

Condition	Manoeuvre	Population
A Recommendations (Do's)		
Child maltreatment	Home visitation by nurses during perinatal period through infancy	First-time mothers of low socioeconomic status, single parents, or teenaged parents
Dental caries	Fissure sealants	High-risk children
Dental caries	Community fluoridation, fluoride toothpaste, or supplement	General population
Dental caries, periodontal disease	Brushing and flossing teeth to apply toothpaste (A) and prevent gingivitis (B) but not cariostatic (C)	General population
Developmental hip dysplasia (DHD)	Timing of abduction therapy (early intervention) - supervised period of observation with detected DHD	Normal- or high-risk infants
Hearing impairment	Hearing exam	Infants
Hepatitis B	Immunization	Infants, children, and adolescents
Household and recreational injury	Public education / legislation on poison control	General population
Immunizable infectious disease	Immunizations, Childhood	Infants and children
Vehicle-related injury	Legislation, restraint use, and control of drinking and driving	General population
Varicella vaccine	Immunization and catch-up immunization with varicella vaccine	12-15 month old children; 1-12 year old children (catch-up)
Varicella vaccine	Immunization with varicella vaccine	Susceptible adolescents
B Recommendations (Do's)		
Adverse consequences, children of alcoholics	Children of Alcoholics Screening Test (CAST)	General population

2.   **Pediatric Quick Table: All Relevant Recommendations (cont'd)**

Condition	Manoeuvre	Population
B Recommendations (Do's)		
All-cause mortality and morbidity	Moderate physical activity	General population
Developmental hip dysplasia	Repeated serial clinical examination by trained examiners	Normal-risk infants
Disorders of physical growth	Serial height, weight, head circumference measurement	Infants
Gingivitis	Brushing teeth	General population
Gonorrhea	Counselling, educational materials	General population
HIV/AIDS	Voluntary HIV antibody screening	Infants of HIV positive women
Household and recreational injury	Counselling on home risk factors, poisoning	Children/parents
Household and recreational injury	Legislation, window and stair guards, smoke detectors	General population
Household and recreational injury	Public education / legislation, fire burn and water (tub and swimming) safety	General population
Household and recreational injury	Legislation, avoidance of alcohol with water recreation	General population
Influenza	Immunization, annual	High-risk sub-groups
Iron deficiency anemia in infants	Iron fortified formula, cereal or supplementation	Infants
Iron deficiency anemia	Routine hemoglobin	High-risk infants, disadvantaged children
Lead exposure	Blood lead screening	High-risk children
Lung cancer	Dietary advice on green leafy vegetables and fruit	Smokers

2. Pediatric Quick Table: All Relevant Recommendations (cont'd)

Condition	Manoeuvre	Population
B Recommendations (Do's)		
Vehicle-related injury	Counselling on restraint use and avoidance of drinking and driving	General population
Periodontal disease	Tooth scaling and prophylaxis	General population
Problem drinking	Case finding and counselling	General population
Skin cancer	Counselling, sun exposure, clothing	General population
Skin cancer	Counselling, sun exposure, clothing	General population
Tobacco-caused disease	Referral to validated cessation program	Smokers
Tobacco-caused disease	Counselling to prevent smoking initiation	Children and adolescents
Unintended pregnancy; STDs	Counselling, sexual activity, contraception	Adolescents
Vehicle-related injury	Legislation, bicycle, motorcycle, or all-terrain vehicle helmet	General population
Vision problems	Visual acuity testing	Preschool children
C Recommendations (Inconclusive)		
Adverse consequences, children of alcoholics	Routine evaluation; some screening options	General population
All-cause mortality and morbidity	Counselling, physical activity; prevent obesity	General population
All-cause mortality and morbidity	Measure body mass index and treat obesity	General population
All-cause morbidity and mortality	Office contact or home-based parenting education programs	Disadvantaged children
Child maltreatment	Comprehensive health care program	Families with children

2.   **Pediatric Quick Table: All Relevant Recommendations (cont'd)**

Condition	Manoeuvre	Population
C Recommendations (Inconclusive)		
Child maltreatment	Parent education and support program	Families with children
Child maltreatment	Combination of home-based services,including case management, education, and psychotherapy	Families with children
Child maltreatment	Sexual abuse, abduction prevention programs	General population
Colorectal cancer	Flexible sigmoidoscopy beginning at puberty	High-risk adults with Familial adenomatous polyposis (FAP)
Dental caries	Counselling, diet, or baby bottle	General and high-risk population
Developmental hip dysplasia	Abduction therapy	Normal- or high-risk infants
Developmental hip dysplasia	Timing of abduction therapy (early intervention) - optimal duration of observation	Normal- or high-risk infants
Developmental problems	Developmental screening questionnaires	Preschool children
Hemoglobinopathies	Screening for carrier status and counselling	Non-pregnant adolescents
HIV/AIDS	History, sexual and drug-use counselling	General population
HIV/AIDS	Voluntary HIV antibody screening	General population including pregnant women
Household and recreational injury	Counselling, household and recreational injury (except some home hazards, poisoning for children)	Children
Household and recreational injury	Public education / legislation, gun control, and use of Heimlich manoeuvre	General population

2.   Pediatric Quick Table: All Relevant Recommendations (cont'd)

Condition	Manoeuvre	Population
C Recommendations (Inconclusive)		
Hypertension	Pharmacological treatment	Adults <21 years, isolated systolic hypertension
Idiopathic adolescent scoliosis	Physical exam, back	Adolescents
Iron deficiency anemia	Routine hemoglobin	Infants
Lead exposure	Universal screening (blood lead level or questionnaire)	General population
Vehicle-related injury	Counselling, helmet, alcohol use	General population
Obesity	Exercise and/or nutrition and behaviour modification	Obese children
Obesity	Height, weight, skin-fold thickness, BMI, etc.	Children
Otitis media	Screening to identify children with clinically important otitis media with effusion (OME) (tympa-nometry,microtympanome-try, acoustic reflectometry and pneumo-otoscopy)	Children up to 4 years of age
Otitis media	Screening to prevent delay in language development as a result of OME	Children up to 4 years of age
Periodontal disease	Flossing teeth	Children
Skin cancer	Counselling, sun block	General population
Suicide	Suicide risk evaluation	General population
Testicular cancer	Physical exam or self-exam	Adolescents

3.   **Women (Including Pregnant Women) and Men 21–64 Years of Age Quick Table: All Relevant Recommendations**

Condition	Manoeuvre	Population
A Recommendations (Do's)		
Breast cancer	Mammography and clinical exam	Women 50-69 years
Colorectal cancer	Multiphase screening with the hemoccult test	Average risk adults >50 years
Dental caries	Community fluoridation, fluoride toothpaste or supplement	General population
Dental caries, periodontal disease	Brushing and flossing teeth to apply toothpaste (A) and prevent gingivitis (B) but not cariostatic (C)	General population
Hearing impairment	Noise control and hearing protection	General population
Household and recreational injury	Public education/legislation on poison control	General population
Hypertension	Pharmacological treatment	Adults 21-64 years with DBP >90 mmHg
Vehicle-related injury	Legislation, restraint use, and control of drinking and driving	General population
Neural tube defects	Folic acid supplementation	Women capable of becoming pregnant
Oral cancer mortality	Smoking cessation counselling	General population
Periodontal disease	Flossing teeth	Adult population
Pneumococcal pneumonia	Single dose of 23-valent pneumococcal vaccine	Immunocompetent patients >55 years in institutions
Progressive renal disease	Urine dipstick	Adults with Insulin dependent diabetes
Tobacco-caused disease	Counselling, smoking cessation, or offer nicotine replacement therapy	Smokers

3.   Women (Including Pregnant Women) and Men 21–64 Years of Age Quick Table: All Relevant Recommendations (cont'd)

Condition	Manoeuvre	Population
B Recommendations (Do's)		
All-cause mortality and morbidity	Moderate physical activity	General population
Breast cancer	Counselling on benefits and risks of using tamoxifen to reduce likelihood of breast cancer	High-risk women
Cervical cancer	Papanicolaou smear	Women
Chlamydial infection	Smear, culture or analysis	High-risk women
Colorectal cancer	Sigmoidoscopy	Average risk adults >50 years
Colorectal cancer	Flexible sigmoidoscopy beginning at puberty, genetic testing	High-risk adults with FAP
Colorectal cancer	Colonoscopy	High-risk adults with hereditary nonpolyposis colon cancer
Congenital rubella syndrome	Screen and vaccinate or universal vaccination	Non-pregnant women of child-bearing age
Coronary heart disease	Diet/drug treatment	Males 30-59 years with elevated cholesterol or LDL-C
Coronary heart disease	General dietary advice on fat and cholesterol	Males 30-39 years
Diet-related illness	Counselling on adverse nutritional habits	Adult population
Gingivitis	Brushing teeth	General population
Gonorrhea	Counselling, educational materials	General population
Household and recreational injury	Legislation, window and stair guards, smoke detectors	General population
Household and recreational injury	Public education/legislation, fire burn and water (tub and swimming) safety	General population

3. **Women (Including Pregnant Women) and Men 21–64 Years of Age Quick Table: All Relevant Recommendations (cont'd)**

Condition	Manoeuvre	Population
B Recommendations (Do's)		
Household and recreational injury	Legislation, avoidance of alcohol with water recreation	General population
Lung cancer	Dietary advice on green leafy vegetables and fruit	Smokers
Vehicle-related injury	Counselling on restraint use and avoidance of drinking and driving	General population
Obesity	BMI measurement	Obese adults with obesity-related disease
Obesity	Weight-reduction therapy	Obese adults with obesity-related disease
Osteoporotic fractures (and side effects)	Counselling, hormone replacement therapy	Perimenopausal women
Periodontal disease	Tooth scaling and prophylaxis	General population
Problem drinking	Case finding and counselling	General population
Skin cancer	Counselling, sun exposure, clothing	General population
Tobacco-caused disease	Referral to validated cessation program	Smokers
Varicella vaccine	Immunization with varicella vaccine	Susceptible adults
Vehicle-related injury	Legislation, bicycle, motorcycle, or all-terrain vehicle helmet	General population
C Recommendations (Inconclusive)		
Abdominal aortic aneurysm	Abdominal palpation	General population
Abdominal aortic aneurysm	Abdominal ultrasound	General population
All-cause mortality and morbidity	Counselling, physical activity; prevent obesity	General population

3.   **Women (Including Pregnant Women) and Men 21–64 Years of Age Quick Table: All Relevant Recommendations (cont'd)**

Condition	Manoeuvre	Population
C Recommendations (Inconclusive)		
All-cause mortality and morbidity	Measure body mass index and treat obesity	General population
Bladder cancer	Urine dipstick or cytology	High-risk males >60 years
Breast cancer	Screening mammography	Women 40-49 years at average risk of breast cancer
Breast cancer follow-up	Follow-up for local recurrence	Women having been previously diagnosed with breast cancer
Breast cancer follow-up	Follow-up for contralateral breast cancer	Women having been previously diagnosed with breast cancer
Cardiovascular disease	Acetylsalicylic acid prophylaxis	General population
Child maltreatment	Sexual abuse, abduction prevention programs	General population
Colorectal cancer	Hemoccult/sigmoidoscopy in combination	Average risk adults >50 years
Colorectal cancer	Colonoscopy	Average risk adults, high-risk adults with family history of polyps/colorectal cancer
Congenital rubella syndrome	Universal vaccination	Young men (living in crowded conditions)
Coronary artery disease events	Screening for total plasma homocysteine levels	General population or those at high risk for coronary artery disease events
Coronary artery disease events	Vitamin therapy (folic acid alone or with vitamin B12) to lower total plasma homocysteine levels	All populations
Coronary heart disease	Diet/drug treatment	Individuals with elevated cholesterol or LDL-C except males 30-59 years

3.   Women (Including Pregnant Women) and Men 21–64 Years of Age Quick Table: All Relevant Recommendations (cont'd)

Condition	Manoeuvre	Population
C Recommendations (Inconclusive)		
Coronary heart disease	Measurement of blood total cholesterol level	General population with case-finding for males 30-59 years
Coronary heart disease	General dietary advice on fat and cholesterol	General population except males 30-69 years
D (Rh) sensitization	Repeat D (Rh) antibody screening and immunoglobin (D Ig) administration	Women undergoing specific obstetric procedures or complications
Hemoglobinopathies	Screening for carrier status and counselling	Adult population
HIV/AIDS	History, sexual and drug-use counselling	General population
HIV/AIDS	Voluntary HIV antibody screening	General population including pregnant women
Household and recreational injury	Public education / legislation, gun control and use of Heimlich manoeuvre	General population
Household and recreational injury	Counselling, household and recreational injury (except some home hazards)	Adult population
Influenza	Immunization, annual	General population <65 years
Iron deficiency anemia	Routine hemoglobin	General population
Vehicle-related injury	Counselling, helmet, alcohol use	General population
Vehicle-related injury	Monitor medical impairment	General population
Obesity	BMI measurement	General populatio

3. **Women (Including Pregnant Women) and Men 21–64 Years of Age Quick Table: All Relevant Recommendations (cont'd)**

Condition	Manoeuvre	Population
C Recommendations (Inconclusive)		
Obesity	Community-based obesity prevention programs	General population
Obesity	Weight-reduction therapy	Obese adults without obesity-related disease
Oral cancer	Physical exam, oral cavity	General population
Prostate cancer	Digital rectal examination	Males >50 years
Protein/calorie malnutrition	Protein/calorie malnutrition screening	Adult population
Skin cancer	Counselling, self-examination	General population
Skin cancer	Counselling, sun block	General population
Skin cancer	Physical examination, skin	General population
Suicide	Suicide risk evaluation	General population
Testicular cancer	Physical exam or self-examination	Men
Thyroid cancer	Neck palpation	Adult population
Thyroid disorders	Thyroid-stimulating hormone test	Perimenopausal women
Tuberculosis	Isoniazid prophylaxis	General population >35 years
Urinary infection	Urine dipstick or culture	Elderly, ambulatory women

4. Elderly Women and Men (>65 years) Quick Table: All Relevant Recommendations

Condition	Manoeuvre	Population
A Recommendations (Do's)		
Breast cancer	Mammography and clinical exam	Women 50-69 years
Cognitive impairment	Follow-up based upon caregiver or informant description of decline	Elderly
Colorectal cancer	Multiphase screening with the hemoccult test	Average risk adults >50 years
Dental caries, periodontal disease	Brushing and flossing teeth to apply toothpaste (A) and prevent gingivitis (B) but not cariostatic (C)	General population
Falls/injury	Multidisciplinary post-fall assessment	Elderly
Household and recreational injury	Public education / legislation on poison control	General population
Hypertension	Pharmacological treatment	Elderly, specific sub-groups
Influenza	Outreach strategies to reach high-risk groups	Specific groups (e.g., diabetics), elderly
Vehicle-related injury	Legislation, restraint use, and control of drinking and driving	General population
Oral cancer mortality	Smoking cessation counselling	General population
Periodontal disease	Flossing teeth	Adult population
Pneumococcal pneumonia	Single dose of 23-valent pneumococcal vaccine	Immunocompetent patients >55 years in institutions
Progressive renal disease	Urine dipstick	Adults with IDDM
Tobacco-caused disease	Counselling, smoking cessation, or nicotine replacement therapy	Smokers

4.   **Elderly Women and Men (>65 years) Quick Table: All Relevant Recommendations (cont'd)**

Condition	Manoeuvre	Population
B Recommendations (Do's)		
All-cause mortality and morbidity	Moderate physical activity	General population
Cervical cancer	Papanicolaou smear	Women
Cognitive impairment	Assessment based upon individual's complaint of memory loss	Elderly
Colorectal cancer	Sigmoidoscopy	Average risk adults >50 years
Colorectal cancer	Flexible sigmoidoscopy beginning at puberty, genetic testing	High-risk adults with FAP
Colorectal cancer	Colonoscopy	High-risk adults with HNPCC
Coronary heart disease	General dietary advice on fat and cholesterol	Males 30-69 years
Diet-related illness	Counselling on adverse nutritional habits	Adult population
Diminished visual acuity	Snellen sight card	Elderly
Gingivitis	Brushing teeth	General population
Gonorrhea	Counselling, Educational materials	General population
Hearing impairment	Enquiry, whispered voice test or audioscope	Elderly
Household and recreational injury	Legislation, safety aids, stairs, bathtubs	Elderly
Household and recreational injury	Legislation, window and stair guards, smoke detectors	General population
Household and recreational injury	Public education / legislation, fire burn and water (tub and swimming) safety	General population

4.   Elderly Women and Men (>65 years) Quick Table: All Relevant Recommendations (cont'd)

Condition	Manoeuvre	Population
B Recommendations (Do's)		
Household and recreational injury	Legislation, avoidance of alcohol with water recreation	General population
Hypertension	Blood pressure measurement	Elderly
Influenza	Immunization, annual	Elderly
Lung cancer	Dietary advice on green leafy vegetables and fruit	Smokers
Vehicle-related injury	Counselling on restraint use and avoidance of drinking and driving	General population
Obesity	BMI measurement	Obese adults with obesity-related disease
Obesity	Weight-reduction therapy	Obese adults with obesity-related disease
Osteoporotic fractures (and side effects)	Counselling, hormone replacement therapy	Perimenopausal women
Periodontal disease	Tooth scaling and prophylaxis	General population
Problem drinking	Case finding and counselling	General population
Skin cancer	Counselling, sun exposure, clothing	General population
Stroke	Anticoagulation if atrial fibrillation detected after stroke	Patients with paroxysmal atrial fibrillation
Stroke	Anticoagulation (warfarin) for intracardiac thrombus to prevent systemic emboli	Patients with stroke and intracardiac thrombus
Stroke	Echocardiography: transthoracic (TTE) or transesophageal (TEE) for detection of intracardiac masses	Patients with clinical cardiac disease and no pre-existing indications for anticoagulation

4.   Elderly Women and Men (>65 years) Quick Table: All Relevant Recommendations (cont'd)

Condition	Manoeuvre	Population
Tobacco-caused disease	Referral to validated cessation program	Smokers
Vehicle-related injury	Legislation, bicycle, motorcycle, or all-terrain vehicle helmet	General population

C Recommendations (Inconclusive)

Condition	Manoeuvre	Population
Abdominal aortic aneurysm	Abdominal palpation	General population
Abdominal aortic aneurysm	Abdominal ultrasound	General population
Adverse consequences, children of alcoholics	Routine evaluation; some screening options	General population
Age-related macular degeneration	Fundoscopy	Elderly
All-cause mortality and morbidity	Counselling, physical activity; prevent obesity	General population
All-cause mortality and morbidity	Measure body mass index and treat obesity	General population
Bladder cancer	Urine dipstick or cytology	High-risk males >60 years
Breast cancer follow-up	Follow-up for local recurrence	Women having been previously diagnosed with breast cancer
Breast cancer follow-up	Follow-up for contralateral breast cancer	Women having been previously diagnosed with breast cancer
Cardiovascular disease	Acetylsalicylic acid prophylaxis	General population
Cognitive impairment	Mental status screening	Elderly
Colorectal cancer	Hemoccult/sigmoidoscopy in combination	Average risk adults >50 years

4.   **Elderly Women and Men (>65 years) Quick Table: All Relevant Recommendations (cont'd)**

Condition	Manoeuvre	Population
C Recommendations (Inconclusive)		
Colorectal cancer	Colonoscopy	Average risk adults, high-risk adults with family history of polyps/CRC
Coronary artery disease events	Screening for total plasma homocysteine levels	General population or those at high risk for coronary artery disease events
Coronary artery disease events	Vitamin therapy (folic acid alone or with vitamin B12) to lower total plasma homocysteine levels	All populations
Coronary heart disease	Diet/drug treatment	Individuals with elevated cholesterol or LDL-C except males 30-59 years
Coronary heart disease	Measurement of blood total cholesterol level	General population with case-finding for males 30-59 years
Coronary heart disease	General dietary advice on fat and cholesterol	General population except males 30-69 years
Elder abuse	Elder abuse questionnaire	Elderly
Glaucoma	Fundoscopy, tonometry, or automated perimetry	Elderly
HIV/AIDS	History, sexual and drug-use counselling	General population
HIV/AIDS	Voluntary HIV screening	General population including pregnant women
Household and recreational injury	Monitor medical impairment	Elderly
Household and recreational injury	Public education / legislation, gun control and use of Heimlich manoeuvre	General population

4. **Elderly Women and Men (>65 years) Quick Table: All Relevant Recommendations (cont'd)**

Condition	Manoeuvre	Population
C Recommendations (Inconclusive)		
Household and recreational injury	Counselling, household and recreational injury (except some home hazards)	Adult population
Household and recreational injury	Public education, non-flammable fabrics, self-extinguishing cigarettes	Elderly
Iron deficiency anemia	Routine hemoglobin	General population
Vehicle-related injury	Counselling, helmet, alcohol use	General population
Vehicle-related injury	Monitor medical impairment	General population
Obesity	BMI measurement	General population
Obesity	Community-based obesity prevention programs	General population
Obesity	Weight-reduction therapy	Obese adults without obesity-related disease
Oral cancer	Physical exam, oral cavity	General population
Oral cancer mortality	Opportunistic screening by clinical examination	Asymptomatic patients
Osteoporosis	Counselling, weight bearing exercise	Pre- and post-menopausal women
Osteoporotic fractures	History and physical examination	Women
Ovarian cancer	Pelvic exam, transvaginal ultrasound, CA 125, or combination	Pre- and post-menopausal women
Pneumococcal pneumonia	Immunization, one dose	Immunocompetent elderly living independently
Protein/calorie malnutrition	Protein/calorie malnutrition screening	Adult population

4.   Elderly Women and Men (>65 years) Quick Table: All Relevant Recommendations (cont'd)

Condition	Manoeuvre	Population
C Recommendations (Inconclusive)		
Skin cancer	Counselling, self-examination	General population
Skin cancer	Counselling, sun block	General population
Skin cancer	Physical examination, skin	General population
Stroke	Ambulatory ECG	All patients presenting with stroke or transient ischemic attack
Stroke	Echocardiography: transthoracic (TTE) or transesophageal (TEE) for detection of intracardiac masses	Patients without clinical cardiac disease
Stroke	Treatment for patent foramen ovale	General population
Suicide	Suicide risk evaluation	General population
Testicular cancer	Physical exam or self-examination	Men
Thyroid cancer	Neck palpation	Adult population
Thyroid disorders	Thyroid-stimulating hormone test	Perimenopausal women
Tuberculosis	INH prophylaxis	General population >35 years
Urinary infection	Urine dipstick or culture	Elderly, ambulatory women

5. **Patients with First Degree Relatives with Disease Quick Table: All Relevant Recommendations**

Condition	Manoeuvre	Population
B Recommendations (Do's)		
Colorectal cancer	Flexible sigmoidoscopy beginning at puberty, genetic testing	High-risk adults with FAP
Colorectal cancer	Colonoscopy	High-risk adults with HNPCC
Cystic fibrosis	DNA analysis for carrier status	Siblings of children with CF
Cystic fibrosis	Sweat test, immunoreactive trypsin; and BM meconium test	Siblings of children with CF
Hemoglobinopathies	DNA analysis, fetal tissue sample/counselling	Families, parents confirmed carriers
Skin cancer	Physical exam, skin	First-degree relative with melanoma
C Recommendations (Inconclusive)		
Colorectal cancer	Colonoscopy	Average-risk adults, high-risk adults with family history of polyps/CRC
Ovarian cancer	Pelvic exam, transvaginal ultrasound, CA 125, or combination	Family history of first-degree relative
Tobacco-caused disease	Counselling on environmental tobacco smoke	Families with smokers

Appendix

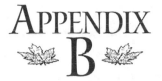

B

Educational Objectives

1. CRITICAL APPRAISAL

i) *Characteristics of study design including sources of bias*
   (a) RCT
   (b) Cohort
   (c) Case-control
   (d) Cross-sectional

ii) *Measurements*
   (a) Characteristics of measurement, distributions, error, reliability, terminology
   (b) Measurement of central tendency, dispersion, variability
   (c) Test validation: sensitivity, specificity, pre-/post-test likelihood, predictive value
   (d) Measurement of health and disease in a population
   • specific rates (e.g., age/sex):
   • incidence, prevalence
   • standardization
   • odds ratio
   • relative risk
   • attributable risk
   • case fatality ratio
   • primary/secondary attack rates

iii) *Sampling, including sources of bias*

iv) *Analysis*
   Tests of significance
   • statistical vs. clinical
   • sample size
   • p value, confidence intervals
   • common tests (e.g., t-test, x^2)
   • intro to multivariate analysis

v) *Efficacy, effectiveness, efficiency, compliance*

2. CONCEPTS OF DISEASE AND INJURY PREVENTION AND CONTROL

i) *Concept of natural history of disease*

ii) *Models of causation*

iii) *Approaches and limitations to classification of health, function and disease*

iv) *Levels of prevention*
   (a) Primary (e.g., immunization, lifestyle)
   (b) Secondary (e.g., screening, periodic health examination)
   (c) Tertiary (e.g., disability, rehabilitation)

v) *Screening, surveillance, case-finding, contact tracing*

vi) *Strategies for control*
   Points of intervention:
   • host/agent/environment

vii) *Prevention in clinical setting*
   Periodic health examination:
   • conceptual approach

---

*Source: Adapted from JS Baumber, ed. *Objectives for the qualifying examination*, Medical Council of Canada, 1992.

• protection packages
• updates of protection packages

3.   DATABASE, VITAL STATISTICS, DEMOGRAPHY, HEALTH STATUS

i) *Uses and limitations of Canadian data sources*
(a) Census
(b) Statistics Canada
(c) Registries
(d) Medical examiners, autopsy
(e) Health surveys
(f) Birth certificates
(g) Death certificates
(h) Hospital, medical services data
(i) Workers' compensation data

ii) *Demographic characteristics of the population*
(a) Age/sex/structure
(b) Compression of morbidity
(c) Mortality
(d) Fertility
(e) Implications to the health care system

iii) *Health indices and health status*
(a) Direct
   • Infant mortality rate
   • Crude mortality rate
   • Life expectancy
   • Causes of death
   • Specific health surveys
   • Potential years of life lost
   • Survivorship
   • Age/sex specific distribution of mortality
   • Disability days
   • Activities of daily living
   • Prevalence of disability
(b) Indirect
   • Percentage of low birth-weight neonates
   • Percentage of communities with potable water
   • Risk factor distribution
(c) Correlates
   • Morbidity and utilization data

• Gross national product
• Socioeconomic status of individual
(d) Descriptive epidemiology of diseases and injuries in Canada
   • Motor vehicle injuries
   • Cardiovascular disease
   • Major cancers
   • Respiratory diseases
   • Common infectious diseases
   • Substance abuse

4A.   HEALTHCARE SYSTEM

i) *Historical development and principles of health services*
(a) British North America Act
(b) Hospital Insurance and Diagnostic Services Act
(c) Medicare
(d) Principles of b and c
(e) Established Programs Financing Act
(f) Canada Health Act
(g) International comparisons
(h) Trends and issues in the evolving health system

ii) *Organization of health services: federal vs. provincial*

iii) *Self-regulation of professions*
(a) Peer review
(b) Audit

iv) *Professional organization*
v) *Methods of physician payment*
vi) *Distribution and projections of health manpower*
vii) *Health resource allocation*
viii) *Institutional organization*
(a) Structure
(b) Accreditation
(c) Audit

ix) *Role of voluntary organizations*
x) *Alternate delivery systems*
xi) *Women's health movement*

4B.   PUBLIC HEALTH SYSTEM

i) *Role of public health system in*
(a) Maternal and child health
(b) Home care

(c) School health
(d) Sexually transmitted diseases
(e) Inspection
(f) Disease surveillance
(g) Mental health
(h) Health promotion
(i) Biological
ii) Role of physicians in public health
(a) Medical health officer
(b) Epidemiologist
(c) Occupational health
(d) Role of the practising physician
iii) Statutory responsibilities of the practising physician
Reportable disease notification
iv) Outbreak investigation
v) National and international health networks as relevant to the public health system
vi) Product regulation
(a) Biologicals
(b) Drugs and pharmaceuticals
(c) Medical devices

5. OCCUPATIONAL AND ENVIRONMENTAL HEALTH

i) Exposure
(a) Long-term/low-dose
(b) Multiple
(c) Mechanisms of toxic action
• Cancer
• Reproductive hazards
• Respiratory diseases
(d) Routes of entry
(e) Types of exposures
ii) Standard setting
(a) Physical
(b) Chemical
(c) Biological
(d) Psychological
iii) Occupational diseases and injuries
iv) Occupational history taking
v) Risk assessment
vi) Ethics and occupational medicine
vii) Workers' compensation board functions
viii) Environmental health
• food, air, water

6. GROUPS WITH SPECIAL HEALTHCARE NEEDS

i) Characteristics and health status
(a) Canadian Indian/Inuit/Métis
(b) Immigrants
(c) Low income/unemployed
(d) Elderly
(e) Disabled
ii) Service needs and availability

7. PSYCHOSOCIAL ASPECTS OF HEALTH

i) Health and illness behaviour and risk perception
ii) Compliance
(a) Barriers to individual
(b) Environmental and behavioural factors in compliance
iii) Family, social network and peer group alternatives to kinship
iv) Biopsychosocial, culture, gender, and age effects on health
(a) Health beliefs
(b) Patients and providers
v) Health education and health promotion
• Individual behaviour vs. social change
(a) healthy public policy
vi) Lifestyle and the environment
vii) Modalities of health education
(a) Behavioural diagnosis and modification
(b) Health marketing
viii) Blaming the victim
• Stigmatization
ix) Professional vs. consumer control of health-related initiatives

INDEX